# Cultural Sociology from Concern to Distance

Lilli Zeuner

# Cultural Sociology from Concern to Distance

*Copenhagen Business School Press*

**Cultural Sociology from Concern to Distance**


Printed in Denmark
1. edition 2003

ISBN 87-630-0112-8



Distribution:

*Scandinavia*
DJØF/DBK, Siljangade 2-8, P.O. Box 1731
DK-2300 Copenhagen S, Denmark
Phone: +45 3269 7788, fax: +45 3269 7789

*North America*
Copenhagen Business School Press
Books International Inc.
P.O. Box 605
Herndon, VA 20172-0605, USA
Phone: +1 703 661 1500, fax: +1 703 661 1501

*Rest of the World*
Marston Book Services, P.O. Box 269
Abingdon, Oxfordshire, OX14 4YN, UK
Phone: +44 (0) 1235 465500, fax: +44 (0) 1235 465555
E-mail Direct Customers: direct.order@marston.co.uk
E-mail Booksellers: trade.order@marston.co.uk

To my husband
Steen
Thank you

# Contents

# Preface

Many years of doing empirical studies in the cultural field have laid the basis for my interest in sociological theory of culture. My empirical studies into youth culture, educational culture and culture among young delinquents have led me to raise the question of what to understand by culture and how we can explain the relationship of culture to other societal phenomena. Originally, I had been much inspired by the Birmingham School and its focus upon youth culture. Later followed 'the cultural turn' and, more recently, contours of 'cultural returns', focussing upon a great number of different cultural expressions. On the one hand, these trends in the research into culture were of great inspiration in my empirical studies. On the other, they left also a sense of inadequacy or perhaps eclecticism in the scientific treatment of cultural phenomena. I needed myself to return to sociological theory of culture in order to clarify the conceptual and theoretical problems, I had run into.

The focus of my research thus changed from cultural phenomena to theory of culture. The problematic of my research became a different one. The issue now became how one can understand the evolution of sociological theory of culture. Habermas' book *On the Logic of the Social Sciences* became an important source of inspiration for the undertaking of this analysis. The distinction between natural scientific and cultural scientific thinking was the basis for his understanding of the evolution of the social sciences. On this background, I decided to investigate what the implications of this distinction have been for sociological thinking about culture. To what extent are the concept of culture and the theory of culture in sociology characterised by natural scientific and by cultural scientific thought, respectively? Have attempts been made to form syntheses between these two forms of thinking in the sociology of culture?

It soon became clear to me that there was another question which was just as important, which is the question of how the sociological understanding of culture has changed over time. Therefore, in my investigation I have included both classical and contemporary sociology to analyse how sociology views cultural phenomena. Here, the issue is tracking down the substantial changes from the time when the classical sociologists founded sociology as a thinking of modernity and to the present time, where sociology struggles to understand the unfolded modernity and what comes after. This book is thus laid out over both a logical and a historical dimension, and the analysis is undertaken as a comparative analysis around these two dimensions.

The idea for this book thus goes some years back in time. As a visiting researcher at the Department of Sociology, University of Warwick in1991, I became much inspired to set out on this project. In the years that followed, different parts of the manuscript have been presented at research seminars at the Department of Sociology, University of Copenhagen and at the Danish National Institute of Social Research. On both occasions

I have received many valuable comments. More recently, I have presented papers while visiting the Department of Sociology, Lancaster University and at a conference about 'Cultural Returns' arranged by the Pavis Centre, Open University, Milton Keynes at the University of Oxford. On this background I would like to thank all those, who I have had the opportunity of discussing sociological theory of culture with. Special thanks are due to Torben Agersnap from the Department of Organization and Industrial Sociology, Copenhagen Business School and to Margareta Bertilsson, from the Department of Sociology, University of Copenhagen. Finally, I would like to thank Steven Harris, who has undertaken the translation of the book into English both meticulously and conscientiously.

*Copenhagen, in October 2002*

*Lilli Zeuner*

# 1

# Introduction: Between Natural Scientific and Cultural Scientific Thought

According to Jürgen Habermas, from its beginnings the development of sociological theory has been bound by a dualism between natural scientific and cultural scientific thought (Habermas, 1967/1988). The question which I want to consider here is whether it is also possible to understand the sociological theory of culture within the same framework. Is it possible to see traces of natural scientific thought and cultural scientific thought in the development of the sociological theory of cultural phenomena? If this is the case, this raises a further question about the extent to which it may be possible to join these two ways of thinking. Is it possible to create a synthesis between a sociological theory of culture characterised by natural scientific thought, and a sociological theory of culture characterised by cultural scientific thought?

As the starting point for a discussion of these questions I will seek, in this introduction, to clarify what is understood by natural scientific thinking and cultural scientific thinking. I will also include contributions to a philosophy which seeks to create theories which are sufficiently general that they can include both forms of thought.

Natural scientific thought is represented by, among others, the Austrian/English philosopher Karl Popper. Popper's theoretical ideas on natural science were based on the search for explanation. A significant representative for cultural scientific thought is the German philosopher Hans-Georg Gadamer. Gadamer's philosophy of science was based on the search for interpretation. The distinction between the two ways of thinking is thus primarily a distinction between explanation and interpretation.

There have been several different attempts to overcome the contradictions between natural scientific and cultural scientific thinking. One contribution is that of the German sociologist Niklas Luhmann. He set himself the goal of developing a sociological theory which is so general that it can include itself as an object of study. This is thus a universal theory. This also means that it is a theory which can cover both natural scientific and cultural scientific thinking. Another contribution to this thinking comes from the German philosopher Ernst Cassirer. He gave himself the task of developing a theory which could cover all symbolic forms. As a result, he developed a theory which is so general that it can cover both natural scientific and cultural scientific thinking. Finally, the Norwegian sociologist, Dag Østerberg, points out that entirely new forms of thought are being developed both within and around sociology. These new forms of thought contain a reconciliation of the contradictions between natural scientific and cultural scientific thinking.

The aim of this introduction is thus to undertake a clarification and discussion of natural scientific and cultural scientific thinking, and a clarification and discussion of the different attempts to overcome the contradictions between them. This raises the question of whether it is possible, within this conceptual framework, to bring clarity to the sociological theory of culture. Is it possible to understand it in the light of these overarching forms of thought? Is it possible understand the sociological theory of culture in the light of the distinction between a natural scientific and a cultural scientific philosophy, and in the light of attempts to create a synthesis between these two forms of philosophy?

## *Natural scientific thought: Karl Popper*

Karl Popper worked on the basis of a philosophical pluralism, and his work was particularly focussed on natural scientific thought. In his book, *Objective Knowledge*, he developed his theory of objective knowledge.

With his philosophical pluralism it was possible for Popper to rise above the classic dualism between the physical world and the world of ideas. Within the world of ideas he introduced a distinction between the mental world and the world of ideas, as objectively understood. Popper thus based his theory of knowledge on the distinction between three worlds. The first world is the physical world. The second world is the mental world and consists of the mental state. The third world consists of ideas in their objective state, and consists of theories, logical relations between theories, and the arguments and problems which they give rise to and which are rooted in the theories themselves. There can only be interaction between the first world and the second world and between the second world and the third world. There cannot be any direct interaction between the first world and the third world. The connection between the physical world and the world of theories can only be made via subjective and personal experience (Popper, 1972/1992, pp. 154-155).

Popper emphasised that the third world should, on the one hand, be regarded as autonomous, and on the other hand, be regarded as being the product of human activity. It is thus both created by humans and it is suprahuman. People can act in relation to the third world, while at the same time it is above the people who create it. This becomes clear when we see the powerful effect which the world of theories has on the physical world when it is mediated through human activity. It also becomes clear when we see how the world of theories grows far beyond what any single person, or indeed all people, can grasp. This growth of the world of theories is due to the challenge which lies in uncovering autonomous problems of the third world. There will always be a challenge in revealing such problems, because there will always be an infinite number of undiscovered problems. It is because of the autonomy of the third world that there will always be a place for original and creative work (Popper, 1972/1992, p. 161).

It was Popper's view that, by and large, any form of understanding has its starting point in the third world, and that understanding consists of operating with the objects which the third world consists of. This means that scientific activities relate to third world objects. Scientific activities thus involve the arguments which are put forward in relation to these objects and their mutual relations. What is said about these scientific activities must thus reveal the objects of the third world to which they relate, and the arguments produced in relation to the problems revealed (Popper, 1972/1992, p. 163).

According to Popper, the solution to the problem is a model which starts by defining the problem. This problem will always be set out against the background of the third world. The problem and its background in the third world together constitute the problem situation. There will be competing and conflicting theories about the problem. Comparisons can be made between the problem and other phenomena, with accompanying contrasts or analogies. A preliminary solution to the problem will be developed on this basis, which will be subject to criticism and the elimination of mistakes. The result of this will be the development of a new problem situation.

If the problem is the understanding of a given theory, then, according to Popper, the solution will use the same model. The starting point here is a problem of understanding. This too must be approached against the background of the third world and the competing theories which relate to the solution to the problem of understanding. On this basis, a preliminary solution must be constructed, which can be subjected to criticism. The result will also be a new problem situation.

On the basis of such general ideas, Popper developed some principles for how to understand or contribute to the understanding of a scientific theory. He formulated these principles under seven headings.

1. If one wants to understand a theory, one must start by reconstructing its problem situation, and this applies whether or not the theory is a successful one. In this context the problem situation is highly complex. It consists of the solutions which the theory produces in relation to a given problem. In addition to this, it consists of the background which forms the basis of the theory, in other words, the pre-existing theories for the solution of the given problem. The problem situation thus also consists of the opinions which have been built up around the existing theories about the given problem. One must thus reconstruct the problem situation from the standpoint in which the creator of the theory in question stood.
2. The reconstruction of the problem situation must be in the nature of a hypothetical reconstruction. One must have an assumption about the problem situation which can be distinguished from other assumptions about the same problem situation. The problem to be solved with such an assumption is a problem of understanding, the problem of understanding a given theory.
3. The problem of understanding which arises is a metaproblem. The theory which is developed to solve such a problem is a metatheory. If one wishes to understand a given theory, one must refer to the theories in the third world which are concerned with the development of theories and with the solution of problems in relation to the development of theories.
4. Any attempt to understand a theory is required to start with a historical investigation of the theory and its problem, so that the problem itself becomes part of the subject of the investigation. The problems which such a historical investigation seeks to solve will be metaproblems which should be clearly distinguished from the problems which are linked to the objects which are investigated.
5. The history of science should not be treated in the same way as the history of theories. It should be treated as the history of problem situations and their modifications through their attempts to solve problems. In this development, failed attempts can be just as important as successful ones.
6. It is necessary to make a clear distinction between the problems of understanding which are linked to the history of science and problems linked to researchers' theories. The problems of understanding are linked to metaproblems and must be dis-

cussed on the basis of metatheories, while the other problems are linked to the objects which the researcher will investigate.

7. If one wishes to explain how and why a theory has a given structure, one must, as an assumption, seek to reconstruct the problem situation or situational logic in which the agent found himself in order to make his actions rationally understandable. Even if it is never entirely possible to explain a creative action, one can at least try to make it understandable. One can attempt to see the creation of the theory as being appropriate for the situation, as the theorist saw it at the time. Here it is necessary to distinguish between an assumption about how the theorist saw the situation, and an assumption about how the situation was in fact. A researcher into theories will not be satisfied with the first assumption alone. He will also develop the second assumption in order to be able to identify the faults of the theory (Popper, 1972/1992, pp. 176-179).

According to Popper's perception of the theory of science, there is an important distinction between the problem which the researcher wishes to investigate, and the problem situation in which the researcher finds himself. There are theories linked to concrete problems, and it is these theories, together with the concrete problem, which create the researcher's problem situation. This problem situation is the starting point for the researcher's scientific action. Therefore, the question of understanding a given theory is really a question of acquiring an understanding of the problem situation in which the researcher found himself, in order to obtain an explanation of the theory. In this way Popper sought to eliminate the whole of what he called the psychological element of the researcher's work. According to Popper, the researcher's work should have its starting point in the logical relations between the different elements in the third world, and not in the psychological conditions. The researcher will put forward arguments in the light of these logical relations. In Popper's view of science, it is thus the logical relations between the elements in the existing world which are the starting point for the arguments which the individual researcher can develop as part of his scientific work. Logical relations and rational arguments are decisive for the explanation which is established in relation to a given problem or a given theory.

However, it is a problem that, in his philosophy of science, Popper based his ideas on examples of problems from and theories about the physical world. His theoretical constructions do not include the social world and theories about the social world. The problem is that, in principle, theories about the physical world deal with unchanging objects. Therefore one can concentrate on considering the continual changing of the theories. In this context it makes sense to set up the third world to be the true starting point for research. However, this situation does not apply to the social world. It is therefore difficult to understand theoretical developments purely as the consequences of problem situations in relation to the third world. They must also be consequences of developments which take place in the social world.

## *Cultural-scientific thought: Hans-Georg Gadamer*

Gadamer worked on the basis of a hermeneutic philosophy, particularly directed towards humanist studies. It was his view that it is not possible to develop a method for seeking after truth; truth must be experienced.

In his book *Truth and Method*, Gadamer linked together the historical development of concepts with a discussion of substantive matters. In terms of the historical development of concepts he paid particular attention to the works of Schleiermacher, Dilthey and Heidegger. The substantive matters he referred to were art, history and language. He considered Schleiermacher to be a major influence on Dilthey, who in turn was a major influence on Heidegger. He also believed that the hermeneutics of art was the basis for the hermeneutics of history, which in turn was the basis for the hermeneutics of language (Gadamer, 1960/1993, p. xxv). That part of his work which is particularly relevant in this context is his development of a hermeneutic view of history.

Gadamer's hermeneutic view of history was based on Heidegger's concept of the hermeneutic circle. It was Heidegger's belief that a person who reads a text approaches it with an existing opinion, and therefore develops a prejudice about the text after reading only a few pages of it. Gadamer emphasised that this did not mean that there was prejudice in the negative sense given to the word in the period of the Enlightenment, but rather that the reader has a pre-existing view. As the reader penetrates further into the text, the pre-existing view will be revised. The result will be an understanding of the text. This is considered to be a circular process (Gadamer, 1960/1993, pp. 265-267).

In this way Gadamer undertook a rehabilitation of the principle of prejudice. There was another principle which was discredited during the Enlightenment, and this was the principle of authority on the basis of tradition. Gadamer also sought to rehabilitate this principle. It was his view that authority is associated with people, and that these people must deserve their authority. They must have special insight. Therefore, authority represents knowledge. Authority must be based on and must be sanctioned by tradition. All forms of education and of moral development are based on this principle of authority through tradition. Since tradition is based on preservation and maintenance, and thereby on the principle of voluntariness, it must also represent common sense. Gadamer supported this view by pointing out that the great gains in the humanist sciences are enduring; they never become obsolete (Gadamer, 1960/1993, pp. 277-285).

When tradition represents knowledge, the classical texts also represent knowledge. For Gadamer, classical texts are characterised by being raised above changing times and tastes. They are constant, and their meanings do not go away. A classical text has meaning in itself and it interprets itself. The classical texts are also characterised by being the basis for classical culture, to which a cultural consciousness and an ultimate community are attached. Therefore, understanding is not a subjective action, but a participation in a tradition. In tradition, the past and the present are in constant communication with each other (Gadamer, 1960/1993, pp. 285-290).

It is a condition for the hermeneutic approach that it should be linked to a tradition. Hermeneutic work is developed out of the mutual influences between the tradition and the interpreter. On the one hand the interpreter will proceed according to the principles which tradition requires. And on the other hand the tradition will be maintained through the work of the interpreter. Gadamer emphasised that this circular movement is not a methodological principle, but rather the ontological structure of understanding.

The ontological structure of understanding is a circular movement in which the interpreter returns to the text and, through his questions, separates productive from non-productive prejudices. In this way, even the distance in time between the text and the interpreter becomes productive.

The questions which the interpreter asks of the text are the result of a consciousness of being influenced by history. This consciousness is a consciousness of a hermeneutic situation. In order to achieve such consciousness, the interpreter must see himself as a part of a situation which he will constantly seek to illuminate. However, this will never be totally successful because the interpreter himself has a historical dimension and can therefore never attain complete knowledge about himself.

What the interpreter can do is to draw up the right horizon for the questions which are to be asked in the meeting with tradition. The interpreter must place himself in the horizon from which the traditional text speaks. This presupposes that the interpreter himself has a horizon. The interpreter must thus bring his own horizon within the historical horizon. In this way understanding becomes a fusion of these two horizons. However, this fusion of horizons implies the possibility that tensions can arise between the text and the interpreter's contemporary conditions. This tension should not be hidden, but should be brought out into the open. The consequence of the fusion can be that the historical horizon fades into the background (Gadamer, 1960/1993, pp. 300-307).

According to Gadamer, one of the most important hermeneutic problems is how to use a text in a new situation. He raises the question of application. In order to understand this situation he refers to the hermeneutics of law and the hermeneutics of religion. In both of these areas there can be tensions between the concrete texts and the view of their application to a given situation. Neither law texts nor religious texts exist with a view to their historical understanding, but rather with a view to being interpreted for their juridical or religious content. As a consequence, such texts must be understood in relation to any concrete situation. To understand the text is thus to apply it. In this way, even the understanding of a text is historical. The text will be understood differently as different situations arise. A reader must accept that future generations will understand a given text differently from the way in which he himself does (Gadamer, 1960/1993, pp. 307-311).

Another hermeneutic problem concerns the structure of consciousness. It was Gadamer's view that consciousness has the structure of experience. In order to study this more closely, he dealt with experience as a concrete phenomenon so that he could then understand the structure of consciousness in the light of the structure of experience. Gadamer saw experience as a process. A person who has had an experience will be open to new experiences. The experienced person will thus be undogmatic. The problem is that experiences must be had and they can be painful. They can involve disappointments and negative events, but they give insight into the surrounding world and to oneself. The truly experienced person will have so much insight that he or she will recognise the limits to their own capabilities. True experience is thus an experience of oneself as being in a historical context. On the basis of this understanding of the structure of experience, Gadamer developed his view of the structure of consciousness. This is where tradition comes into the picture. According to Gadamer, hermeneutic consciousness must necessarily have its starting point in tradition so that a reflexive relationship can be developed between the tradition and the interpreter. This reflexive relationship requires mutual recognition in the same way that a relationship between two people requires mutual recognition. The problem is that the relationship between tradition and interpreter can lead to tensions. In the worst case there can be domination and repression. It is not possible to reflect oneself out of one's own relationship to tradition without destroying the meaning of the tradition. One must place oneself within the tradition and retain an openness towards it. Consciousness must therefore experience tradition and be open to the truth which is embodied in it. Hermeneutic consciousness is developed first and foremost by having a readiness to experience tradition. Hermeneutic consciousness must be open to receive the experiences which tradition can give in the same way that a person must be open to receive the experiences which life can give. It is this readiness which characterises both the experienced person and hermeneutic consciousness (Gadamer, 1960/1993, pp. 346-362).

A third hermeneutic problem concerns how this experience takes place. Gadamer believed that it was possible to experience things by asking questions. It is necessary to have the ability to ask questions. This requires, on the one hand, openness and, on the other hand, a recognition of one's own limitations. In fact Gadamer believed that the question asked was more important than the answer given. The question must be asked so as to allow multiple possibilities for answers. Something may be asked about in one way or another way. There is no method for asking questions. It is not anything which can be learnt. The only requirement for asking is a recognition that there is something one does not know. If one recognises this, the questions will come of themselves. They will push themselves forward. The art of questioning thus consists in continuing to question. It consists in being able to think. Gadamer considered the art of thinking as being a dialectical process. It is a process which takes the form of a dialogue and is therefore structured as questions and answers (Gadamer, 1960/1993, pp. 362-369).

Against the background of these ideas about the dialogue between questions and answers, Gadamer returned to the question of the interpretation of a text. It was his view that the starting point is that it is the text which asks questions of the interpreter. It is therefore the interpreter's job to understand the horizon which lies behind the questions asked. The meaning of the text extends beyond what is said in the text. If one is to understand the meaning of a text, one must first reconstruct the questions which it tries to answer. Next, one must understand that the relevance of the text is continually renewed by developing circumstances. As a result, the reconstructed questions of the text can never be understood exclusively from the standpoint of its original horizon. The text is put into the contextual environment of the interpreter who confronts the text. In this way the questions originally asked by the text are merged together with the questions of the interpreter. The horizon of the text and the horizon of the interpreter merge together (Gadamer, 1960/1993, pp. 369-379).

The consequence of asking questions is not just that one obtains an understanding of the text. When one asks questions, this gives the possibility of finding a meaning, and this meaning can be absorbed into one's own thinking. To obtain understanding through dialogue is to be changed and transformed into a community in which we are no longer what we were.

According to Gadamer's philosophy of science, it is the interpretation of texts which is central to scientific work. Interpretation takes place through a circular movement, which involves a constant re-assessment of pre-existing views of the text. However, interpretation presupposes a link with tradition and respect for the authorities which communicate this tradition. Interpretation must thus take place within the context of existing tradition. According to Gadamer, the work of interpretation consists of asking questions of a text. This leads to a fusion between the horizon which the author was in when he wrote the text, and the horizon of the interpreter. Gadamer saw scientific work as a question of interpretation of texts on the basis of a given tradition. This interpretation takes place by asking questions of the text both from one's own and the author's social horizon.

The consequence of Gadamer's hermeneutics is that any text may represent a fusion of the traditional and the contemporary. In this way, the text will always reflect its own time. However, the question is whether this fusion between traditional and contemporary is an entirely simple process. For instance, Gadamer did not concern himself with the fact that tradition contains disagreements and conflicts, of which his own works give clear evidence. This means that the process through which the two contexts are fused may not be so simple. It is possible that tensions and contradictions will arise during this process.

It is also possible that the status of authority as truth can give rise to problems. Authority may prevent the formation of new contexts for interpretation. Thus, it may be that tradition alone influences the interpretation of a text. The result can be that knowledge is not developed.

There is a further question about the necessity for texts of previous ages to ask questions of the readers of today, and whether these readers must necessarily seek the text's original horizon. Maybe the contemporary reader is not at all interested in reconstructing the questions which the text originally tried to provide answers for. Maybe only some scattered remnants survive in the texts of succeeding generations.

Finally, one can ask how the fusion of the horizon of the text and the horizon of the interpreter is to come about. A reading of Gadamer's writings does not provide a very concrete idea of this. How does such a fusion happen? Is it entirely without problems for the interpreter?

## *The development of a universal theory: Niklas Luhmann*

The basis of Niklas Luhmann's writings was functionalist thinking. His aim was to develop a universal theory which has not only the social systems, but also itself as a field of study. It is thus both a theory with universal claims and a self-referential theory.

I his book, *Social Systems*, Luhmann stated that the field of study for his theoretical programme was the entire world, and that it should be understood in the light of the difference between system and environment. The consequence of this view, according to Luhmann, is that there are no epistemological criteria. One can start from the point of a naturalistic epistemology. The beginning is random.

Luhmann's inspiration for the development of a universal theory was the theory of self-referential, autopoietic systems. Organisation theory, computer theory and information theory, *inter alia,* form the basis of the theory of self-referential systems. Luhmann transferred the idea of self-referential systems to sociology. General systems theory is thus a common designation for very different kinds of research projects.

The starting point for the general systems theory is concepts formulating problems. It is thus formulated as problems and as different types of solutions to problems. Thus, general systems theory formulates problem encounters. Luhmann linked his theory to the formulation of such general problem encounters and related them to sociology.

On the basis of systems theory's problem encounters, and the associated attempts to formulate them, Luhmann established the basic concepts which contribute to the change of the scientific landscape. As a start, he argued that the difference between system and environment acts as a point of departure for any system analysis (Luhmann, 1984/1995, pp. 16-17). What matters for the system is that it is structurally oriented towards its environment, and that it cannot exist without its environment. It maintains itself by the establishment of differences in relation to its environment and by drawing borders in relation to that environment. What matters for the environment is that it maintains its unity through the system. It is surrounded by open horizons, and it is therefore not a system. It has no self-reflexivity and no capacity to act. Within a given system there can be a further differentiation into sub-systems. The consequence of this increasing differentiation is that the system gains in systematisation. Such systematisation can, for example, take the form of a hierarchy or of centre/periphery relations.

Apart from the difference between system and environment, there is also a difference between elements and relations. In many ways, the circumstances which apply to the system/environment difference also apply to the element/relation difference. Just as there is no system without an environment, there are no elements without relations. Just as there is a constitutive unity in the difference between system and environment, there is a constitutive unity in the difference between element and relation. The contrast between the two types of difference lies in the fact that the system/environment difference leads to further differentiation of the system, while the element/relation difference leads to further system complexity (Luhmann, 1984/1995, p. 21).

With increasing complexity, the system must undertake a selection of the relations between its elements. Even if the system consists of relatively few types of elements, through selection it will be possible to form many different types of systems. The consequence is further complexity. At the same time, the environment is more complex than the system, apart from anything else, because it consists of several systems. As a result, the system is forced to make a selection, not just in relation to itself, but also in relation to its environment. The true form-giving principle will always be the difference between two complexities.

The elements contained in a system are constituted through the system. It is thus the system which determines the elements. This means that systems theory has no need of the concept of subject. The concept of subject is replaced by a concept of self-referential systems. Units within this system are constituted by the system itself.

For each element, system or process it is the case that it functions as a unit in itself. The fact that they function as units in themselves is designated as self-reference, reflection or reflexivity. The consequence of such self-reference can be the emergence of paradoxes. Systems which act self-referentially can arrive at a position where they have to get rid of such paradoxes.

According to Luhmann, a system can be called self-referential if it, itself, constitutes the elements which it consists of as functional units. Self-referential systems thus operate in relation to themselves, and they have no form of contact with the environment other than contact with themselves. Self-referential systems are thus closed systems which operate through self-observation. This means that the elements in the system connect up by referring back to one another. This creates coherence and processes. However, it is a precondition that the elements should be of more or less the same character (Luhmann, 1984/1995, pp. 33-37).

New events may occur within a self-referential system, from which new differences may arise. This means that new forms of causality may arise within a closed system. In other words, the system generates its own history and its own causal basis. This also means that it is possible to resist causal pressure from the environment. It becomes possible to ward off control from outside.

Following this general discussion of systems, Luhmann introduced the question of time in relation to systems. Luhmann considered time to be the difference between the future and the past. The problem is that there can be time differences between system and environment. There will not necessarily be continuity of development between them. The system can foreshadow reactions or delay reactions in relation to the environment.

The introduction of the element of time means that elements are linked to each other in a temporal perspective. When elements are linked to each other in a temporal perspective, this means that it can create new situations at any time. Consequently, complexity is also set in a temporal perspective. The system is formed of unstable elements with short duration. It is not the elements which ensure stability, but rather the system itself.

For the system this means that it must ensure the continuous renewal of the elements of the system. There must be dynamic stability. All elements disappear, and there must be an ongoing production of new elements. This production has the nature of reflexive production. Production takes place made on the basis of products (Luhmann, 1984/1995, p. 49).

A system which must constantly change itself in this way, needs to gather information from the environment. Thus, the system is more sensitive to the environment. Another problem is that constant change causes internal disturbance, which requires the system to set limits to this disturbance.

Starting from the basic concepts described and from the time factor which relates to these basic concepts, Luhmann sought to establish a functional analysis. It was his view that functional analysis is a kind of theoretical technique. It uses relations with the aim of understanding the existing as contingent and similarities as comparable. It relates the given to the points of view of the problem, and it seeks to make it understood that the problem can be solved in one or more ways. The relation between the problem and the solution functions as a guideline for the solution of other problems.

The fruitfulness of the functional method depends on how the relationship between the problem and the solution can be specified. It is thus necessary to narrow down the scope of possibilities. The gains in cognition in the field of empiricism lie in being able to compare causalities. The functional method is primarily a comparative method, which opens up the existing for the benefit of other possibilities. In other words, it studies the relations between relations. A functional explanation is thus a general investigation and segregation of functional equivalents (Luhmann, 1984/1995, pp. 53-54).

According to Luhmann, the true yield of the theory lies in the construction of problems. Through the construction of problems one must reveal the possibilities of analysis and comparison. However, he emphasised that it is not yet settled whether self-referential systems are able to observe and describe themselves, and thereby reveal functional conditions.

When it comes to science, Luhmann believed that the functional condition is the truly fruitful principle for the selection of scientifically relevant data. One can imagine the analysis of both personal and social systems within the scientific system, just as one can imagine a dialogue between the scientific system and other systems of functional analysis.

The problem is that the system which science observes is subject to a process which it is not, in itself, capable of producing. This is due, *inter alia,* to science's use of abstract concepts. The functional method allows its objects to be seen as more complex than it is itself. This is a substantial challenge for the self-referential ordering of its objects. It irritates, disturbs and eventually ruins the observed system, if it is not able to protect itself against scientific observation.

When a system is made subject to functional analysis, on the one hand there will be a clarification of structures and functions which are not visible to the system itself. On the other hand there will be a displacement of the known and familiar. They will be subject to comparison, through which previously unknown relations will come to light. In this way the analysis will surpass its object.

The last of the reference problems which functional analysis is directed towards, is the unity of the difference between knowledge and object. In both cases this is a matter of demonstrating connections. According to Luhmann, these connections can be understood as indicators of truth. The result of functional analysis is therefore that it grasps reality, and that it is reliable as a system of ordering.

Luhmann subjected sociology to this understanding of problems and functional analysis. It was his view that sociology is in a theoretical crisis. It has not been able to develop a unified theory. The problem is that theoretical work is often characterised by referring back to the classics. Theoretical texts are legitimised by reference to those texts which have already been considered as theoretical. The task is to dissect and recombine the existing texts. One can create something new by making new combinations of existing theories (Luhmann, 1984/1995, pp. xlv-xlvi).

The consequence of this is a rapid increase in complexity. Sociology appears as nothing but complexity. Meanwhile, the problem according to Luhmann is that sociology has not been able to observe or understand what has been happening. It has had to concern itself with self-produced data and self-produced classics.

Luhmann's theory should be seen as an attempt to solve this problem. Starting with functional analysis, he sought to create a sociological theory with a claim to universality, i.e., a theory which, *inter alia,* has itself as an object.

With his systems theoretical approach for the understanding of both empirical and theoretical phenomena, Luhmann sought to create a theory which would be so universal that it could contain all previous forms of thought and all kinds of empirical phenomena. All types of phenomena should be understood in the difference between system and environment and in the difference between element and relation. The system is self-referential and seeks to avoid influences from the environment. Nevertheless, the environment will be a constant irritation for the system which will thus be forced constantly to renew its elements. The result of this will be internal disturbance of the system and steadily increasing complexity. Luhmann believed that it is the task of functional analysis to study the relation between problem and solution and make a comparative analysis of this relation. This leads to the opening up of further potential solutions.

One of the problems of Luhmann's functionalist theory is that he dismissed the subject. The subject is replaced by the self-referential system. This means that human action is the consequence of the need for renewal when the system is exposed to the environment. In the final analysis, this must mean that the individual subject is not responsible for his actions.

Another problem with Luhmann's theory is that it is presented as being an eternal truth. The basic concepts which he developed apply to all theories at all times. On the other hand, the theories which can be developed within the framework of these basic concepts are temporary. Only the theory which encompasses this process, functional analysis, continues to exist.

Luhmann regarded references back to the classics negatively. This was because of his view that theories are temporary. In this way the classics lose their value. They have no inherent value. Luhmann did not believe that they had anything to say to the present. They have no substantive significance. They can only be regarded as a link in the theoretical development which can be understood by means of functional analysis.

Finally, in relation to Luhmann's scientific criteria, one may ask why comparison should be the decisive element in the search for the connection between problems and solutions. What is the basis for the idea that, because one system gives rise to some specific relation between a problem and a solution, another system should be understood in the light of the same relation? Why will the relations between problems and solutions in biology and computer technology be of the same character as relations between problems and solutions in the social world? And why will we necessarily be able to learn from them in relation to the social world?

## *A philosophy of all symbolic forms: Ernst Cassirer*

Ernst Cassirer based his ideas on the philosophy of Kant. In his major work, *The Philosophy of Symbolic Forms*, he attempted to develop a general philosophy of all symbolic forms. He moved from linguistic forms, into mythical thought and on to the philosophy of science. His aim was to develop a general theory about how these different symbolic forms developed. At the same time he wanted to throw some light on those characteristics which separate them from each other. What he was looking for was a general rule to govern the concrete differences of symbolic forms.

According to Cassirer, the common principle for the establishment of knowledge is that the particular must be put in a context where it is presented as part of a logical structure. It is through the epistemological process that the particular is articulated within a universal law or order. This law binds the individual elements together. The consequence of this principle is that the universal can only be understood through the particular, while the particular can only be understood by reference to the universal. Other forms of intellectual activity must follow corresponding rules. Every authentic function of the human spirit contains an original formative force through which a given phenomenon is given meaning and conceptual content. Cassirer believed that this applies to all forms of knowledge, even if these are mystical or religious. We all live in our own world view which does not mirror the empirical world, but which rather presents it in accordance with independent principles. Each of these functions create their own symbolic forms which, to the same extent, must be recognised as products of the human spirit. They must all be considered as ways by which the human spirit progresses towards its objectification. Art, language, myth and knowledge thus present a common problem which open the way for a universal philosophy of the cultural sciences (Cassirer, 1921-1929/1955, pp. 77-80).

Cassirer thus starts from the position that there is a complex system of forms of knowledge, within which each form has its place and develops its own special character. When all these forms of knowledge are put together as a whole, then analogies and typical relations will become apparent. Such typical relations will be able to be characterised through their qualitative expression, by which Cassirer meant their type. For example, there can be temporal relations, spatial relations or causal relations. The typical relations can also be characterised through their formal qualities, by which Cassirer meant the context in which they appear. For example, this can be a mathematical theory or an artistic form of expression. All contexts for relations have their own constitutive principle which leaves its mark on the relations. This means that there are countless different forms of relations.

Cassirer believed that both the forms and contents of elements and relations mutually constitute each other (Cassirer, 1921-1929/1955, p. 98). For example, a series of points in time constitute a temporal relation, while the temporal relation constitutes the individual point in time. A point in time cannot be understood without the concept of a temporal relation, and conversely, there would be no temporal relation if there were no actual points in time in the past, present and future.

When Cassirer expressed his general principle for the development of knowledge, he used the mathematical concepts of differentiation and integration. There must be differentiation in the epistemological process, through which the individual element is expressed through its different types of relations. Thereafter there must be an integration so that the specific becomes transformed into the whole.

It was Cassirer's view that all forms of cultural expression must be able to be understood on the basis of one principle, which is the principle of constituting the particular by the general. In order to demonstrate this principle, he looked for a common medium which lies behind the different forms of cultural expression. He found this common medium in language. Therefore, the logic of language is decisive for the logic which is found in other forms of cultural expression.

Cassirer believed that language is built up on the basis of substantive terms which can be differently linked together by means of relational concepts. Cassirer showed, through his studies of language at different stages of development, how substantive terms for objects, phenomena, people etc. are developed first. Thereafter the relations between them are noted through suffixes, relative pronouns and so on. The substantive terms thus operate as the basis for expressing relations (Cassirer, 1921-1929/1955, Vol. I, p. 307).

On the basis of the construction of language, Cassirer studied the construction of myths. When he explained the development of myth, Cassirer started with anthropology. In the development of myths, anything can be derived from anything . One kind of substance can lead to another kind of substance. The cause of a change is a substance which can move from place to place and from person to person. Mystical powers are independent, substantial realities. The cause of change can be an animal. When animals come, they bring the seasons. The cause can be a part of a whole, because the whole and the parts are the same phenomenon. If one possesses a part of a person, one has power over the person and can cause changes to that person. The cause can also be a demon. Illness is a demon which resides in its victim (Cassirer, 1921-1929/1955, Vol. II, p. 57). In myth, the cause is a substance, and change consists of a change from one form of substance to another form of substance. In myth, everything is a substance.

Finally, Cassirer believed that ideas about numbers and the development of higher mathematics and natural sciences is based on relational thinking. He showed how the structuring of numbers is based on serial relationships. This was the starting point, and the relationships between phenomena were established first. Once the starting point has been established, and the distance between the individual elements of the series of numbers has been established, all the other elements of the series of numbers can be added infinitely. It is on this basis that negative and irrational numbers can be developed. The relations between positive and negative numbers and between rational and irrational numbers are laid down as an assumption in the creation of each number. Multiplicity becomes infinite. Relational structures constitute the true object of mathematical research. Cassirer also pointed out that in the world of the natural sciences there has been a development of general laws on the basis of which all individual examples of change can be understood. The law of gravity explains the falling of the individual body. Natural science thus tries to distinguish between different kinds of relations through which the complex universe can be understood. Thus, what matters for science is to distinguish relations from substance. Relations are freed from substance (Cassirer, 1921-1929/1955, Vol. II, p. 53).

By reviewing these different forms of thinking Cassirer supported his idea of a common constitutive principle and a common medium for the development of cultural forms, but at the same time he emphasised the specific in the different cultural forms. He followed his own ideas of cultural forms. He allowed individual cultural forms to be constituted by the whole, while allowing them to be presented as individual elements in their own right.

Thus, with his philosophy of symbolic forms, Cassirer created a philosophy which can contain all kinds of phenomena and all kinds of thinking. The fundamental principle for all symbolic forms is that they can generally only be understood through the specific and that the specific can only be understood by reference to the general. The common medium behind all symbolic forms is language. The syntactical distinction between substantive terms and relational concepts forms the basis for the development of symbolic forms from myths, which are characterised by substantive thinking, to science, which is characterised by relational thinking.

The problem with this approach is that language is ascribed such decisive importance as the medium and structuring principle behind all symbolic forms. The consequence is that the symbolic forms become a mirror image of the structure of language, rather than being the result of the actions of human beings. Thus, it will be seen that in Cassirer's philosophy, too, the subject tends to disappear.

## *The search for a synthesis: Dag Østerberg*

Dag Østerberg also bases his thinking on Kant's philosophy. In his book, *Metasociology*, he distinguishes between substance and form when presenting the basis for his analysis. On the one hand he presents the substantive idea of the book. And on the other hand he presents the conceptual distinction which is the guideline for the book's analysis.

When considering the substantive part, Østerberg presents his basic idea of sociology as being a science which arises as a counterpart to political thinking. Sociology's ideas about society are developed as a counterpart to political science's ideas about the state. According to Østerberg, sociology is developed in opposition to liberal and to statistical/economic thinking.

When considering form, Østerberg presents two basic distinctions. It is his view that the analysis of the development of sociology should take place by distinguishing between external and internal relations, on the one hand, and between facticity and project on the other hand.

The distinction between internal and external relations is a distinction between two forms of thinking. The fact that the relation between two unitary things is external means that it is conditional and thus can take place. The fact that the relation between two unitary things is internal means that it is mutual, and that together they constitute a unity so that the one unitary thing is what it is by virtue of the other. The view of relations as being external is derived in particular from the Scots philosopher, David Hume, and it is still current in contemporary realism. The view of relations as being internal was put forward by the English philosopher, Francis Herbert Bradley. Kant adopted a middle position in this argument about the understanding of relations. Kant was largely indifferent to the external relations which were, to him, much the same as empirical relations. His interests were focussed on *a priori* categories in mathematics and transcendental logic (Østerberg, 1988, pp. 8-11).

The distinction between facticity and project is a distinction between two qualities of a phenomenon. With reference to Heidegger and Sartre, Østerberg makes this distinction as a division between the actual existence of a given phenomenon, and the process by which people transfer the given phenomenon to their consciousness. However, behind the project, by which people transfer the actual phenomenon to their consciousness, there lies a second form of facticity, which consists of the circumstances of the person in question. This involves that person's personal history, language and capacities. According to Østerberg, internal relations apply between facticity and project. Facticity and project require each other. A phenomenon has no actual existence unless it has been transferred to human consciousness, and vice versa. With reference to Cassirer, he emphasises that facticity becomes a phenomenon in itself, but it can only be experienced through the formative activity of human beings. There must thus be some symbolic forms through which humans can experience the world, but if the world is to be experienced, it must be by means of these forms. In this connection, the greatest threat is the destruction of forms and thus of the possibility of experiencing the world (Østerberg, 1988, pp. 11-12).

Østerberg then undertakes an analysis of sociology on the basis of this presentation of content and conceptual distinctions. In his analysis he contrasts different ideas about interpersonal relations.

The starting point for his analysis is ideas about social statistics and liberal philosophy. Østerberg argues that ideas about social statistics are based on external relations and on the view that everything is conditional. At the same time, he points out that its results consist of facticity, without this being mediated through any form of project or cultural form. Østerberg says that another problem is that the probability calculations used by social statisticians assume that the future will have the same form as the past and the present. Finally, Østerberg points out the problem that, in social statistical thinking, theory is subordinate to empirical data. Østerberg argues that the strange view of this form of thinking is that the individual can be considered as being in external relations to other individuals and to the state. While social statistics regards the individual as something which must be monitored and controlled, liberal thinking sees the individual as a citizen trying to protect himself against the state and its exercise of power. Østerberg says that the basis of liberal thinking is the defence of the freedom of rights of property and the state's defence of this freedom. Østerberg sees it as a problem that liberal thinking looks on economic activity as a purely utilitarian relation. The problem is that it ignores tradition in the sense of culture and morality. Emphasis is put on decision-making rather than tradition. Another problem is that liberal thinking sees production and consumption as purely individual affairs. This disregards the fact that these are frequently collective undertakings. Finally, Østerberg argues that liberal thinking tends to ignore the conflicts which are apparent within the economy (Østerberg, 1988, p. 86).

Sociology and Marxist thought are a reaction to these two forms of thought. Østerberg sees sociology as a science of social integration, and as a science which, in essence, is concerned with entireties and with internal relations. The starting point for sociology is a concern for social disintegration and the consequent anomie (Østerberg, 1988, p. 118). Its theoretical development is therefore based on concepts for understanding social integration. Durkheim underlined the necessity of education and the socialisation of the individual. Using modern knowledge in the fields of mechanics and biology, it is possible to distinguish between the mechanical and the organic. This is seen in the distinction between society and community, between a society regulated by laws and a community regulated by rituals. In this way sociology functions as a science which positions society in between the individual and the state. Social cohesion occupies the central role. Marxist philosophy argues that it is a basic principle that man and man's rights are changeable. In essence, they are historical. The state is considered to be an instrument for domination and repression. Therefore, the decisive relationship is between the class struggle and the bourgeois state. In Marxist philosophy there is a connection between socialisation and class structure. There is a socialisation within each class in such a way as to strengthen the existing class structure (Østerberg, 1988, p. 142).

In conclusion, Østerberg puts forward some current attempts to solve the tensions which contradictory modes of thinking have led to. He distinguishes between the thinking which can still be characterised as sociological, and thinking which no longer has the characteristics of sociology.

Within the thinking which still has the basic characteristics of sociology, three attempts at syntheses have been developed, and these are the theoretical contributions of Adorno, Habermas and Bourdieu. Adorno argues that we live in an age in which it is impossible to live without social statistics. Therefore we must accept this and its opposite, both sociological thinking and Marxist philosophy. According to Østerberg, both human intellect and reason were re-introduced by Habermas. Reason forms the basis for human interaction. It is reason which is constitutive for human relations, and it is reason which must operate as a yardstick for established institutions. Østerberg says that Bourdieu sought to combine both social statistics and the philosophy of the classical sociologists (Østerberg, 1988, p. 173). He saw social life as being constituted by individuals who pursue their own goals through considered actions, but he also saw it as being constituted by collectives which have intentions which are independent of individuals.

As examples of thinking which has moved beyond sociological thinking, Østerberg refers to the theories developed by Sartre, Foucault, Touraine and Luhmann. Østerberg says that the underlying theme in Sartre's work was the question of human freedom. In this respect, Sartre had a view which was in common with liberal thinking. Nevertheless, Sartre disagreed with liberalism. In Sartre's thinking, the relations between people were seen in two dimensions, first as the consciousness of being an object, and secondly as the consciousness of being the other (Østerberg, 1988, p. 203). This means that one cannot have an instrumental relationship with the other, but must respect the other's freedom. Sartre regarded human beings as individuals who are not motivated by utilitarian principles. The consequence of his views, says Østerberg, is that the truth about human co-existence is that it is a form of anarchy. Foucault denied the contradiction between the state and the individual. For him there were neither individual nor society. What there are, are bodies which can no longer be objectified and thus cannot be separated from one another (Østerberg, 1988, p. 225). Individualisation takes place against the will of the individual. Individualisation is like branding as deviant and abnormal. The separation between normal and abnormal is a matter of the exercise of power. The abnormal becomes apparent through definition, discourse and patterns of behaviour. According to Touraine, there has been a shift from the meta-social to the social. There is no longer a supreme judge. Human behaviour should be understood in the light of the values which are created through human behaviour. Touraine sees human behaviour through a fusion of Parson's and Sartre's theories of action. On the one hand human action is the outcome of norms. On the other hand it is historical. It is Touraine's view that society has changed from being an industrial society to become a programmed society. It is no longer the relations between classes which determine development, but rather the insight into these relations. This means that society's development is influenced by the knowledge of the conditions for its development. Consequently, there must be a new historical subject. According to Touraine, this could be the student movement or the women's movement. In Touraine's thinking, the historical subject does not consist of individuals, but of collective actors (Østerberg, 1988, p. 249). Finally, Østerberg includes a review of Luhmann's thinking. It is Østerberg's view that the individual disappears in Luhmann's theory. Social life no longer consists of individuals. Instead, social systems with self-referential communication exist (Østerberg, 1988, p. 264). Ideas of social integration are replaced by inclusion and exclusion in relation to the social systems.

Østerberg's meta-perspective of sociology thus gives a review of the development of sociology. With its distinction between external and internal relations he arrives at a division between social statistical and liberal thinking on the one hand, and between sociological and Marxist thinking on the other hand. In this perspective, sociology is presented as an alternative to the ideas which distinguish between the individual and the state. Sociology becomes the science which puts social coherence on the agenda. It is Østerberg's view that many of the newer theories are a reaction to the tension which has arisen in the field of study generally described as the social sciences. Adorno, Habermas and Bourdieu are among those sociological theorists who seek to combine the two types of thinking. Østerberg says that these theorists seek to maintain sociological ideas about society and integration, while focussing on the individual and the state. Then there are those theorists who go beyond the original separation of individual and state and social integration. These theorists include Sartre, Foucault, Touraine and Luhmann. For Sartre, the individual and his relation to the other was central. For Foucault, the individual first becomes apparent when he is labelled as abnormal. For Touraine, the individual becomes non-existent, and is replaced by the collective as historical actor, and with Luhmann, the individual and subject disappear completely. Østerberg admits that he is most attracted by Touraine's and Sartre's attempts to rise above the original tensions. Touraine's ideas seem promising because we still live in a society with a capitalist mode of production. Here there must be a historical subject. Sartre's thinking is promising because it makes it possible to develop emotional relations which differ between different individuals.

Østerberg's meta-sociological view can be objected to because, by separating internal and external relations, he arrives at a very crude classification of social scientific thinking. It is not possible to exclude the consideration of sociology as a philosophy which is based on internal relations. From Durkheim and up to the present there are many examples of causal thinking in sociology where relations between phenomena are conditional.

Furthermore, one must question whether sociology solely consists of a theory of social integration. Durkheim, and a number of prominent sociologists who followed him, took this point of departure, but if one takes one's point of departure in Weber's sociology, integrationist ideas are not at the centre. Here the focus is primarily on the individual and its cultivation.

## *Theory of culture between natural and cultural scientific thought*

From this overview, presenting and discussing examples of natural scientific and cultural scientific ideas, and attempts to overcome their contradictions, I will now move on to the question of how far it is possible to understand the sociological theory of culture within this formal framework.

The main problem is whether it is possible to understand the sociological theory of culture within the distinction between natural scientific and cultural scientific thought. This problem raises the question of whether it is possible to make a synthesis of these two forms of thought within the sociological theory of culture.

In order to investigate whether such a conceptual framework is relevant over time, I have chosen to include representatives of both classical and contemporary sociology. In this way it becomes possible to study whether this conceptual framework has enduring qualities in relation to the sociological theory of culture.

I will include three key theorists from classical sociology: Émile Durkheim, Max Weber and Georg Simmel. Likewise, I will include three key theorists from contemporary sociology: Margaret Archer, Robert Wuthnow and Pierre Bourdieu. It is my view that the theories of the three classical sociologists constitute some of the most important contributions to the development of sociology as a science, and that it is therefore of great importance to investigate how these thinkers have understood and worked with cultural phenomena. It is also my opinion that the theories of the three contemporary sociologists are some of the most central contributions to the current development of cultural theory.

Given the problem to be studied, it will be important to investigate how the selected theorists have approached methodological questions. It is in these methodological considerations that it becomes most clear whether a theory is based on natural scientific or social scientific thought. Therefore, each of the six following chapters starts with a clarification of the methodological principles of the theorist in question. In these sections there will be a discussion of the thinkers' attitudes to natural and cultural scientific approaches.

Against the background of this clarification of the methodological principles, there is an investigation of the attitudes of each theorist to culture. How is the concept of culture dealt with in their analyses? What do they understand by 'culture' and how, in their analyses, do they relate cultural phenomena to other kinds of social phenomena? This clarification of concepts and contents is based on those works in which each author deals with the question of culture. Each work will be presented on the basis of its own premises, after which the understanding of culture, which is more or less explicitly set out in the work, will be distilled.

However, the clarification of each theorist's methodological approach and their understanding of and theoretical ideas about culture, raises the question of what influences lie behind this understanding. To answer this question, the social context and the intellectual context for the development of the theory are discussed. The question is whether we can see the chosen texts as contributions which are both affected by the intellectual debate which was current at the time when the text originated, and by the contemporary social development. I will consider how this double context may have affected the content and conceptual development of each of the theories.

Finally, with each of the six writers, I will investigate how other sociologists have interpreted their theories on culture. In this way, my own understanding will be related to the available literature on the writings of each of the six. On the other hand, there will not be a relation of an overarching thesis of the sociological theory of culture to existing literature for the simple reason that no other overarching thesis of the sociological theory of culture has yet been proposed.

# Part I
# Classical Sociology of Culture

# 2

# Émile Durkheim: Culture as System

In his major biography of Durkheim, Steven Lukes hardly mentions the word 'culture'. Culture does not appear to be one of the concepts which Durkheim was very much concerned with. According to Lukes, Durkheim's work lay in the fields of education, the division of labour, the family, suicide, law and punishment. He considers Durkheim's most significant contribution to be in the fields of the sociology of morality, the sociology of knowledge and the sociology of religion (Lukes, 1973). Any attempt to establish a view of Durkheim's understanding of culture must therefore start with these contributions to the development of sociology. By studying Durkheim's contributions to theories about morality, knowledge and religion it becomes possible to develop an understanding of how Durkheim regarded the phenomenon of culture.

In this connection, the most important of Durkheim's works is *The Evolution of Educational Thought*, which is taken from a series of lectures given in 1904-5 (Durkheim, 1938/1977), *Moral Education*, which is from a series of lectures given in 1902-3 (Durkheim 1925/1968) and *The Elementary Forms of Religious Life* (Durkheim 1912/1995). This last named work was written as an independent study and it must be considered as one of Durkheim's major comprehensive works. In each of these three titles there are analyses of phenomena which he himself considered to be cultural phenomena, namely the intellect, morality and knowledge. Others of his works, including *The Division of Labor in Society* (Durkheim, 1893/1997) and *Professional Ethics and Civic Morals* (Durkheim, 1950/1992), include further contributions to his studies of morality, but do not add anything new to help interpret Durkheim's understanding of culture. These works are therefore omitted from the further discussions.

It is helpful to start by looking at the methodological principles which underlie Durkheim's sociology. These principles are set out in his book *The Rules of Sociological Method* (Durkheim, 1895/1966). In the Preface to the first edition of the book Durkheim emphasised that he had a rationalist approach to sociology. He was of the view that past behaviour can be reduced to the relations between cause and effect, whereafter these relations can form the basis of rules for future behaviour.

The basic concept in Durkheim's discussion of methods is the concept of 'social facts':

> "A social fact is every way of acting, fixed or not, capable of exercising on the individual an external constraint; or again, every way of acting which is general throughout a given society, while at the same time existing in its own right independent of its individual manifestations." (Durkheim, 1895/1966, p. 13)

The methodological problems which concerned Durkheim were: how is it possible to study social phenomena, and how can they be explained? What was important for him was to develop a scientific method which would command the same kind of respect for the social sciences as had been achieved by the natural sciences. Social facts should therefore be studied as 'things', which means that they should be isolated from everyday ideas about them. When social facts are studied, they must be considered independently from their individual circumstances, and should instead be studied as groups of phenomena with common characteristics. It was Durkheim's view that it was possible to explain a social fact in all its complexity by following it through all the stages of its development. He called this a 'genetic' method (Durkheim, 1895/1966, pp. 138-139).

## *The intellectual aspects of culture*

Durkheim developed his genetic method while researching the development of educational ideas in France. He emphasised that it is only through the study of the past that it is possible to understand the present and go forward into the future (Durkheim, 1938/1977, p. 9). He considered it necessary to go back in time to find the nucleus of the idea and the first germination of academic institutions.

> "But this nucleus, this original germinative cell, where is it to be found?" (Durkheim, 1938/1977, p. 19).

In seeking the nucleus of the idea that formed the basis for the development of educational ideas, Durkheim looked to the intellectual culture which was transferred from the Roman Empire to France. This cultural transfer did not take place without some resistance. The backward and barbarous Franks were initially not at all receptive to literature, art and philosophy.

> "The entire substance of our early intellectual culture came to us from Rome. .... The Germanic peoples (i.e. the Franks) ... attached no value at all to literature, the arts or philosophy. We know that even the buildings and sculpture of the Romans inspired in them only hatred and contempt." (Durkheim, 1938/1977, p. 19).

The institution which succeeded in overcoming this resistance was the church. It was the church's desire to bring the Christian gospel to the Franks which was the basis for the idea of education.

What made it possible for the Christian church to establish a foothold among the barbarous and uncivilised Franks was that it could offer them spiritual comfort in their poverty. Christianity glorified the humble poor and offered salvation. The Franks accepted this spiritual comfort and with it received a culture. The problem was that the dissemination of Christian belief made it necessary to educate people, so they would be able to preach and teach. Education presupposes the existence of a culture, and at that time there was no culture other than paganism. The church therefore had to assimilate this.

> "Now, teaching presupposes a culture, and at that time there was no culture other than pagan culture. It was therefore necessary for the church to appropriate it. Teaching and preaching presuppose in him who is teaching or preaching certain linguistic skills, a certain capacity for dialectic, and a certain familiarity with man and with history. All this knowledge was only to be found in the works of the ancients." (Durkheim, 1938/1977, p. 23).

It was the same for both clergy and laity that they had to acquire a certain amount of culture. This could only be obtained by reading the classical writers. The culture of antiquity was absorbed together with the classical texts. At the same time there was a fundamental problem arising out of the contradictions between Christian faith and paganism. These contradictions were to be the source of conflict through many centuries.

> "There was on the one hand the religious element, the Christian doctrine; on the other, there was classical civilisation, and all the borrowings which the church was obliged to make from it, that is to say the profane element. In order to defend and propagate itself, the Church, as we have seen, was forced to rely on a culture and this culture could not but be pagan since there wasn't any other." (Durkheim, 1938/1977, p. 25).

What this meant for education was that right from the very start it contained the germ of the conflict between the religious and the secular. In the course of time it was the secular ideas which came to predominate over the religious ideas.

Durkheim's analysis moved forward through history in order to see how this original contradiction between the religious and the secular affected the development of educational ideas. He showed how ideas about education were influenced by the church's attempt to eliminate the secular content of the classical texts and concentrate on their form. Thus, from the start, the emphasis was on the formal and abstract aspects of the ideas. To begin with the grammatical aspects of the language were studied. Later, more emphasis was put on logic and dialectic, which were necessary for reasoning. Thus, the study of man's intellect was at the core of all forms of education. It was during the Renaissance that humanism began to come to the fore and importance was attached to the substantive content of the texts, but it was not until the French Revolution that natural sciences and mathematics were included in the curriculum of the French educational system.

It was Durkheim's opinion that educational ideas change in parallel with developments in society. In his analysis, he pointed out that changes in living conditions, increased integration between the social classes and the establishment of the European nation states all contributed to the development of ideas. At the same time he emphasised that the development of ideas is not a clear path along some pre-determined course. It is the result of skirmishes and battles between conflicting ideas. In his analysis he referred to the ideological battles between the different centres of religion in Europe. Such battles have meant that some ideas, which were fundamentally good and which ought therefore to have survived, have been suppressed, while other good ideas have only achieved ephemeral success. The problem is that adherents of new ideas tend to believe that there is nothing of the earlier ideas which is worth preserving. Although new ideas are developed on the basis of earlier ideas, the adherents of new ideas have a tendency to be bitter opponents of previous ideas. They reject them in their entirety and are blind to what they themselves have in common with their predecessors. This can result in regrettably destructive actions, so that elements of earlier cultures are expunged. In this way, earlier ideas are wiped from the record of history, so they do not become part of the inheritance of ideas.

> "Here as elsewhere the struggle for survival has led to results which are only crude and approximate. In general it is the best adapted and most gifted which survive." (Durkheim, 1938/1977, p. 13).

In this work on the development of educational ideas, Durkheim did not give any definition of what he understood by the word culture, even though he used a concept of culture. It is clear that human intellect is associated with his concept of culture. He spoke of the intellectual culture which originated with the Roman Empire. Culture thus concerns man's understanding and ability to reason. This is not necessarily an exhaustive definition, but it does at least establish one element of culture.

In the text culture is presented with two facets. On the one hand culture is linked to texts, and on the other hand it is acquired by people. When Durkheim referred to the intellectual culture of the Roman Empire, he was referring to literature, art, sculpture and architecture. When he referred to pagan culture he was referring to the writings of antiquity. On the other hand, he asserted that both clergy and laity had to acquire a certain level of culture in order to understand the scriptures. For Durkheim, acquiring culture meant acquiring certain linguistic skills, developing the ability to think and obtaining knowledge and insight. For the time being it can be concluded that Durkheim's concept of culture covered man's intellectual activities as they become deposited in cultural products and from there acquired by the individual.

It is thus possible to distil a concept of culture from Durkheim's analysis of the development of educational ideas. The next question is whether it is also possible to deduce a theory of culture from this analysis. Such a theory must be able to explain first what it is that affects people's intellectual activities, and thus the creation of cultural products, and second how these cultural products affect people. On the face of it, one can say that *The Evolution of Educational Thought* does not contain any such theory. Nowhere did Durkheim explain what it is that affects the development of culture or how culture affects people. However, if thinking about education is taken as an example of man's intellectual activities, then it is clear that this work is one long theory of what affects culture. On the one hand Durkheim pointed to the social changes in living conditions and relations between social classes as factors which can affect and bring about changes to educational ideas. On the other hand he pointed to the conflicts between ideas as factors which are significant in determining which ideas emerge triumphant. Using ideas from biology, he concluded that in the battle for the survival of ideas it is the fittest that win. In the long run there is a steady development which is only disturbed by conflicts and revolutions to a limited extent. If one takes the other part of the question, about how culture is transferred to people, then Durkheim supplies us with a long list of ideas concerning this question from religious and secular institutions, but nowhere do we obtain his view of how culture is transferred to people. However, we obtain this in the book *Moral Education*.

## *The moral aspects of culture*

In *Moral Education* Durkheim pursued the question of what affects people's morality, and especially how children's morals can be affected through education. Here, his rationalist approach is apparent. In the introduction to the book he stressed that morality must be considered as a rational phenomenon, as a fact that can be observed and analysed. He gave himself two tasks: to find the forces which are the basis for a moral life, and to find a rational expression for this morality (Durkheim, 1925/1968, p. 20).

> "Thus, we can say that morality consists of a system of rules of action that predetermine conduct." (Durkheim, 1925/1968, p. 24).

Such a system of rules of conduct is external to the individual and must be communicated by older persons being models of behaviour in applying the rules. There are thus rules of conduct which we are not free to change according to taste. The rules dominate us and carry a significant element of authority. The rules cannot exist without some acknowledgement of the authority which lies behind them. If there is no such acknowledgement, then there is no morality. Conversely, if there is acknowledgement of the authority behind the morality, the consequence will be regularity of action. In this connection Durkheim referred to biology. He considered regularity of action to be a phenomenon which is analogous to periodicity in biology.

> "Regularity is the moral analogue of periodicity in the organism." (Durkheim, 1925/1968, p. 34).

Durkheim discussed the question of what affects morality, and how morality is absorbed by human beings by reviewing its three elements: the formal element of morality, as a discipline, the substantive element of morality, which is subordination to groups, and morality as an element of understanding, which enhances self-determination or autonomy.

The formal element of morality, discipline, leads to the regulation and restriction of the behaviour of the individual. The consequence of discipline is thus that the individual is restricted and must suppress certain needs and moderate certain tendencies. Therefore, moral behaviour is orderly behaviour. It is behaviour which follows enduring principles and which overrides impulses and urges.

Durkheim stated that the substantive element of morality, subordination to the group, is an external factor in relation to the individual. In other words the field of morality begins where the field of society begins. This means that man is only a moral creature to the extent that he is a social creature. This in turn means that to act morally is to act in accordance with collective interests (Durkheim, 1925/1968, p. 59).

If one is to understand the essence of this view, it is necessary to understand that, according to Durkheim, collective interests are not merely the sum of individual interests. Society is an independent phenomenon which the individual is attached to. Man must learn to communicate with the source of the mental and moral life which society consists of.

According to Durkheim, it is society which produces morality. It requires of us that we should develop ourselves as ideal types. It does this because it can only exist if its members are sufficiently uniform, in other words if they all reflect, to a certain degree, the characteristics which are essential for a given ideal type and thus for a collective ideal. If it is society itself which has created the moral rules, it must also be society which has given them authority.

> "For it follows from all that we have said that society infinitely surpasses the individual, not only in material scope, but beyond that, in moral power. Not only does it command incomparably greater power, since it derives from the mutual reenforcement of all the individual forces, but in it is found the source of that intel-

> lectual and moral life to which we turn to nourish our thought and our morality." (Durkheim, 1925/1968, p. 88).

When a new generation is formed it must assimilate the cultural milieu. This happens gradually as the individual child absorbs elements of culture and in this way becomes a human being. Since it is society which accumulates and protects the cultural values and passes them on from one generation to the next, these values must come to us through society. Therefore we have duties towards society.

> "For the fashioning of a newly born generation implies the assimilation, little by little, of the cultural milieu; it is only gradually as the animal – as we are born – incorporates the elements of his culture that the human being emerges. For it is society that is the repository of all the wealth of civilization; it is society that accumulates and preserves these treasures transmitting them from age to age. It is through society that these riches reach us." (Durkheim, 1925/1968, pp. 88-89).

It was Durkheim's view that the content of morality has a double aspect, that on the one side it is an imperative and on the other side it is an ideal. Morality thus involves both a sense of duty and an ideal about what is good.

> "For there is only one method for eliciting such ideas and sentiments in the child's mind ... This is to link the child as directly as possible with that to which these ideas and feelings refer. It is only this that, through its influence on the consciousness, can stimulate those mental states expressing it. Education through direct experience affects the moral as well as the intellectual elements of culture." (Durkheim, 1925/1968, p. 97).

Morality can thus be derived from empirical conditions, being those empirical conditions which the duty and the ideal relate to. Therefore, education is just as important for moral development as for the intellectual facets of culture.

> "... morality can be completely derived from empirical realities and ... consequently education is in the nature of things as applicable to the moral as to the intellectual elements of culture." (Durkheim, 1925/1968, p. 105).

The third element of morality concerns people's understanding of morality and the autonomy and self-determination which this understanding gives. According to Durkheim this development has two stages. The first stage concerns understanding the rules, and the second stage concerns an explanation of the rules. Both stages lead to autonomy and self-determination.

Durkheim believed that if people are to understand the world and act in relation to it, they must be able to understand what is happening within themselves. This is the first step towards autonomy. We emancipate ourselves through understanding. Therefore knowledge is the source of autonomy. Development of knowledge about morality will mean that we come to master morality so that it is no longer an external factor. We can thus create our own autonomy by acquiring a more and more complete knowledge of things. This does not mean that man is able to avoid the world and its laws. We are an integral part of the world, and it operates in relation to us and works its way into every part of us. But:

> "... we can, through science, use our understanding to control both the things that exert an influence upon us and this influence itself. In this way we again become our masters. Thought is the liberator of will." (Durkheim, 1925/1968, p. 119).

The second step towards autonomy concerns the symbolic explanation of rules and thus the reasons for their existence. Education about morals is thus not a question of preaching or indoctrination. It is a question of explanation. The child should not only know what its duties are, it must also know the explanation for its duties. The moral development of a child means enabling it to understand its country and getting it to accept responsibility. The child must be prepared to take its part in the collective tasks which await it.

Durkheim gave some thought to the methods which can be used for developing the moral elements in children.

> "To influence the child morally is ... to develop and even to constitute completely, by appropriate methods, those general dispositions that, once created, adapt themselves readily to the particular circumstances of human life." (Durkheim, 1925/1968, p. 21).

The child's tendency to develop habits and its openness to ideas are dispositions which may form the starting point for the moral education of the child. It is possible to develop regularity of behaviour by using the child's disposition to form habits. When a child registers regularity in the behaviour of adults it will come to view such regularity as being the general rule. The child's disposition to openness to ideas means that each new idea meets very little resistance. By using this disposition it is possible to develop the child's understanding of the moral forces which surround it (Durkheim, 1925/1968, p. 143). In the last part of the book Durkheim discussed how it is possible, by using the pedagogical tools of punishment and reward, to develop such a nucleus of morality and create a defined and complex feeling of morality.

In this work on moral education, Durkheim expanded his concept of culture in relation to his work on the development of educational thinking. Here it is not only man's intellect which is part of culture. He also included morality as part of culture. In several places he spoke of the intellectual and the moral aspects of culture.

When Durkheim defined morality, he used the concept of a system. Morality is a system of rules. In this connection he drew his inspiration from biology and compared regularity of behaviour with periodicity in biological phenomena. Thus, at least one aspect of culture, namely morality, was to be regarded as a system.

This understanding of culture was also reproduced in *The Evolution of Educational Thought*. Culture is regarded as treasures and wealth which are accumulated and preserved by society and from there passed on to individuals.

With *Moral Education* we have come a step further towards identifying a theory of culture in Durkheim's work. According to Durkheim there is no doubt that both the moral and the intellectual aspects of culture are created collectively. If we are to explain culture we must look to its origin, which is society. It is society which is the basis of culture. Morality is a reflection of culture. At the same time it is society which preserves the cultural treasures and from there culture is conferred on the individual.

The transfer of culture takes place through experiences, but it also takes place through active pedagogical measures which use the child's natural tendency to form habits and to be open to ideas. However, culture is not merely transferred to passive recipients. If people create a scientific understanding of culture they will be able to control it. Man can become the master of culture through his insight and understanding.

## *The scientific aspects of culture*

In *The Elementary Forms of Religious Life* Durkheim gave a more detailed presentation of his entire theoretical construction. This was one of Durkheim's later works and so it is the work where all the elements of his theory are present.

The genetic method which was the basis for his study of the development of educational ideas also characterised this work on the development of religion. Durkheim reached back to that religion which he believed was the most elementary, the religion of the aboriginal Australian tribes. Durkheim believed that the germ of all forms of religion is to be found in the most simple and primitive form, from which it has developed into its contemporary and complex form. For Durkheim the aim of the study of primitive religion was therefore to obtain an understanding of the omnipresent causes of religion. These causes are easier to observe in primitive societies than in more complex societies (Durkheim, 1912/1995, pp. 3-7). Durkheim's objective was not only to understand religion, but also to understand its function. His view was that, from its very beginning, religion has served as both science and philosophy. It has not merely contributed to the enrichment of man's intellect, it has also helped to shape it. Religion has thus prepared the way both for the substantive and the formal aspects of knowledge. Therefore, for Durkheim, his study of religion was also a study of knowledge.

According to Durkheim, the most fundamental categories of intellectual life, such as time, space, number, cause, substance and personality, originate from religious thought. It applies both to religion and to these general categories that they must be considered as collective realities, as social things (Durkheim, 1912/1995, pp. 8-9).

According to Durkheim, knowledge consists of two elements: empirical knowledge, which is based on the experience of the individual, and categorical knowledge, which is based on the way the collective is organised. Collective representations are the products of extended co-operation and accumulation over many generations.

> "Collective representations are the product of an immense co-operation that extends not only through space but also through time; to make them, a multitude of different minds have associated, intermixed, and combined their ideas and feelings; long generations have accumulated their experience and knowledge." (Durkheim, 1912/1995, p. 15).

Categorical knowledge is, according to Durkheim, much richer and much more complex than individual experience. Therefore reason has much greater power than empirical knowledge. This power is due to the duality of human nature. On the one hand it consists of the physical person, based within his own body, and on the other hand it consists of the social person which represents the highest observable intellectual and moral reality, which is society. As a consequence of this, morality cannot be reduced to motives and reason cannot be reduced to individual experience. Because he is a part of society, the individual must go beyond his own self, both when he thinks and when he acts (Durkheim, 1912/1995, pp. 14-16).

The categories on which thinking is based cannot be the subject of free choice, according to Durkheim. There must be a certain consensus both about morality and logic. Society cannot, therefore, accept that an individual should try to depart from the norms of thinking. Because of this we can feel internal restraint against moving away from the fundamental categories, and feel external opinion which judges us. The authority, which is in-built in thought and which is the basis for action, is the authority of society (Durkheim, 1912/1995, p. 16).

Durkheim undertook his discussion of primitive religions on the basis of making a fundamental distinction between belief and ritual, which corresponds to his fundamental distinction between thought and action. In his view, belief is based on a further distinction between the sacred and the secular. This distinction contains a fundamental categorisation of the universe, in which sacred things are protected while secular things can be subject to prohibitions. Religious beliefs are the representatives which express the nature of sacred things and the relations they have with other sacred things and with secular things. Rituals are the rules of behaviour which prescribe how human beings should behave in relation to sacred things. When a given number of sacred things relate to each other, they form a system with a special collective force. This system constitutes a religion which is associated with an organisational centre, a cult (Durkheim, 1912/1995, p. 38).

Durkheim discussed the religion of the Australian tribes starting with their totem. A totem is a mark which is put on sacred things and it is at the same time associated with a given social organisation, the clan. A totem is thus a tangible expression, a material representation of the clan, and it is from this that the sacred develops. The clan's totem is linked to its name, its members and a number of natural phenomena such as the weather, plants and animals. A clear distinction thus arises between different totems and the things and phenomena which are associated with them. In extension of each totem there can be a development of sub-totems, leading to a hierarchical system of totems. Durkheim suggested that this is the first form of classification which is seen in history. It is shaped by social organisation. It adopts the structure of society as its own.

> "The purpose of a classification is to establish relations of subordination and coordination, and man would not even have thought of ordering his knowledge in that way if he had not already known what a hierarchy is. … Hierarchy is exclusively a social thing. Only in society do superiors, subordinates, and equals exist. Therefore, even if the facts were not sufficiently conclusive, the analysis of those notions would be sufficient in itself to reveal their origin. We have taken them from society and projected them into our representation of the world. Society furnished the canvas on which logical thought has worked." (Durkheim, 1912/1995, p. 149).

Apart from the collective totem there is also an individual totem. While the collective totem is determined from birth, the individual totem requires a series of rituals. The individual totem must thus be acquired or allocated.

Society has its own character and its own aims, and it is thus distinct from its individuals. This can mean that the individuals must be subordinated to its requirements. The individual must thus subordinate himself to rules of thinking and acting which he may not have desired for himself. This happens when society's requirements enter into us and are organised within us. Its power then becomes an integrated part of our being. This is possible because:

> "In all kinds of acts that express the understanding, esteem, and affection of his neighbour, there is a lift that the man who does his duty feels, usually without being aware of it. But that lift sustains him; the feeling society has for him uplifts the feeling he has for himself. Because he is in moral harmony with his neighbour, he gains new confidence, courage, and boldness in action …" (Durkheim, 1912/1995, p. 213).

The feeling of belonging is further strengthened by tradition. We speak a language which we have not ourselves created, we use tools which he have not ourselves invented, and we claim rights which we have not ourselves established. Each generation inherits a treasury of knowledge which it has not itself discovered. We owe all these benefits to society.

Subordination by the individual to rules can only take place if the individual has developed a sense of being elevated. This can be by the development of a feeling of harmony with other people. However, such feelings cannot be developed in relation to society because it is too complex. Therefore these feelings must be developed in relation to something which represents society, and for the aboriginal Australians this was their totem. Without such symbols, the feelings towards society would be unstable. As a consequence, social life is only possible if there is a considerable degree of symbolism.

Durkheim believed that his theory on totemism was the key to understanding how religious development shaped logical development, and how both phenomena are based on social conditions. This has led to an established practice which is based on scientific culture with a tendency to distinguish between the different areas of nature, and within these to distinguish between different classes.

> "Long-established practice, which scientific culture has rooted even more deeply in our minds, taught us to set up barriers between realms of nature. ... Within each realm, the same barriers separate different classes." (Durkheim, 1912/1995, pp. 236-237).

The rituals which are associated with Australian totemism can, according to Durkheim, be divided into positive and negative rituals. The purpose of the negative rituals is to prevent secular things polluting sacred things. Thus they take the character of prohibition and isolation. The positive rituals have the aim of enabling sacred animals procreate. They therefore take the character of mimicking these animals. The problem is that if the sacred animals do not procreate, the clan is doomed. This means that the clan cannot leave such things to chance. It must stage a ritual which initiates procreation. In this way a link is made between the idea of procreation and the action which is required to bring it about. An axiom is established, i.e., a fundamental assumption of a causal connection, and the authority for this is society. The category of causality is thus created by the collective. It operates as a framework for the individual's empirical observations and makes it possible to think about these observations. It becomes possible for us to view these observations from a particular angle and to understand each other with regard to these observations. The reason for the existence of the category is that society needs it.

> "... if the framework can be applied to the content, that is because it is not without relationship to that content, but ... it is made, first and foremost, to satisfy the needs of life in common." (Durkheim, 1912/1995, p. 372).

Durkheim concluded that man supplements the secular world with a sacred world, which only exists in thought and which is more highly regarded than the secular world. Human beings create an ideal version of the real world which they are part of. The individual's ideal of the world is added to this collective ideal. This individual ideal can differ from the collective ideal. The basis of the common ideal is the feeling of belonging which is obtained by social gathering. However, these principles for religion are no different from the principles for science. In both, there is an attempt to link phenomena with each other, to establish their inner relations, to classify and systematise them. And in both of them the categories are derived from society. First, they are institutionalised by society, and second, their content expresses different aspects of society.

> "... the categories are ... social in another sense and ... to a higher degree. Not only do they come from society, but the very things they express are social. It is not only that they are instituted by society but also that their content is various aspects of the social being." (Durkheim, 1912/1995, p. 441).

This work on the religious life of primitive societies introduces yet another element of culture, the element of knowledge. In several places Durkheim wrote about scientific culture. The scientific element of culture is now added to the intellectual and moral elements of culture which were dealt with in the previous discussion of the two works.

In Durkheim's definition of knowledge we find again the perception of intellectual culture as expressed in *The Evolution of Educational Thought*, namely that it is a treasure which is inherited by each succeeding generation from the generations that went before. Categorical knowledge is an expression of intellectual work which has been developed through co-operation and accumulated over generations. It is thus that the categories of thinking have been developed over generations and are a part of culture.

According to Durkheim the explanation of this knowledge is to be found in society. It is the organisation of the collective which determines which categories of thought are developed. This is effected in two ways. First, society is reflected in the categories. The collective knows its own organisation and uses it as a basis for developing the content and hierarchical order of the categories. Second, it is society which constitutes the categories. For social life to function, the collective needs categories and establishes them through the development of feelings of belonging in the collective.

In this work we thus get a theory about how scientific culture is formed, but we do not in fact get any real explanation of how these categories have been developed from being belief-based categories to become scientific categories and as such to remain unaltered through time. It remains a postulate.

Compared with the two works of Durkheim previously discussed, in his work on religion we obtain a number of novel elements to explain the question of how culture is conferred on the individual. Here the question of feelings is of key importance. The feelings of elevation and of belonging in relation to culture make it possible on the one hand for the individual to subordinate himself to the rules of thought which have been established by the collective, and on the other hand, to appropriate to himself individual symbols which can differ from the collective symbols. These feeling are generated through ritual actions.

## *Discussion*

According to Steven Lukes, Durkheim's theory has not been the subject of heated debate. However, some criticism has been made both of his empirical basis and of his theoretical approach. Lukes refers to criticisms made by Bronislaw Malinowski and Arnold van Gennep, among others. They point out that the empirical basis for his *The Elementary Forms of Religious Life* is so poor that the whole of his theoretical construction falls to the ground (Lukes, 1973, pp. 520-529). Others criticise Durkheim for failing to include individual and psychological aspects in his theory. Lukes points out that he has been criticised for putting too much emphasis on society (Lukes, 1973, pp. 500-510). In the following these questions are not taken further, but the focus is on clarifying Durkheim's understanding of culture and on discussing the internal logic of this understanding.

In the development of his theory, Durkheim was influenced by two kinds of factors, the scientific factors and the social factors. On the one hand he was influenced by the growing recognition accorded to the natural sciences. This gave him an alternative to the historical method which was his original influence. In his biography of Durkheim, Lukes writes that he was strongly influenced by the German historical school, at the same time as being critical of them because they had a tendency to describe rather than explain (Lukes, 1973, pp. 397-404). On the other hand he was also influenced by social and cultural developments. He wrote in *The Elementary Forms of Religious Life* that his own time had been characterised as being a period of transition and moral mediocrity (Durkheim, 1912/1995, p. 429). In *Moral Education* he wrote that secularism was triumphant and that this made it necessary to replace the religious basis for morality with a scientific basis (Durkheim, 1925/1968, p. 11). In his introduction to *Professional Ethics and Civic Morals* he wrote that European societies were in a state of crisis because of the dominance of economic life which is without moral rules (Durkheim, 1950/1992, pp. 11-12). His aim was thus to develop a science so as to form the basis for understanding morality and the effects of morality. The inspiration of the natural sciences is meant to safeguard the authority of this science of morality and to give it impact.

Among the natural sciences it was particularly biology which was a source of inspiration for Durkheim. This can be clearly seen in his choice of language, which includes biological terms such as cells, germs, genes, systems, periodicity, evolution, survival etc. Also, his concept of social facts was inspired by natural scientific thinking.

Under the influence of biology, Durkheim developed his genetic method, which lead him back to the social phenomena of cells and germs. He sought the original source and most simple forms of social phenomena, in order to be able to explain their later and more complex forms. We can see two very different results of this method in the works discussed. In the study of educational thought we see a development from the contradictory approach of the sacred and secular elements of education towards a predominantly secular thinking about education. In this case there have been some notable changes over time. In the study of religion, Durkheim identified the original categories for thinking and made these the basis for all forms of thought right up to modern scientific thought. The categories are the same. It is only complexity which grows. The explanation for these differences is presumably to be found in the actual methods used. In his study of educational thinking, Durkheim followed the actual historical development. He did not do this in his study of religion. Here he only studied the primitive religions and postulated the existence of some connection between the forms of thinking he found in their beliefs and the modern forms of scientific thinking. The study of educational thought is thus influenced by actual contradictions, disagreements and strife, while his study of the development from religious thinking through to scientific thinking has the character of a theoretical construction. In any case, the consequence of the use of the genetic method was that questions of change or stasis remain unanswered. The reason for this presumably is that *The Evolution of Educational Thought* is still characterised by the influence of historical research on Durkheim, while *The Elementary Forms of Religious Life* are more influenced by his natural scientific thinking.

If one is to explain Durkheim's understanding of culture, it is necessary to start by stating that he did not himself provide any definition of culture. His concept of culture seems capacious and, at a higher level, in line with his concept of society. If we are to get closer to Durkheim's understanding of culture, we must therefore look at those aspects of culture which he dealt with, in particular the intellectual, moral and scientific aspects. In his treatment of these aspects, culture appears to have two facets: first it appears as an external culture of the treasures which are preserved by society, and second there is an inner culture of personal characteristics linked to the individual. With these two facets of culture there is immediately a theoretical problem of how these two facets can be linked together into a cohesive theory. This problem can be solved by borrowing ideas from biology. Durkheim confronted the system and the individual with one another. Culture is considered as a system which the individual must be in a dialogue with. There can be a system of rules of conduct, a system of rituals or a system of categories which can affect the individual. Culture is made 'scientific' by being ordered as a system. Nevertheless, in all three works, Durkheim retained an enthusiasm for the culture which contains cultural treasures which are preserved by society. These treasures are the concrete works which can be studied and acquired by generation after generation. In the same way, Durkheim had a scientific approach to the acquisition of culture by the individual. Using the concept of periodicity, the concept of regularity is an expression of the transfer of culture to people. Personality is developed consisting of systems of ideas, feelings and habits. As a consequence, the behaviour of human beings becomes regular and orderly. Here too it must be said that Durkheim had a more concrete opinion of the individual's acquisition of culture. The individual acquires linguistic skills, an ability to think and knowledge and insight. It can be said that in his understanding of both the external and the internal culture, Durkheim developed both a natural scientific understanding of culture, characterised by concepts of system and periodicity, as well as by a more historically based understanding of culture, characterised by concepts of cultural treasures and human skills.

There is no doubt that, for Durkheim, culture is created by and influenced by society. It is the collective which creates the rules of conduct and the categories. However, his different writings contain differing kinds of explanations as to how this influence makes itself felt. In his analysis of religion Durkheim explicitly stated that there are two kinds of influence: the reflecting and the constituting. In his analysis of the development of educational thought, there are likewise two kinds of explanation: the development of resources and conflicts. The explanation of reflection is based on the view that the collective creates the categories which are already known from its own social organisation. In this way the social organisation is reflected in the culture. The constituting explanation is based on the view that society needs categories and therefore establishes them through rituals. This is done by engendering feelings for the symbolic representations of society. The explanation of resources is based on the view that when welfare increases, a surplus is created for intellectual work. In the same way, increased social integration allows peaceful conditions for intellectual work. There is thus the creation of a surplus and resources for the development of culture. Finally, there is the explanation of conflicts which is based on the view that culture is generated through struggle and by conflicts between different groups in society. There are thus no less than four different kinds of explanation for how society influences culture.

The question of how culture can be transferred to the individual was clearly a very important one for Durkheim. His concerns about social development led him to study how culture can be transferred to the individual as rules of conduct, categories, knowledge and insight, and thereby create a basis for greater social cohesion. In this connection we also find a number of different explanations. In the analysis of religion, he pointed to rituals as a means of transferring culture. In his analysis of moral education, he pointed to pedagogy as a means of transferring culture. Rituals can transfer culture to the individual because they can engender feelings in society about its symbols. It is thus the feelings of individuals which ensure the continued existence both of the symbols and of society. Pedagogy can ensure the transfer of culture to the individual because of its potential for using the child's natural disposition to develop feelings of duty and ideals and the possibility of associating these duties and ideals with empirical conditions. Duties and ideals can thus be explained. When Durkheim wanted to explain the transfer of culture to the individual he used two types of explanation: the explanation based on feelings, and the explanation based on understanding.

When the transfer of culture to the individual is based on understanding, it gives the explanation, in particular the natural scientific reasoning, a special role. The science of cultural phenomena - without doubt, Durkheim had sociology in mind - is the basis for the development of the morality, thinking and knowledge of the individual. When one can understand these cultural phenomena and can explain them, it is also possible to influence them. Thus thinking can liberate the will.

Durkheim's understanding of culture was thus very open. There are several kinds of view and several kinds of explanation. The reason for this multiplicity seems to be that his study of social phenomena was inspired by ideas from biology. This use of the terminology and thinking from biology ran up against Durkheim's own historical ideas. The biological categories reflect biology and not society. By introducing biology into a theory of society Durkheim came into conflict with his own theory that categories reflect society. He thus created a sociological contradiction of the same kind which he had himself analysed in *The Evolution of Educational Thought*. In order to study cultural phenomena scientifically, it is necessary to introduce natural scientific methods into the study of cultural phenomena.

The question is whether sociology still struggles today with this contradiction between systems thinking and historical thinking, in the same way that the church struggled with the contradictions between the sacred and the secular, and what the consequences of this will be.

# 3

# Max Weber: Culture as Meaning

In their selection of Weber texts, *From Max Weber*, Gerth and Wright Mills gave an introduction to the life and work of Max Weber (Weber, 1948/1970). From this introduction it appears that Weber directed his studies towards bureaucracy and charisma, methodological problems, ideas and interests, social structures and the conditions for freedom. Weber's sociology is thus presented as a sociology with a material and a conceptual content. The word 'culture' does crop up in a few places, but it is not apparent that culture was a phenomenon that was the subject of Weber's theoretical developments. This view appears to be supported by the biography which Weber's wife, Marianne Weber, wrote of him. She considered the problems of cultural logic as being a sideline to his work. It was general sociological studies which constituted the core of Weber's work (Weber, 1926/1995, pp. 305-355).

In more recent works on Max Weber, the cultural aspects are presented as being much more significant. For example, in his book *Max Weber and the Sociology of Culture* Ralph Schroeder writes that Max Weber's project should fundamentally be seen as a contribution to the sociology of culture. It is Schroeder's view that Weber's work is bound together by a desire to illuminate the relations between cultural and social life. According to Schroeder the question which occupied Weber was the question of how belief can be transformed into social reality, and how we can understand the cultural significance of different views of the world (Schroeder, 1992, p. 2).

As a starting point there are thus two sharply contrasting views about the position of culture in Weber's collected theoretical work. One view is that culture is virtually absent from Weber's work. The other view is that culture was the overwhelmingly important topic in Weber's theoretical work.

The question of how Weber considered culture and how he saw it in relation to other social phenomena is complicated. Weber's views on culture are interwoven with his methodological thinking. The treatment of these methodological questions cannot therefore be considered as only concerning discussions of method. His views on culture are thus buried within this discussions of method. Weber's understanding of culture also turns up in his analyses of empirical conditions.

The task of distilling Max Weber's understanding of culture must therefore start with some of his articles on methodological problems, specifically the articles which Shils and Finch have collected in the book *The Methodology of the Social Sciences*. These articles were written in the period from 1903 to 1917 and were published in *Archiv für Sozialwissenschaft und Sozialpolitik* and in *Logos* (Weber, 1904-1917/1949, iii-iv). In addition, the task must be based on *The Protestant Ethic and the Spirit of Capitalism.* This work was also originally published in *Archiv für Sozialwissenschaft und Sozialpolitik* in the years 1904 and 1905 (Weber, 1904-1905/1970, ix). Parts of Weber's great work, *Economy and Society*, must also be taken into account. This last work was assembled after Weber's death by his wife Marianne Weber and Melchior Palyi and published in 1922 and 1925. This work was later re-edited by Johannes Winckelmann and published in 1956 (Weber, 1956/1968, lx). Finally, the collection of Weber texts edited by Gerth and Wright Mills and published in 1948 under the title of *From Max Weber* should be included. This collection contains selected texts from *Economy and Society* and articles from, among others, *Archiv für Sozialwissenschaft und Sozialpolitik.* These works are far from covering all of Weber's very extensive production, but they may be taken as being the most important documents for an understanding of his views on culture.

By way of introduction, it is necessary to look at the methodological questions which Weber discussed in the three articles in *The Methodology of the Social Sciences.* In these articles Weber discussed three significant methodological problems. First, he considered the question of how it is possible to study the question of the values which lie behind existing research. Second, he considered the question of how it is possible to explain the value content of a given phenomenon, whether it be a research phenomenon or an empirical phenomenon. Third and finally, he discussed the question of how it may be possible to develop concepts which can capture value phenomena. Weber's discussion is thus primarily directed towards a clarification of the significance of value-relevance for research and towards the methodological principles that can be derived on the basis of this significance.

In the article "The Meaning of 'Ethical Neutrality' in Sociology and Economics" from 1917, Weber discussed two important questions in relation to values. On the one hand he discussed the question of the value-judgements of researchers. On the other hand he discussed the question of the significance of the relevance of a given phenomenon for a researcher's values. This distinction between value-judgement and value-relevance concerns first and foremost the distinction between the researcher's ability to assess his research results and the researcher's basis for choosing his research topics.

> "By 'VALUE-JUDGMENTS' are to be understood, where nothing else is implied or expressly stated, practical evaluations of the unsatisfactory or satisfactory character of phenomena subject to our influence." (Weber, 1904-1917/1949, p. 1).

When Weber spoke of value-judgement, he referred to a researcher's evaluation of whether a given phenomenon was satisfactory or not.

As the starting point for the discussion of value-judgement Weber introduced a decisive distinction between establishing empirical results and evaluating those results.

> "What is really at issue is the intrinsically simple demand that the investigator and teacher should keep unconditionally separate the establishment of empirical facts ... and his own practical evaluations, i.e. his evaluation of these facts as satisfactory or unsatisfactory ..." (Weber, 1904-1917/1949, p. 11).

What was important for Weber was to distinguish between factual information and the value-judgement of those facts. According to Weber it is not the task of the researcher to undertake a value-judgement of the empirical facts he has collected. The factual information should not be judged by the researcher; it must speak for itself.

Even though the researcher's value-judgement ought not to appear in relation to the empirical results, it will nevertheless be significant for the research carried out. It is therefore important to analyse the values which lie behind the research.

According to Weber, the discussion of the value-judgements of existing research can have two purposes. First, it can establish the axiomatic values which lie behind the research, and second, such analysis can have practical consequences for the value-judgements. In order to identify the axiomatic values it is necessary to follow a fixed procedure. One should start with concrete, specific value-judgements and the analysis of the significance of these judgements. Thereafter one should proceed to the more general level of non-reductive evaluations. In this process one must follow the rules of logic. The result will thus be consistent axiomatic values. The consequences of value-judgements can thus be derived both logically and empirically. The practical consequences of given value-judgements can be that the researcher is restricted to certain means and certain conclusions (Weber, 1904-1917/1949, pp. 20-21).

In practice, the problems which social scientists are concerned with can be selected on the basis of the value-relevance of the given phenomena. What Weber meant by 'value-relevance' was the scientific interest which determines the choice of a given topic and the choice of the problems with which the empirical analysis is concerned.

> "... the problems of the social sciences are selected by the value-relevance of the phenomena treated. ... It should ... be recalled that the expression 'relevance to values' refers simply to the philosophical interpretation of that specifically scientific 'interest' which determines the selection of a given subject-matter and the problems of an empirical analysis." (Weber, 1904-1917/1949, pp. 21-22).

According to Weber, it is the value interests which determine the direction of empirical sciences. These interests can be made explicit and differentiated through a discussion of values.

Weber exemplified these principles by discussing research into the development of music. Here it is necessary to distinguish between the actual technical development of music and the aesthetic values which lie behind the choice of which music to study with reference to this technical development. It is thus necessary to study the values which lie behind the scientific interest in music. It is necessary to identify the axiomatic values which are the basis for the choice of research topics in music (Weber, 1904-1917/1949, pp. 30-31).

The same principle applies to research into economic and social developments. Here it is possible, for example, to study economic progress as technological progress, but even the value interests which lie behind research into such progress must be investigated. The identification of the axiomatic values which lie behind the research interests is a much more complex task than the research into the progress itself. Religious and ethical values, for example, can affect the value interests (Weber, 1904-1917/1949, pp. 35-38). At a higher level Weber points out that economic theory is an axiomatic discipline (Weber, 1904-1917/1949, p. 43).

According to Weber, a researcher should abstain from giving value-judgements of his results. On the other hand, he should investigate the value-judgements which have been significant for the choice of topics which are researched. The axiomatic values which have been the motive force of the existing research should also be made clear.

In his article "Critical Studies in the Logic of the Cultural Sciences" from 1905, Weber discussed the question of analysing the values which are hidden within research. His argument not only concerned the question of explaining the creation of a text, it also concerned how it is possible to explain the historical development of the matter. What Weber highlighted here was how to explain value-phenomena.

In this article Weber operated with a basic distinction between value analysis and causal analysis. The two analyses should not be conflated, but each should be carried out independently. Value analysis is a necessary prerequisite for causal analysis.

If the object of research is a text, one should start by carrying out a value-interpretation of the text. The value-interpretation means an evaluation of the content of the given work by which we obtain an understanding of its intellectual and spiritual content. This produces an attitude towards the text. The result will be an evaluating opinion.

> "Interpretation can and does become first 'value-interpretation' (*Wertinterpretation*), i.e., it teaches us to 'understand' the intellectual, psychological and spiritual (*geistigen*) content of that correspondence; it develops and raises to the level of explicit 'evaluation' that which we 'feel' dimly and vaguely. For this purpose, interpretation is not at all required to enunciate or to 'suggest' a value judgement. What it actually 'suggests' in the course of analysis are rather various possible relationships of the object to values (*Wertbeziehungen des Objektes*)." (Weber, 1904-1917/1949, p. 143).

To carry out a value-interpretation of a given text, the task is thus not to undertake a value-judgement of the text, but rather to investigate its value-relevance. How does it relate to values?

Weber emphasised that value-interpretation should not be confused with the linguistic interpretation which is the basis for all types of scientific treatment and use of source materials. The linguistic interpretation is thus the means of verifying facts. It is a tool for history and other scientific disciplines.

When a value-interpretation of a work is carried out, one must look for an explanation for the existence of the work. This explanation should be sought in its historical context. This context will include both the personal circumstances as well as the wider cultural environment. As an example of such a causal analysis, Weber states that Karl Marx's *Das Kapital* was historically determined. It was the historically given 'problem situation' which was the basis for the creation of the work. Another example is Goethe's love letters, where the social environment and the concrete events of the time were the basis for the creation of the letters. However, the causal analysis is of less significance in itself. Value analysis must be the starting point for causal analysis, so it is value analysis which directs causal analysis.

> "... that type of 'interpretation' which we have alone called 'value analysis' functions as a guide for this other 'historical' i.e. causal type of 'interpretation'. ... The former creates the points of attachment from which there are to be regressively traced the web of causal connections and thus provides causal analysis with the decisive 'viewpoints' without which it would indeed have to operate, as it were, without a compass on an uncharted sea." (Weber, 1904-1917/1949, p. 149).

The purpose of value analysis is thus to explain what important viewpoints are hidden in a given text. Starting from these viewpoints it is possible to regress to the circumstances which can have influenced the creation of a given work.

The procedure sketched out here does not only apply to written works. It also applies to historical events or historical characters. Value analysis must explain what ideas are incorporated in or are expressed by the phenomena in question. One must construct the phenomenon by making explicit the key points for the possible attitudes which it reveals and which give it meaning. The meaning which is revealed by this must be kept quite distinct from the causal significance.

> "... in constructing historical individuals I elaborate in an explicit form the focal points for possible 'evaluative' attitudes which the segment of reality in question discloses and in consequence of which it claims a more or less universal 'meaning' – which is to be sharply distinguished from causal 'significance'." (Weber, 1904-1917/1949, p. 151).

It is the researcher who finds an interest in the phenomena in question and sees the unique intellectual content of a work or the qualities in a historical event. The historical interest which guides the researcher is linked to many different forms of values.

The evaluation of a historical event is based on an abstraction. There must be a conceptual isolation of the components of the data which may be assumed to form a complex of possible causal relations. The mere fact of making this abstraction transforms a given part of reality into a conceptual construction and in this way it operates as a historical fact. Referring to Goethe, Weber wrote that theory is involved in facts (Weber, 1904-1917/1949, p. 173).

The conclusion is thus that, as distinct from the natural scientist, when the historian attempts to explain a phenomenon, he must first interpret it and then understand it. He must first find the values in the matter and thereafter understand it on the basis of its historical context. However, both of these steps occur as a conceptual construction.

The third methodological problem which Weber discussed is the question of the creation of the concepts of the social sciences.

In the article " 'Objectivity' in Social Science" written in 1904, we meet again the idea that the researcher is guided by value-judgements and that these value-judgements are significant for the researcher's development of concepts. In this way he makes explicit the value-relevance which lies behind the research. The principle which Weber developed in this article is the principle of the development of ideal types as a means for understanding unique historical phenomena.

In this article Weber introduced another important distinction, that between the development of concepts and the use of concepts. Weber pointed out that the values which lie behind the choice of topics for research are the guiding points of view in the development of the concepts which will be used in research. When the concepts are used, this part of the task will be subject to the conventions for thinking which otherwise apply (Weber, 1904-1917/1949, p. 84).

The question which Weber pursued here was, what logical structure and function can we find in the concepts which social science uses, or put differently: What is the significance of theory and the development of theoretical concepts for our knowledge of cultural reality?

In providing an answer to this question Weber distanced himself from the idea of adopting the thought processes of natural sciences for the social sciences. In Weber's view, the transfer of the biological theory of evolution to the field of the social sciences had led to historical development being reduced to laws, of which actual events are examples. For Weber what was most important was to study unique historical events. He therefore attached importance to the construction of concepts which make it possible to study such phenomena. It was his aim to be able to develop an ideal picture of events under specific conditions.

Weber's method consisted of constructing a conceptual framework on the basis of an analytical emphasis on certain elements of reality. By creating such an ideal type there is a clarification of specific phenomena under specific conditions.

> "An ideal type is formed by the one-sided accentuation of one or more points of view and by the synthesis of a great many diffuse, discrete, more or less present and occasionally absent concrete individual phenomena, which are arranged according to those one-sidedly emphasized viewpoints into a unified analytical construct (*Gedankenbild*). In its conceptual purity, this mental construct (*Gedankenbild*) cannot be found empirically anywhere in reality. It is a utopia." (Weber, 1904-1917/1949, p. 90).

Once the ideal type has been constructed, it is the task of historical science to investigate the extent to which it approximates to reality or departs from it. Weber referred to the capitalist culture as an example of such an ideal type.

For empirical science the ideal type is a guideline that can help the researcher in the construction of hypotheses. It is not itself a hypothesis. The ideal type is thus a concept which can be used to formulate relations which can afterwards be transferred to objective situations (Weber, 1904-1917/1949, pp. 90-93).

Weber then introduced yet another distinction, which was that between the ideal type and the historical idea which can direct people's behaviour. While the ideal type is a concept, the idea is a concrete phenomenon. However, there is a question whether there is a causal relationship between the idea and the ideal type. Here Weber pointed out that the idea can be formulated in the manner of an ideal type because it exists concretely in the minds of an unlimited and constantly changing number of people. This can take place by including a varied quantity of material such as, for example, religious doctrines, norms laid down in church laws, rules of conduct etc. The formulation in the manner of an ideal type becomes even more important when the ideas are no longer present in the minds of people, but when they still direct their behaviour. In such a case a comparison between the ideal type and reality will be of great importance. (Weber, 1904-1917/1949, p. 97).

The ideal type is a tool for the systematic characterisation of unique concrete patterns which are significant in their uniqueness, such as Christianity or capitalism. However, the ideal type can also be used to determine classifications or kinds of concepts. This occurs through abstraction and through the emphasis on conceptually essential elements. In reality, each ideal type contains elements both for classification and for describing the unique. The aim in forming the concepts of ideal types must always be to emphasise the unique character of a cultural phenomenon, and to distinguish it from the typical.

The problem is that the concepts which have been developed according to the principles described will always appear to be inadequate as a form of scheme into which reality can be integrated. The concepts, which are developed on the basis of knowledge and interests, will always conflict with the new knowledge which we can and are interested in extracting from reality. The result is a continuing reconstruction of the concepts through which we understand reality (Weber, 1904-1917/1949, pp. 100-105).

Together the three articles supply us with insight into some of Weber's most important methodological principles for social science. It is first and foremost the question of values which is discussed. On the one hand it is clear that the researcher ought not to undertake value-judgements of his own empirical results. On the other hand it is equally clear that research cannot be undertaken without some relevance to values. The researcher's assessment of values is significant for the topics which he chooses for his research, and for the point of view he brings to such topics. The consequence is that the researcher can only develop his own concepts in the light of his own values. In fact, there will only be a development of a concept if, in the light of his own values, the researcher applies a particular point of view to the phenomenon he wishes to study. It can be said that the researcher's consideration of values can be an asset for making possible the development of concepts for understanding the social world. If there were no values there would be no social science research. Another consequence is that one must assess existing research with regard to how it relates to values. One must identify the axiomatic values which have directed it, and the consequences which these have had for the choice of subject matter, of approach, and of formation of concepts. One must interpret the value-content of a text and then explain its historical origin.

Against this background, Weber considered social science to be a part of cultural science. It is not possible to practice or to study social sciences without involving the question of values. This relation to values makes social science a cultural science. As a result, it is possible to make a preliminary definition of Weber's understanding of culture on the basis of these articles. In a manner of speaking this is implicit in the articles and in places it even becomes explicit.

## *Culture as value-related reality*

It is especially in the earliest of the three articles, " 'Objectivity' in Social Science", written in 1904, that Weber's views on culture were presented. This article gives an idea of what Weber meant by culture and how he related culture to other social phenomena.

In fact, in this article Weber gave a definition of culture.

> " 'Culture' is a finite segment of the meaningless infinity of the world process, a segment on which human beings confer meaning and significance." (Weber, 1904-1917/1949, p. 81).

Weber explained how this culture is formed. He stated that empirical reality becomes culture for us to the extent that we connect it to value-ideas.

> "The concept of culture is a value-concept. Empirical reality becomes 'culture' to us because and insofar as we relate it to value ideas. It includes those segments and only those segments of reality which have become significant to us because of this value-relevance. Only a small portion of existing concrete reality is colored by our value-conditioned interest and it alone is significant for us." (Weber, 1904-1917/1949, p. 76).

Culture can be formed in this way because human beings are cultural creatures. Human beings are equipped with the ability and the desire voluntarily to adopt attitudes to the world, and to give it meaning. When the meaning of an empirical phenomenon first becomes clear, it will prompt us to evaluate specific human phenomena in the light of it, and it will make us react to it as a meaningful phenomenon. The attitudes which are developed will have cultural significance for us.

From this point of view, phenomena such as prostitution, religion and money may be regarded equally as cultural phenomena. They are all three cultural phenomena insofar as their existence and their form affect our cultural interest, either directly or indirectly (Weber, 1904-1917/1949, p. 181).

Weber emphasised that culture is changeable. The cultural problems which shape human beings are continuously reshaping themselves in different colours. In the unending stream of concrete events, the boundaries to the area which achieve meaning and significance for us, i.e. which are historically unique, are constantly subject to change. As an example, Weber referred to the cultural significance of a normatively regulated legal system, where the norms themselves can undergo fundamental and revolutionary change even within the terms of the ruling legal norms (Weber, 1904-1917/1949, pp. 83-84).

In this article we also see the beginnings of a theory about how culture should be related to social conditions. Weber thus suggested that the social relations, including institutions and groups of people with common interests, have an indirect influence on culture.

> "The indirect influence of social relations, institutions and groups governed by 'material interests' extends (often unconsciously) into all spheres of culture without exception, even into the finest nuances of aesthetic and religious feeling." (Weber, 1904-1917/1949, p. 65).

On the other hand, all the activities and situations which constitute a given historical culture will affect the material needs and the way in which they are satisfied, just as they will affect the integration of interest groups and the kind of powers which they exercise.

If cultural science is to understand the relationship between culture and social relations, then on the basis of the argument set out about the relationship between socio-economic and cultural conditions, it must undertake a scientific investigation of the consequences of the socio-economic structure which arises out of human society for culture in general, and what general culture means for the socio-economic structure.

After having specified the relationship between culture and social relations, Weber stressed, however, that cultural phenomena should not be deduced as a product of or a function of a given constellation of material interests. Social and cultural phenomena should rather be analysed with special reference to their economic preconditions (Weber, 1904-1917/1949, pp. 65-68).

Finally, the article gives us insight into what Weber's understanding of culture meant for his views of cultural science. Weber pointed out that, first and foremost, science is a product of culture. In the same way that human consciousness has been cultivated and refined by culture, so science must also have been affected by culture (Weber, 1904-1917/1949, p. 55).

Weber's definition of culture as being the segment of reality to which human beings attach meaning and significance, leads to the view that cultural science is the science which deals with events in human life with regard to their cultural significance. On this basis he included social science as a cultural science. The task of cultural science is thus to understand the cultural significance of and origins of unique events (Weber, 1904-1917/1949, pp. 67-72).

In the article " 'Objectivity' in Social Science" we thus get a definition of Weber's concept of culture and an impression of how culture is related to the social world. The decisive element in Weber's understanding of culture is value-ideas. Human values are a prerequisite for enabling social phenomena to be transformed into culture. In this way, culture becomes those segments of reality which humans endow with meaning and significance through their thoughts. The criteria of meaning or significance are therefore decisive for whether or not something is culture. It is not possible to determine in advance whether specific types of phenomena are cultural or social. They become cultural to the extent that people ascribe significance to them.

On this basis, any form of social science is a cultural science, regardless of its substantive content. Any social phenomenon will be a cultural phenomenon as soon as any researcher ascribes meaning to it on the basis of his own values. It is therefore not possible to point to any specific research topics as being matters of cultural research. Cultural research is research which is directed by opinions and values.

The consequence of Weber's understanding of culture is that the effect of social relations on culture is an unconscious effect. Those parts of reality, which have not been ascribed meaning and significance through human thought, can very well affect the content of culture, but it will be an unconscious influence.

Based on Weber's article on objectivity in social sciences there thus appear to be two decisive views on the question of culture. On the one hand there are value-ideas which are the basis on which social phenomena can be transformed into culture. On the other hand there is the unconscious, which is the basis on which social relations can affect culture. Both views involve humans. On the one hand humans are cultural creatures who have values, and on the other hand they are subject to unconscious influence. Humans act both consciously and unconsciously.

## *The capitalist culture*

In his study, *The Protestant Ethic and the Spirit of Capitalism*, Weber used methodological principles which he had discussed and developed in his articles on methodology. Here we see the question of values and principle of the development of the ideal type discussed and applied.

The question of values is touched upon in the introduction to the book. Weber stressed that he would not take sides on the question of the relative values of different cultures. It was his view that those who undertake research into the fates of humans cannot avoid being influenced by them, but that it is wisest to keep one's personal comments to oneself. (Weber, 1904-1905/1970, p. 29). He would absolutely not assess the ideas of the Reformation as social or religious values. The form of evaluation which Weber would undertake, when he studied religious dogmas, was an evaluation of a phenomenon's historical significance as a causal factor. Weber would thus not evaluate dogmas as values, but he would study their historical and cultural significance (Weber, 1904-1905/1970, pp. 98-99).

For Weber what mattered was not to form an opinion on the religious values, but to investigate what roles these values played in the complex interaction between countless factors which have formed our modern culture. He emphasised the need to liberate ourselves from the idea that the Reformation can be argued to be some historical necessity on the basis of some specific economic developments. His aim was to investigate which concrete aspects of the capitalist culture could be traced back to the religious forces. On this basis it would become possible to evaluate the extent to which modern culture can be explained by these religious forces, and the extent to which they were due to other forces (Weber, 1904-1905/1970, pp. 90-92).

The principle of the ideal type was especially used in developing the concept of the capitalist spirit, in other words the development of a concept of a unique phenomenon. Weber also used the principle of the ideal type in his study of class phenomena. He used it in developing the concept of the capitalist entrepreneur as being the class which was the standard bearer of the capitalist spirit. He also used it in his study of religious ideas, in which the Protestant ethic was expressed. It was his opinion that, in order to understand the significance of religious ideas, it is necessary to study them in their most logical and consistent form.

In developing the concept of the capitalist spirit, Weber argued that one cannot directly define this concept. The problem is that it refers to a unique historical phenomenon consisting of a complex of interrelatedness in historical reality. It is this complex which the researcher unites into a conceptual unity, starting from the question of its cultural significance. The concept of the spirit of capitalism must be developed gradually by taking the elements which form it from historical reality. Weber thus reasoned that in the course of the argument he must develop the best possible concept from the point of view he was interested in establishing.

The point of view which Weber chose to establish at a general level was the question of the influence of religious ideas on the development of the economic spirit, in other words on the moral attitude of the economic system. More specifically it was a question of the relation between the spirit of the modern capitalist economy and the rational ethic in ascetic Protestantism. Weber emphasised that this point of view is not the only possible characterisation of the capitalist spirit. Other viewpoints will highlight other characteristics as being essential. With the point of view chosen by Weber, he sought to establish the significance the capitalist spirit had for him (Weber, 1904-1905/1970, pp. 47-48).

Weber himself said that his approach to the question would be to undertake an initial description of what he believed to be the spirit of capitalism. Thereafter there was a clarification of the phenomenon itself. The initial description was made on the basis of a text which contained the classic opinions for illuminating the spirit of capitalism. After having clarified the content of the spirit of capitalism, Weber investigated which factors restricted its development and which factors promoted it. It was his view that tradition was what most restricted the development of the capitalist spirit, while religion and the conduct which it encouraged supported the development of the capitalist spirit.

It was Weber's view that in reality the capitalist spirit was an ethic, and in particular an ethic which required the individual to work in such a manner that his economic capital was increased. On this basis Weber raised the question of the intellectual roots of this ethic:

> "It will be our task to find out whose intellectual child the particular concrete, form of rational thought was, from which the idea of a calling and the devotion to labour in the calling has grown, which is, as we have seen, so irrational from the standpoint of purely eudæmonistic self-interest, but which has been and still is one of the most characteristic elements of our capitalist culture." (Weber, 1904-1905/1970, p. 78).

The starting point for this search for the intellectual background for the calling and devotion to work is Luther's concept of a calling. It was Luther's view that man should hold fast to that which he was called to do. The calling was part of God's ordinance with which man had to comply. Men had to go about the tasks which God had set before them. According to Weber this was the traditional view of a calling. However, for Calvin and the other leaders of Protestant sects, a calling was a logical consequence of their religious doctrines.

Weber emphasised that the leaders of the Protestant sects were not the founders of a specific ethical culture nor the proponents of a humanitarian project of social reform or cultural ideals. It was the saving of souls which lay at the heart of their lives and their work. Their ethical ideals were all based on this work and were the consequences of purely religious motives. The cultural consequences of the Reformation were thus unforeseen and undesired. They were often the opposite of what the religious leaders themselves wanted.

Weber suggested that there were four main sources of inspiration for the Protestant ethic of asceticism, and these were Calvinism, Pietism, Methodism and Baptist teachings. These four movements were interwoven with one another, just as their doctrines were combined in a complex way. What interested Weber was not so much the struggle between the movements and the ideas, but more the influence of the ideas on the way people behaved. What interested him was the psychological sanctions which, on the basis of religious belief and practice, gave direction to people's behaviour in practice and made people keep to the path laid out before them.

> "We are interested ... in ...: the influence of those psychological sanctions which, originating in religious belief and the practice of religion, gave a direction to practical conduct and held the individual to it." (Weber, 1904-1905/1970, p. 97).

The psychological sanctions were to a great extent derived from the basic specific religious ideas. Therefore it was important for Weber to look at the abstract dogmas which so concerned people at that time. His starting point was the religious ideas, as laid down in the texts.

According to Weber, the Calvinist doctrine of predestination was the most consistent of the Protestant doctrines. It also had a powerful psychological effect. The belief, that who should have eternal life and who should be damned was predestined, led to an inner loneliness in the individual. No-one could help. One had to follow the path one trod alone. The magical elements of religion and the emotional aspects of culture were excluded. Warnings were given against friendship between people. Burials were without ritual. The individual had to work out his own salvation with his God.

This meant that it was essential to find out whether one was one of the chosen or not. This answer had to be looked for in the works of the individual, because God worked through his chosen. This meant that for a Calvinist it was important to show evidence that he belonged to God's chosen. He had to work for the glory of God in order to be able to show that God worked through him. Throughout his life he had to do something which was compatible with the universal system. In this way moral behaviour had to be supported by consistent behaviour as a whole. Behaviour was rationalised and subject to constant self-control. The result was that a broad group of Calvinists had a strong incentive to be ascetic.

The Pietists, too, had a doctrine of predestination. Here too the doctrine concerned evidence. This meant that the question of whether or not one was one of the chosen was made clear by a sign from God. What mattered was that one waited patiently and methodically. Here again there was emphasis on methodical behaviour, but there was also an emphasis on satisfying an immediate emotional need. There was a possibility of obtaining certainty of salvation.

The Methodists had the same emotional element in their religion as the Pietists. This concerned obtaining proof that one belonged to God's chosen. This meant that one could obtain a feeling of conversion through methodical behaviour. When this feeling was awoken it could be directed into a rational struggle for perfection. The rational nature of behaviour was not broken by the awakening.

For Baptists there was no predestination. Here the Holy Spirit could speak to anyone who was willing to listen. One should not work to deserve God's mercy, one had to wait patiently until the Holy Spirit spoke to one. When this happened one could be born again and, at a symbolic level, baptised. The systematic waiting led to the same result as the Calvinist doctrine of predestination, which was systematic behaviour.

In Weber's view, despite their differences, what the Protestant sects had in common was their seeking after the religious grace which would give them eternal life. As a consequence of this, they also had a common development of systematic and rational behaviour. Initially, the sects shut themselves off from the outside world, but over time they left their monastic existence and moved out into the world. They took their rational behaviour with them. In this way Christian asceticism came to penetrate life's daily routines with its methodical behaviour.

Weber studied the links between religious ideas and the rules for everyday economic life through the texts written by Protestant clerics. By studying these texts he was able to identify the Protestant ethical guidelines for economic behaviour. In his texts the Calvinist preacher, Richard Baxter, stressed that wealth is dangerous. On the other hand the elect must never rest, but serve their God through hard systematic work, both in mind and in body. It was the same for the Baptists. Here the requirement was that one should work to be rich for the sake of God, not for the sake of enjoying temporal and sinful life.

For Puritans the impulsive enjoyment of life was unacceptable. It could entice the saved away from religion and the calling to work. Rational asceticism was thus hostile towards those aspects of culture which did not have any immediate religious value. However, Puritanism did not lead to a narrow-minded disdain for culture. In their sermons and in their theological arguments they often revealed their classical learning.

> "Its attitude was thus suspicious and often hostile to the aspects of culture without any immediate religious value. It is not, however, true that the ideals of Puritanism implied a solemn, narrow-minded contempt of culture. Quite the contrary is the case at least for science, with the exception of the hatred of Scholasticism. Moreover, the great men of the Puritan movement were thoroughly steeped in the culture of the Renaissance." (Weber, 1904-1905/1970, p. 168).

On the other hand, if one looks at non-scientific literature and at art, the Puritans clearly distanced themselves from them. The same applied to decoration of the person, including clothing. Above all it was clear that the enjoyment of culture must not cost anything. It was the duty of people to look after their property. The more one owned, the greater was the feeling of responsibility to keep it undiminished for the glory of God. This was the consistent ethic which was so significant for the development of capitalism.

The practical outcome of this ethic was the accumulation of capital. The problem, according to Weber, was that this increasing accumulation of wealth also increased temporal wants and needs. As a result, religion was diminished and the economic ethic, to which it had given birth, grew. Rational behaviour grew out of Christian asceticism. This rational behaviour was based on the idea of a calling which Weber regarded as one of the fundamental aspects of modern capitalism and all modern culture. This led to specialisation of work and the loss of the universality of human beings.

> "This fundamentally ascetic trait of middle-class life, if it attempts to be a way of life at all, and not simply the absence of any, was what Goethe wanted to teach … For him the realization meant a renunciation, a departure from an age of full and beautiful humanity, which can no more be repeated in the course of our cultural

> development than can the flower of the Athenian culture of antiquity." (Weber, 1904-1905/1970, p. 181).

As asceticism penetrated into everyday life and began to dominate secular morals, it came to play a role in the growth of the modern economic order. This order now requires industrial production which determines the lives of all the people who are born under these conditions. What was originally thought of as a light cloak has become an iron cage.

Following this analysis of the significance of Protestant asceticism for the development of capitalist culture, Weber stressed that if we really want to evaluate the cultural significance of Protestant asceticism for other elements of modern culture, it is necessary to study the actual historical development within all parts of ascetic religion. One must also study its significance in a large number of other areas. One must study what it meant for practical social ethics, and for the function and organisation of social groups. It is also necessary to investigate its relation to humanistic rationalism, including its ideals of life and cultural influence. Finally, it is necessary to analyse what it means for the development of philosophical and scientific empiricism, for technical development and for the development of spiritual ideals (Weber, 1904-1905/1970, p. 183).

In this work, we are not given any definition of the concept of culture, but we are given a theory about how a specific cultural phenomenon has developed. This phenomenon is the capitalist culture. According to Weber this culture is characterised by the sense of calling and devotion to work. Weber thus gave a substantive characteristic of the cultural phenomenon which he studied. He then sought an explanation of the preceding cultural phenomenon which was the Reformation.

In his theory on the connection between the Reformation and capitalist culture Weber operated with two separate problems. On the one hand he looked for a link between the ethical culture of the Reformation and the culture of capitalism. On the other hand he looked for a link between the ethical culture of the Reformation and behaviour under capitalism. He thus looked at both the cultural and the behavioural consequences of the ideas of the Reformation. These two problems run side by side throughout his text.

In explaining the concept of calling in the capitalist culture, Weber followed the threads back to the thinking of the Reformation. He started with Luther's thinking and then followed it through to Calvin and the other religious thinkers in other Protestant sects. Rational thinking was developed out of their religious doctrines, and this in turn formed the basis for the idea about a calling to work. On the way Weber also introduced other forms of thought, for example Jewish ideas and the Old Testament. He demonstrated which elements of the earlier thinking had survived this process, which elements had been changed, and which elements had been disposed of. In this way Weber presents a theory on how the sense of a calling in capitalist culture has been developed on the basis of other cultural phenomena. He shows whose intellectual child it is.

When Weber explained the devotion to work in the capitalist culture, he equally followed the threads back to the thinking of the Reformation. He showed how these religious ideas had certain psychological consequences. These included feelings of loneliness, patience and the joy of feeling oneself to be one of the elect. These psychological consequences led to rational behaviour in striving to show that one belonged to God's elect. This rational behaviour involved devotion to work, acceptance of scientific thinking, rejection of art and literature, and the rejection of all forms of pleasure. The consequence of this was the accumulation of capital and the development of a new economic order. Weber thus put forward a theory of how, in capitalist culture, devotion to work is the consequence of religious ideas. He explained the direction taken by practical behaviour and what it is that makes people maintain that direction.

If one tries to distil Weber's understanding of culture on the basis of this analysis, one would have to say that culture appears through its intellectual and spiritual content. It thus appears as the result of the meaning and significance which human beings confer on concrete phenomena in their thinking. It appears in the texts which people have written and which can now be subject to value-interpretation.

Culture is significant for the further cultural development. Luther's ideas formed the basis for the ideas of the Protestant sects, which in turn formed the basis for rational thinking under capitalism. Culture can also be the basis for the development of an economic order. The concrete ideas which constitute culture form the basis for the psychological conditions which in turn influence people's behaviour. The result of this is a new social order. Culture affects both culture and the social order.

Apart from this general understanding of culture, Weber's analysis of the link between the Protestant ethic and the capitalist culture gives some more concrete suggestions about what culture is. Weber spoke about Renaissance culture, about humanist culture and about a modern capitalist culture. The content of these cultures is science, classical learning, the holistic view of mankind, a calling and devotion to work, and finally rational thinking. Culture thus comes to consist of a view of human nature, ethics, science and thinking. On the basis of this concrete thinking we shall now look at some of the works in which Weber's understanding of culture was shown in more concrete detail.

## *Cultivation*

In a few places in his major work, *Economy and Society*, Weber included some consideration of cultural phenomena. However, there is no definition of culture or systematic consideration of the relation of culture to other phenomena. When one considers that *Economy and Society* is a systematic sociological work with a definition of important sociological concepts, this is remarkable. The same applies to the selection of Weber's texts published by Gerth and Wright Mills under the title *From Max Weber*. One part of this selection is taken from *Economy and Society* while others are articles from periodicals. By studying these texts, it is possible to obtain some further insight into Weber's understanding of culture. This applies in particular to national questions, culture in relation to education and social strata, and finally culture in relation to the individual. A reading of these texts also gives some insight into some of Weber's concerns about cultural developments.

When in "Structures of Power", which is part of *Economy and Society*, Weber gave a concept of a nation, it is clear that culture plays a significant role in the foundation of a nation. Among people who consider themselves as members of a nation one should expect a certain feeling of solidarity. This solidarity can exist side by side with differences in other major cultural values, for example religion, and side by side with ethnic differences and social conditions. The idea of a nation must include feelings of shared origins and homogeneity. If a population group wishes to belong to a specific nation it must cultivate memories of a shared political destiny.

According to Weber the idea of a nation is connected with a cultural mission. The importance of a nation is normally rooted in some overriding cultural values and a desire to protect these values through the cultivation of the people who are part of the nation. Those who have the task of promoting the idea of the nation are the intellectuals.

> "By 'intellectuals' we understand a group of men who by virtue of their peculiarity have special access to certain achievements considered to be 'culture values' and who therefore usurp the leadership of a 'culture community'." (Weber, 1948/1970, p. 176).

Among the cultural elements which are particularly significant for the engendering of national feelings is a shared language. Language, and the literature which is based on it, is the only cultural value which is accessible to the masses. The appreciation of art requires a much higher level of education, so that this enjoyment is reserved to the aristocracy.

In this discussion of the national question the cultural foundations of a nation appear to be both shared and divided. On the one hand there is the common cultural basis of solidarity. On the other hand there are differences in people's access to the cultural values. Some of these values are restricted to those who are educated. In this way, Weber raised the question of differentiation between people in relation to culture. In discussing this differentiation Weber used the two concepts of class and social status.

A status group is defined by its consumption of goods, its lifestyle and its honour, while a class is defined by its relation to production and its access to goods. The social order thus expresses divisions according social honour, while the economic order expresses divisions of property and service.

> "We have seen above that the market and its processes 'knows no personal distinctions': 'functional interests' dominate it. It knows nothing of 'honor'. The status order means precisely the reverse, viz.: stratification in terms of 'honor' and of styles of life peculiar to status groups as such." (Weber, 1948/1970, p. 192).

The status group is a community within which a certain lifestyle is to be expected. Here the boundaries are set by whom one is accustomed to socialise with. This can be relevant with regard to marriage, choice of where to live and personal appearance. The status group is based on exclusivity, but there are also different forms of monopoly. Finally, Weber stated that status groups are often based on specific types of occupation, which means that there can be some overlap between status group and class.

If we go from here to Weber's discussion of education, it is clear that education and cultivation are linked to status. In his article "The Chinese Literati", which is from *Archiv für Sozialwissenschaft und Sozialpolitik*, Weber states that there are two opposing aims for education: to awake charisma and to develop specialisation. However, these two aims are not entirely separate from each other. There are many intermediate forms, including the aim of cultivation of people's conduct of life. Such conduct of life belongs to a distinct status group.

The charismatic education is directed towards awakening and testing the charismatic capacity. Such a capacity is considered as being something a person is born with. Specialised education aims to train the pupil to prepare him for specific functions. Anybody can be given such training. The pedagogic aim of cultivation is to educate a cultivated person. The content of this cultivation depends on the ideals of cultivation of the specific stratum. This means that people can be educated for distinct purposes both in relation to attitudes and behaviour.

As an example of cultivated education Weber referred to the Chinese Mandarin education and the education of German civil servants.

> "In Germany, such an education, until recently and almost exclusively, was a prerequisite for the official career leading to positions of command in civil and military administration. At the same time this humanist education has stamped the pupils who were to be prepared for such careers as belonging socially to the cultured status group." (Weber, 1948/1970, p. 427).

In the section in *Economy and Society* which concerns bureaucracy and education, Weber pointed out that within the modern educational system there is a struggle between two of the three named ideals: the ideal of the specialised man and the ideal of the cultivated man. This struggle is very important for the cultivation of the individual.

Weber's view was that the modern European educational systems aimed at producing experts and that they were therefore dominated by the ideal of the specialised man. Such an education brings with it privilege and status. The educational ideal of the cultivated man is known from feudal relations of authority. This form of education too generated social respect. The aim of this education was to lead to a cultivated way of life. Thus the special qualities of the ruling classes consisted in their special cultural qualities (Weber, 1956/1968, pp. 998-1002).

The question of the cultivation of the individual was further discussed in the article "Religious Rejections of the World and Their Directions" which was published in 1915 in *Archiv für Sozialwissenschaft und Sozialpolitik*. Here Weber argued that the cultivated person must strive after cultural values throughout his life and strive continuously to perfect himself. The man who lives in a cultural environment must always be moving forward towards perfection, in the same way as cultural values.

> "... the perfectibility of the man of culture in principle progresses indefinitely, as do the cultural values." (Weber, 1948/1970, p. 356).

The problem is that the segment of culture which the individual can acquire in a lifetime becomes less and less significant as the cultural values and aims for self-perfection become more and more differentiated and multiply. This means that a human being's striving for the internal and external world of culture will hardly enable him to acquire culture as a whole or even the essence of culture. Added to this, there is no possibility for judging whether this happens in fact.

> "The 'culture' of the individual certainly does not consist of the quantity of 'cultural values' which he amasses; it consists of an articulated selection of cultural values." (Weber, 1948/1970, p. 356).

On this basis, Weber's assessment of the steady progress of culture was very negative. He believed that for each step which culture took forwards, it would lead to an increasingly ruinous meaninglessness.

> "The advancement of cultural values, however, seems to become a senseless hustle in the service of worthless, moreover self-contradictory, and mutually antagonistic ends. The advancement of cultural values appears the more meaningless the more it is made a holy task, a 'calling'. Culture becomes ever more senseless as a locus of imperfection, of injustice, of suffering, of sin, of futility." (Weber, 1948/1970, p. 357).

If we take an overall view of the texts referred to here, it is clear that they do not contain any definition of the concept of culture. Weber presented us with some cultural elements, such as language, literature and art, and some cultural values, such as solidarity and religion. We therefore meet some formal and substantive aspects of culture. The most important is Weber's identification of the individual's culture as being a selection of values. On the basis of the continual development of culture, the individual must make some choices about the content of his culture.

By making a review of the texts referred to it is possible to sketch some elements of a theory of culture. If culture is understood as cultural values, these are constantly developing. There is a progressive development whose most significant consequences are contradiction and the loss of meaning. This progressive development in itself has negative consequences.

Access to culture is reserved to those who are educated to it, and who can, on that basis, undertake cultural leadership. On one hand they can promote certain cultural values, and on the other they can ensure the cultivation of the next generation through education. This cultivation takes place with a view to membership of a particular status group and is therefore distinct from educational specialisation which is for all.

The people who have been cultivated must relate to the cultural progress and the general loss of cultural meaning. In the light of this development the cultural person must strive after perfection just as the cultural values strive after perfection. At the same time it must be acknowledged that, in the light of the continual development, this task becomes more and more impossible. Thus the individual's culture will always consist of a selection of values. However hard he strives after perfection the cultural person will never be perfect. He must choose.

## *Discussion*

Max Weber has been the subject of wide ranging debate, so it will be impossible to include all contributions to the debate in this connection. Here we will only look at some of the contributions which concern his methodological principles, and some of the contributions which discuss his understanding of culture.

In his book *Max Weber's Methodology*, the American sociologist Fritz Ringer (1997) argues that Weber's methodology consists of a union of cultural science and social science, and of explanation and interpretation. He highlights a number of essential principles in Weber's methodology, in particular the principle of seeking the individual, the principle of causality and the principle of objectivity. He suggests that these principles emphasise the rationality and value-freedom of Weber's work.

It is possible to interpret Weber's scientific principles as being a union of cultural science and social science. It is in this sense that Weber transferred ideas from cultural science to the social science, thereby making them cultural sciences. However, this does not mean that Weber followed a strictly rational methodology. Ringer's emphasis on Weber's rationality, objectivity and value-freedom means that he underplays the value aspects of Weber's methodology. For Weber value-relations are a methodological principle which comes before causality. Weber stressed the importance of finding the values which lie behind a given phenomenon before one can begin to explain it. And he also stressed that research must necessarily be guided by the researcher's relations to values. There was thus no question of Weber approaching the social sciences from the angle of natural sciences. Weber rejected this kind of social science.

The Danish political scientist, Hans Henrik Bruun, carried out a detailed analysis of the whole of Max Weber's value teaching in his book *Science, Values and Politics in Max Weber's Methodology*, with the special aim of understanding the significance of

Weber's value teaching for political science. Those aspects of Weber's methodological principles which Bruun highlights are value-freedom, value-relevance, value-analysis and the ideal type as a conceptual tool.

Bruun believes that it is especially the principle of value-analysis which is relevant for an understanding of Weber's view of political science. Bruun points out that Weber distinguished between axiomatic and teleological value-analyses, in other words, between value-analysis which focuses on the fundamental values and value-analysis which focuses on goals. Bruun's view is that Weber had a tendency to allow teleological value-analysis to push axiomatic value-analysis into the background, and that this tendency can be traced all the way through Weber's views on political science, where there is a tendency for an ethic of responsibility to carry more weight than an ethic of conviction. (Bruun, 1972, p. 271).

It is also Bruun's view that the principle of the ideal type as a conceptual tool was influential on Weber's political science understanding. He points out that Weber's ideal type is characterised by being expansive. Given its plasticity, inner consistency and self-evident nature, it has a tendency in practice to sweep aside all theoretical reservations such as warnings against generalisations. According to Bruun this can be especially dangerous in the field of political science because political science analyses can be understood as practical political recommendations and thus be the basis for political propaganda. (Bruun, 1972, pp. 235-236).

In my view, Bruun's analysis has clarified different aspects of Weber's value teaching and set it in a wider context. As such it contributes to understanding the development of the methodological background to Weber's view of culture. The question is whether the warnings, which Bruun gives about the consequences of the methodological principles in relation to political science, apply equally to culture.

With regard to the tendency to allow teleological value-analysis to push axiomatic value-analysis into the background, it is my opinion that this does not apply to the field of culture. In the analysis of religion, there is a clear axiomatic analysis of the religious values, but at the same time there is an analysis of their purpose. It is also open to doubt whether this applies to political science analyses. In his analysis of politics as a profession Weber pointed out that politics requires both an ethic of responsibility and an ethic of conviction. (Weber, 1948/1970, p. 127).

As for the warning about the expansive tendency of the ideal type, this should be taken seriously. If generalisation on the basis of a particular ideal type is too dominant, then there is without question a risk that it will distort the understanding of the given phenomenon. On the other hand it should be said that Weber's emphasis on the possibility of considering one specific aspect of a given phenomenon while excluding other aspects makes it possible to emphasise significant value-relevant aspects of the phenomenon, rather than giving a more descriptive and impersonal impression of the whole. It is precisely in relation to the study of cultural phenomena that it will be important that such principles should predominate.

In 1996 the periodical *Dansk sociologi* (Danish Sociology) published a special issue on Max Weber. This issue dealt largely with the methodological issues of Max Weber, but the question of his understanding of culture was hardly touched upon. Mogens Blegvad (1996) raises the question of how far Weber's principle of value-freedom in research could be combined with his ideas on value-relevance. The question is whether the researcher can both be influenced by values in his choice of research topics and at the same time claim to have value-freedom. Blegvad argues that this can only apply to a limited extent. As long as it only concerns the value-based influence on the choice of research topic, Blegvad argues that value-freedom is possible, but he questions whether it is possible to maintain value-freedom when it comes to the choice of scientific direction and questions of classification. In this context he argues that in such cases there would be a problem with objectivity if the researcher were to be influenced by what he himself found valuable. Thus, according to Blegvad, it is not easy to combine value-relevance with Weber's requirement for value-freedom in research.

The same question is touched upon in an article by Manni Crone (1996) in which she refers to Leo Strauss's critique of Weber. Strauss equally believed that it is not possible to combine the requirement for value-freedom with the idea of value-relevance. However, for Strauss it is first and foremost the requirement for value-freedom which gives rise to problems. According to Crone, Strauss argued that it is necessary to have a view about the social phenomena which one studies. Here it is more of an ethical question than a logical question which is raised.

Finally, Finn Collin (1996) discusses the question of the use of Weber's concept of the ideal type. Collin does not believe that it is possible to use the ideal type to create *a priori* valid causal relationships as Weber did. Collin believes that the use of the ideal type should be limited to the purposes of description, classification and exposition.

The question of logic raised by Blegvad, whether value-freedom can be combined with value-relevance, seems highly relevant. If the choice of research topic is influenced by the values of the individual who makes the choice, then these values must also influence the choice of theoretical approach and thus the results which are arrived at. This need not necessarily mean that the researcher holds some explicit opinion about the content of his results. It merely means that one must put a question mark against the value-freedom of the research. In any case, value-relevance is such an essential element in Weber's methodological thinking that it cannot be ignored. The whole of Weber's understanding of science is based on the idea that the researcher acquires knowledge starting from his own point of view.

When Collin argues that Weber's ideal type can only be a tool which can be applied to description, classification and the exposition of empirical phenomena, he is reducing it to cover those phenomena which were of secondary importance to Weber, the class phenomena. Thus what was important for Weber, the development of a method for studying unique historical phenomena, in their full complexity, vanishes. In effect, Collin empties the concept of its original content.

The question of Weber's view of culture is discussed by Ralph Schroeder in the book *Max Weber and the Sociology of Culture* (1992). In relation to Weber's methodological thinking, Schroeder argues that cultural sciences are the sciences which concern human behaviour, and what was special about Weber's theory was that he wished to work with those parts of reality which possess cultural significance. His view is that the social sciences, and especially Weber, are concerned with a particular part of reality. It is also his view that the whole of Weber's project was first and foremost a contribution to a sociology of culture. The aim of Schroeder's theoretical analysis is to clarify Weber's theory on cultural change. He believes that this theory is based on three elements: the fact that culture is influenced by the development of ideas about the world, the ability of charisma to triumph over routine, and the differentiation between different spheres of life and the conflicts which are the consequence of such differences.

The problem with Schroeder's interpretation of Weber is that he makes Weber's methodological approach into a theoretical approach. Weber did not concern himself particularly with phenomena which have a cultural significance, but he believed that, by becoming engaged with a given phenomenon a researcher endows it with significance and thereby makes it part of our culture. The same consideration applies when Schroeder argues that, according to Weber, cultural change is caused by ideas becoming world images, acting like switchmen (Weber, 1948/1970, p. 280). For Weber culture was not the outcome of the development of ideas. Ideas are one of many phenomena which can contribute to the foundations for creating new concepts and in this way promote cultural change. For Weber cultural change was due to changes in society and the consequent need for creating new concepts for understanding this world. Cultural change in fact has the character of constant revision and new thinking.

In what follows I shall attempt to clarify my own view of Weber's understanding of culture, but to start with I shall look in more detail at the social and intellectual background to Weber's work.

In his book, *The Decline of the German Mandarins* (1969), Fritz Ringer gives a picture of the social and intellectual conditions in Germany at the time when Weber developed his ideas. It is Ringer's view that the period from the end of the 19th century and up to the fall of the Weimar Republic was characterised by radical changes in society and a breakdown of the special position of intellectuals. Ringer makes it clear that his concept of the German mandarins was inspired by Weber's own analysis of the social and intellectual significance of the Chinese mandarins. German intellectuals had previously had a status as mandarins, but this status was now threatened and had to be defended.

On the social level the German mandarins were threatened by an increasing social, and thus also intellectual, specialisation which made it impossible to maintain the concept of man as a unity and the general cultural education. On the intellectual level the mandarins were threatened by French positivism and the natural scientific thought immanent in their epistemology. Both these threats meant that not only was German cultivation and its attendant world view threatened, but the position of social monopoly, which the mandarins had enjoyed in German society as civil and military administrators, was also threatened.

Ringer divided the German mandarins into two groups, according to their reaction to this situation. On the one side there were the orthodox who defended German culture to the end, and on the other side there were the modernists who acknowledged the necessity of re-conceptualising German culture in the light of modern society. According to Ringer, Weber belonged to the latter group (Ringer, 1969 and 1992).

There is some evidence for such a view in Weber's writings, but there is also, perhaps, the basis for a more balanced view, especially with regard to the intellectual background. It was clearly Weber's view that specialisation and the desire for the education of specialists in the world of European universities was a threat to the concept of the holistic view of the cultivation of man. He was thus quite conscious of this social development. The consequence was that his theory was pessimistic in its content. As for Weber's intellectual position, it is clear from his works that he defended himself against two intellectual standpoints and leaned towards a third. The two positions he distanced himself from were historical materialism and the influence of natural sciences on the social sciences. The tradition which he took as his starting point was the historical school. Weber clearly saw himself as being in the German cultural tradition, while distancing himself from Marx's materialist explanations and French positivism. Max Weber's contribution to sociological thinking thus appears as a defence of German cultural thinking, not as a dogmatic defence, but as a defence which is capable of reforming traditional thinking. This defence is especially evident in his philosophy of scientific theory.

On the methodological front Weber reformed the historical school by distancing himself from its highly objectivist approach. On the one hand he maintained the idea of value-freedom and neutrality towards the topic studied. On the other hand he was more open to the interpretative approach. It is here that value-relevance comes into the picture. The researcher can only raise his research above the highly descriptive level by choosing a personal point of view. The contradiction between the requirement for value-freedom and the need for value-relevance can thus be interpreted as a result of the contradiction between wanting to defend and at the same time to reform the historical school which was his starting point.

Since Weber's concept of culture was methodologically determined, his methodological position is relevant to the whole of his thinking on culture and to those elements of a theory of culture which we find in his works. Weber's methodological principles form the basis for his definition of culture. When a researcher is to develop concepts, he must start from the basis of his own values and apply his personal point of view to a phenomenon. It is this view which is the basis for Weber's definition of culture. For Weber, culture is the segment of the world to which human beings relate their values and thus give it meaning and significance. Once man has first understood the significance of an empirical phenomenon, its significance operates as a means of helping to understand other empirical phenomena. As a result, human beings develop attitudes, interests and reactions to these phenomena.

This concordance between social science methods and the view of culture does not, of course, mean that social science and culture are identical with each other. It means that social science is part of culture. Other parts of culture are literature, art and philosophy. All these forms of expression are related to values and they create meaning and give significance. Among the values which can help to constitute culture are ethics, purposes, feelings, belief and aesthetics. Without such values there would be no possibility for creating culture, nor any social science.

In the discussion on culture Weber undertook some categorisation of culture. He referred to cultures which were typical of an age, for example, classical culture, the Renaissance, humanist culture and the capitalist or modern culture. In addition to this there are national cultures. Weber referred to German culture, French culture, and so on.

In Weber's view of culture there is also a view of the relation between culture and human being. What he meant was that culture is available in different degrees to different categories of human beings. Access to culture and to cultural values requires cultivation through education. However, it is not all forms of education which lead to cultivation. Those kinds of education which aim at specialisation do not have this aim of cultivation. Cultivation is not the same for all. Cultivation takes place with reference to specific status groups.

If we look at culture in a wider perspective it is clear that, according to Weber, it is changeable. Culture is developed in time and space. It is influenced by a multiplicity of forces, including socio-economic structures, interest groups, institutions and ideas.

Culture also affects social and spiritual development. It affects people's needs, the ways in which these needs are satisfied, and integration, power, behaviour and the whole economic order. It also affects spiritual values, ideals, philosophical principles and so on.

The consequence of cultural development is, as Weber analysed it, that culture becomes more and more specialised and gets more and more conflicting aims, so that it develops towards loss of meaning.

For those who have to relate to this culture the consequence is that they cannot achieve the cultural perfection they strive for. Culture simply becomes too extensive and cannot be acquired by a single individual. The cultivated human being must relate selectively to cultural values.

On the basis of this discussion of Weber's cultural philosophy it appears that his concern for intellectual and cultural development leaves its imprint on his view of culture. Culture should not be understood in a natural scientific or in a materialist perspective. According to Weber, it should be understood in a value-related perspective. Culture is the outcome of the value-based thinking about empirical phenomena by human beings. Empirical phenomena become culture when they are related to values and thus acquire meaning and significance. The problem is that Weber transferred this view of culture to cultural science. This, too, is supported by values. When an empirical phenomenon is looked at from a specific point of view, a concept is developed so that the empirical phenomenon acquires some significance. However, this view of cultural science comes head to head with Weber's maintaining the requirement for value-freedom in research. The question is, what this very open and interpretative formation of concepts of culture, combined with the requirement for value-freedom in cultural research, has meant for sociology.

# 4

# Georg Simmel: Culture as Form

It is characteristic that the question of culture appears to be a theme with very different meanings in the writings on Georg Simmel. In one of the earliest works on Simmel, *The Social Theory of Georg Simmel* by Nicholas Spykman, published in 1925, the word 'culture' is hardly used. Spykman's object was rather to investigate Simmel's contribution to distinguishing sociology as an independent science. In *Sociological Impressionism* (1981), David Frisby deals to a certain extent with Simmel's ideas about culture. His discussion of Simmel focuses particularly on Simmel's works on the aesthetic aspects of culture. In *Sansernes Sociologi* ('The Sociology of the Senses') (1991), Niels Gunder Hansen gives a relatively short review of Simmel's theory of culture and analysis of urbanisation. In *Experience and Culture* (1960), Rudolph Weingartner includes Simmel's discussion of the tragedy of culture in his assessment of Simmel's philosophy of life. In this way, he gives culture a relatively central role in Simmel's philosophy. In a special issue of *Theory, Culture and Society* on Simmel (1991), Birgitta Nedelmann's article summarises the different aspects of Simmel's theory of culture. Culture is thus a theme which has enjoyed a variable status in the literature on Georg Simmel's writings.

When one looks into Simmel's writings, he did in fact make explicit contributions to ideas about culture and to the clarification of the concept of culture. This discussion is carried on first and foremost in a number of minor essays, of which the most important are collected in Peter Etzkorn's collection of Simmel texts, *The Conflict in Modern Culture and Other Essays* (Simmel, 1968). In addition to this, in Simmel's major work, *The Philosophy of Money* (1907/1978), the economic discussion includes questions about lifestyle and culture. Finally, collections of Simmel texts have been edited by Donald Levine (Simmel, 1971), P.A. Lawrence (Simmel, 1976) and Guy Oakes (Simmel, 1984). These texts also deal with the question of culture to a certain extent. The works identified here will be referred to in the following discussion of Simmel's thinking on culture. On the other hand, some of Simmel's core sociological works will not be referred to. These do not really deal with the question of culture. This concerns *Grundfragen der Soziologie* (Individuum und Gesellschaft) and *Soziologie, Untersuchungen über die Formen der Vergesellschaftung*. These are included in Kurt Wolff's edited collection of Simmel texts (Simmel, 1950/1964; 1959).

Simmel's thoughts on methodology are taken as the starting point for a discussion of the cultural thinking that can be seen from Simmel's texts referred to above. These thoughts are mainly to be found in his philosophical works. Therefore these works are drawn on to the extent that they are judged to be relevant for Simmel's thinking on the theory of culture. However, this will not include a discussion about Simmel's substantive contribution to philosophy itself. Such a discussion would lie outside the scope of this book.

In *The Problems of the Philosophy of History*, which was first published in 1892 and revised and re-published in 1905, Simmel discussed the question of historical knowledge and he touches on some of the general methodological principles which can be important for understanding his later contributions to cultural thinking.

Simmel undertakes this discussion of the methodological principles of history writing in a dialogue with historical realism which, according to him, sees history as holding up a mirror to reality. Simmel disagreed with this view and saw it as his task to develop an alternative understanding of the science of history.

Simmel was primarily concerned with the question of how one should perceive and understand historical knowledge. He approached this question from two angles, considering the significance of the historian's general assumptions and the use of raw facts. The question which he constantly returned to was how historical knowledge arises in the gap between the historian's general assumptions and the available raw facts. The historian's general assumptions include on the one hand some general *a priori* categories and on the other hand the historian's own personality. Simmel therefore sought to clarify how one should understand the establishment of *a priori* categories and how one should understand the subjective element in historical research.

In this work on the philosophy of history, Simmel was clearly influenced by the contemporary progress in psychology. He thus saw the same relation between history and psychology as there is between astronomy and mathematics. The topics of history are man's thoughts, intentions, desires and feelings.

> "The mental status of historical processes ... seems to require the following ideal for historical enquiry: history should be a form of applied psychology." (Simmel, 1905/1977, pp. 39-40).

This understanding of history was of decisive importance for Simmel's methodological considerations. The psychology of perception came to form the basis not only for his understanding of history, but also for his methodological principles for historical research.

One of the questions which concerned Simmel was that of how *a priori* categories are developed for the understanding of concrete historical phenomena, and what the consequence is of working with such *a priori* categories. As a starting point for this discussion, he advanced Kant's view. According to Simmel, Kant believed that there are *a priori* categories which can function as the most general conditions for experience. These *a priori* categories are clearly distinguished from the empirical. However, it was Simmel's view that when one looks at the most abstract of statements, they are in reality empirical in the sense that they use the most general form of thinking about some specific material circumstances. Even though the most abstract of statements are empirical, they can also function as *a priori* categories for whole areas of knowledge.

> "The Kantian *a priori* ... is only the most highly abstract stage in a sequence of *a priori* propositions, ... Consider propositions insofar as they are ... seen from the top of this sequence, its most abstract level. They are empirical in the sense that they represent an application of the most general forms of thought to specific mate-

> rial. However, these same propositions can function in an *a priori* fashion for entire provinces of knowledge," (Simmel, 1905/1977, p. 43).

Statements in the character of *a priori* categories can thus function as relational forms which can be used for the special thinking that classifies, defines and emphasises a given mental content in such a way that it can be adapted to suit the most differently constituted forms. What was important for Simmel was that there was some content and that it was this content which was constitutive for more concrete thinking. In other words, it was Simmel's view that even the most abstract statements are empirical, and even though they are so, they operate as *a priori* statements with constitutive power in relation to specific areas of knowledge.

According to Simmel, that which is given *a priori* has a significant influence on the knowledge which is produced. If, for example, we wish to obtain knowledge about a specific individual, this will be done by using our *a priori* knowledge about personality. Such *a priori* knowledge is acquired through a long process in which each person's personality is clearly a link. The consequence of this process is that a structure is created which is the basis for the knowledge we can obtain about an actual person's personality. It is this structure which makes it possible for us to understand the mental structures which lie behind what we directly observe in the actual person.

The problem is that, in using *a priori* structures, we add something to the observable facts. We try to make these observable facts fit into the general structure which is our starting point. The psychology of perception teaches us that we add something to what we observe so that it fits our *a priori* view. This form of spontaneous supplementing of what we in fact register shows us that mental processes can only be understood as a combination of registered facts and general assumptions. When it comes to more complicated mental processes, this combination of facts and general assumptions leads to great uncertainty with plentiful opportunities for wrong conclusions.

> "In accordance with experiential laws governing the relation between the mental and the physical, the external processes produce a continuous parallel series of mental processes. Precisely this spontaneous supplementation is one of the strongest proofs of the following proposition: these mental processes are not simply deduced from the facts ... On the contrary, they are correlated with the facts on the basis of general presuppositions." (Simmel, 1905/1977, pp. 46-47).

If this is transferred to historical thinking it means that this emphasis on the combination of facts and general assumptions must take place as a combination of the processes we can observe and our general assumptions, including our view of mental processes. The historian must have a general idea of the psychological premises for the actions of human beings in order to be able to explain the concrete registered action. Without such a general understanding of mental processes, it would be impossible to establish explanations and thus make the effects of historical phenomena understandable. However, it is possible to conceive of many different mental processes behind a given action. It is therefore important to identify the general assumptions which lie behind a given historical text. Simmel suggested that this task is complicated, but essential.

What does it mean for historical science that it forces its material into such *a priori* categories? Simmel said that the consequence will be that historical knowledge will be created as a mental reconstruction or transformation process. Thus history will be presented in a new form.

> "... every form of knowledge represents a translation of immediately given data into a new language, a language with its own intrinsic forms, categories and requirements. In order to qualify as a science, the facts ... must answer certain questions, questions which they never confront in reality and in their form as brute data. In order to qualify as objects of knowledge, certain aspects of the facts are thrown into relief and others are relegated to the background." (Simmel, 1905/1977, p.77).

Science presupposes such a selection. Some specific qualities are emphasised and given inherent relations are established on the basis of ideas and values. All this exceeds reality.

Historical truth thus becomes an intellectual activity. Historical truth produces something new out of its raw material. History is developed by questioning this raw material, and endowing individual phenomena with meaning. History reveals the meaning and value of its raw material. These meanings and values structure the past in such a way that a new construction is produced which can satisfy all the criteria which we establish. Knowledge is thus a consequence of *a priori* forms. (Simmel, 1905/1977, p.78).

These methodological principles put the historian in a special role in relation to history. Through his choice of point of view he will affect the development of knowledge. Simmel thus believed that in history we find elements of a structure which are only partly or discontinuously interwoven. The only way in which it is possible to make a synthesis of these disjointed elements is by the historian imposing a certain problematic on them. These fragments can only constitute history from the perspective of the historian. He must therefore impose the problematic on them which he believes is right. This is the only way in which it is possible to create a synthesis out of the fragments.

On the basis of this methodological principle, Simmel had to recognise that there is no such thing as knowledge, pure and simple. Knowledge is only possible insofar as it is produced and structured by constitutive concepts, and these constitutive concepts must be qualitatively determined.

> "There is no knowledge as such: knowledge is possible only insofar as it is produced and structured by constitutive concepts that are qualitatively determined. Because these concepts are qualitatively determined, they are inevitably partial and biased. Given a criterion for knowledge that is perfectly general, it would be impossible to identify or distinguish any element of reality. This is the deeper reason why there are only histories, but no history as such." (Simmel, 1905/1977, pp.82-83).

Simmel was primarily concerned with the methodological principles for research into the historical personality, in other words research into the individual. As a starting point for this discussion, he established that individuality cannot be understood by logical deduction. Individuality can only be understood psychologically by another person who has the same quality of individuality. The requirement for methodological norms was therefore transferred to a form of understanding which inevitably had to be subjective (Simmel, 1905/1977, p. 90). Objectivity cannot thus be separated from its subjective basis, in the same way as these elements of subjectivity cannot be eliminated from the results of historical knowledge. It is only possible to criticise and to structure them in accordance with standards, supplemented with methodological and substantive categories.

Simmel believed that these methodological principles had consequences for when it is possible to say that one has developed knowledge about some specific phenomenon. In this discussion Simmel again takes his point of departure in the views of Kant. Sim-

Simmel stated that Kant believed that we acquire knowledge about an object when we have first developed an entity out of a multiplicity of perceptions. Kant developed this view especially in relation to the natural sciences. For historical research this view means that the historian's consciousness becomes the source of the entity of the historical person. Simmel did not believe that this view is tenable for historical science. Against the background of his methodological principles he was of the opinion that behind the historian's consciousness there is a pre-ordained entity, which is the entity which is found in the concrete historical personality. The cohesive force of the historical personality thus becomes the ultimate source for the cohesive force of the historical content.

> "In the case of history ... the content ... is more clearly and definitely performed or prefabricated than is the case in the natural sciences. This is because the basis of the coherence of historical content, or even its origin, is already there – even though it is not immediately accessible – in the historical personality. This is the ultimate source of the coherence of its elements or aspects." (Simmel, 1905/1977, p.98).

It was Simmel's view that these methodological principles for research into historical individuals can be transferred to research into more general social conditions. He believed that the social structures and movements, the legal systems of civil society, the hierarchical relations of groups and the formation of collective life can be reconstructed on a personal basis. This is a prerequisite for being able to identify, describe and understand them. Even the qualities of these movements, which we believe we can identify through simple observation, can in reality only be identified if we refer to these mental processes. Both the necessary conditions for psychological understanding and the necessary conditions for objective scientific simplification are thus allied in the general simplification (Simmel, 1905/1977, p.102).

It is possible to trace some general methodological considerations in these historico-philosophical works. For Simmel, establishing historical knowledge is an intellectual activity. Knowledge thus appears as a process of mental reconstruction. Knowledge of history is produced by a combination of, on the one hand, the historian's general assumptions and, on the other hand, historical facts. The general assumptions have the character of *a priori* categories which, in origin, are empirically based, and the historian's personality. As for the historical facts, they must answer the questions put by the historian. Knowledge is thus created by the historian using *a priori* categories and his own personal point of view to make a conscious selection from a range of given observations. It is on this basis that Simmel argued that each historian creates his own history.

For Simmel these methodological principles not only apply to studies of empirical conditions. They also apply to the study of philosophical works. He sets this out in the introduction to his work on Schopenhauer and Nietzsche. He argued that the picture which can be formed of a person's life in a cultural-theoretical context can never be an exact copy of the whole life. Depending on the point of interest which prompts the study much must be excluded while other aspects must be the point of focus. The most essential aspects must be brought together in a cohesive picture, but this picture will not have any direct counterpart in reality. It is more in the nature of an ideal interpretation with the meaning derived by means of the method and even by the aim of the presentation. Out of the totality of the statements of philosophers, one must choose those that create a cohesive, uniform and meaningful context of thoughts, and it does not matter if this totality includes inconsistencies, weaknesses and ambivalence. It was Simmel's belief that when a philosopher moves between ideas which are mutually exclusive, this says something about his psychological state or his lack of self-criticism, but it does not exclude the possibility of these ideas being correct or at least useful (Simmel, 1907/1986, pp. liv-lv).

Simmel's criticism of Schopenhauer and Nietzsche, which I shall not try to reproduce here, was based on these methodological principles. However, it is of interest to understand the culture-historical context in which he positioned the two philosophers. This is relevant to the starting point for his own understanding of culture.

> "It is a paradox that all higher cultures of our type are structured so that the more they evolve the more we are forced, in order to reach our goals, to proceed along increasingly long and difficult paths, filled with stops and curves. Man is the indirect being and becomes more so the higher his cultural development." (Simmel, 1907/1986, p. 3).

According to Simmel, the problem is that the relationship between the end and the means has become more complicated. For primitive man there was only a short distance between the end and the means, but for people who live in a developed culture, a whole chain of means must be constructed in order to reach a particular end. This increased complexity means that the end disappears in the swirling mists of different means. This leads to an angst-ridden search for sense and meaning. Simmel believed that this problem first arose in Greco-Roman culture, especially at the beginning of the Christian era.

> "At that time (at the outset of the Christian era) the systems of living had become so complicated, the units of acting and thinking so complex, and the interests and movements of life so manifold and dependent on so many conditions, that in unconscious mass tendencies as well as in the self-reflection of philosophical consciousness a disquieted search for the goals and the meaning of life was ignited." (Simmel, 1907/1986, p. 4).

Christianity brought a solution to this problem by offering an absolute meaning in life, which was the salvation of the soul and the Kingdom of God. Such absolute goals were presented as being what should come after the meaninglessness of the fragmented and individualised life. In more recent times Christianity has lost its magnetism and its power over many people, but the need for an absolute goal still exists. The desire for an absolute goal is thus an inheritance from Christianity. This is the background against which one should understand both Schopenhauer and Nietzsche.

For Schopenhauer the problem was that a general will exists behind all phenomena, which on the one hand cannot be identified, and on the other hand affects man's seeking for a certain goal. The will exists as a general driving force behind all human actions so that, as soon as a man has achieved one goal, he must strive after another. Schopenhauer's philosophy thus appears to be very pessimistic, where man is driven by such general will and where life is without value. Schopenhauer saw various possibilities for escaping from the will and from meaninglessness. One possibility was to seek salvation though aesthetics, a second possibility was to seek salvation through morality, and a third possibility was to withdraw and thus avoid the onward march of the general will. In his criticism of Schopenhauer, Simmel pointed out that, among other things, the concept of the will had been developed as an ideal without any empirical basis, and that Schopenhauer's philosophy did not allow any room for personality.

Between Schopenhauer and Nietzsche came Darwin, and it was the inspiration of Darwin which gave Nietzsche the basis for a more optimistic philosophy, which was an evolution-oriented philosophy. Simmel believed that Nietzsche had a programmatic approach to the question of life. Nietzsche wanted to develop an alternative to the pessimistic cognition of Schopenhauer, so that it became more valuable. With Nietzsche, it was progress itself that was the aim in life. Life thus begets more life. Man can and should develop himself beyond his present level. As soon as the task which now confronts man is completed, a new task must be revealed (Simmel, 1907/1986, p. 174). The consequence of this view was that life only has meaning through its high points. What matters most is what man contributes, rather than how he has lived his life. On the basis of this view, Nietzsche was led to reject all democratic social movements as being decadent. An individual can only represent a step forward in human development if he ranks above the others in a given group. Simmel criticised Nietzsche for his dogmatic thinking which is in marked contrast to Schopenhauer's seeking after truth. The consequence of this dogmatic thinking was that Nietzsche declared himself to be a moral legislator, rather than a seeker after truth.

In this work on Schopenhauer and Nietzsche, Simmel highlighted the problems posed by the two philosophers concerning the question of the ever increasing complexity of means, and the consequent loss of meaning in life. He looked into how the two philosophers looked at this fundamental question. In this way he established a platform for his own understanding of cultural and metaphysical questions.

By reading these philosophical works, it is possible to establish both a methodological and a thematic starting point for revealing Simmel's cultural understanding. As for methodology, Simmel understood historical knowledge to be the result of the selection of raw facts produced by the researcher applying some *a priori* categories to some given material, together with a personal point of view. In terms of substance, he starts with a discussion on meaninglessness as a consequence of constant development and the increasing degree of complexity. It is cultural development itself which gives rise to meaninglessness and pessimism.

## *The tragedy of culture*

The methodological principles which Simmel developed for historical science were also used in his discussions on culture, not merely as a principle of scientific theory, but also as a general development from science to culture. His ideas on historical science's *a priori* categories and the historian's personal viewpoint are extended to apply to the forms of culture in general.

On the one hand we see how his thinking about culture was coloured by his ideas about *a priori* categories and by his own personal point of view on cultural matters. He sought to establish a concept of culture by using these categories and principles. On the other hand we see an understanding of culture as being these categories and principles. Culture consists of general forms and these forms are a product of a personal point of view, which in turn is a product of an inner psychological condition. In this way, he used his methodological principles in a double sense.

Simmel's most significant contributions to cultural thinking are the articles in Etzkorn's collection of Simmel's texts, consisting of some articles on culture on a general level and some articles for the understanding of more concrete cultural phenomena. It is especially the first category of articles which will be dealt with here, though some of the other articles will be drawn into the discussion.

In his article "The Conflict in Modern Culture", which was published in 1918, Simmel defined culture in such a way that it has virtually the same content as the *a pri-*

*ori* categories he defined for research into historical phenomena. He believed that it was possible to speak of culture when life presents specific forms through which it expresses or realises itself. This can be through art, religion, science, laws and so on.

> "We speak of culture whenever life produces certain forms in which it expresses and realizes itself: works of art, religions, sciences, technologies, laws and innumerable others. These forms encompass the flow of life and provide it with content and form, freedom and order. But although these forms arise out of the life process, because of their unique constellation they do not share the restless rhythm of life, its ascent and descent, its constant renewal, its incessant divisions and reunifications. These forms are frameworks for the creative life which, however, soon transcends them." (Simmel, 1968, p.11).

However, the forms which grow out of life's dynamic develop a fixed identity and their own logic and legality. This new fixity creates a distance between the forms and the spiritual dynamic which creates them. In this way the forms become independent.

In this definition of culture, we thus see a principle about general forms and we meet again Simmel's methodological principle of *a priori* categories. What is common to these two types of concept is their relation to the factual content. The foundation for culture's forms is life itself, while the foundation for historical science's *a priori* categories is empirical conditions. In both cases it is possible to trace a line back to real conditions. Another thing they have in common is distance and independence. When cultural forms are used as a framework for the further development of life, they obtain their own independent logic and significance. We saw this same independence in the discussion of scientific categories. As a result, culture and science are considered as being similar phenomena.

Also in the discussion of what culture is, we meet again the question of the continual development of categories. Simmel said that culture has a history. This is because, as soon as they are created, the forms of culture are influenced by the forces of life.

> "Each cultural form, once it is created, is gnawed at varying rates by the forces of life. As soon as one is fully developed, the next begins to form; after a struggle that may be long or short, it will inevitably succeed its predecessor." (Simmel, 1968, p.11).

This constantly changing content of culture is a sign of life's endless fruitfulness. At the same time, this constant change expresses a fundamental contradiction between life's constant development on the one hand and the validity of the forms through which it makes progress, on the other. This means that life struggles against those products of which it is itself the basis, because these are fixed and do not move forward together with life. There is thus a constant conflict between form and life.

> "Life as such is formless, yet it incessantly generates forms for itself. As soon as each form appears, however, it demands a validity which transcends the moment and is emancipated from the pulse of life. For this reason, life is always in a latent opposition to the form ... Thus life perceives 'the form as such' as something which has been forced upon it." (Simmel, 1968, p. 12).

Simmel sought to give concrete expression to these general thoughts, by giving a number of examples. With these examples he gave some insight into how the forms are developed in a number of different areas. He also sought to characterise the specific placing of his contemporary circumstances within this development.

As examples of forms, Simmel referred to the forms of production, art, metaphysics, religion and ethics. In the course of history, all these forms will experience a general development in which old forms will be replaced by new. For example, religious cultures develop according to a general pattern. According to this pattern, a particular form of religious life, which may originally have been relevant, will in time become locked into superficiality and narrow specialisation. It will be succeeded by new forms within which religious impulses can experience a dynamic development. In this way a new religious form, with its attendant beliefs, will replace an obsolete form.

In his own time, Simmel observed some entirely new tendencies. It was not merely that life produced new forms, but that life sought to liberate itself from these forms. It was necessary to fight against the forms as such. This was happening in painting, where attempts were being made to break the previous forms, in ethics, where attempts were being made to break with the previous rules for living together, and in religion, where attempts were being made to escape entirely from having an object for religious feelings. If we look again at Simmel's example of religion, he said that the consequence of the struggle against form would be a movement towards mysticism. The problem is that one can abolish the supernatural object, i.e. the god which is the basis of the religion, but one cannot abolish the religious impulse. When one removes the aims of religion, the result is that one can no longer see any meaning in life, and one therefore turns to mysticism.

In this article, which Simmel wrote at a relatively late stage in his life, we get some understanding of what culture is. He wrote that there can be culture when life produces the forms through which it expresses and realises itself. Culture is thus a form which should be regarded as a relatively fixed phenomenon, but in another way it is also a production which must be regarded as a dynamic phenomenon. We also get an idea of what it is that makes culture change. It is life's continual development. As life develops, categories become obsolete and seem to limit the realisation of life. They must be replaced by new categories. Life is thus the driving force for cultural development and change. But Simmel also pointed out that in this modern age people can try to fight against this development if they so choose. People can act and try to limit cultural development. If they do so, then a conflict will develop between cultural forms and life. Life is dependent on forms in order to be able to develop, but at the same time life will try to liberate itself from these forms in order not to be limited by them. Simmel's article thus gives both an understanding of culture as a general phenomenon, and an understanding of the relation of culture to life as differing, according to whether it relates to previous ages or the modern age.

In the article "On the Concept and the Tragedy of Culture", which was published in 1911, Simmel pursued the question of the relations between the objective spirit and the subjective soul. In this article he wrote that culture is created through a meeting between the subjective soul and the objective product, which is created through spiritual activity.

> "... culture comes into being by a meeting of the two elements, neither of which contain culture by itself: the subjective soul and the objective spiritual product." (Simmel, 1968, p.30).

Man can only be cultivated by moving through the existing objective forms of, for example, art, morality, science, religion, laws and social norms.

> "... subjective life ... can become truly cultivated only through forms which have become completely alien and crystallized into self-sufficient independence." (Simmel, 1968, p.30).

Conversely:

> "... objectively spiritual realities ... represent cultural values only to the extent that they interpenetrate the path of the soul from itself to itself, from what might be called its natural state to its cultivated state." (Simmel, 1968, p.34).

In other words, man cannot be cultivated without possessing the objective spirit, and the objective spirit only has a cultural function if it is in fact used to benefit man's cultivation.

On the basis of this statement of the relationship between the objective spirit and the subjective soul, Simmel discussed the objective spirit's tendency to become independent and the consequent possibility for specialisation and multiplicity. The problem which concerned Simmel was that the objective spirit's specialisation and multiplicity make it difficult to cultivate the subjective soul.

The basis for the independence of objects lies in their own logic. They have two kinds of values. On the one hand they have a substantive value and on the other hand they have a cultural value. These two forms of values do not necessarily operate on the same scale. A work of art, an economic product, the result of research and so forth are judged by some internal laws, by which they are accorded value as a good or a bad product. Compared with this substantive value, there are cultural values which express whether the product in question has a high or a low value with regard to the cultivation of man. These two forms of values need not have anything to do with each other. An objective product with small cultural value may have great significance for the cultivation of the individual, while an objective product with high cultural value can be almost inaccessible for people (Simmel, 1968, pp. 36-37).

With this distinction between a substantive value and a cultural value, it is clear that the cultural products can be developed in such a way that they create their own substantive value without thereby creating a better basis for man's cultivation. As an example of such a development, Simmel referred to the use of the word 'culture'. Here there is a distinction between religious 'culture' and artistic 'culture' etc. This distinction does not express any of the qualities of the individual personality, but rather general spiritual conditions. Within this objective spirit there are grades of difference, without this necessarily improving man's cultivation. This differentiation within the objective spirit means that there will always be a large number of spiritual products through which the individual has the possibility of being cultivated. However, this wealth of cultural possibilities can be a threat to culture because it leads to people's over-specialisation. A person can thus acquire a remarkable degree of competence or knowledge within a particular area without truly becoming cultivated (Simmel, 1968, pp.38-39).

Simmel gave further examples of this development. One example is our knowledge, whose form is determined by *a priori* measures. This knowledge is constantly added to with new elements. However, there is no guarantee that these new elements will contribute to the perfection of our souls. Another example is our practical or technical relation to things. Even though we may form these relations to suit our own purposes, they need not necessarily function according to our aims. They have their own logic and powers. The problem is thus that objective elements which are technical, moral, artistic or legal have their own internal logic. We cannot control the direction they take. Even though it may be we who create them, they must follow the direction which is determined by their own internal necessities. The consequence of this development will be that friction can easily arise between impersonal cultural forms on the one hand and the internal norms and driving force of the personality which seeks to fulfil itself through culture on the other hand. The objective cultural forms can thus be separated from the cultural elements which surround the ego and reshape them in accordance with their own requirements. There can be religious conflicts between man as a being who is subject to a divine order, and man as a free individual, and there can be social conflicts between man as a member of a social group, and man as a total being (Simmel, 1968, pp. 39-40).

Simmel believed that culture's independent logic and power was underlined by the fact that parts of most intellectual products are not produced by ourselves. Any finished product will contain emphases, relations and values which the producer of them has not himself put into it. An object will contain some spiritual meaning which the producer will not have put into it, but which is due to the form of the object. The objective spirit thus has an independent opportunity of being transferred to a new subject, though this opportunity need not be taken. The special quality of culture is the metaphysical basis for its general independence, by means of which cultural products grow as if by some inner necessity (Simmel, 1968, p.42). The result of this development will be that the cultural products move away from the direction which would have made it possible to unite them with people's personal development.

> "Here ... we are dealing with the immanent logic of cultural phenomena. Man becomes the mere carrier of the force by which this logic dominates their development and leads them on as if in the tangent of the course through which they would return to the cultural development of living human beings ..." (Simmel, 1968, p. 43).

Simmel said that this corresponds to the process through which our thoughts are led by the rules of logic into theoretical consequences which may be far from the original intention. This is the true tragedy of culture. That there is a tragedy means, wrote Simmel, that the destructive forces which are directed towards a being arise from the deepest levels within that being itself, or that the destruction is a logical consequence of the structure by which it has created its own form.

Against this background Simmel painted a gloomy picture of cultural development. He pointed out that the nature of objects to accumulate is incompatible with personal life. The ability of the self to receive is limited not just by the strength and length of life, but also by its unity. The self must therefore choose between different substances which are offered as a means for its individual development. The ever-growing offering of objectified spirit creates desires in him, strikes him with feelings of inadequacy and makes it impossible for him to escape from relating to them. The quantity of products makes him depressed because he is not able to assimilate them all, but he cannot reject them because they belong, potentially, to the sphere of his cultural development. Simmel also pointed out that the tendency of objects to become specialised leads to specialisation in people. This makes the division of labour possible which draws the energies of a whole complex of people into a single product, without necessarily contributing to the individual's personal development. With the division of labour, the product is divorced from its individual contributors. It thereby loses the inner life which can only be given to a whole work by a whole person. This lack of unity in the objectified spirit allows for a speed of development which the individual is unable to keep pace with. At the same time, the individual must protect his own entity against the effects of all these things, and thus against constant stimulation.

> "The situation is tragic: even in its first moments of existence, culture carries something within itself which, as if by an intrinsic fate, is determined to block, to burden, to obscure and divide its innermost purpose, the transition of the soul from its incomplete to its complete state." (Simmel, 1968, p. 46).

As we have seen, Simmel's article also gives a view of what culture is. Simmel wrote that culture is created by a meeting between the subjective soul and the objective spiritual product. Here too we see a dynamic understanding of culture. Culture is something which is created by a meeting between a subjective and an objective phenomenon. Neither of these phenomena can be absent if there is to be culture. We also get an idea of cultural change. It is the inner logic of the objective elements which determine the change of culture. When the products' substantive values are separated from their cultural values, the consequence is that the substantive values can be increased infinitely. There can be infinite differentiation, infinite relations, infinite emphases, without this benefiting man's cultivation. Nevertheless, people must relate to new spiritual products because they can potentially affect their cultivation. As a consequence, man must choose and thus have to accept some specialisation which Simmel did not believe to be an expression of true cultivation. One does not create a whole person through the division of labour. In this article we thus find an understanding of culture as a meeting between objective and subjective phenomena and an understanding of cultural change as being the consequence of the inner logic of the objective products. The source of this change lies in objective products' separation of the substantive values and the cultural values.

In the other articles in Etzkorn's selection of Simmel's texts there are discussions about different aspects of culture, including geometry, painting, music and drama. Here only one of these articles will be discussed in brief, and this is "The Dramatic Actor and Reality", which was published in 1912. In this article, Simmel compared the art of acting with other forms of culture. He wrote that it is just as valid to present elements of life through dramatised action as through painting or poetry, or by recreating them through epistemology or religion. All these different forms of culture have the same function, which is to present or recreate elements of life (Simmel, 1968, p.95).

Simmel emphasised that it can never be the task of the actor to imitate a concrete person, but rather to create a cohesive idea of the person in question. It is the actor's task to create different dramatic elements on the basis of his own personality.

> "... dramatic acting represents an inner unity produced from the diversity of all those great elements of which the dramatic impressions seem to be composed. ... The decisive point is the fact that the dramatic actor creates within himself a complete unity with its unique laws." (Simmel, 1968, p. 96).

It is this personal force which is important for the artistic product. It is the personal viewpoint, with the force of personality, which creates the unity in the product and is thus what makes art become art.

In this article we see an example of the culture which man creates. The criterion for whether something is a cultural product is the unity of the product. There is thus only a cultural product if it has inner coherence. The source of this inner coherence is the personality of its creator. Cultural products are thus related to their creators, but not to other social phenomena.

## *Lifestyle*

*The Philosophy of Money* must be considered as Simmel's most important work. It was first published in 1900, but revised and published in a new edition in 1907. In this work he sought to establish money as a superior category in line with logical categories. It was his view that money and intellect have the same form (Simmel, 1907/1978, p.440). Money, as an abstract category, rules the economic world, while logical categories rule the world of thought. What is common to both these categories is that they are both independent and abstract.

Simmel's idea, that even the most abstract categories have an empirical basis, is apparent in this work. Money is presented as a general category and at the same time it is defined through its historical development. Historically, money has developed from substance to function. Whereas money originally had value by virtue of the metal it was made of, it later came to have value by virtue of its function in relation to its ability to achieve a given purpose (Simmel, 1907/1978, pp. 168-169).

The aim of this analytical and historical definition of money is to look at its significance for people's way of life. With the development of money man obtained personal freedom. He was no longer required to perform service in the form of slavery or the provision of goods in kind, but he could instead receive money as a reward for the work which was put into a specific product. However, hand in hand with this increased freedom there was also a loss of rights and influence and a development towards impersonal and demeaning relations. The problem was that there was freedom from something, but not freedom for something. The consequence of the freedom which can be bought for money was that people were released from being bound to other people and to things, but thereby they lost the sense of direction which other people and things had given them. People began searching after the meaning of existence, and this came to be expressed through a constant search for new styles and forms of expression (Simmel, 1907/1978, pp. 400-404).

The true purpose of this work on money was to clarify the relationship between the modern form of money economy and the modern form of lifestyle, and it is in this connection that culture comes into the picture. Culture operates as a link between money and lifestyle. Culture has this status because of its division into objective culture and subjective culture. It was Simmel's belief that, because of its general nature, money is disinterested and it presents itself as a suitable link between people and objects. Money is thus able to create a connection between the subjective and the objective elements of culture. At the same time, it is this relation between the objective and subjective elements of culture that are decisive for the general lifestyle of people.

Simmel introduced this discussion of culture and lifestyle with a statement of the general relationship between subjective and objective culture and with a statement about the nature of this relationship in his own time. This discussion corresponds largely to the discussion he put forward in the earlier named articles. What is important is to see how he established the relationship between culture, money and lifestyle.

According to Simmel, the entire lifestyle of a society depends on the relationship between the objective culture and the subjective culture. The decisive question is whether the individual's inner life is close to or far removed from the objective cultural development of his time.

> "The relationship between objectified mind and its evolution to the subjective mind is of extreme importance to every cultural community and especially with refer-

> ence to its style of life. ... The general way of living, the framework that the social culture offers to individual impulses, is circumscribed by the following question(s): is the inner life of the individual close to or estranged from the objective cultural evolution of his age?" (Simmel, 1907/1978, p. 467).

In a society with a low level of cultural development this relationship between objective and subjective culture will be more equal, in the sense that the objective cultural potential will not exceed the cultural reality of the subject. The question which Simmel then sought to explain was why the elevation of the cultural level causes disharmony between the two levels (Simmel, 1907/1978, p.452).

The most significant explanation for the disharmony, between objective culture's possibilities and the cultural situation of the individual, is to be found in the division of labour, and thus in the money economy which has made this division of labour possible. The problem with the division of labour is that it displaces the relationship which would otherwise exist between a product and the person who creates it. For example, if we consider art, an object's wholeness is created by the artist investing his personality into the product. But, when there is a division of labour, the product has a fragmentary nature, and it loses the spiritual influence which can be given to it by a single person. This objectification and depersonalisation of products mean that they are suitable for use by many different people. The objectification of products thus runs parallel with the spread of consumption (Simmel, 1907/1978, pp. 454-455).

The division of labour, with its potential for increased differentiation of products, leads to an increased quantity of products, so that it is impossible for an individual person to relate to all of them. The division of labour therefore leads to an estrangement between people and objects. Thoughts, the capacity for work and qualifications are thus objectified in the form of books and goods and can be freely moved around (Simmel, 1907/1978, p. 460). For the individual, the consequence is that his cultural development falls behind this development.

With this separation between people and products there can be a greater or lesser distance between them, and according to Simmel it is this difference in distance which makes different lifestyles possible. As an example of the differing distances between people and products he refers to different styles of art. It is a characteristic of art that it brings us closer to things while at the same time creating a distance from them. It is the tension between these two tendencies which gives a specific character to an artistic style.

> "The inner significance of artistic styles can be interpreted as a result of the differences in distance that they produce between ourselves and objects." (Simmel, 1907/1978, p. 473).

Simmel gave the examples of symbolism and naturalism as opposites within art. With symbolism the distance between people and the product is increased because the artistic product expresses a psychic experience which does not in itself have any visible correspondence with the artistic product. It is the opposite with naturalism which seeks to come as close to its subject as possible, though without being able entirely to remove the distance between people and product (Simmel, 1907/1978, p. 474).

In general, Simmel believed that the modern age is characterised by two opposing tendencies with regard to the distance between people and objects. This distance can be both great and small at the same time. If we look at the scientific world, the distance between people and things is diminished through the use of technical aids such as microscopes and telescopes. At the same time, the better insight which these technical aids give also gives an understanding of the true immensity of the distance to things. The problem is that the more that man overcomes the distance to the physical world, the greater is his distance from the spiritual world.

The consequence of this cultural development is thus that, over time, what previously appeared to be instinctive or unconscious, becomes more sure but fragmented. On the other hand, what previously required attention and conscious care has been replaced by mechanisation and instinctive factual knowledge. What was distant before now comes closer, at the cost of a greater distance to what was previously closer. Simmel believed that this tendency not only applies to cultural phenomena, but also to relations between people, where the dissolution of the concept of common ownership means that family ties are loosened, while life in big cities makes it possible for strangers to come closer together (Simmel, 1907/1978, p. 476).

Simmel's work on the philosophy of money does not give us any clearer picture of the concept of culture. On the other hand we see Simmel's cultural ideas in a wider context, in which on the one hand we get an explanation of culture's development, and on the other hand we see the consequences of culture. Culture is thus related to money and the division of labour, as well as to people's lifestyles. It is money and the division of labour which gives cultural objects their own dynamic and separates from the individual's cultural development. The distance which is thereby created between cultural objects and individuals becomes the basis for people's lifestyles. Differences in distance between people and products create differences in styles. The general tendency of modern cultural development is for the distance between people and objects to become both greater and smaller. What was previously distant becomes closer, and what was previously close to becomes more distant.

## *Female culture*

Among the more concrete questions which Simmel considered was female culture. He considered this in the article "Female Culture", originally published in 1911, in *Archiv für Sozialwissenschaft und Sozialpolitik*, which is included in Oakes's selection of Simmel texts (Simmel, 1984). The starting point for his discussion of the relationship of the two sexes to culture is that the two sexes are different in nature. It was Simmel's belief that masculine energies are expressed by initiative, by the ability to distinguish, and by the ability to create. In the case of women, they lack the ability to differentiate, and as persons they are more whole, integrated and homogeneous. These differences in nature mean that the two sexes have different attitudes to culture. Man's distinctive characteristics mean that he is predisposed to the division of labour, which is a prerequisite for the development of the differentiated objective culture. The objective culture is thus masculine in form. Woman's homogeneous nature means that differentiation, and thus objective culture, is foreign to her.

Against this background Simmel asked whether there are areas of culture in which the female nature could have an advantageous influence on culture.

> "However, if objective culture is to exist, and if women are to accommodate themselves to its form, then new nuances and a new extension of its limits are to be expected from women only if they accomplish something that men cannot do. This is the core of the entire problem, the pivotal point of the relationship between the women's movement and objective culture." (Simmel, 1984, p. 75)

Simmel pointed to a number of areas of knowledge in which he believed women could make a valuable contribution. One of the areas in which advantage could be taken of women's special characteristics is medicine, where their ability to see the whole would make them better at making diagnoses. Another area is historical science where, by using applied psychology, women could bring different interpretations as a consequence of their different natures. A third area is mathematics, which is a science which is characterised by the wholeness of its approach.

In literature, Simmel believed that the genre where women could make the most impact is the novel. This is because the novel is the least formalised form of literature and can therefore be expected to be the most female form of expression. In the field of art, acting is assumed to be the most suited to women. This is because of women's ability to transmit the inner processes and create a more direct expression.

The conclusion is that men externalise themselves so that they give meaning to things which are independent of themselves. Whereas women are characterised by the harmony of their natures. This means that men represent the becoming, while women represent the being.

In this article, Simmel gave clear definitions of the concept of culture. However, these definitions do not add anything to the texts previously discussed. On the other hand, here it becomes quite clear that objective culture is dependent on the nature and psyche of human beings. The individual person's psychic condition is decisive for the extent to which and the method by which he can contribute to the development of objective culture. Whether a person is disposed towards the division of labour and differentiation, or towards wholeness and cohesion, is decisive for his or her potential in the field of culture.

## *The war as life in revolt*

The last question to be looked at here, drawing on Simmel's texts, is the significance of war on culture. He discussed this in the article "The Crises of Culture", which is included in the collection of Simmel's texts made by P.A. Lawrence. It was originally published during the First World War in 1917 (Simmel, 1976). The question which Simmel asked was whether there was any connection between the crises of culture and the war, or more specifically whether there was any connection between the growing distance between subjective and objective culture and the World War. The connection which he could see was that the war could be understood as an expression of the revolt of life against the disintegrating effect of culture.

One of the consequences of war was that it turned ends and means on their heads. Over time, money becomes an end rather than a means, but the war meant that money again became a means. This was due to isolation from the international market and the consequent lack of food etc. When there is scarcity of goods, they will again become the ends of human activity. For a while it will therefore be seen that money cannot be substituted for the true value of the goods (Simmel, 1976, pp. 261-262). Another consequence of the war was that it gave the population a common goal and a shared danger, giving rise to a sense of community. The war thus gave some new objective elements to culture which could replace the fragmentary and chaotic situation within culture (Simmel, 1976, p.264). Simmel did not see any hope for solving the general crisis of culture in this way, but the war would, for a time, slow down the tempo of development.

It was thus Simmel's view that the war would halt the development of some cultural elements and accelerate others. The unifying, simplifying and concentrating forces of war would be an expression of the revolt of life against the disintegrating and destructive function of culture.

> "... the disintegration and perversion of cultural life has reached an extreme, and life has risen in revolt against it in the shape of this war, with its unifying, simplifying and concentrated force." (Simmel, 1976, p.266).

According to Simmel, the war was thus the factor which could put a brake on the process by which objective culture was developed and fragmented in an ever increasing tempo, leaving subjective culture behind.

This article also defined and applied the concept of culture in accordance with the previously discussed texts. What was new in this article was that Simmel introduced a factor which could put a brake on cultural development and the consequent cultural tragedy. It is not possible to stop cultural development, but it can be slowed down for a while. When life takes on the concentrating, unifying and simplifying forces of war, cultural development can be slowed down.

## *Discussion*

As early as 1918, György Lukács, who was a pupil of Simmel, made the criticism of Simmel that his writings are too pluralistic and unsystematic. They are too impressionistic. According to Lukács, the problem is that Simmel neither analysed the great works of Goethe, Kant and Rembrandt in the manner of a historian nor in the manner of a systematist. It was Lukács's opinion that Simmel neither sought to place these works in the chain of cultural development, nor to define them against normative criteria. They are simultaneously unique and *a priori* categories. They are both unique and absolute. (Lukács, 1918/1991, p. 149).

More recently, the same kind of criticism has been made by David Frisby. Directly influenced by Lukács, Frisby suggests that Simmel lacked a methodical, systematic or scientific approach. He believes that Simmel, to a quite remarkable degree, failed to take into account methodological reflections, and that not only was his approach unsystematic, it was virtually anti-systematic. Frisby claims that the lack of scientific approach can be seen by the form which Simmel chose for his works, which was that of an essay without a scientific context and without the customary references and links to existing literature (Frisby, 1981, pp.69-73). In Frisby's opinion, Simmel undertook an aestheticisation of social reality. He believes that Simmel considered the relationship between sociology and society to be of the same kind as that between the art critic and the work of art. The distance which develops between people and things, also develops between people and society (Frisby, 1981, pp. 151-153). Frisby called his first book on Simmel *Sociological Impressionism*, suggesting by this that there is some connection between Simmel's sociology and a specific artistic school. Simmel's sociology is considered as an unsystematic series of impressions without any form of systematic theoretical development.

In his introduction to Simmel's book *The Problems of the Philosophy of History* (Simmel, 1905/1977), Guy Oakes declares his absolute disagreement with this point of view. He believes that all of Simmel's mature works were produced using the same basic tool, which was the concept of form. An investigation of Simmel's use of the concept of form will thus bring order and cohesion to the apparent chaos of his works. However, Oakes had to acknowledge that Simmel's concept of form was a rather vague and imprecise concept. According to Oakes, it is both an epistemological and an ontological concept. On the one hand form is a classifying or conceptual system which includes categories, criteria, principles and distinctions, and on the other hand it is a necessary condition for the existence of a given category of objects, in other words for objects which are constituted in a particular way (Simmel, 1905/1977, p. 19).

Rudolph Weingartner also disagreed with the view that Simmel's writings were an expression of sociological impressionism. The theme which he identified as running through Simmel's work was life and its products, in other words, culture. Weingartner's attempt to rebuild Simmel's position takes its starting point in Simmel's philosophy of life and definition of life. Weingartner points out that Simmel had a double definition of life. Life is thus both 'more life' and 'more than life'. On the one hand life is a process through which life produces something living and is thus more than itself. It thus creates 'more life'. On the other hand life is expressive in the sense that it produces things which are not life. It thus creates 'more than life'. (Weingartner, 1960, pp. 69-70). According to Weingartner this double definition of life is a problem for Simmel's philosophy and theory of culture.

As a consequence of these two definitions there must be two opposing and conflicting developmental tendencies. Life as more life is a process which pushes onwards in an attempt to fulfil its own law of development, while life as more than life produces forms and products which are independent of life. The problem is that life as a process must be supported by forms, which conflicts with the principle of development. Therefore life runs the risk of being restricted by the forms which it produces. (Weingartner, 1960, p.83). Life's forms are both a prerequisite for and a restriction to life's further development. This is the problem which makes itself felt in relation to culture.

Weingartner identifies three components in Simmel's concept of culture. First, there is culture as a process, a cultivation through which the individual is transformed from one stage to the next. Second, there is culture as development, which involves the unfolding of the individual's potential. And third, there is culture as the use of external objects through which the transformation takes place (Weingartner, 1960, p. 73). With this exposition of Simmel's concept of culture, Weingartner arrives at a parallel between life and culture. According to the first two definitions, culture is a process, a cultivation, and according to the third it is the use of forms, of objective products. In the same way as with life, the consequence is that cultivation can only take place with the help of cultural products, and at the same time the cultural products threaten to restrict cultivation. With his double definition of life, Simmel has, according to Weingartner, unleashed an insoluble conflict for life and for culture.

Weingartner makes another criticism of Simmel, that his philosophy is marked by subjectivism (Weingartner, 1960, p.171). Weingartner argues that the basis for this subjectivism was that Simmel regarded *a priori* categories as being the fruit of experience, They are changeable and dependent on the personal point of view (Weingartner, 1960, p. 132). This means that the interests and meanings of historical topics vary from person to person and from age to age (Weingartner, 1960, p. 138).

Birgitta Nedelmann seeks, like Weingartner, to create a system out of Simmel's cultural analysis. She does this by pointing out three cultural problems: first, cultural poverty, where individuals rebel against the forms as such; second, cultural ambivalence, where consumers use art and handicrafts to create their own style; and third, the cultural tragedy, in which the subjective and objective culture are no longer in harmony with each other. There is a cultural concept for each of these problems. For the first problem there is the view of culture as being cultural forms, for the second problem there is the concept of culture as being an aesthetic, and for the third problem there is the concept of culture being a dualism between subjective and objective culture (Nedelmann, 1991, p.

172). Nedelmann thus seeks to bring order to the various views of culture and cultural problems which she identifies in Simmel's writings. However, she does not attempt to merge these concepts into a unifying principle, as we have seen in the case of Oakes and Weingartner.

Finally, reference should be made to Gunder Hansen's work on Simmel in which he confronts Simmel's cultural pessimism. He believes that Simmel's cultural pessimism was rooted in his over-emphasis on the concept of cultivation. Cultivation should form the basis both for individual freedom and the concrete historical reconciliation between the individual and the general. Gunder Hansen believes that it is impossible to sustain freedom and reconciliation together in such a way, and that there is therefore no basis for cultural pessimism. Gunder Hansen therefore believes that Simmel was mistaken when he argued that modern culture had become so overwhelming and fragmented that it was no longer possible to maintain the classical idea of cultivation. On the contrary the individual must, as Simmel himself argued, make choices (Gunder Hansen, 1991, pp. 157-158).

There appear to be two tendencies in discussions on Simmel: there is a tendency to view his writings as being non-cohesive, and a tendency which seeks to find a unifying principle in his works. When a review is made of Simmel's methodologically oriented works and his culturally oriented works, there seems to be good reason to seek a cohesive principle in these works. In fact there is a clear agreement between the principles which Simmel used when thinking about method and the principles he used when considering culture, money and other more concrete phenomena. There is thus good reason to follow the tradition which seeks to establish order in Simmel's works. The question is whether the attempts made here are the most relevant in the discussion of Simmel's understanding of culture. In his own presentation of it, Oakes's view of form as the constituting principle for Simmel's theory is particularly ambiguous. To this can be added that he entirely disregards the personality and the subject as being the unifying principle in Simmel's thinking. Weingartner's view of Simmel's double definition of the concept of life, as being the starting point for the whole of his philosophy, seems to capture a significant problem in Simmel's theory of culture. However, the problem is that none of these attempts to reconstruct Simmel's position is aimed at his theory of culture. In contrast, Nedelmann does consider Simmel's theory of culture, but she stops at the triad of cultural problems, without bringing together the three elements which she seeks to define.

In what follows, I shall attempt to clarify my own view of Simmel's understanding of culture. The starting point for this discussion is the social and intellectual background for Simmel's theoretical work.

The social background, which we have seen in Ringer's description in relation to Weber, also applies to Simmel's work. In Ringer's picture of the social and intellectual conditions in Germany at the start of the twentieth century, there is an increasing degree of specialisation and a threat to general cultural education. According to Ringer, the problem was that at an intellectual level the German intellectuals were threatened by French positivism and scientific thinking, while at the social level their monopoly of administrative functions was under threat.

If we look more closely at Simmel's work it is clear that differentiation and specialisation give rise to concerns and theoretical deliberations. It is equally clear that neither positivism nor natural-scientific thinking were part of the basis for his theoretical deliberations. Likewise, he distances himself from historical materialism. His theory was developed in dialogue with the German historical school and its belief that it is possible to make a photographic reproduction of reality.

The theoretical construction for illuminating and discussing the question of development and differentiation was developed by Simmel under the influence of German philosophy. His point of departure was Kant and his concept of *a priori* categories. The problem is that Kant considered these *a priori* categories as being always valid, but it was clear to Simmel that even the most general forms are empirically based and thus changeable. If the categories can change and be differentiated, Simmel needed some element for creating cohesion. Simmel solved this problem by using ideas from psychology.

The influence of psychology clearly leaves its mark on Simmel's introductory methodological considerations. When Simmel explained why historical science cannot consist of a photographic reproduction of reality, he highlighted history's general preconditions for making selections of empirical material. *A priori* categories and personality are a part of these general preconditions. The categories should create order in the empirical material, while personality should create cohesion. Here Simmel was faithful to Kant's ideas, while including ideas from psychology. This combination gives rise to the question of how far it is possible to allow the selection of empirical data be guided by both *a priori* categories, which are empirically based, and personality. Can history be guided by both at the same time?

When Simmel maintained that the categories are changeable he also needed some way of bringing this question into the discussion. This need was supplied by more recent German philosophy, in particular the works of Schopenhauer and Nietzsche. These philosophers particularly focus on development and change.

When we come to the theory of culture we can clearly see how the ideas of Kant have been supplemented with these two new sources of inspiration, psychology and more recent German philosophy. The problem is that these two sources of inspiration drew Simmel in two different directions. Psychology made it possible to put personality and the unified whole in focus, while more recent German philosophy put change and differentiation in focus. In this way, the basis for Simmel's theory of culture is Kant's *a priori* categories and the conflict between unity and differentiation.

The core of Simmel's understanding of culture is the concept of form. This concept is present in all his work. It is the central epistemological concept. It stands at the centre of art, science, literature, religion, economics and it stands at the centre of the way in which life is lived and organised. Simmel looked for forms and categories in all parts of culture. With the inspiration from Schopenhauer and Nietzsche he related form to life, and with the inspiration of psychology he related form to personality.

The relationship between form and life is one part of Simmel's theory of culture. It is life's continuous development that creates new forms and is the reason why, in time, forms become obsolete and come into conflict with life. The result is a conflict between form and life.

The relationship between form and personality is the other part of Simmel's theory of culture. As a consequence of life's development, forms have been subjected to value-differentiation so that they contain both substantive values and cultural values. When these two forms of values are separated from one another, the substantive values can be developed according to their own rules, without regard for whether they have any value for the human beings who are to be cultivated. In this way distance is created between forms and people which causes problems for the cultivation of the individual person. In view of this, the individual must develop his own personal relation to the forms. On the other hand, he has to understand about the forms in order to acquire culture, while he must also add his own personal point of view to these forms. The individual must both choose between existing forms and add something personal to the chosen forms.

Thus for Simmel culture consists of forms which are one the one hand related to life and on the other hand to personality. Culture's development is due to life's continual development as well as to the division of the forms into substantive values and cultural values which allows the forms to develop their own logic. The development of culture is due both to the development of life and to its own inner dynamic. The consequence of this is that it is a problem for the individual to keep up with developments and ensure his own cultivation, while at the same time the individual's active relation to culture is an indispensable precondition for the further development of culture.

The consequence of Simmel's theory of culture is that personality should predominate over the differentiation of the forms which are created by life and over the forms themselves. It is personality, with its basic cohesive force, which must create the unity which is lost in the careering development of life. Personality must create unity in art, in science, in literature, in acting and so on. The problem is that, when personality creates unity in its own product, it also increases the distance to other products, so that a new differentiation arises. Simmel has thus not created the unity which he sought. On the contrary, he created a new differentiation in culture.

This criticism of Simmel's theory of culture is also a criticism of his methodology. When science and epistemology are a part of culture, they will be increasingly differentiated. When scientific products are imbued with the personality of the person who has created them, this means that each person produces his own scientific products. There will therefore be an infinite number of scientific products.

Simmel's attempt to interweave German philosophy and psychology does not seem to lead to a solution of the problem he identified, which is the problem of the ever increasing level of differentiation and the division of labour. What does this unsolved problem mean for sociology? What does it mean for sociology that it must take its point of departure in a theory whose attempt to create a unified whole has merely resulted in new differentiation? Has Simmel's problem with differentiation been passed on to contemporary sociology?

# Part II
# Contemporary Sociology of Culture

# 5

# Margaret Archer: Culture as Logic

In the works of Margaret Archer culture is presented as an explicit sociological phenomenon which can be made the subject of independent theoretical considerations. Her theory of culture is also part of a wider theoretical construction of both cultural and structural phenomena.

In this connection Margaret Archer's most important work is *Culture and agency*, which was first published in 1988. This work was later revised and published in a new edition in 1996. Between these two editions Archer published *Realist social theory: the morphogenetic approach*. This work, which was published in 1995, contains a fundamental sociological theory, bringing together cultural and structural relations. These two books are thus central to a discussion of Margaret Archer's view of culture.

At an earlier stage of her career Archer was concerned with the study of the development of educational systems. This work resulted in two important books, *Social Conflict and Educational Change in England and France: 1789-1848* (co-author, Michalina Vaughan) published in 1971, and *Social Origins of Educational Systems*, published in 1979. Together with Salvador Giner she has also edited two books on European topics, *Contemporary Europe: Class, Status and Power*, published in 1971, and *Contemporary Europe: Social Structures and Cultural Patterns*, published in 1978.

Finally, Margaret Archer has published numerous articles, of which only a few will be referred to here. In 1982 she published the article: "Morphogenesis versus structuration: on combining structure and action" in *The British Journal of Sociology*. And in 1985 she published "The Myth of Cultural Integration" in *The British Journal of Sociology*. This article was included in her book *Culture and agency*.

In *Realist social theory* Archer lays out the principles which she thinks must be the basis of sociological research. She includes not only methodology, but also ontology and practical theorising about social conditions. It is her fundamental belief that there must be consistency between these three elements. Ontology is thus significant for the explanatory methodology which is used, and this methodology is in turn relevant to the practical theories which can be developed. It is thus necessary to know what a society is and how it can be explained before investigating a specific problem. Methodology is therefore a necessary link between ontology and the formation of practical theories.

> "In short, methodology, broadly conceived of as an explanatory programme, is the necessary link between social ontology and practical theory." (Archer, 1995, p.5).

Archer's ontological starting point is realism. She puts a great deal of emphasis on the study of social phenomena as objective phenomena. Her starting point for a basic understanding of society is that one must distinguish between structure and action. These two levels must not be reduced so as to become dependent on one another. The principle of emergence applies to both levels, so that new properties can emerge on the basis of pre-existing properties. According to Archer, such new properties can develop over time, they have relative autonomy and they have independent causal significance.

> "... social realism ... accentuates the importance of emergent properties at the levels of both agency and structure ..." (Archer , 1995, p.14).

> "When applied to structure and agency, the realist social ontology *entails* the exploration of those features of both which are prior or posterior to one another and of which causal influences are exerted by one stratum on the other, and vice versa, by virtue of these independent properties and powers." (Archer, 1995, pp. 14-15).

With this ontological basis, Archer's methodological starting point is analytical dualism. This principle underlines the necessity of studying the mutual influence of two levels on each other, without allowing them to conflate. For example, this applies to the mutual influence between the social and the systemic, between structure and action, between culture and action, etc.

> "... social realism implies a methodology based upon analytical dualism, where explanation of why things social are so and not otherwise depends upon an account of how the properties and powers of the 'people' causally intertwine with those of the 'parts'." (Archer, 1995, p. 15).

The guidelines which Archer develops for practical theoretical work are constructed on the principles of morphogenesis versus morphostasis, i.e. the principle of origin and development of forms versus the principle of stagnation of forms. Morphogenesis is like a cycle which develops in three phases: structural conditions, social interaction and structural change.

> "The social analyst needs practical guide-lines ... Here the morphogenetic/morphostatic framework is put forward as the practical complement of social realism because it supplies a genuine method of conceptualizing how the interplay between structure and agency can actually be analyzed over time and space." (Archer, 1995, p.15).

> "It constitutes a distinctive linkage between social ontology, explanatory methodology and practical social theorising." (Archer, 1995, p.16).

With these basic principles for ontology, methodology and guidelines for practical theoretical work, Archer approaches the study of structural and cultural phenomena. It is Archer's basic belief that theoretical work must be directed towards its practical sociological application.

## *Culture and agency*

*Culture and agency* is quite clearly the most important work for obtaining an understanding of Archer's view of culture. Here it is possible to see unfold, from the start, her basic ideas on ontology, methodology and guidelines for practical theoretical work.

It is Archer's fundamental view, in other words her ontological standpoint, that it is an inevitable part of everyday life to feel both free and bound. On the one hand one is free to create one's own future, but on the other hand one is confronted with impersonal limitations. This also applies to the world of ideas, where one can feel free to accept or reject an idea, while the stock of ideas itself is limited or restricted.

This point of departure makes it necessary for Archer to distinguish between relations which exist between ideas and the ideational influences that exist between people. As for the relations between ideas, Archer says that these can be characterised by their degree of logical consistency. Ideas can either contradict or complement each other. As for the ideational influences between people, she says that they can be characterised by the degree of causal consensus. Ideational influences between people can take the form of manipulation, mystification, legitimisation, persuasion etc. Causal consensus is thus linked to power and influence, while logical consistency is independent of such factors.

Archer develops two concepts for understanding the two levels in her analysis; one is cultural system integration, which expresses the degree of consistency between ideas, and the other is socio-cultural integration, which expresses the degree of causal consensus between people.

On this basis, Archer arrives at her definitions of the main elements of her theory of culture; on the one hand there is culture, including the cultural system, and on the other hand there is socio-cultural interaction. In this way we obtain a clear definition of culture as being everything which can be made subject to understanding. The cultural system is thus that part of culture which is subject to the law of contradiction, meaning propositions which can be true or false and which can thereby be contradictory or compatible.

> "... culture as a whole is taken to refer to all intelligibilia, that is to any item which has the dispositional capacity of being understood by someone. Within this I then distinguish the Cultural System, which is that sub-set of items to which the law of contradiction can be applied. These are propositions, for only statements which assert truth or falsity can be deemed to be in contradiction or to be consistent with one another. In turn this means that the Cultural System is restricted to the propositional register of society at any given time." (Archer, 1988/1996, p. xviii).

Opposed to the cultural system there is socio-cultural interaction which consists of the influences which people have on each other with regard to culture.

> "... we generate myths, are moved by mysteries, become rich in symbolics and ruthless in manipulating hidden persuaders. But all of these elements are precisely the stuff of Socio-Cultural interaction. For they are all matters of interpersonal influence, whether we are talking at one extreme of hermeneutic understanding (including religious experience at the furthest extremity) or of the manipulative assault and battery of ideas used ideologically." (Archer, 1988/1996, pp. xviii-xix).

The methodological question, which follows from this distinction between the cultural system and socio-cultural interaction, is the question of how these two levels affect each other. Here Archer uses her principle of analytical dualism, as she considers the two levels to be analytically separate so it is possible to investigate their effects on each other.

For Archer, the question of mutual influence concerns how contradictory or compatible propositions in the cultural system affect the ordered or conflicting relations between people, and it goes on to deal with how socio-cultural relations affect the reactions of agents in relation to the cultural system.

When Archer develops her views on the mutual influences between the cultural system and socio-cultural interaction, she starts with the ideas which are supported by some people at a given moment. It is her opinion that it is a prerequisite for the logical relations between these ideas that they affect people. The deciding issue is whether the ideas are compatible, or whether they contradict one another. These two types of logical relations will thus give rise to different kinds of situational logic and thus to differing frameworks for action.

> "In short, analysis opens by examining the effects of holding ideas with particular logic relations (of contradiction or complementarity to others) ... It is then maintained that to uphold ideas which are embroiled in a contradiction or enmeshed in complementarities places those who do so in different action contexts where they are confronted with different situational logics." (Archer, 1988/1996, p. xxii).

The basic idea is that if ideas conflict with one another, in other words, if the logical propositions contradict each other, then the agents will be in a problematic situation, where they can either choose to maintain their ideas dogmatically, or solve the problem of inconsistency by adjusting their ideas. It will be the reverse of this if the ideas are compatible. In this case the agents are in an unproblematic situation where they can investigate the existing ideas. The consequence of this can be the reproduction of ideas and a lack of will to change them.

Confronting these situational logics, determined by the logical relations between ideas, are the causal relations between groups or individuals on the socio-cultural level. These relations affect what the agents actually do in relation to culture. Thus the differences in material interests produce differences in social conditions, and thereby differences of ideational interests and actions.

> "The other part is made up of the causal relations operating between groups and individuals at the Socio-Cultural level. Such relationships have their own dynamics, rooted in different material interests, producing various forms of social stratification and different ideal interests, such as ethnic, religious or linguistic divides (which are ideational but not propositional). ... They form the other side of the interface and are thus co-determinants (with Systemic conditioning) of what actually takes place there." (Archer, 1988/1996, p. xxii).

The dynamic, which comes from the mutual influence between the cultural system and socio-cultural interaction, depends on how the situational logic and socio-cultural interaction fit together. The systemic conditions are only decisively important if the socio-cultural influences pull in the same direction. It does not matter if the situational logic points towards the need for change of the culture, if the power and interests pull in the opposite direction. Conversely, it does not matter if the situational logic points towards cultural stasis, if the power and the interests pull in the direction of cultural change.

> "Again, fundamentally and universally no corrective formula (generated to repair contradictions) and no reproductive scheme (elaborated to protect complementari-

> ties) can be made to 'take' in society when the contemporaneous distribution of interests and power do not gel with it." (Archer, 1988/1996, p. xxiii).

From this methodological starting point Archer includes the morphogenetic principle as the basis for developing a theory of cultural change. Her purpose is to reveal the conditions under which the structure of the cultural system can be changed, and the conditions under which it remains unchanged. Archer introduces sequential thinking, in which time is always the decisive element. Over time the morphogenetic/morphostatic cycle has three phases: cultural conditions, socio-cultural interaction and cultural development/stasis.

Morphogenetic thinking is based on the principle that the cultural system predates the socio-cultural interaction which transforms it, and that cultural development follows the socio-cultural interaction which has created it. With this sequential thinking Archer links together aspects of the past, the present and the future. It is her view that both the past and the future exist in the present and influence how people act in the present. This is because we are all born into a given cultural context. This means that we start with given cultural knowledge, given interests in maintaining or changing culture, and given possibilities for influencing culture. All these circumstances contribute to determining our cultural actions.

> "For we are all born into and can only live embedded in an ideational context which is not of our own making. Our very knowledge about it, our vested interests in rejecting it or retaining it and our objective capacities for changing it have already been distributed to us *before* the action starts." (Archer, 1988/1996, pp. xxv-xxvi).

For Archer this position should not lead to cultural determinism. The agents can exploit their varying degrees of cultural freedom. On the one hand they have material interests which pull them in different directions, and on the other hand they have reflexive abilities to fight against the given conditions and confront them with originality.

> "... actors can exploit their degrees of cultural freedom to great (elaborative) effect. ... the structural conditioning of material interests is also operative in the same 'present' and pulling in different directions. More importantly, however, is the quintessential reflective ability of human beings to fight back against their conditioning ..., giving them the capacity to respond with originality to their present context." (Archer, 1988/1996, p. xxvi).

Archer's theory of culture is based on the view that the past creates the conditions for whether there *can be* cultural development in the future, but whether there *is in fact* any cultural development depends on the material interests and the originality of people in the present.

On the basis of this statement of ontology, methodology and principles for practical theorising, Archer unfolds her theory of cultural change. The unfolding of this theory follows the morphogenetic cycle.

The theory starts with the first phase of the morphogenetic cycle, which is cultural conditions. Archer defines the cultural conditions as being the relations between ideas which people associate with, and the possible actions which these conditions give rise to. The issue revolves around the relations between the ideas which people associate with. Do they contradict or complement each other? What situational logic do these mental relations lead to? Are there restrictions or possibilities for the cultural agents? (Archer, 1988/1996, pp. 144-145).

Archer starts with two possible cultural conditions. She characterises them as constraining contradictions and concomitant complementarities, respectively. If the conditions are characterised by constraining contradictions, this means that the theories or beliefs conflict with each other. If the conditions are characterised by concomitant complementarities, this means that the theories or beliefs are compatible.

If the cultural conditions are characterised by constraining contradictions this means, says Archer, that there is a necessary connection between two ideas. One is dependent on the other and cannot operate without it. If one associates with one of the ideas, it is impossible to avoid the other, even though they conflict with each other. As an example of such a constraining contradiction, Archer refers to Christian belief and classical civilisation. Christian belief grew out of the civilisation of antiquity, while being in conflict with it. Archer takes this example from Durkheim's analysis in *The Evolution of Educational Thought.* She points out that, according to Durkheim, the Christian church could only explain the holy texts by making a closer study of pagan literature. Thus, both ways of thinking are bound to each other in spite of their contradictions. This brought Christianity to a position where it constantly had to combat the thinking of antiquity, without being able to dismiss it entirely (Archer, 1988/1996, p. 151).

For cultural agents, constraining contradictions mean that they must try to repair the relations between ideas which conflict with each other. This can only be done by correcting one of the conflicting ideas or both of them. If, in Durkheim's example, cultural agents supported Christian beliefs, they had to do whatever they could to correct classical culture and thus overcome the inconsistency between the two philosophies. This is the situational logic presented to them. The consequence of the correction of ideas is syncretism, which is an attempt to reconcile conflicting ideas by drawing a veil over some of their differences (Archer, 1988/1996, pp. 157-158).

If cultural conditions are characterised by concomitant complementarities, then according to Archer this means that two ideas are linked to each other without conflicting with each other. One idea is dependent on the other and, as a consequence of their supplementing each other, there can be an ongoing clarification, strengthening and confirmation of the ideas. As an example of this, Archer refers to ancient China and India, in which religious beliefs, and their stratification of social status, harmonised with the economic ethic. On this basis, ideas and actions could develop without problems (Archer, 1988/1996, p. 153).

For cultural agents, the presence of concomitant complementarities means that they are in a problem-free situation. Here it is worth investigating the idea which is the basis for the idea which one has associated with. The consequence of this situation is that there is no renewal. The situational logic points towards protecting ideas rather than correcting them (Archer, 1988/1996, p. 158). On the conceptual level there will be a systematisation, in other words, a strengthening of existing relations between ideas and the addition of ideas which have not previously been included. In the longer term this systemisation will lead to increasing cultural density. After a while, as more and more ideas have been gathered and systematised, it becomes more difficult to add new ideas. Therefore it will be necessary to erect a barrier against new ideas. They must be repressed and rejected. In this way culture is protected (Archer, 1988/1996, pp. 171-178).

Having discussed two different kinds of cultural conditions, Archer goes on to discuss the second phase of the morphogenetic/morphostatic cycle, which is socio-cultural interaction. Archer's view is that socio-cultural interaction, the actions which the agents in fact carry out, is dependent both on cultural conditions and on socio-cultural conditions. Thus it is not only relations between ideas which determine what agents in fact do, but also the relations between agents. These relations can be characterised by an unequal distribution of interests and different possibilities for exercising power. Archer says that the combination of systematic relations between ideas on the one hand, and socio-cultural relations between people on the other hand, determine whether there will in fact be cultural development.

> "... it is how the contradictory or complementary relations between parts of the Cultural System map onto orderly or conflictual Socio-Cultural relationships which determine morphostasis or morphogenesis. Cultural Elaboration is therefore completely at the mercy of the *combination* between the two levels of analysis." (Archer, 1988/1996, p. 187).

Here Archer again follows the basic division between constraining contradictions and concomitant complementarities on the systemic level. Taking this basic division as her starting point, she develops that part of the theory which concerns how people interact and influence each other and thus contribute to determining whether culture is developed or not. The basic division between constraining contradictions and concomitant complementarities gives rise to two types of interaction processes.

One interaction process starts from a cultural system which is characterised by constraining contradictions. From here the relation between the cultural system and socio-cultural interaction is in turn characterised by two types of relations. On the one hand socio-cultural relations can be less conflictual than systemic relations. On the other hand socio-cultural relations can be more conflictual than systemic relations.

If the socio-cultural relations are less conflictual than the systemic relations, this means that peaceful socio-cultural conditions can be used to obscure conflicting conditions between cultural ideas. It is possible to try to repress, with force, the cultural ideas which conflict with those which one supports oneself.

One possibility for obscuring conflict between cultural ideas is to arrange that there may only be access to a restricted part of the heretical ideas. Such cultural repression can take many forms, for example, partial censorship, prohibition of certain books, use of sanctions, forced confession of errors etc. The problem is that such cultural repression can lead to a reaction and be self-defeating. The ruling ideas are dependent on the heretical ideas, so there must still be some access to the heretical ideas. Here Archer refers again to the example of Christianity's dependence on the ideas of antiquity. The earliest Christian writings contained commentaries and explanations relating to classical ideas. The question therefore is, where should one draw the line between Christian ideas and classical ideas? If the reading of the early Christian writings were permitted, the door would be opened to the study of the works of antiquity. Thus, the portion of classical writings which one was allowed to read becomes greater.

A second possibility for obscuring the contradictions between cultural ideas is to limit the number of people who have access to heretical ideas. Such a strategic restriction can ensure socio-cultural order for months, years or even centuries. The problem is that even if people of low status in the socio-cultural hierarchy are kept away from the heretical texts, the elite will still be confronted with the contradictions in the cultural system. The question is, who shall censor the censors? Nothing can guarantee their immunity against infection from constant contact with the heretical texts. If, in this situation, external interest groups gain ground, the elite will be vulnerable, because they will long have had knowledge of the contradictions.

The consequence is that if there is clear exercise of power and effective repression, then even though the cultural system may be characterised by constraining contradictions, there can be morphostasis for long periods. However, in the longer term it will be impossible to retain constraining contradictions within the cultural system. In time the clear exercise of power will be undermined by the contradictions which those in power seek to hide, and morphogenesis will result (Archer, 1988/1996, pp. 189-197).

If the socio-cultural relations are more conflictual than the systemic relations, there will be no-one with the resources to undertake the cultural repression necessary for hiding the contradictions in the cultural system. In this situation the cultural agents can act on the cultural contradictions. One possibility is to desert. They can leave the group which persists in trying to repair the cultural system with a view to syncretisation. And deserters seldom go in silence. They will most often bring the forbidden ideas into the full light of day. Another possibility is the formation of factions. In this case, different factions will focus upon different parts of the forbidden ideas. This means that different parts of the heretical ideas will be presented in different contexts, so the overall result will be that heretical ideas will be even more the centre of focus. Thus, the result of the lack of socio-cultural integration is that it becomes difficult to repress the agents who will no longer co-operate in the repression of contradictions. They will come forward and reveal the contradictions, and morphogenesis will result (Archer, 1988/1996, pp. 197-203).

Regardless of whether the contradictions are stronger on the systemic level or the socio-cultural level, the consequences in the longer run will be that the contradictions will come to light, and a situation will arise in which the two conflicting ideas compete with each other. Archer referred to this systemic situation as competitive contradictions. Archer emphasised that competitive contradictions are not the only possible form of development. Apart from this development from constraining contradictions there is also the possibility that an entirely different group may propose ideas which are opposed to the prevailing ideas. This requires that such other group can have access to the fund of ideas, though this can be difficult if the ruling group is determined to restrict their access (Archer, 1988/1996, pp. 205-207).

When competitive contradictions are developed at the systemic level, competing groups will attempt to eliminate each other's ideas. They will use the power of the communicative system. In order to discredit others, attempts will be made to brand the competing idea as a primitive belief, false consciousness, old wives' tales, pseudoscience etc. Such discrediting only seriously affects the weakest of competitors. What is more effective is preventive discrediting, which consists of denying competitors the opportunity to formulate their antitheses. If this is unsuccessful, then more extreme measures will be used, such as murder, political persecution, or the less brutal denial of research grants, denial of publication of research results etc. (Archer, 1988/1996, pp. 207-209).

The other interaction process starts from a cultural system characterised by concomitant complementarities. Here the starting point is a high level of integration at the systemic level. Here too the clear and monolithic exercise of power can ensure morphostasis for long periods. However, in the longer term it will be impossible to maintain such socio-cultural integration. This is because at the systemic level the concomitant complementarities contain in themselves the seeds of socio-cultural change. In the longer term this will result in morphogenesis.

The fact is that compatibility of ideas at the systemic level leads to ever-increasing cultural density. More and more elements are added so that an increasing degree of systematisation becomes necessary. With this systematisation it becomes difficult for all cultural agents to acquire an equal share of the cultural fund. In this situation a socio-cultural hierarchy will develop. This hierarchisation leads to differences of interest and this creates the basis for socio-cultural disintegration. Archer refers to Weber's analysis of the Chinese mandarins as an example of this. There, cultural density was so great that it took a lifetime for a person to acquire culture. When this is the case very great differences will arise with regard to insight into culture which ought to be common to all.

According to Archer, such a development will prompt the formation of three interest groups. First there is a socio-cultural elite which knows all the byways of the cultural system and therefore has an interest in preserving the systematised unity against any socio-cultural disturbance. Second, there is a marginalised group which has received education, but which finds that this brings it fewer and fewer advantages. They have made a personal investment in education without it bringing them the expected privileges. The consequence will be that they will regard the situation as rigid and they will turn to opportunism. And third, there are the masses. These consist of the residue which has not acquired its share of cultural insight. They are the object of the exercise of cultural power.

There are several possible strategies for the elite. One of them is the naturalisation strategy which consists of manipulating and structuring desires and expectations. The problem is that this strategy cannot persuade the marginalised. They can see through it and see that they do not gain anything by this naturalisation. Therefore the elite must often use direct cultural repression of the marginalised, to prevent them from presenting alternative ideas. Repression can consist of depriving them of honours, professional degradation etc. It is easier in relation to the masses, towards whom it is possible to use non-decision making. Here it can be enough to use ridicule or other ways of showing that attempts to develop an alternative are ridiculous.

If such strategies are insufficient, the elite can use other strategies. They can close off the ultimate sources of cultural inspiration. For the marginalised this means that they are deprived of the necessary tools and opportunities for developing alternatives.

The marginalised thus find themselves in a situation in which they are dissatisfied with their culture because it does not give them the expected advantages, and if they are cut off from the sources of culture, they have every possible reason to desert and seek new ideas. As migrants they will be able to link new ideas to their previous ideas. This new situation will appear highly advantageous for them. They will be able to continue to exploit their investment in education, but by taking in new areas which do not conflict with the old, they will be able to develop new ideas without resistance. The morphogenetic process becomes a reality (Archer, 1988/1996, pp. 209-219).

Archer refers to the situation which arises from this at the systemic level as contingent complementarities. It is a situation in which the cultural system is characterised by the linking together of ideas which do not really have anything to do with each other, but which are complementary. Archer emphasises that this development of contingent complementarities is not the only possible form. It is also possible that new elements can develop without them being looked for. They can develop through gradual distancing from the original thinking. For example, research can always lead to unexpected results (Archer, 1988/1996, pp. 219-223).

The consequences of contingent complementarities will be a higher degree of specialisation and a lower degree of consensus. For cultural agents, certainty will be replaced by choice, common communication will be replaced by specialised forms of communication, and detailed information will be replaced by more generalised points of view. This will lead to greater freedom and increased individualism (Archer, 1988/1996, pp. 223-224).

From here Archer proceeds to the third stage of the morphogenetic/morphostatic cycle, which is the development of the cultural system. It is evident that both constraining contradictions and concomitant complementarities contain the seeds of cultural change which socio-cultural interaction must generate in the longer term. What happens is that constraining contradictions give rise to competitive contradictions, while the concomitant complementarities develop contingent complementarities. These are the two outcomes which Archer investigates in the third phase of morphogenesis.

In her presentation of the part of the theory which concerns the third stage of the morphogenetic cycle, Archer distinguishes between competitive contradictions and contingent complementarities within the cultural system. From these two starting points she discusses cultural conditions, socio-cultural interaction and cultural development.

In one systemic process, the cultural system is characterised by competitive contradictions. This need not in itself be decisive for whether there is any development or not. If no socio-cultural groups take a view on the competing ideas, the situation will be one of morphostasis. If there is to be morphogenetic development, there must be socio-cultural groups which have an interest in taking a stance on the competition between ideas, and in encouraging others to do likewise. It is therefore human action which activates the competitive contradictions. As an example of competitive contradictions, Archer refers to scientific theories where there is competition as to which theories are the most tenable. Competition between different scientific theories is also part of this struggle. Another example is ideologies, where the supporters of each ideology fight over which ideology has the greatest universal value (Archer, 1988/1996, pp. 229-235).

For the cultural agents, the competitive contradictions mean that they have to make a choice. As soon as contradictions become apparent, the agents must take up one of the ideas and simultaneously try to eliminate the others. If one chooses to support one scientific theory, one must attempt to eliminate the other. If one has chosen to support one ideology, one must attempt to eliminate the other (Archer, 1988/1996, pp. 239-242).

Competition between different groups has consequences for the development of the cultural system. The constant debate between two competing ideas will lead to these ideas being dissected by their opponents, while being more clearly defined by their supporters. These opposing expositions of the ideas will mean that they become more visible. Archer refers to the competition between classical political economy and socialist economy as an example of such a development.

Another consequence of competition between contradictory ideas is that there will be increasing refinement of their arguments. The ideas will be more and more sharply defined. To illustrate this, Archer refers to the debate on the significance of nurture and nature in relation to intelligence. This continuing debate led to an increasingly sharp argumentation and the instruments for measuring intelligence became ever more refined. With this constant refinement of arguments, splintering can easily occur within the groups which support either of the two competing ideas, so there is effectively competition between those who originally supported the same idea.

A third consequence can be that an idea must be withdrawn and wait for more propitious times. This is a very defensive attitude and does nothing to convince opponents.

Finally, it is possible that some agents may try to establish peace between opposing parties. This will most often be by trying to take the best from each idea. The problem is that it is not possible to solve the problem of contradictions in this way. What happens is that this produces a new idea which people have to take into consideration.

The overall result of these different developments is not, therefore, the intended suppression of ideas, but rather the evolution of pluralist thinking. Ideas become more and more visible, they become fragmented into splinter groups, they hibernate and wait for better times, or they are bolted together by compromises. The end result of competitive contradictions is a pluralism of ideas (Archer, 1988/1996, pp. 245-258).

In the other systemic process, the cultural system is characterised by contingent complementarities. This systemic situation need not, of itself, lead to cultural change. If there are no socio-cultural groups which will take on the task of linking together complementary ideas, there will be morphostasis. If a morphogenetic process is to be initiated there must be socio-cultural groups which can identify possibilities for joining together complementary ideas, and see an advantage in doing so. This is where the marginalised people come into the picture. They have the least to lose by setting such a process in motion (Archer, 1988/1996, pp. 235-239).

For cultural agents, the contingent complementarities mean that they are free to make a choice. There is no socio-cultural manipulation. For the cultural system this means that there is wide variation. There is room for extreme doctrines and daring of theories. At the socio-cultural level this leads to divisions, specialisation, new formations etc. (Archer, 1988/1996, pp. 242-245).

This complete freedom means that there can be fusion of ideas. The example which Archer gives of this is the development of radio-astronomy, which resulted from linking ideas from radio-physics and astronomy. Such fusions of ideas increase systemic variation. Such fusions are not always productive. If the linking together of ideas takes place without a proper synthetic basis it will result in ineffective syntheses. The fusion of ideas can thus lead to the boldest new ideas, but it can also lead to ineffectual intellectual flights of fancy.

Such linking together of ideas can lead to the creation of a network and in the longer term to institutionalisation. This is especially the case if the ideas attract formal recognition, including the establishment of professorial chairs, the awarding of Nobel prizes and so on.

Such formal recognition also leads to visibility, and visibility can in turn lead to further linking of ideas. The more ideas that are developed, the more it will be possible to create fusions of ideas. Increased variation creates the basis for further variation. The overall consequence for the cultural system will be specialisation. For the social agents the consequence will be division into sections. There will be specialists in their own fields of study who will have less and less to say to each other. They must separate the professional from the social so as to prevent social isolation. There is an obvious concern about the lack of social cohesion (Archer, 1988/1996, pp. 258-269).

Archer has thus developed four kinds of cultural systems, of which two can, under certain circumstances, be evolved out of the other two through a morphogenetic process. Each of these systems is characterised by the situation within the cultural system. Furthermore, they are looked at with regard to their situational logic, their development in the cultural system and their development in socio-cultural interaction.

The constraining contradictions imply that there is a situational logic that requires the correction of the cultural ideas. This leads to the syncretisation of the cultural system and unification at the socio-cultural level.

This gives the basis for the development of competitive contradictions, which involves a situational logic characterised by the elimination of ideas. This leads to pluralism in the cultural system and cleavages in socio-cultural interaction.

The concomitant complementarities involve a situational logic that requires the protection of cultural ideas. From this follows the systemisation of the cultural system and reproduction in socio-cultural interaction.

This gives the basis for the development of contingent complementarities which involves a situational logic characterised by opportunism. Within the cultural system this leads to specialisation, and at the socio-cultural level it leads to sectionalism (Archer, 1988/1996, p. 270).

## *Culture and structure*

In her book *Realist social theory: the morphogenetic approach*, Archer links her theory of culture to her theory on structure. This linking together is part of the further development of the principle of morphogenesis/morphostasis. The true purpose of the book is thus to develop her ideas on the morphogenetic principle. The basic elements of the book are her ontology, her methodology and her principles for practical theorising.

Also in this book, Archer expresses her fundamental view of human beings as being both free and bound. The ontological standpoint is therefore a basic distinction between structure and agency and between culture and agency. Within each of these levels, the principle of emergence applies, which is the principle of creative development according to which new characteristics can arise on the basis of preceding characteristics. This principle of emergence is of fundamental importance to Archer's overall theory. It applies both to structure and to culture, and it also applies to human agency.

At the methodological level Archer again lays out her basic principle of analytical dualism. One can investigate the mutual influences between two analytically separate levels without conflating them. This principle is concretised both for the structural and the cultural part of the analysis. It is Archer's opinion that culture and structure can be analysed on the basis of the same principles. The same mechanisms apply in both areas.

> "Culture is approached analytically in exactly the same way as structure, for it is just as appropriate to speak of cultural as of social structures." (Archer, 1995, p. 179).

Within the structural domain it is necessary to undertake an analytical separation between structure and agency, with a view to investigating their influences on each other. It is necessary to distinguish between the relations which are dominant within social structures, and the reactions which people have towards these structures.

According to Archer, relations between the structural components can either be internal and necessary, or external and contingent. If the relations are internal and necessary, Archer characterises them as emergent properties. These emergent properties have relative autonomy and can have causal effects. If the relations are external and contingent, Archer characterises them as aggregated properties. The first kind of relations are those which *must* be present, while the second kind of relations are those which *can be* present.

> "To focus upon internal and necessary relations between components as constitutive of an emergent property is to set them apart from relations which are external and contingent. In the latter case, two entities or items can exist without one another and it is thus neither necessary nor impossible that they stand in any particular relation to one another, for the nature of either does not depend upon this." (Archer, 1995, p. 173).

Archer expands on her view of internal and necessary relations. She emphasises that emergent properties which are developed at the structural level must necessarily be materially based. This is the whole basis for their existence and for their ability to operate as causal factors.

> "What differentiates a *structural* emergent property is its *primary dependence upon material resources*, both physical and human. In other words, the internal and necessary relations between its constituents are fundamentally material ones: these make it what it is and without them it could neither exist as such nor possess the causal powers which characterize it." (Archer, 1995, p. 175).

It further applies that structural emergent properties must be kept separate from the people who live in relation to them.

> "... *structural* emergent properties (and also cultural ones), are defined and identified independently of their occupants or incumbents and of the social interaction taking place between the latter." (Archer, 1995, p.176).

For Archer it is thus of the greatest importance that an analytical separation should be made, on the one hand, between structural components, which can have the character of systems, institutions, roles and positions, and on the other hand the people who stand in relation to them, and this can be the population at large, organised groups (corporate agents), individual actors or collectives (primary agents) (Archer, 1995, p. 190). Only by making such a separation is it possible to investigate each in turn and study the influence they have on each other.

> "As with every other type of SEP [structural emergent properties] (roles, institutions and systems), it is crucial to distinguish between structural conditioning and the emergent powers of different categories of people (primary and corporate agents, as well as individual actors). For it is the interplay between the powers of the 'parts' and the powers of the 'people' which is decisive for the outcome and not merely whether this can be characterized as reproduction or transformation but in order to explain the precise form of structural elaboration to take place." (Archer, 1995, p. 179).

The decisive principle is thus the mutual influence between structural relations on the one hand and agents or actors on the other hand. This mutual influence is decisive for whether there will be any development, and if so what the character of the development will be.

Within the cultural domain it is necessary to make an analytical separation between culture and agency. Here again we meet Archer's distinction between the cultural system and socio-cultural interaction. The same definitions are put forward, but they are included in the overall thinking which Archer has developed in this work.

The relations within the cultural system are logical relations, which can either be internal and necessary, which means that purely logically they must relate to each other, or external and contingent, which means that they may be related to each other. If the relations are internal and necessary, they constitute the cultural emergent properties and, as such, are relatively autonomous and able to operate as causal effects. If they are external and contingent, then they are aggregated phenomena.

As opposed to the cultural system, there is socio-cultural interaction as a relation between people with regard to culture. The mutual influence between the cultural system and socio-cultural interaction is decisive for whether there will be a change or stasis within the cultural sphere.

The principles for the development of practical theorising, which Archer develops on the basis of her methodological principles, are the same for structure and for culture.

She develops the principle of morphogenesis or morphostasis for both domains by following developments over three phases: structural or cultural conditions, interaction or socio-cultural interaction and structural or cultural development.

When Archer presents her theory on structural change, she starts with the first phase of the morphogenetic cycle. The starting point for Archer's structural theory is thus structural conditions. However, she emphasises that these conditions do not in themselves give rise to change. Something happens only if these conditions are understood and realised by people, and this will occur through the situations which people experience. These situations form the basis for different kinds of action.

> "… *all* structural influences (i.e. the generative powers of SEPs [structural emergent properties] and CEPs [cultural emergent properties]) work through shaping the situations in which people find themselves. It is the situations to which people respond which are mediatory because they condition (without determining) different courses of action for those differently placed, by supplying different reasons to them." (Archer, 1995, p. 201).

The situations which people find themselves in are characterised by being involuntary. People are born into them and they are enduring. The consequence is that from the start people are given different rights. Their positions determine the degree to which their rights are secured. If they want to change their position, this will have a price. The price is greater for some people than for others. It costs less for the rich man than for the poor to try to change his position. The degree of freedom to choose is thus also unequally distributed.

According to Archer, structural conditions can be characterised by different relations between the structural elements. As previously referred to, these relations can be internal and necessary or external and contingent. To this can be added that they can be complementary or incompatible. They can either support each other or obstruct each other. In this way Archer has four possible relations between structural elements: necessary complementarities, necessary incompatibilities, contingent compatibilities and contingent incompatibilities. Each of these structural relations will generate a different situational logic and give rise to different strategies for the people who are confronted with them.

If the starting point is necessary complementarities, the social institutions are bound to one another and support each other. As an example of this, Archer refers to ancient India where the Brahmins were given greater rights than any other group. However, the high level of cohesion in the system meant that everyone had something to lose by changing it. The king was dependent on the Brahmins and vice versa. Craftsmen were protected by rules against the free movement of workers etc. A situational logic of protection was created. As a consequence, renewal and variety were suppressed, while tradition was maintained by protection against the loss of secured rights (Archer, 1995, pp. 19-21).

If the starting point is necessary incompatibilities, the relations between social institutions are enforced but they are incompatible. This situation contains the potential for change. As an example of this, Archer refers to Weber's analysis of patrimonial bureaucracy. Here there was an internal and necessary relation between the bureaucracy and taxation because the bureaucracy could not exist without the basis for taxation. The incompatibility existed between an effective tax system, which favoured the bureaucracy, and a subsistence economy, which favoured decentralisation. For the bureaucracy this situation meant that, while they had an interest in maximising the tax base, they had to be careful not to impose too great a tax burden on the big landowners. This situation led to compromises. Even though the tax collectors were interested in collecting as much tax as possible, so as to gain as large a commission for themselves as possible, they had to recognise that if they pushed the big landowners too hard, this would weaken the central princely power which they themselves represented. They therefore had to compromise with the big landowners. This resulted in the tax burden being displaced downwards onto the farmers. Here too there was a need for a compromise. The farmers could either ally themselves with the local landowners against the prince, or with the prince against the local landowners, depending on which of them oppressed the farmers least. All parties had to weigh up the claims for the redemption of certain promised rights against the risk of loss by asserting these rights. Such a situation was highly unstable and could only be temporary. Without the existence of a money economy the bureaucracy had to undergo significant changes or develop into a totally different kind of structure (Archer, 1995, pp. 222-225).

If the starting point is contingent incompatibilities, there will be possible but incompatible relations. For example, if there is a war, even the most integrated society may find itself in the situation where it is no longer in a position to protect previous rights. What now matters is to inflict as much damage as possible on the enemy. The situational logic points towards elimination. Old protected rights must be surrendered, and this often has effects beyond the duration of the war. As an example of such a situation Archer refers to Weber's analysis of ancient Palestine, in which war leads to territorial separation, institutional splits, social movement and finally the settlement of Jews outside Palestine. The result is thus social division (Archer, 1995, pp. 225-226).

If the starting point is contingent compatibilities, there will be possible and compatible relations. For example, there can be new groups who move in and ally themselves with certain interest groups. These can be groups on the margin which can see an advantage in allying themselves with the new groups. Contingent compatibilities thus lead to a situational logic which is characterised by opportunism. There is nothing to lose, only something to gain. As an example of this situation, Archer refers to Marx's analysis of mercantilism. The quantities of gold and silver which flowed from the new world to the old led to price rises which were damaging to the big landowners. Trade with the colonies gave large profits. This gave further incentives to trade, which damaged the old craftsmen. The accumulation of capital, together with the mobility of the work force, made it possible to create new manufacturing industries. Thus, new interests arose and new material possibilities for satisfying these interests. Here the situational logic points towards opportunism, and the structural consequences are institutional restructuring (Archer, 1995, pp. 226-227).

As with structural conditions, cultural conditions can be affected by different relations between cultural elements. Relations can be internal and necessary, or external and contingent. At the same time they can be contradictory or compatible. There are thus four possibilities, corresponding to the relations already discussed between cultural elements: necessary incompatibilities (corresponding to constraining contradictions), necessary complementarities (corresponding to concomitant complementarities), contingent incompatibilities (corresponding to competitive contradictions) and contingent complementarities. These different types of relations between the cultural elements shape the situational logic, and are thus the starting points for people's strategies and actions (Archer, 1995, pp. 230-245).

The second phase of the morphogenetic cycle is social or socio-cultural interaction. However, it is Archer's view that this interaction itself consists of a morphogenetic cycle. At the moment when agents are interacting in relation to structural or cultural morphogenesis, a change occurs in the agents' basic grouping. A morphogenesis of the agents occurs. When collectives hinder the development of structures or cultures, they undergo a development as agents. There is a double morphogenesis. The interaction which creates a cultural or structural morphogenesis is itself a morphogenetic process with three phases: conditions, interaction and development.

> "... the self-same sequence by which agency brings about social and cultural transformation is simultaneously responsible for the systematic transforming of social agency itself. In other words, a 'double morphogenesis' is involved: agency leads to structural and cultural elaboration, but is itself elaborated in the process." (Archer, 1995, p.247).

The conditions under which action takes place are created by previous generations. They are not created by the agents themselves; they are rather the unintended results of the interactions of the past. However, what matters is whether the agents are interested in maintaining or changing these conditions. These interests relate to whether they are in a privileged or an unprivileged position, and whether their situation appears to be advantageous or disadvantageous.

The given conditions need not in themselves initiate change. The existing conditions have to be mediated through the agents' situation. If there are no agents whose conditions give them an interest in and make them believe that they can gain by acting in the conditions, then nothing will happen. The result will be a morphostatic cycle. If, on the other hand, there are agents who have such interests and who expect to be able to make changes to their own advantage, then a morphogenetic process can be initiated. Thus, even if there are objective grounds for acting, each individual must make a subjective assessment of the advantages and disadvantages of an action which can initiate change.

The development resulting from the morphogenetic cycle is the product of human action, but usually it is not a result which anyone has wished. It is more likely to be the result of compromises and the unintended consequences of interaction between people. The result is either emergent or aggregated properties which are relevant for the next morphogenetic phase within the structural or cultural domain.

To explain the morphogenesis of this action, Archer makes distinctions between agents, actors and persons. When agents go through a morphogenetic process there will be some re-grouping. This will lead to new roles and thus new kinds of actors. Here there is another morphogenetic process, and this is the actors' morphogenesis. But neither the agents nor the actors must be regarded as dehumanised elements. They are both rooted in persons.

> "Both Agents and Actors, however, remain anchored in Persons ... they concern real people ..." (Archer, 1995, p. 256).

The position is that both actors and agents are anchored in persons, but where the agents are directly anchored in persons, the actor's anchoring on the person must be through the agents. The agent is thus the link between the actor and the person. The role of the actor must be mediated through the agent. This is because the person in himself has no interests which can be transferred to a given role and thus give rise to renewal. However, the agent has such interests. On the other hand the person has an energy which can be transferred to the actor and thus give rise to actions. This means this energy must be mediated by the agent. It is the agent who can give a purpose to the activities, and it is the agent who helps to decide which persons shall be actors. The influence thus goes from person, through agent to actor.

> "If Persons furnish activity-potential for Actors, then Agency is a necessary mediator between them in order to supply activity with a purpose. Furthermore, Agency is also the mediating mechanism which accounts for who, out of the total population, acquires which role(s) within the total role array ... Agency stands as the middle element linking Persons to Actors ... Hence the genealogy, Human Being - Agent – Actor." (Archer, 1995, p. 256).

When discussing how the morphogenesis of agency is linked to structural and cultural morphogenesis, one must include not only the agent, but also the actor and the person. The extent to which there will be structural or cultural change depends on all three links in the chain, person-agent-actor. Archer thus discusses the second link in the morphogenetic process, which is social or cultural interaction, by discussing the morphogenesis of agency, the morphogenesis of the actor and the anchoring of both of these processes in the person.

Archer defines agents as collectives with the same life opportunities. Agents are thus, by definition, plural. They are groups or collectives. Archer further distinguishes between corporate agents and primary agents. Corporate agents can, for example, be interest groups with vested interests, groups which try to promote their own interests, associations for mutual protection, or social movements. Agents are able to exercise power by articulating common interests, organising with a view to collective action, initiating social movements and exercising influence on decisions. Primary agents are groups without influence. They do not represent any interests, and they are not organised with a view to strategic efforts.

It is corporate agents who create frameworks. Primary agents must operate within these frameworks. It is thus corporate agents which set the framework for primary agents, but it is the reactions of primary agents which are decisive for whether there is change.

If corporate agents maintain a distance from primary agents, there will be a morphostatic situation. If the corporate agents maintain their position as the elite, everyone else will be excluded from exercising influence. Conversely, if there is a morphogenetic process, there will be a re-grouping between corporate and primary agents. As an example of such a morphogenetic process, Archer refers to the development of the educational system. In a historical perspective, it initially had a strong corporate agent, the church. This corporate agent had its vested interests which made it possible for it to determine the content and form of education. Within this system individual schools operated as primary agents without any influence on the education. Over time the schools combined and, in alliance with the state, they could operate as new corporate agents. They could take action and influence education. They became broader and accepted more pupils. In this new system of corporate agents it was the pupils who were the primary agents. They were more concerned with education as a path to social elevation. As a result many of these educated people combined in professional groups. In this way they could also operate as corporate agents in relation to education. Thus in the long term there has been a re-grouping between corporate and primary agents. The consequence has been an increase in the number of corporate agents and a corresponding reduction in the number of primary agents. The result of the morphogenesis of agency has been this re-grouping.

When there is re-grouping among agents, this must have an effect on the actors. The morphogenesis of agency thus leads to another morphogenesis, the morphogenesis of the actor. When agents, understood as collectives, operate in relation to social or cultural structures, this will also affect the individual actor. There will be potential changes to the roles which people play. The total number of possible roles will be increased.

There is thus a triple morphogenesis. The morphogenesis of the actor springs from the morphogenesis of agency which springs from the structural or cultural morphogenesis.

What applies to both agents and actors is that they must be anchored in persons. According to Archer, the basis for this anchoring is the division between the social self and the personal self. The personal self has relative autonomy in relation to the social self. This relative autonomy is due to the person's ability to reflect and be creative and to have authentic inner experiences. Thus the person also has the possibility of making decisions.

The consequence of this division between the personal self and the social self is that, even though we are born into social conditions which we do not ourselves determine, within these social conditions there are possibilities for making personal choices. As persons, within our given circumstances, we can choose whether we accept or reject what is different, whether we use or abuse the environment, whether we live in harmony or in competition with other people. The morphogenetic cycle thus consists of conditions, choices and consequences.

> "... our choices as to whether to acknowledge or repudiate Otherness, to use or to abuse the natural environment, to live in mutual concern or competitive conflict with one another are the processes shaping society – not once and for all after the Fall – but continuously throughout all time, by that combination of circumstances, choices and consequences which has been called morphogenesis." (Archer, 1995, p. 293).

After having deduced this interaction which can take place in the second phase of cultural or structural morphogenesis, in other words the morphogenetic processes in relation to agents and actors, and the anchoring of these in persons, Archer moves on to the third phase, which is structural and cultural development.

The starting point for the development of this third phase of the morphogenetic cycle is the mechanisms which combine the interaction with actual development. These mechanisms are exchange and power. It is Archers fundamental belief that exchange transactions and power relations are decisive for the direction of actual development.

Exchange processes and power processes are linked to each other. Together they can influence whether mutuality or control will exist between groups. In all exchange and power processes there must be a resource transaction. For example, there can be a transaction of wealth, expertise and sanctions (Archer, 1995, p. 296).

The allocation of resources can be decisive for which exchange or power processes take place, and thus the result of the morphogenetic process. The difference in degrees of access to resources is the basis of exchange and power processes. Agents who have poor access to resources will have weak negotiating positions, while agents who have good access to resources will have strong negotiating positions.

The allocation of resources can also affect the actual development. If a number of agents have ready access to resources, there will be many who will take part in resource transactions. Conversely, if there are only few agents who have ready access to resources, there will be few who will take part in resource transactions.

The negotiating strengths of different agents are thus dependent both on their own access to resources and on the total distribution of access to resources. The negotiating strength of a given group is thus dependant on its own access to resources and on its relationships to other corporate agents. In other words, their negotiating strength is relationally determined.

How negotiating strengths are used depends on how the structural relations are presented to the agents. Here the decisive question is how structural development and cultural development fit together. At the systemic level culture and structure together form a whole set of developments, which form the situational logic for the agents. As against this, the agents will react with different strategies, which in turn can lead to re-groupings within both the social and the cultural domain (Archer, 1995, p. 304).

According to Archer, the starting point for the discussion of these processes is that cultural and structural processes can influence each other through socio-cultural or social interaction. The question is thus how culture can influence structural interaction, and how structure can influence socio-cultural interaction. Here Archer refers to two basic mechanisms.

Culture can lead the way to social interaction if a material interest group endorses a given doctrine with a view, for example, to increasing its influence or acquiring legitimacy. As soon as it has done so, it has placed itself in the centre of the cultural situational logic.

> "The basic mechanism by which cultural factors find their way into the structural field through the intersection is extremely simple. Let any material interest group ... endorse any doctrine (theory, belief or ideology) for the advancement of those interests (that is their articulation, assertion or legitimation), and that group is immediately plunged into its situational logic." (Archer, 1995, p. 306).

The problem is that such an endorsement of a given doctrine is a public matter. This means that the material interest group must, to some extent, study the theoretical basis for the doctrine. When it does this, it affects all the structural relations of the group. It affects its allies and opponents, those it supports and so on. These other material interest groups will also be drawn into the situational logic. Before they know where they are, they find themselves in a more or less advanced cultural struggle.

Structure can lead the way to culture if the adherents of one doctrine ally themselves with a material interest group and thus make themselves dependent on the fate of that group.

> "Thus, let the advocacy of any doctrine (theory, belief or ideology) become associated with a particular material interest group and its fate becomes embroiled in the fortunes of that group *vis-à-vis* others. For all such attachments immediately enmesh cultural discourse in power play." (Archer, 1995, p. 307).

The advantage of this alliance is that resources are transferred from the material interest group to the socio-cultural group. The socio-cultural group will have found itself a sponsor. The disadvantage is that the doctrine which the socio-cultural group espouses loses some of its universality in the light of the particular interests of the material interest group. What happens is that as soon as the material interest group has given its support to the socio-cultural group, other socio-cultural groups will seek support from other material interest groups. They too need sponsors. Socio-cultural groups will thus be drawn into the power struggles which exist in the structural domain.

On the basis of these general remarks on the development of culture and structure, Archer outlines four developmental processes. These developmental processes are based on four different combinations of cultural and structural developments. The four possible combinations of development are: cultural morphostasis and structural morphostasis, cultural morphostasis and structural morphogenesis, cultural morphogenesis and structural morphostasis, and finally cultural morphogenesis and structural morphogenesis.

If there is both cultural and structural morphostasis, this means that there is stasis within both domains. Within the cultural domain the ideas are systematised or syncretised, and there is no apparent alternative to the dominant ideas. In this way the cultural forces promote a homogeneous population which does not have many possibilities for formulating alternatives, nor for creating disturbances in the structural domain. In the structural domain there is cohesive social organisation with a clearly distinct elite and highly concentrated resources. There will be no marginal or rebellious groups which are able to disturb the social order. Nor are there any material groups which can come and disturb the social order. As a consequence, by far the largest part of the population have to accept their role as primary agents. For the cultural elite this situation means that, as an intellectual group, it enjoys social distinctions. It becomes a corporate group which can exchange its intellectual expertise for material advantages. For the structural elite this situation means that it finds itself in an intellectual environment which ensures that it is able to maintain structural conditions. The two elites thus have every possible reason to support one another, as a bishop does the king. This situation can last a long time, but not for ever. There are internal cultural dynamics which can disturb traditional thinking. These can be let loose by structural disturbances or kept in check by structural routines (Archer, 1995, pp. 309-312).

If there is cultural morphostasis and structural morphogenesis, this means there is stasis within the cultural domain and development within the structural domain. Within the cultural domain there will still be systematisation or syncretisation, and there will be one dominant cultural agent. But within the structural domain new agents will come forward with new forms of material interests. This can arise as a consequence of war, mercantilism, political alliances, colonialism, urbanisation etc. These new groups will be concerned to define themselves and get themselves noticed and to promote their own interests, all of which takes place within a cultural context. However, in this they will feel themselves to be censored, sanctioned and subject to force. In this situation the new agents will react by pointing out the contradictions which lie behind the synrcetisation, or by bringing in new ideas so as to distance themselves from the traditional systematisation. This will lead to cultural development. In this situation, through the development of new corporate agents, the structural development will influence cultural development. (Archer, 1995, pp. 312-315).

If there is cultural morphogenesis and structural morphostasis, this means that there is development in the cultural domain and stasis within the structural domain. One strong agent will still dominate within the structural domain, while within the cultural domain a number of cultural agents will be developed. This can happen as a consequence of the cultural domain's own dynamic. This means that there will be pluralism or specialisation in the cultural system. In the structural domain the dominant agent will attempt to eliminate non-orthodox groups in order to avoid the formation of new material interest groups. However, with cultural change such structural change cannot be prevented, it can only be delayed. If new ideas are developed, as, for example, during the Renaissance or the Age of Enlightenment etc., these will be present not only for the cultural actors, but also for the structural actors. This is because the cultural actors are also structural actors. The structural actors will then begin to think of alternatives. Frequently the corporate agents in the structural sphere will be those who can gain most from espousing such new ideas. It will be the same if there are competitive contradictions. In this situation, too, corporate agents will be best placed to think and to act according to the new ideas simply because they will gain the most from doing so. It can be costly for them to hang on to the old ideas because of the declining returns from them. Thus, when corporate agents find themselves in a situation characterised by fragmentation and conflict, they can either choose to maintain the old ideas and oppose the new groups, or they can choose to absorb the new ideas, and find themselves in conflict with those who hang on to the old ideas. Thus, cultural change leads to structural reorganisation and the formation of new groups. There can either be a gradual differentiation of new groups, or there can be an intensification of conflicts with associated polarisation within the structural domain (Archer, 1995, pp. 315-318).

If there is cultural morphogenesis combined with structural morphogenesis, this means there will be change within both domains. Within both domains there will be a development towards competing groups each pulling in their own direction. The question is how the material and structural interests will affect one another in this situation. On the one hand there will be certain material interest groups which look at a number of different ideas with a view to finding the one that best fits their structural interests. Against this there are a number of cultural interest groups which only regard the material interest groups as potential sponsors. If one starts by looking at the situation from the angle of cultural agents, it is possible to imagine that a cultural agent will be able to obtain sponsorship from a structural agent. This means that they will obtain resources and be stronger within the cultural sphere. For the other cultural agents this means they must try to obtain corresponding sponsorship, in order not to lose ground. They must thus seek to ally themselves with other structural groups. In this way cultural diversity comes to influence the structure in the direction of diversity. The problem is that if cultural agents are to obtain support, they must refine their ideas towards the material interests of the structural agents in question. If one looks at this situation from the point of view of structural agents, one can imagine that a structural agent will decide to sponsor a cultural agent. As soon as this is done, the agent will have bound the socio-cultural dimension to the structural interaction. The socio-cultural situational logic, with its fund of conflicting ideas, will also apply to them. This means that other structural agents cannot choose freely which agents or ideas they will support. They must choose in the light of the cultural situational logic. The problem is that the cost of not having some ideas as a source of legitimacy is too high for the structural agents. The result is that all must seek ideas for their own legitimation, which in turn means that more and more ideas are drawn in, and cultural diversity becomes greater and greater. In this way social interaction and socio-cultural interaction reinforce one another. After competition between themselves, conflicts and re-orientation, they lead to morphogenesis (Archer, 1995, pp. 318-322).

Archer emphasises that the theory she presents should be understood as an explanatory format which is to form the foundation for analytical histories of emergence. As an example of such history she refers to the development of the state educational systems in England and France. These analytical histories are part of her earlier work on *Social Origins of Educational Systems*.

## *Analytical histories*

*Social Origins of Educational Systems* is a comprehensive work on the development of educational systems in England, Denmark, France and Russia. The book, which primarily consists of empirical studies, was published in 1979 and thus preceded the two theoretical works, *Culture and agency* and *Realist social theory*. This is a study which lies within what Archer would call the structural domain. The book does not look at the cultural aspects. Nevertheless it is worth mentioning briefly here because it can serve as an example of an empirical study carried out within the theoretical framework which she developed in *Realist social theory*. It is an example of an analytical history of emergence.

Already in *Social Origins of Educational Systems*, we see the birth of the principles which are made more explicit in *Realist social theory*. The principle of analytical dualism is hinted at as a principle which shall be used to explain why some relations lead to change while others lead to stability.

> "The practical and analytical advantages of such a macro-sociological approach ... consist in the capacity to distinguish conflictual interaction likely to produce change (because related to lack of systems integration) from that which simply reflects group antagonisms (lack of social integration). Its advantage ... consists in the capacity to distinguish those relations between systems parts which make for change from those which make for stability ..." (Archer, 1979, p. 33).

The principle of the morphogenetic cycle was defined without actually being named as such. It was clear from the start that Archer analysed developments in educational systems as being a process with three phases, consisting of: conditions, interaction and development. The book is in two parts, of which the first follows this cycle, which led to the formation of the state educational systems in England, Denmark, France and Russia. The second half deals with the cycle which is developed on the basis of the conditions which the first cycle led to.

> "The two parts are continuous, and in fact represent two analytical cycles each of (a) structural conditioning, (b) social interaction, and (c) structural elaboration. (Cycles are analytic in the sense that the historical sequence is an unbroken series of interaction – structural development – structural conditioning – interaction – structural elaboration etc.)." Archer, 1979, p. 44).

The first cycle in the analysis of the development of the four educational systems starts with the conditions which were the basis for the systems arising. In all the countries the starting point was a monopoly situation in which the church or the religious orders owned and controlled the educational institutions. However, the processes of interaction which developed against this background were different. In England and Denmark the forces which were opposed to the church developed a strategy which Archer calls the substitution strategy. This meant that the oppositional forces invested their efforts in establishing educational institutions which could replace the ecclesiastical educational institutions. In Russia and in France the forces which were opposed to the church developed a strategy which Archer calls the restriction strategy. This meant that the oppositional forces invested their efforts into limiting the powers of the ecclesiastical educational institutions. The development of the educational systems which followed from these different forms of interaction were thus also different. In England and in Denmark development took the course of state educational systems, characterised by decentralisation. This meant that negotiations on changes to the educational system were dealt with de-centrally. In France and Russia development took the course of state educational systems, characterised by centralisation. This meant that negotiations about changes to the educational system were dealt with centrally.

The second cycle in the analysis of the four educational systems starts from the conditions which were created as the result of the first cycle. Two different types of conditions now existed. In England and Denmark there were state educational systems characterised by decentralisation, while in France and Russia there were state educational systems characterised by centralisation. Since the educational systems were a state matter, interaction in relation to the educational systems had the character of negotiations. In this connection Archer distinguishes between three kinds of negotiation: political manipulation, internal initiating and external influencing. These negotiation strategies had differing potential strengths within centralised and decentralised educational systems, respectively. Social interaction in relation to decentralised educational systems had scope for all three kinds of negotiation. Here there could be negotiation with and influence from the holders of political power. In addition to this there could also be both internal and external influencing. Professional educators could initiate change from within, while external interest groups could influence developments from without. This was not how it worked in centralised educational systems. Here there was no possibility for internal initiating or external influencing. Here there was solely the possibility of negotiation with and influencing from the holders of political power. This meant that the development processes in the two educational systems were very different. In the decentralised educational systems there was a constant stream of change, while in the centralised educational systems alternated between long periods of stasis and sudden change. While decentralised educational systems were characterised by differentiation and specialisation, centralised systems were characterised by the constant pursuit of uniformity and systemisation.

Archer's study of the four educational systems is thus an empirical study, and a very thorough study, which forms the basis for her general theoretical work. She includes the results of *Social Origins of Educational Systems* towards the end of *Realist social theory*. In this way she puts her own results from the study of education into the conceptual framework which she developed later. She emphasises that practical theorising must always produce such analytical histories of emergence when it wishes to explain why the conditions of structure, culture or action develop in a certain way. So these analytical histories of emergence are explanatory and operate with retrospective and correcting histories. The analytical histories of emergence can thus never be grand histories. What is related by them must necessarily alternate between the necessary and the contingent.

The question of the relation between the theoretical and the empirical was also discussed in the two books about Europe which Archer edited together with Salvador Giner. These two books were published under the common title: *Contemporary Europe*. The first, *Class, Status and Power*, was published in 1971, while the other, *Social Structures and Cultural Patterns*, was published in 1978. In the first book Archer wrote the introduction together with Salvador Giner, while in the second she wrote it on her own. Archer's thinking is thus most clearly presented in the introduction to the second book.

In the introduction to *Social Structures and Cultural Patterns*, Archer discusses the relation between abstract theoretical thinking and comparative study. Here she advances her opinion that there must be mutual influencing between theoretical and comparative analysis of social structures. It is thus her opinion that the ultimate criterion for theoretical explanation is how far it is empirically satisfying. There must thus be a continual scientific dialogue in which comparative investigation and theoretical formulation are woven together.

> "... it involves acceptance of empirical adequacy as the ultimate criterion of theoretical explanation ... and also a continuous scientific dialogue in which comparative investigation and theoretical formulation are inextricably intertwined ... " (Archer in Giner and Archer, 1978, pp. 23-24).

## *Discussion*

There is not much written commentary on Archer's published work. There are diverse references to her work but no comprehensive presentation or discussion. In his book, *Globalization*, Roland Robertson discusses the question of how far sociology has come in its development of a theory of culture. He adopts Archer's view of the situation. He stresses that it is Archer's view that the concept of culture is one of the concepts of sociology which is relatively poorly developed and has played a changeable role. Thus far he agrees with Archer. But, when it comes to Archer's approach to the sociological debate on the concept of culture, he criticises her for ignoring the most significant contributions which sociology has in fact developed, for example Bourdieu's contribution (Robertson, 1992, pp. 35-36).

Another sociologist who has briefly commented on Archer's theory is the American sociologist, George Ritzer. The problem which he discusses is Archer's methodological principle of analytical dualism. Ritzer does not believe that it is always necessary to split the two elements. He believes that it is quite possible that in some cases the two elements can be regarded as indivisible (Ritzer, 1992, pp. 574-576).

Looking at these two rather sporadic discussions of Archer's theory prompts questions about Archer's views on the other sociological theories of culture and about her fixed principle of analytical dualism. I will state my view on both these questions in the following discussion (cf. also Zeuner 1999; 2001).

The questions which I shall deal with are first and foremost how to summarise Archer's understanding of culture, how she defines culture and how she relates this to other sociological phenomena. The background for this understanding of culture should be looked for in her opinion of the most significant social problems, and the inspiration which she draws from existing theory.

When one reads Archer's works it is difficult to see any concerns about society. Some of the cultural constellations which she develops can give rise to actions which can cause concern. Repression, violence and manipulation are included in the theory. The cultural constellations can give rise to so much specialisation and divisions between people that it becomes difficult for society to cohere. However, such concerns do not appear to be the driving force behind her theory. Archer's concerns are more directed towards sociology.

Most of Archer's works are introduced with a highly systematised critique of sociology. This is the case right from her introductions to the anthologies on Europe and up to her most comprehensive theoretical works. She uses the principle of analytical dualism to criticise large parts of sociology. She believes that sociology, and for that matter parts of the philosophy of science, have a tendency to break with this principle. As a consequence, different levels become conflated.

In her article "The Myth of Cultural Integration", which is later included as an introduction to *Culture and agency*, Archer accuses sociology of allowing the cultural system and socio-cultural interaction to conflate (Archer 1985). It is her view that the myth of cultural integration comes from the anthropological studies of traditional societies and from there it has spread to sociological studies of modern society. According to Archer, this myth means that cultural patterns are considered as being fundamentally linked together, and that these linked patterns form the basis of uniform actions and thus for social homogeneity. Integrated culture thus becomes the basis for social integration. This is where the thinking short-circuits, according to Archer. It is here that there is a conflation of the cultural system and socio-cultural interaction.

In *Culture and agency* Archer expands her criticism of the conflation of the cultural system and socio-cultural interaction (Archer, 1988/1996, pp. 25-96). She directs her criticism towards sociology's various forms of conflation. She distinguishes between three forms of conflation: downwards conflation, upwards conflation and central conflation. In that part of sociology which Archer thinks undertakes downwards conflation, culture's cohesive force is significant enough to ensure socio-cultural cohesion. Thus, socio-cultural interaction is a phenomenon which is derived from culture. Socio-cultural interaction is an appendix to culture. Archer says that the foundations for this thinking were laid down by Pitrim Sorokin (Sorokin, 1957), the foundations for functionalist thinking were laid down by Talcott Parsons (Parsons, 1951) and the foundations for structuralist thinking were laid down by Claude Levi-Strauss (Levi-Strauss, 1958/1969). In that part of sociology which Archer thinks undertakes upward conflation, the socio-cultural cohesive forces are considered to have the ability to create cultural cohesion. Here culture is derived from socio-cultural interaction. In this way culture is reduced to being an appendix to socio-cultural interaction. Here, Marxist thinking in particular is subject to criticism. This applies both to the instrumentalist version, as represented by Antonio Gramsci (Gramsci, 1932/1975) and Ralph Miliband (Miliband, 1969), and to the technocratic version represented by Herbert Marcuse (Marcuse, 1964) and Jürgen Habermas (Habermas, 1971). Where central conflation occurs, there is a confounding of culture and socio-cultural interaction, so that both phenomena have a tendency to disappear. The two phenomena are considered to be inseparable. Archer identifies this form of conflation in the structuration theory represented by Anthony Giddens (Giddens, 1979).

Archer also finds a lack of analytical dualism in two kinds of philosophy of science which she labels methodological individualism and methodological collectivism. She puts forward this criticism most explicitly in *Realist social theory* (Archer, 1995, pp. 33-64), but it is also present in the introduction to *Social Origins of Educational Systems* (Archer, 1979, pp.5-25). The problem which she points out is that the two forms of thinking do not make an analytical separation between structure and agency. According to Archer, methodological individualism considers that the individual and his actions have decisive importance, so that structures become derived phenomena. In this way structures have a tendency to disappear as independent phenomena. Archer considers this thinking to be downwards conflation. As representatives of methodological individualism, Archer refers to the scientific philosophers J.W.N. Watkins (Watkins, 1968) and F.A. Hayek (Hayek, 1973). With methodological collectivism the structures are decisive for the actions of the individual. Here actions are derived from a phenomenon which has a tendency to disappear. Archer refers to this as upwards conflation. As representatives of this kind of thinking Archer refers to the scientific philosophers Ernest Gellner (Gellner, 1968) and Maurice Mandelbaum (Mandelbaum, 1973).

In more recent developments of sociological theory, Archer considers two attempts to develop a theory which can overcome both methodological individualism and methodological collectivism. One tendency is structuration theory represented by Anthony Giddens. The other is the morphogenetic approach represented by herself. Archer puts these ideas forward in *Realist social theory*, but already in *Culture and agency* and in the article "Morphogenesis versus structuration: on combining structure and action" she laid out the opposing views of Giddens and herself (Archer, 1995, pp. 93-134; Archer, 1988/1996, pp. 72-96; Archer, 1982). She points out that what is common to Giddens and herself is that they both maintain the necessity of distinguishing between structure and agency. The differences between them arise from their methodological principles. On the one hand there is Giddens's principle of duality, and on the other hand there is

Archer's principle of analytical dualism. Giddens's principle of duality means that structure and agency mutually constitute each other. They are thus bound to each other. It is this principle to which Archer takes strong exception. For her, structure and agency are two independent phenomena which are separated by time. The structures which form the basis for a given action can have been created by earlier generations and must thus be independent in relation to the actual actions. It is against this background that Archer so firmly maintains the principle of analytical dualism. According to this principle, structure and agency must be considered as two separate phenomena which can influence each other.

After this criticism of large parts of sociology and the philosophy of science for their lack of dualist thinking, Archer finds inspiration in David Lockwood's article "Social Integration and System Integration" (Lockwood, 1964). This small article, of just 10 pages, published in 1964, is a decisive source of inspiration for Margaret Archer. Her analysis of the development of educational systems is inspired by Lockwood's thinking. She herself wrote that she would attempt to develop her theory of culture on the basis of Lockwood's theory. She later developed her theory on structural conditions so that it could be understood in the same way as cultural conditions. It is thus this coupling together of conflict theory and general functionalism which is the starting point for Archer's theory. The question of social integration is imposed over socio-cultural interaction and social interaction, while the question of system integration is imposed over the cultural system and social structures. The requirement for analytical dualism as the methodological basis thus seems to be satisfied by Lockwood's distinction between social integration and system integration.

The second decisive element in Archer's thinking, the morphogenetic approach, seems to stem from Walther Buckley's ideas on systems theory. Buckley's attempt to develop a general model for a morphogenetic process is the basis for Archer's theoretical work on structural and cultural development processes. In his book *Sociology and Modern Systems Theory*, Buckley distinguishes between morphostasis and morphogenesis. The aim of this book was to develop a general model for a morphogenetic process. In this process there are elements which correspond to Archer's view of morphogenesis, including the ability of systems themselves to generate change, tension in the system, transaction processes in the form of exchanges, negotiation etc. (Buckley, 1967, p. 160). Archer's division of the morphogenetic phases into three parts can also be seen in Buckley, though not identically.

In *Realist Social Theory*, which contains Archer's more recent theoretical thinking, it is also possible to see the influence of critical realism, represented by the philosopher Roy Bhaskar. Even Bhaskar's basic idea, that science must be realistic and thus bound to materialist thinking, is reflected in Archer. More specifically, Bhaskar develops the idea that a context consisting of contradictions between differentiated and stratified units forms the basis for emergence and thus for totality. Totality in turn forms the basis for reflexivity and thus for the development of a self that can undertake evaluations and thereafter take action (Bhaskar, 1993, pp. 303 and 382). For Bhaskar, emergence is coterminous with a relation between two links, in which one link is developed by the other link, diachronically or synchronously. The second link is able to work backwards on the first link, but it cannot be reduced to the first link (Bhaskar, 1993, p. 397). Archer thus develops Bhaskar's philosophy of development further, but she emphasises that it must be accompanied by analytical dualism.

When we come to the more substantive part of Archer's theory of culture and her definition of the concept of culture, we see that her source of inspiration is Karl Popper. Her definition of culture corresponds to Popper's definition of the third world. In *Objec-*

*tive Knowledge* Popper distinguished between the first world (the physical world), the second world (the mental world), and the third world (ideas in objective form). The connection between the first world and the third can only pass through the second world. The third world thus consists of theories, their logical relations, the arguments of the theories and the problem situations which lie in the theories themselves (Popper, 1972/1992, pp. 154-155). The third world is thus ideas in objective form, in other words, ideas as presented in books or in other accessible forms. These materials have an objective existence which can be the subject of other people's understanding. It is this objective world which Archer understands as culture.

Archer thus develops her theory of culture on the basis of a wide range of different sources, of which those she refers to are only the most important. What is the significance of these sources for the development of her theory? And to what theory of cultural change do these sources lead?

The influence of Lockwood means that analytical dualism stands at the centre of Archer's theoretical construction. However, Lockwood's theory was developed in relation to structural conditions. It is also notable that Archer initially builds on Lockwood's theory in her analysis of the development of educational systems. Thereafter she asks how far it is possible to develop a theory of culture on the same theoretical basis. This means that Archer considers culture and structure to be phenomena which are developed by the same kinds of mechanisms.

The influence of Lockwood therefore means that both the theory of culture and structural theory are based on a combination of general functionalism and conflict theory. Therefore, both in her theory of structure and in her theory of culture, Archer must develop her views both on the systemic development and human interaction.

In developing her view of the systemic development of culture, Archer draws on the ideas of Popper's theory of the third world. This means that, for Archer, culture consists of ideas which have an objective existence. However, only a limited part of the culture is included in a cultural system. The cultural system consists of logical propositions which can be true or false and thus either contradictory or compatible. By narrowing down culture like this, Archer creates a universe in which the laws of logic predominate. Where the rules of logic predominate, situational logics can be created and these situational logics can move people.

When Archer develops her view of human interaction with regard to culture, she draws on Lockwood's use of conflict theory. This means that socio-cultural interaction is guided by material interests. People's actions in relation to culture are thus guided by the material advantages they can obtain. To explain this point of view in more detail, Archer introduces the distinction between agents, actors and persons. As agents, i.e. collectives, we live under material conditions which we have not ourselves determined. As actors we are offered roles that are determined by the agents. And as persons we have the possibility of reflection in order to arrive at a choice within the given conditions. Socio-cultural interaction starts from the material conditions which we, as collectives, must live with.

The aim of Archer's theory is to be able to explain cultural change or cultural stasis. To do this she introduces Buckley's morphogenetic cycle. Using this, Archer creates three phases: conditions, interaction and development. It is the relationship between the systemic conditions and the socio-cultural conditions which is decisive for whether there can be change. However, it is human interaction, which itself goes through a morphogenetic cycle, which is decisive for whether any change in fact occurs. Furthermore, structural morphogenesis can also give rise to cultural change. The social interaction which occurs as a step in structural morphogenesis can take effect and influence cultural interaction and thus initiate cultural morphogenesis. In this way culture, structure and action are bound together in three morphogenetic processes.

Archer combines considerable theoretical elements in her theoretical construction. The question is whether the combination of these theoretical elements causes any problems. Are all these widely differing elements compatible?

The two most important elements in Archer's theory are the principle of analytical dualism and the principle of morphogenesis. Analytical dualism has its roots in Lockwood's linking of general functionalism and conflict theory. The principle of morphogenesis has its roots in Buckley's system theory. Analytical dualism leads to the requirement that culture and action should be kept separate and analysed separately in order to understand their effects on each other. According to this principle, system and interaction should be kept separate. The problem is that over time Archer allows morphogenetic thinking, and thus the system theoretical approach, to take priority over interactional thinking. This is because action thus itself becomes a morphogenetic process. It becomes a system in itself. Here the question is whether this development of Archer's theory breaches with her principle of analytical dualism. The system prevails over the action and turns it into a system. The interaction is no longer separated from the system. Analytical dualism is not maintained.

Another significant link in Archer's theory is the combination of Popper's theory of knowledge with analytical dualism. According to Popper, one must distinguish between the physical world, the mental world, and the world of objective ideas. It is the third of these worlds, that of the objective ideas, which is the starting point for Archer's concept of culture. However, Popper assumed that the mental world connects the physical world to the world of objective ideas. This mental world is virtually absent from Archer's theory of culture. On the other hand, she allows analytical dualism, as developed on the basis of Lockwood's article on social integration and system integration, to apply not only to the structural domain, but also to the cultural domain. This was certainly not the aim of Lockwood's article. It was intended as a new sociological perspective in which general functionalism and conflict theory are combined, and it was directed towards the analysis of the societal elements which Archer calls structural conditions. By assuming that culture and structure are guided by the same mechanisms, Archer transfers the mechanisms of the structural domain to the cultural domain. She thus assumes that socio-cultural interaction is guided by material interests. It is her view that socio-cultural actions occur with a view to maintaining or promoting vested interests. As a consequence, in her theory on the mutual effects of structure and culture, she arrives at the position where culture confers legitimacy on structure. The structural world's most significant benefit from the cultural processes is thus that it can legitimise itself. By imposing analytical dualism over both structure and culture, Archer in fact turns culture into a reflection of structure. When material considerations control the cultural domain, this domain is, in effect, subject to the structural domain. The autonomous cultural dynamic in Popper's theory, where the mental processes constitute the relation between the objective culture and its material foundations, is eliminated by Archer. On the other hand she allows that material interests are the link between objective culture and its material foundations. Thus, it is not ideas which are decisive for how culture is developed, but the material benefits to which the thinking can give rise. In this way culture is subordinated to structure.

With the premises which Archer propounds for the development of her theory, that culture consists of objective ideas, that the cultural system consists of logical propositions, that culture and structure operate according to the same mechanisms etc., she creates a universe which is very limited. The problem is that her theory of culture does not present any analytical history which can challenge this theory. She herself writes that her theory is in the nature of an analytical format that can be used in practical sociological work. However, this is not the case in the cultural domain. When she seeks to give concrete examples to substantiate her theory, she refers to her own research into the development of educational systems. The development of these systems is used as an analytical history of emergence. It is thus not merely her premise that culture is developed on the basis of the same mechanisms as structure. Her historical foundation for the theory is also a history which lies within the structural domain. In this way Archer's theory of culture is without any analytical history. It lacks any real historical content. It remains a format.

www.reading.ac.uk/library

# 6

# Robert Wuthnow: Culture as Discourse

Robert Wuthnow is primarily concerned with cultural phenomena, but he has also worked on the theory of culture and he has had ongoing discussions about how one should understand and analyse cultural phenomena. The aim of this chapter is to extract his understanding of culture from his extensive writings. There will also be an investigation of how he relates culture to other social phenomena.

Robert Wuthnow's writings are focused around three themes: culture, religion and voluntary organisations. This chapter will focus on his contribution to the first of these themes, but it will be impossible to avoid touching on the other two themes. In his overall sociological view, cultural phenomena can probably be considered as being more important than the two more concrete phenomena of religion and voluntary organisations.

The works which are most relevant to a discussion of Wuthnow's understanding of culture are *The Consciousness Reformation* (1976), *Cultural Analysis* (1984), *Meaning and Moral Order* (1987), *Communities of Discourse* (1989a), *Producing the Sacred* (1994a), *God and Mammon in America* (1994b) and *Poor Richard's Principle* (1996a). These works will be considered in the following discussion.

The following works are among those which deal with religion: *Experimentation in American Religion* (1978), *The Restructuring of American Religion* (1988), *The Struggle for America's Soul* (1989b), *Rediscovering the Sacred* (1992), *Christianity in the 21st Century* (1993), *Christianity and Civil Society* (1996b), *The Crisis of the Churches* (1997) and *After Heaven* (1998). In addition, there are works on voluntary organisations, including: *Acts of Compassion* (1991), *Sharing the Journey* (1994c) and *Learning to Care* (1995). Finally, Wuthnow has edited a number of books on these same topics, which need not be named here.

So Robert Wuthnow has written extensively on these topics. Many of his works are based on empirical data about the values and behaviour of the American people. His favoured method is survey research, but he also uses in-depth interviews widely. Most of his works include appendices with a presentation of the methodology used. Wuthnow's works do not, to any great extent, include extensive methodological discussions. However, he does include certain methodological discussions in *Meaning and Moral Order* and *Communities of Discourse*.

In *Meaning and Moral Order*, Wuthnow writes that his epistemological starting point is interpretive sociology.

> "Throughout, the epistemological stance taken in this volume is that of *interpretive sociology*. The very business of sociology is assumed to be one of interpretation, not one of discovering objective facts ... The hermeneutic circle, and all that it implies about the limitations of positivistic knowledge, is taken for granted." (Wuthnow, 1987, p. 17).

In extension of this attitude, Wuthnow writes in *Communities of Discourse* that his starting point is a theoretical scaffold, a loose net of concepts. It is his view that such a loose-fitting framework of concepts can contribute to structuring empirical research, without tying it down. It then becomes possible to revise it in the light of empirical results.

> "There is also an implicit theoretical scaffold ... It is in fact a scaffold more than it is either a foundation or an inner system of girders and beams. It provides a loose-fitting framework from which an edifice of many particular details and architectural refinements can be constructed. It can be torn away so that the empirical contours of this edifice can be seen unobstructed. It does, however, affect the way in which these contours are arranged." (Wuthnow, 1989a, p. 6).

Wuthnow's methodological considerations are thus primarily directed towards the establishment of a loose-fitting framework which can be used to direct empirical research. His preferred approach is to use interpretation rather than fixed systems of concepts. This means that he is not tied down to using specific methods. He uses both quantitative and qualitative data in his work, and carries out both empirical and theoretical studies.

## *Meaning systems*

In one of his very early works, *The Consciousness Reformation* (1976), Wuthnow's understanding of culture is presented as being meaning systems. He frequently uses the term 'cultural meaning systems'.

> "... our concern is ... with the overarching symbolic frames of reference, which we shall refer to as *meaning systems*, by which people come to grips with the broader meaning and purpose of their lives." (Wuthnow, 1976, pp. 2-3).

The aim of *The Consciousness Reformation* is to examine the links between the development of cultural meaning systems and experimental behaviour. More specifically, it is to examine the relationship between, on the one hand, meaning systems associated with religion, individualism, social sciences and mysticism, and on the other hand, the experimental behaviour of people in the San Francisco area at the end of the 1960s and the beginning of the 1970s. In this connection Wuthnow puts forward this basic view:

> "... we are siding with a perspective on human behaviour that assumes that people seldom act solely on the basis of objective social circumstances, but rather according to the meanings they attribute to their circumstances." (Wuthnow, 1976, p.2).

In specifying the concept of meaning systems, Wuthnow makes a clear distinction between meaning systems and values and consciousness of everyday phenomena. Meaning systems are thus different from, and more than, what is normally understood as consciousness, attitudes, values or beliefs. Meaning systems go beyond everyday realities. Meaning systems have a significance beyond the more specific meanings about everyday realities.

> "We shall here be concerned with those meaning systems that transcend everyday reality. There is need, therefore, at a conceptual level to establish that these transcendent meaning systems have significance over and against the more specific meanings of everyday reality and to indicate generally what this significance is." (Wuthnow, 1976, p. 59).

In his conceptual definition of meaning systems Wuthnow starts with a discussion of the concept of consciousness. He considers consciousness to be a construction of reality. His view is that reality presents itself as factual and true, but it does this because we construct it in this way. The existence of reality thus depends on human consciousness. On this basis he defines consciousness as the ongoing process through which reality is constructed on the basis of symbols and experience. Even this process, through which reality is constructed, consists of repeated selection and organisation. In this way reality becomes a product of the culture in which one lives, and its definition varies according the symbols which dominate different cultures. In addition to this, reality is formed through the actions through which the symbols are used. However, Wuthnow emphasises that we have not each constructed our reality, but we share certain common definitions in the construction of reality (Wuthnow, 1976, p. 64)

From the discussion on consciousness, Wuthnow moves to a discussion on conscicusness about everyday life. In everyday life reality is first and foremost a 'here and now' reality. It is divided up according to the past, the present and the future, according to relevance and irrelevance, according to public space and private space, according to suffering and dreams and so on. From this a need arises for wholeness for the individual. Wholeness tends to be manifested subjectively, as the realisation of well-being, inner harmony and fulfilment. It is the need for wholeness which forms the basis for the experiences and symbols which constitute a level of consciousness which goes beyond everyday life, puts it in a better perspective and gives it greater meaning (Wuthnow, 1976, pp. 70-71).

Behind the consciousness of everyday reality lies a system of symbols and ideas which call forth a wider context and meaning than can be found in everyday reality. In order to sense such wholeness in everyday life, there must be some common element which cuts across experiences. For centuries archetypal expressions have existed for the most basic elements of all spheres of reality. For example, there are symbols of being, life, karma, nature and will. Such symbols can be a common basis for resolving the tensions and inconsistencies in different spheres of reality, and for organising them into more meaningful patterns.

There must thus be some symbols which express wholeness and transcendence. This does not mean that they deny everyday life, but rather that they connect what happens here and now with what exists beyond the here and now. By using transcendental meaning systems each of life's spheres will be considered as being linked with and having a significance for other spheres of life.

> "Within such overarching 'systems of meaning' each realm of life is no longer discrete, but perceived as connected with and as having significance for other realms." (Wuthnow, 1976, p.74).

The symbolism which creates an overarching meaning system for the individual is shown to have the same function for society. In a society divided up into different institutions, each institution will have specific assumptions about that part of reality with which it has dealings. Each of these assumptions may, however, be rooted in more general understandings of reality. There must be some standards of behaviour which can control the mutual relations of institutions in following wider social goals. There must be symbols, such as fate, luck, will, power, God and development which can transcend the different sectors of society.

> "Such symbolism tends to integrate collective behavior by pointing to some broader, or more basic, order of reality which crosscuts as well as permeates the institutional sectors of society." (Wuthnow, 1976, p. 77).

Meaning systems have an integrating function. Because they are able to provide reality with a perspective of wholeness, they have a tendency to achieve a special status in society. They achieve a special authority, and much energy is used in protecting them and using them under changing circumstances. They are given a sacred status in society. It is the ability of meaning systems to give social reality its fundamental definition and meaning that gives them their sanctified status. This status is supported by the enduring nature of meaning systems.

However, Wuthnow points out that unavoidable pressure for change of these transcendental symbols can arise. This pressure can come from changes in the existing philosophy, scientific or aesthetic ideas. There can also be changes to the social conditions in which these are rooted. It is therefore necessary to be alert to the forces of conservation and change which can affect these symbols. It is also necessary to investigate whether the transcendental meaning systems themselves operate to conserve or have the ability to create visions showing how it is possible to overcome the limitations associated with the existing social conditions (Wuthnow, 1976, p. 81).

Through his empirical analysis, Wuthnow shows that there are in fact changes to the meaning systems in American society, which are exemplified by the San Francisco area. It is his view that adherence to the religious meaning system is in decline. The same applies to adherence to the individualist meaning system. On the other hand there is growing adherence to the scientific meaning system, and to the mystical meaning system. Using his analysis of the survey data gathered, Wuthnow demonstrates that these trends promote the tendency to carry out political, economic, religious, family and lifestyle experiments. The consequence of these experiments is increased diversity within these spheres of life. Several different types of lifestyle will emerge. It is Wuthnow's view that this situation is well adapted to the social scientific meaning system and the mystical meaning system. It is harder to combine diversity and choice between many different types of lifestyle with meaning systems characterised by religion or individualism.

This book, which is one the earliest of Wuthnow's works on cultural phenomena, thus contains an understanding of culture as consisting of meaning systems. Such meaning systems are transcendental in relation to everyday meanings. They are overarching and enduring, though without being unchangeable. They can be altered by changes to ideas and changes to social conditions. For the individual these meaning systems create wholeness, since they establish a connection between what is happening here and now with something which is bigger and more cohesive. For society they create integration between different institutions, since they set standards of behaviour for pursuing wider social goals. Culture thus helps to create cohesion both for the individual and for society. At the same time, it is Wuthnow's view that people take action on the basis of the meaning which they ascribe to phenomena. Therefore, meaning systems can help influence people's behaviour, including their experimental behaviour.

### *The symbolic-expressive aspect of behaviour*

In his book, *Cultural Analysis*, published in 1984, Wuthnow looks at the question of what is understood by culture, and how it is possible to analyse cultural phenomena. The book was written with James Hunter, Albert Bergesen and Edith Kurzweil. The book is presented as a collective work, but those parts of it which are selected for discussion here were, according to the book's preface, written by Wuthnow. The four authors base their discussions, of how to understand and analyse culture, on a review of the works of Peter Berger, Mary Douglas, Michel Foucault and Jürgen Habermas. The book is arranged in such a way that all the discussions about these four theorists are aimed at clarifying the definition and content of culture, the construction of culture, the relationship of culture to social conditions and how culture can be changed (Wuthnow et al., 1984, p. viii).

In the introduction to the book, which was written by Wuthnow, culture is defined as being the symbolic-expressive aspect of human behaviour.

> "… culture may be provisionally defined as the symbolic-expressive aspect of human behavior. This definition is sufficiently broad to take account of the verbal utterances, gestures, ceremonial behaviour, ideologies, religions and philosophical systems that are generally associated with the term culture." (Wuthnow et al., 1984, p. 3).

Starting from this provisional definition of culture, the authors discuss the state of cultural analysis within sociology. It is their view that, since the Second World War, sociology has made very little progress in this area. They find the cause of this in a number of limiting assumptions. First, it has been assumed that culture consists of thoughts, moods, feelings, beliefs and values. In this way culture becomes the residue, which is left when one has taken into account all human behaviour. Culture has been reduced to the most fluid, floating and least observable category of non-action. On this basis the authors do not find it surprising that it has been difficult to make progress in cultural analysis (Wuthnow et al., 1984, p. 5).

A second of the assumptions which restricts the progress of cultural analysis follows from the first. When culture is held to consist of thoughts and feelings rather than actions, it becomes obvious to investigate the relations between these two areas. A connection is made between the subjective view and the objective conditions. Attitudes are linked with actions. The consequence of this is that culture is not regarded as a phenomenon to be studied in itself. Culture is thus reduced so that it can only be understood in relation to social structures.

A third assumption which has a limiting effect on the progress of cultural analysis is the assumption that only individuals have culture. This is another form of reductionism. The problem is that if one concentrates solely on the feelings and thoughts of individuals, one loses sight of some of the broader dimensions of social life, including institutions, classes, social movements and organisations. Another problem is that if one looks for consistency in the thoughts and feelings of the individual, one will miss the potential for clarifying actual patterns in cultural phenomena. These are not always logically consistent. In fact, individuals have a quite remarkable ability to maintain inconsistent attitudes.

According to the authors, such assumptions about culture and cultural phenomena have pushed cultural analysis into the background. These assumptions have reduced culture to being merely the thoughts and feelings of individuals. Culture has been explained away, rather than being studied for its more systematic patterns. It has been more misunderstood than understood.

The aim of the review of the four theories is thus to re-establish the premises for culture. How is culture defined, what is its relation to social structures, and how is it changed? These questions are asked of Berger, as the representative of the phenomenological tradition, of Douglas as the representative of cultural anthropology, of Foucault as the representative of neo-structuralism and of Habermas as the representative of critical theory.

The result of the review of these four theories is that the authors are able to show both differences and parallels between the four theories. They regard the differences as being a consequence of the four theorists starting from widely differing theoretical and national traditions. This leads to different epistemological assumptions, different views about the aims of cultural analyses and different ideas about the job of a social scientist. In their cultural analyses they have focused on different phenomena. Berger has looked at the individual interpretations by means of which the individual adapts to everyday reality. Douglas has looked at the meaning of ritual and material artefacts in defining conceptual limits. For Foucault, power and its impact through categories of knowledge are most important. And for Habermas the epistemological basis of communicative action is most important. In their methods, they range from empirical studies to philosophical reasoning.

When the authors explain the similarities between the four theorists, they look at their use of earlier thinkers. To a large extent, all four have the same intellectual forefathers, including Marx, Weber, Durkheim, Freud, Mead, Nietzsche and Heidegger. Their similarities also include the fact that all four theorists attach importance to language and communication, systems and classification, to symbolic-expressionism, and to culture. They wrestle with the problem of subjectivity and perception. They reject the idea that social sciences should be modelled along the lines of the natural sciences. Therefore, they are concerned with the underlying assumptions and aims of the social sciences. They look at the important problems in modern culture, which lead to their critical reflections (Wuthnow et al., 1984, p. 18).

In particular, there are two marked developmental tendencies which are repeated in the works of all four theorists, though perhaps less so with Berger than with the other three. One is the tendency to break with the dichotomous approach to human behaviour, in other words the traditional split between objective social structures and people's thoughts, beliefs and ideas. The second tendency is to emphasise the observable and objective aspects of culture and investigate their patterns. Language, ritual and categories of classification have replaced subjective opinions as the focus of cultural analysis. In this way, culture is considered as a behavioural phenomenon or, more precisely, as an analytical aspect of behaviour.

The analyses of the four theorists arrives at a conclusion, also written by Wuthnow. In this he discusses some of the recurring themes. One of these themes is the problem of subjectivity. This problem is discussed from the premise that Berger is the only one of the four theorists who attaches importance to the subjective aspect of cultural analysis, while the other three consider this aspect to be less important. On this basis, there is an investigation of the advantages and disadvantages of including or omitting subjectivity in cultural analysis.

In Berger's writings the perspective of culture rests on the view that there is a constant dialectic between subjectivity and socio-cultural objectivity. Human subjectivity is externalised in objectified social products, and the objectified reality operates reciprocally on subjectivity. According to the authors, the advantage of this view is that culture must necessarily be rooted in human subjectivity, and that it affects human consciousness. The problem with this approach is its methodology. Cultural analyses which includes subjectivity require access to the inner thoughts of the actors. For each social situation they must reconstruct the actors involved in it. Another problem of including subjectivity is that it presupposes that, by interpreting cultural artefacts, it will be possible to say something about the subjective intentions of those who have produced them. However, the authors debate whether there can be great differences between cultural objects and the desires and intentions that lie behind them.

The authors say that there is a clear distinction between culture and subjectivity in the writings of Douglas, Foucault and Habermas. Here it is possible to investigate the relationship between cultural elements, without being concerned with subjective meaning. According to the authors, Habermas is interested in human behaviour in his cultural analyses. Douglas is interested in objective, symbolic classifications, the ritual dramatisation of their patterns and their function in the social order. Foucault focuses on categories, concepts, relations and rituals, which can be conceived as objectified growths in the social interaction, and not as subjective elements. A clear advantage of this separation of culture and subjectivity is, say the authors, that the cultural elements are, by definition, observable. Culture attains the status of a reality, as an autonomous object, which can be the subject of investigation. Another advantage of this separation is that it becomes possible to use a more flexible theoretical perspective. It becomes possible to analyse cultural patterns in the light of the limitations imposed by social interaction, the state or by patterns of communication. Finally, the authors suggest that there is an advantage in separating subjectivity and culture, as it becomes possible to use a broader perspective in cultural analysis. It becomes possible to include, not just the meaning of symbols, but also the conditions, patterns and rules for use which make the symbols meaningful.

Another recurring theme, which is revealed by these conclusions, is the question of the relationship between culture and social structure. The authors point out the limitations of the sociological tradition, which lets social structures be determining for the development of ideas. They regard the sociology of knowledge, among other things, as being an expression of this tendency. Among the four theorists studied, they see a tendency to attach more importance to the patterns, rules and relations within culture itself. The authors say that, of the four theorists, Berger is the one who most strongly maintains the distinction between culture and social structures. This is because of his dialectical view of the relationship between these two levels. However, in this dialectic, it is clear that the social structures are the determining factor. Also, when Berger considers cultural change, this change is due to the development of the social infrastructure. The whole of this approach is based on his heavy reliance on the classical sociologists, including Marx, Weber and Durkheim. Nevertheless, Berger has an understanding of culture as an independent entity. This culture gets its form from the individual's needs for meaning and order. These needs are so powerful in relation to human thinking and action, that they leave their mark on the pattern of culture. It is Berger's opinion that culture can best be understood by reference to these needs. On this basis, it is clear that culture has identifiable structures which can be researched and made the subject of systematic empirical analysis. Culture comes to consist of relatively rational, or at least ordered, sets of classifications which enable the individual to understand his surroundings and to operate actively in relation to them (Wuthnow et al., 1984, p. 251).

Douglas too, according to the authors, is more interested in identifying patterns at the symbolic-expressive level than of relating culture to social structures. She considers culture as being the dynamics of social interactions, as it is dramatised in rituals, speech and in social arrangements. She considers these arrangements to be phenomena which are used to transmit the information which is necessary for carrying on the ordered behaviour of social life. However, her theory is distinguished from Berger's in two ways. First, she does not make any analytical separation between culture and social structures. According to the authors, she considers culture to be an object which can be observed, and which exists more at the social level than the individual level. In this way, culture is woven into social life. Second, Douglas emphasises the moral aspect of culture, as distinct from its psychological functions for the individual. The aim of culture is to ensure predictable behaviour, which is necessary for social interaction to occur. A moral order implies that it is possible to reckon with certain relations, and take them for granted.

According to the authors, Foucault also distanced himself from the dualistic approach to culture. He looked more at cultural patterns, rather than trying to explain their roots in social structures. He focused on written and verbal discourse. He implicitly distinguished between discourse and social arrangements. He could thus interpret discourse by studying larger social arrangements. However, the authors do not believe that there is a clear distinction between discourse and social arrangements. They believe that the most important task for Foucault was to explain the co-existence of mutually existing arrangements, whether or not these are in the nature of discourse or social interaction. This must occur by revealing the underlying rules for cultural construction. In this way social arrangements become a form of discourse.

In the discussion on Habermas, the authors emphasise that, of the four theorists, it is he who is most explicitly concerned with the relations between culture and social structures. For Habermas, the social pattern is useful for determining what constitutes meaningful expressions at a cultural level. He thus relates the development of cultural patterns to social conditions. For him, culture consists of the patterns of relations between actors which arise out of their efforts to engage in communication.

On the basis of this discussion, the authors arrive at the view that the four theorists share an opinion of cultural analysis as being the investigation of symbolic-expressive elements of behaviour. This definition of culture thus comes to cover not merely verbal discourse, but also the dramatised everyday life and the ritualised aspects of social arrangements. Having defined culture like this, the authors believe that the most important task for cultural analysis is to identify the underlying patterns which give culture form and substance. In the light of this task, there is still a possibility of relating social structures to culture. This must take place by relating aspects of behaviour which have a mutual effect on each other.

> "Having defined culture in these broad terms, a primary task of cultural analysis is to identify recurring features, distinctions, and underlying patterns which give form and substance to culture. ... possibilities for relating culture and social structure continue to exist ... as mutually influencing aspects of behaviour." (Wuthnow et al., 1984, pp. 255-256).

On the basis of this discussion, the authors put forward some conclusions on cultural analysis. They identify that there is a framework for cultural analysis which arises out of the discussion of the four theories. They identify culture as being a distinct aspect of social reality, whose patterns can be observed and subjected to theoretical interpretation. They look upon cultural analysis as the study of the symbolic-expressive dimensions of social life. Thus the contents of cultural analyses are objective actions, events, expressions and social interactions. The level of analysis is the patterns between these artefacts of interaction.

The authors conclude their book by discussing different analytical strategies based on the framework for cultural analyses. They point out the possibility of focussing on deviance, with the aims of viewing standard behaviour as less evident. Both Foucault and Douglas looked at mental illness, illness, torture, imprisonment and sexual deviation. Such studies in deviation have a theoretical purpose because deviant behaviour helps to dramatise cultural limits. At the same time, these limits help to dramatise order. Therefore it is a task for cultural analysis to investigate symbolic limits and how they constitute cultural order. These limits are the basis of cultural differentiation. When culture is considered as an observable aspect of human behaviour, this means that symbolic limits acquire considerable significance. They are visible in the way in which social interaction takes place, in discourse and in physical objects. Many social activities must be understood as attempts to reinforce the limits, redefine cultural distinctions and as symptoms of ambivalent frameworks. The real task for cultural analysis is to identify these activities. According to the authors, the bulk of such work must be guided by metatheoretical perspectives.

In this work on cultural analysis, Wuthnow and the other authors arrive at a definition of culture as being the symbolic-expressive aspect of human behaviour. Culture is thus an element of human behaviour. The purpose of the book is to discuss how cultural analyses can be carried out. Through their studies of Berger, Douglas, Foucault and Habermas, they conclude that culture should be studied as an objective and distinct phenomenon. Culture must be studied so as to reveal its own patterns and relations. The authors point to some strategies for analysis, such as studies of deviance, by which it will be possible to throw light on how normal behaviour has been ritualised, and studies of social activities, which aim to dramatise and maintain existing limits.

This study of four theories on cultural phenomena will be seen to be significant for a number of Wuthnow's later works.

## *Levels of cultural analysis*

In his book *Meaning and Moral Order*, Wuthnow continues his discussion of the existing sociological theory of culture, while establishing a structure for his own view of how cultural analysis should be carried out. This book is thus a link between his earlier studies of existing theory and his later studies of different cultural phenomena.

The problem which interests Wuthnow, in his discussion of existing theory, is how different theories relate to the question of meaning. It is his thesis that, by focusing on the question of meaning, existing theories have been held back from the further development of cultural analyses. The aim of his book is thus to contribute to a reformulation of cultural analysis, focussing beyond the question of meaning.

> "... opportunity will be taken to indicate some of the ways in which the study of culture may have been hindered by its concern with the problem of meaning." (Wuthnow, 1987, p. 22).

In pursing this thesis, Wuthnow divides the development of theories into three phases: the classical approach, the neo-classical approach and the post-structuralist approach.

According to Wuthnow, it was classical sociologists who put the question of meaning on the agenda. They did so out of a recognition that there is an increasing split between the self, as subject, and the external world, as object. In view of this split, finding a meaning for existence became pressing. It is Wuthnow's opinion that Marx directed his concerns towards alienation, that Weber directed his concerns towards meaninglessness, and that Durkheim directed his concerns towards the process through which the individual is cut off from the normative order. According to Wuthnow, the consequence was that the classical writers had a tendency to look upon culture as having only a subjective dimension, so culture could be explained on the basis of social structures. Culture became a question of meaning (Wuthnow, 1987, pp. 23-36).

Wuthnow identifies Berger, Bellah and Geertz as belonging to the neo-classical tradition. These theorists carried further the classical focus on the question of meaning. For them, meaning is a symbolic property and a function of the context in which the symbol or the individual finds himself. Here, both the subjective and the objective reality are symbolically constructed. In this way, everything is referred to the symbolic world. The neo-classical tradition thus looked on the problem of meaning as being a question of creating a meaning of wholeness in a world of divisions. The key to creating this wholeness is symbols. Such symbols can express deeper meanings in life, can link the individual to his cultural inheritance, give value to art and nature, etc. The neo-classical tradition therefore raises up culture, understood as symbols, so that it occupies a prominent position.

Wuthnow categorises Douglas, Foucault and Habermas as belonging to the post-structuralist school. What these three theorists have in common is that they are inspired by structuralism. They seek patterns or relations in cultural material. For the post-structuralist, the human drama no longer consists of the split between subject and object or in a fragmentation into many parts. The problem here is that people are cut off from one another and must therefore rely on communication. Only through communication can people clarify their shared values. In this way concerns about meaning disappear, indeed even the individual vanishes. The consequence of this is that emphasis is put on how symbols communicate, rather than on what they communicate. Wuthnow suggests that the post-structuralist approach is more concerned with the relations between symbols than with their meaning. The most notable development is in the works of Douglas, who focuses on schemes of classification. It is also observable in the work of Foucault, who focuses on the origin and development of categories. Habermas investigates what makes verbal communications meaningful, but is not concerned with their meaning.

For Wuthnow, the question which arises from this is whether this development is a satisfactory answer to his search for a cultural analysis which rises above the question of meaning. Wuthnow points out that sociology's focus on the question of meaning is contingent on cultural constructions, rather than being an inherent part of culture. All this focus on the question of meaning is due to the fact that there are some broader definitions of the human condition, including the sharp division between subject and object and the fragmentation of reality into many parts. The consequence of this view is that it must be possible to study culture without making meaning the central question. For Wuthnow it means that he does not focus on the question of meaning, but rather seeks to make phenomena meaningful.

> "We do not in fact explicate 'the meaning' of an event … but only try to render it meaningful by putting it in a clear interpretive framework. In a sense, then, we retain much of what has been seen to be of value in discussions of meaning, but we consciously try to move away from focusing cultural analysis itself on the radically

> subjective beliefs, attitudes and meanings of the individual." (Wuthnow, 1987, p. 65).

In his search for a new interpretive framework which is to make events more meaningful, Wuthnow develops four levels for cultural analysis: the subjective, the structural, the dramaturgical and the institutional. The subjective level includes beliefs, attitudes, subjective dispositions, moods, motivations, meanings, mentalities, norms and values. At this level the question of meaning is central. The structural level includes cultural structures, including categories of, boundaries between and associations of cultural elements. Emphasis is put on the cultural patterns and the mutual relations between the cultural elements. At the dramaturgical level, clarification is sought of the relations between culture and broader social relations. The cultural pattern is assumed to play an important role in the dramatisation and confirmation of the moral order. At the same time, it is assumed that the cultural pattern is formed by social relations. At the institutional level it is assumed that all the above assumptions are operative, but that special emphasis is put on the meaning of the social resources for the production and maintenance of cultural forms.

Having put forward the task which he means it is important for sociology to tackle, and having sketched the four levels of cultural analysis which he believes are relevant, Wuthnow runs through a number of topics in which he has the opportunity of discussing the advantages and disadvantages of carrying out analysis at the four levels.

Among the themes which Wuthnow looks at are moral order, ritual dramatising, selection of ideologies, institutionalisation of science and the social foundations of religion. For each of these topics he tries to make a cultural analysis at one or more of the four levels. However, it is his opinion that the subjective level has been thoroughly discussed in sociology, so he focuses mainly on the structural level, the dramaturgical level and the institutional level.

The first theme which Wuthnow looks at is the moral order and the possibility for throwing light on it at the structural level. To understand the moral order, it is necessary to identify the moral codes and distinctions on which it is based. Here, Wuthnow emphasises three significant distinctions. The first distinction concerns the separation between the moral object and the real programme. As an example of this, he refers to the father who says to his son that he must follow a university education for the sake of himself and his people. Here the real programme is the education, but the people is the moral object. The second distinction concerns the separation between the self and the actor. With this separation it is possible for the individual to separate his true self from the role which he plays. It is possible to keep a certain distance from the role played. The third distinction concerns the separation of the unavoidable from the intended. There is a distinction between circumstances over which the individual has no control and circumstances which he has the possibility of influencing. These types of distinction form some of the underlying boundaries within cultural constructions. At the structural level it is thus possible to find the underlying structures for moral codes. The problem with this approach, according to Wuthnow, is that the analysis of the cultural constructions takes place in a social vacuum. If one wishes to relate cultural constructions to social structures, one must involve the dramaturgical level.

> "Cultural constructions ... can be viewed ... as codes that consist of many symbolic elements with an underlying structure involving boundaries between moral objects and real programs, selves and actors, and realms of intentionality and inevitability." (Wuthnow, 1987, p. 75).

The second theme which Wuthnow deals with is rituals and the possibility of illuminating them at the dramaturgical level. According to Wuthnow, rituals are an aspect of culture, and their function is to communicate meaning. However, one must not regard ritual as a special form of action. Ritual is rather a dimension of all forms of social activity which leads to the regulation of everyday life. As an example of a ritual contributing to the communication of meaning and the creation of relations between people, Wuthnow refers to the TV series on Holocaust, the Nazi persecution of the Jews during the Second World War. According to Wuthnow, this series, which was seen by a vast number of people, helped to dramatise evil at a time of social and moral uncertainty.

> "... the ["Holocaust"] program was a symbolic-expressive event that communicated something about social relations in a relatively dramatic way." (Wuthnow, 1987, p. 125).

The third theme which Wuthnow looks at is ideologies and the possibility for analysing them at the dramaturgical level. Here Wuthnow draws a parallel between rituals and ideologies. In the same way that rituals can be understood as symbolic-expressive actions that help to dramatise the moral order, ideologies can be understood as symbols which help to dramatise the social order (Wuthnow, 1987, p. 145). Wuthnow suggests that the relations between ideologies and the broader social environment should be understood by using a model consisting of three phases: production, selection and institutionalisation. In each of these three phases, ideology will be affected by both the moral order and social resources. Both these conditions are significant for determining which ideologies can arise and develop.

At the dramaturgical level, the decisive question is which types of ideology are suited to which types of social conditions. Wuthnow seeks to clarify different forms of ideology in order to investigate which forms of social environment they will flourish in. As an example he refers to popular piety, which is a relatively informal ideology. It flourishes best in small and unstable social environments. Another example is fundamentalism, which consist of relatively few elements which are strongly linked to each other. This form of ideology flourishes best in relatively homogeneous social environments. A third example is individualism, which is characterised by the tendency to disconnect the links between substantive basic beliefs and formalised doctrine. This type of ideology flourishes best in a social environment characterised by individualisation. The last example applies to rationality which is characterised by a high degree of universality. The procedures which are developed to make a link between means and ends must be regarded as being sufficiently general to apply to many different types of situations. Rationality flourishes best in a society characterised by a high degree of heterogeneity.

These relations between ideologies and social conditions must not, according to Wuthnow, be understood as a simple reflection. Apart from the form of an ideology, its ability to dramatise existing social relations will also be important for how it affects a given social context.

> "The connections drawn between ideologies and their environments, therefore, depend primarily on assumptions about the formal structure of ideological systems and the capacity of these systems to withstand changes in the environment, on the one hand, and to facilitate necessary kinds of communication about social relations, on the other." (Wuthnow, 1987, p. 214).

In his search for social conditions which are significant for cultural change, Wuthnow includes world systems. It is his view that there are different kinds of dynamic world systems. As examples, he refers to expansive systems, polarising systems and systems characterised by reintegration. As an example of an expanding system, Wuthnow refers to the 19th century English free trade system. This led to the breaking up of established moral communities. As an example of a polarising system, Wuthnow refers to periods characterised by colonial wars of liberation and de-colonisation. In such systems, militant movements develop on the periphery. These adopt earlier ideological forms in order to legitimise their use of force against the central powers. Finally, there are systems characterised by reintegration. As an example of this Wuthnow refers to the period after the Second World War. Here there was a shift towards mainstream values while sectionalism developed within groups whose possibilities had been reduced.

Following these different thoughts about how social relations and culture can relate to one another at the dramaturgical level, Wuthnow goes on to consider analysis at the institutional level. He exemplifies this by using the institutionalisation of science. Thus, the fourth theme is science and its possibility for being analysed at the institutional level.

In order to speak of the institutionalisation of culture, a number of conditions must be satisfied. The given culture must have acquired a certain degree of autonomy. There must be sufficient social resources for both creative and administrative tasks. There must be an internal system for communication and organisation. There must be sufficient legitimacy for developing good relations with the holders of central power.

In discussing the institutionalisation of science, Wuthnow builds on his view of world systems as determining cultural development. It is his view that the institutionalisation of science took place in 17th century Europe. This world systems was characterised by having many small sovereign states. So the overall system was characterised by decentralisation, while the individual parts of it were characterised by a high degree of centralisation. The multiplicity of small sovereign states made it difficult for individual rulers to control science. Scientists could move to another state if the control became too strict. Therefore the possibility arose of the autonomy of science. At the same time, the small states were rivals of each other. Therefore they needed to develop knowledge which could strengthen their power in relation to the other European rulers. Science was seen as a useful tool. This increased the possibility of scientists obtaining resources from the rulers. This utilitarian approach to science gave it legitimacy in relation to the European rulers. Finally, the overall European system of many small states meant that there was a structure of communication which could be transferred to the scientific community. There was a cross-border community of scientists. At the same time they organised themselves in competing associations. In the 17th century, science came to satisfy the conditions of autonomy, allocation of resources, legitimacy and organisation. Thus, according to Wuthnow, institutionalisation became a reality.

The last theme which Wuthnow deals with is religion and the possibility of analysing it at the institutional level. Here too the question is, how the institutionalisation of religion occurred. Again, Wuthnow emphasises that there is no direct reflection between the impact of religion and of social conditions. As an example he looks at the relation of the English state to Protestantism compared with the French state and Catholicism. During the period in which Protestantism emerged and became institutionalised, the English state was characterised by being strongly centralised, while the French state was marked by rivalry between different regions. According to Wuthnow, the reason why Protestantism succeeded in England, but not in France, was that the English king challenged the Pope's authority over his state and fought against the economic power of the church, while the French king supported educational reforms at both popular and state levels. So it is Wuthnow's opinion that the precondition for the Reformation, understood as belief and moral order, being able to succeed was the existence of favourable social conditions (Wuthnow, 1987, p. 325).

In general, Wuthnow asserts that an ideology needs social resources in order to be realised and maintained. On the other hand, ideology defines the moral duties which affect the allocation of social resources. Over time ideologies become institutionalised in organisations, professional roles, collective rituals and in relation to the state.

Having completed the discussion of the different levels of cultural analysis in relation to a number of themes, Wuthnow concludes with the question of the advantages and disadvantages of using this approach.

If we look first at the subjective level, Wuthnow points out that the approach has its limitations because of the methodological difficulties in revealing the meaning which an individual attaches to a specific phenomenon. This is because the individual will form his meaning in an immediate context, influenced by his own biography and intellectual experiences. This means that new experiences, connections and memories will change the meaning which a person attaches to a phenomenon. At a theoretical level the limitation consists of an underestimation of the significance of social conditions for cultural development. The advantages of the subjective approach are, according to Wuthnow, that it is easier to get an intuitive feeling for what is happening. It makes it possible to investigate the degree of an individual's adherence to a given idea. It makes it possible to find out whether the individual is willing to defend and fight for a specific ideology. It makes it possible to clarify the relationship between symbol and person.

Wuthnow says that the limitations of analysis at the structural level are that this approach has a tendency to operate with structures consisting of pairs of opposites. The advantages of this approach are that it is possible to study deviations from normality, developments in cultural patterns over time and the possibility of studying moral order, including ambivalence towards the moral order. Finally, Wuthnow emphasises that the structural approach gives good possibilities for studying culture as an objective phenomenon.

The limitations of analysis at the dramaturgical level are, says Wuthnow, that with this approach there is a lack of a theoretical specification of the central concepts in relation to the moral order. From this it follows that there is theoretical uncertainty about how one should understand the dramatisation of social relations by cultural forms. The advantages of the dramaturgical approach consist in seeing ideology as a response to social conditions, seeing the cultural dramatisation of the moral order as a response to moral uncertainty and ambivalence, and finally, in stressing that ideologies help to strengthen moral duties.

Finally there is the institutional level. The limitations of analysis at this level are that one can too easily ignore analysis of the content and form of culture because the institutions are themselves very complex. It is therefore necessary to ensure lower levels where cultural variations can be subject to more detailed analysis. The advantages of analysis at the institutional level are that social resources are regarded as necessary preconditions for cultural production, that social movements are recognised as fighting for a given ideology, and that the importance of the role of the state is recognised.

In conclusion, Wuthnow stresses that culture should not just be understood as a cultural form. It must be understood more broadly:

> "Institutional analyses of culture run the danger of focusing too heavily on deliberately produced cultural forms … culture also needs to be considered more broadly as the symbolic-expressive dimension of social life generally, as an aspect of behavior that communicates implicitly as well as explicitly. Keeping in mind the

> structural and dramaturgic levels of analysis is, therefore, likely to be a useful corrective in pursuing institutional analyses of culture." (Wuthnow, 1987, p. 348).

Wuthnow's conclusion is that institutional analysis is important, but that it must be supported by analyses at the dramaturgical and structural levels. The subjective level fades into the background.

In this work on meaning and moral order, Wuthnow maintains the definition of culture which he put forward with the other authors of *Cultural Analysis*; that is, the view of culture as the symbolic-expressive aspect of human behaviour. At the same time, he distances himself from the view he put forward in *The Consciousness Reformation*, that culture should be understood as meaning systems. It is clear that Wuthnow wishes to go beyond the very subjective approach which he started using as a guide to his cultural research. For this reason *Meaning and Moral Order* is a decisive book for Wuthnow's later work. It is here that he comes to terms with his own and sociology's past. He introduces the neo-structuralist approach in order to move on to structure-oriented analysis. The wish to include social conditions as the background to culture also leads him to include the dramaturgical level and the institutional level. His view is that concrete analysis can contain all the levels referred to.

The work also includes the beginnings of a theory of culture. Culture consists of elements which can be investigated in themselves, as well as relations between them which can be investigated. Culture has a function, which is the ability to dramatise both the moral and the social order. The function of ritual is thus to communicate the moral order, while the function of ideology is to dramatise the social order. Wuthnow stresses again and again that, when explaining culture, there is no direct reflection between social conditions and culture. What is decisive, for whether an ideology gains a foothold in a specific social environment, is whether the form of ideology is suited to the social environment and whether the ideology is able to communicate something about the social relations in the environment in question. Even the process through which an ideology obtains a foothold requires a social movement which can acquire the resources necessary for ensuring the dissemination of the ideology. Wuthnow says that such a process must pass through three phases: production, selection and institutionalisation. It is through this process that a relationship is created between the social conditions and the ideology.

## *Communities of discourse*

In his book *Communities of Discourse*, which is probably his most significant work so far, Wuthnow maintains and deals in more depth with the theory which he developed in *Meaning and Moral Order*. *Communities of Discourse* contains an analysis of the development of the Reformation, the Enlightenment, and of socialism in Europe. Wuthnow considers these three ideational fields as ideologies, and the main aim of his work is to explain the articulation of these ideologies.

In the introduction to the book he establishes some of the concepts which are most important for his analysis. These are the concepts of culture, discourse and ideology.

> "Culture is understood here ... as a form of behavior itself and as the tangible results of that behavior. In the present context it is distinguished ... as religious discourse, sermons, theological writings, instruction in the ways of worshipping, literature, plays, newspapers, philosophical treatises, political tracts, party platforms

and propaganda. ... The important point is that culture is explicitly produced ..." (Wuthnow, 1989a, p. 15).

Culture can thus be observed in the actions of the producers and in the artefacts that are produced by these actions. However, culture exists in a dynamic context, so Wuthnow introduces the concept of communities of discourse. Discourse combines the written with the verbal, the formal and the informal, the gestural or ritual and the conceptual. This discourse is carried on within a community of competing producers, interpreters, critics, listeners, consumers, patrons and other significant actors who are themselves the object of communication. Then Wuthnow introduces the concept of ideology. This concept refers to the identifiable constellation of discursive elements which, to one extent or another, articulate the social context in which they exist.

As a starting point for empirical analysis of the three ideologies, Wuthnow establishes some sequences of concepts. He calls this his theoretical scaffold or loose-fitting framework for the ensuing empirical analysis. To start with, he creates three sequences of concepts: a sequence for social conditions, a sequence for social processes and a sequence for cultural articulation.

In his investigation of social conditions, Wuthnow distinguishes between the environmental conditions, the institutional contexts and action sequences. The environmental conditions consist of the most general social, cultural, political and economic contours. The task is to investigate how these conditions develop and change. Such changes will very probably affect the resources which are needed to bring about new cultural movements. The institutional context consists of the organisational situations in which a given ideology is created and disseminated. Such situations usually include power, economic support, persons and legitimacy. The institutional context includes schools, universities, churches, scientific academies, newspapers, government bodies, political parties etc. Within this framework, it is possible for cultural producers to obtain access to the necessary resources. And finally, there are the action sequences. These include the behaviour of producers and consumers, and the decisions taken by patrons, censors and political leaders. These actions take place within the institutional context and are a necessary condition for cultural development. In order for there to be cultural development there must be action sequences, and for these actions resources must be provided through the institutional contexts, and there must be a development of the environmental conditions which make it possible to transfer resources to new cultural movements.

The relationship which must exist between the social conditions and a given ideology must be studied as a process. It is a process which involves mutual influence and adaptation. The study of this process requires a distinction to be made between production, selection and institutionalisation. Production concerns formulating ideas, initiating discourse, writing books and articles, arranging courses, publishing newspapers etc. This production is often manifold and overwhelming. There must therefore be some selection. There must be a choice of genres, styles, schools, etc. Some forms obtain greater support than others. Some forms obtain more resources than others. Some forms of discourse start to adapt to particular environments. Finally there is institutionalisation. Some mechanisms become routine, some styles predominate, certain forms of communication become standard, organisations obtain control over access to resources. The result becomes relatively stable institutional structures.

Then there is the question of the articulation of a given ideology. Here, Wuthnow's view is that the articulation of an ideology will never fit perfectly with its environment. There must be a certain element of disarticulation. The ideology must, to some extent, free itself from its environment. The concepts which Wuthnow distinguishes here are the social horizon, the discursive field and figural action. The social horizon consists of the properties of the real world in which the ideology has been produced. These elements consist of both the context for the ideology and the elements of text which the ideology consists of. The world, as experienced, will thus be incorporated in the text, but this is a selective transformational process. The text and the social world will be only partially in agreement with each other. The discursive field refers to the symbolic space or structure of the ideology itself. Such a symbolic space can consist of pairs of opposites, but it can also be more complex. The discursive field supplies the fundamental categories within which thinking can take place. It sets the limits and defines the topics which can be considered. Following this, articulation becomes a question of including in the discursive field special themes from the social horizon. Disarticulation becomes a question of developing a conceptual space within which creative reflection can take place. In this way it is possible to identify theoretical questions of more enduring significance. Figural action refers to representative behaviour and forms of thinking within the discursive field. Figural action contributes to the solution of the problems defined within the discursive field. They thus give direction to behaviour. It is figural action which is abstracted from concrete social situations but set in a more general framework for discourse. Articulation here consists of identifying the problems in the social horizon which are incorporated in figural action. Disarticulation consists of making figural action representative and adapting it to a more general conceptual field. If figural action is to function as a model for behaviour, it must be both concrete and general.

> "... the question of articulation becomes one of identifying features of the social horizon that are incorporated directly into the depiction of figural action, or that limit the ways in which that action can be depicted. And the question of disarticulation is a matter of determining the ways in which figural action is indeed representative and confined within more abstract conceptual fields ... For figural action to provide an effective model for behavior it must demonstrate both concreteness ... and generality and openness ..." (Wuthnow, 1989a, p. 14).

The aim of these sequences of concepts is, says Wuthnow, that they should give a better understanding of the relationship between social conditions and ideologies. The concrete ideologies which the concepts relate to are the Reformation, the Enlightenment and socialism.

The first ideological movement which Wuthnow focuses on is the Reformation. The starting point for his discussion of the Reformation is its contemporary context. Wuthnow describes rural life in Europe and sees a clear connection between the agrarian class structure and religion at the beginning of the 16th century. To start with, there was clear support for the Catholic church by the land-owning classes, which in turn gave material and symbolic advantages to the agrarian upper class. The growth of economic activity, with increased internal trade, a growing population, and rising prices all led to a higher living standard in Europe. In particular, it led to the growth of towns, both in population and in importance. The towns were thus the social environment in which the Reformation was able to take root. With their growing economic importance, the towns could free themselves from the domination of the powerful landed aristocracy. They were able to achieve a level of autonomy. The way to secure this autonomy was via religious innovation. The local authorities in the towns thus had a clear incentive to support the Reformation.

Wuthnow also takes up again the discussion of the connection between the structure of the state and the development of religion in different parts of Europe. Central Europe was characterised by decentralised states with towns which, because of their growing trade, achieved an increasing degree of autonomy. This was the point of departure for the Reformation. Northern Europe was less fragmented. Here it was not only the increasing strength of the towns, but also the growing power of the rulers who wanted greater autonomy in relation to the landed aristocracy. It was therefore particularly the rulers and the townspeople who espoused the new religious ideas. It was the same in England, where the king was the decisive actor for implementing the Reformation. The most important event was that the Catholic church stood in the way of the king's desire for a divorce. This led to the king breaking with the Catholic church and, together with the townspeople, carrying through the Reformation.

In eastern Europe, the increased economic activity consisted of increased agricultural production, rather than increased trade. This meant that the landed aristocracy was strengthened while the position of the townspeople was weakened. Against this background the new religious ideas had difficulty in gaining a foothold. It was the same in France. Here, because of its economic progress, the landed aristocracy was able to keep its control over the state. The consequence of this was that the Reformation was repressed and existing religious customs were maintained. Another consequence was that the clergy continued to be recruited from the ranks of the nobility and it was expected that their families would continue to give material support to the church. In Spain, the state was heavily dependent on the landed aristocracy, both in relation to taxation and loans etc., and because of the extensive military activity. There was no development of a bourgeoisie. Here too there was no basis for the establishment of new religious ideas.

Altogether, Wuthnow argues that it is the institutional context and its channelling of economic progress which was decisive for the extent to which there was or was not religious renewal. Economic progress did not, in itself, give rise to religious renewal. On the basis of this discussion, Wuthnow looks in more depth at the institutionalisation and articulation of the Reformation.

Within the geographical areas where the Reformation gained ground, there were differing developments. Where there was most fragmentation, there was the greatest religious diversity. The local authorities had different interests with regard to reform and control of doctrinal development. In England, it was the state which stood behind the reform of who should have access to the scriptures. The institutional framework was thus decisive for which reforms and which ideas predominated. Relations between the head of state, the landed aristocracy, the church and wider society influenced the direction which the Reformation took. However, the content of the Reformation was not determined by this institutional framework, it was determined by the creative processes of the reformers (Wuthnow, 1989a, p. 130).

Wuthnow's opinion is that the close relationship between the social context and discourse, was due to the fact that the discourse primarily had the character of a sermon. This meant that there was a strong identification between the narrator and the narrative, that there was a strong identification between the preacher's public role and his text, and because the preacher was a figural actor. The actions of the preacher were an example to his flock. In addition to this, the preacher was just as interested in the practice of religion as he was in doctrine. This was rooted in ordinary life and referred to local history. In the writings of Luther, there was a constant dialectic between references to the social environment and references to biblical characters. In this way, Luther created an ideology which, on the one hand, articulated practical conditions, and, on the other hand, set them in a critical light. He created a discursive field. Within this discursive field the actors were given certain moral duties, including discretion, responsibility, to serve the purposes of God, to follow ethical standards of behaviour etc. These moral instructions were in the nature of a framework within which the individual could operate as one who was morally responsible. Because of their content, and because of the form in which they were disseminated, which was through preaching, the figural roles which were disseminated through the Reformation were sufficiently open so that they could speak to the individual long after the concrete circumstances had changed.

The second ideological movement which Wuthnow focuses on is the Enlightenment. Here too, the contemporary context must be the starting point of the discussion. 17th century Europe was characterised by stagnation and a declining population. Wars, rebellions and revolutions were part of everyday life at the start of the century, but from the middle of the 1600s mercantilism began to influence relations between states and establish more peace and growth.

Mercantilism was first and foremost a method for creating incomes for states. Mercantilism therefore expressed a high degree of regulation of the relations between states, while being the basis for competition between the same states. In this situation, states needed to acquire powers not just impinging on social, economic and political life, but also on cultural life. Cultural production was a way in which the state could display its wealth and power. By sponsoring cultural activities, states could demonstrate their strength to competitors. At the same time, mercantilism opened the way for cross-border communication. This meant that scientists, authors, artists and philosophers could communicate with greater ease and exchange ideas, regardless of where they came from. Finally, mercantilism and growth in agricultural and industrial production opened the way for the growth of the bourgeoisie, and thus the development of a market for cultural products.

The intellectual background for the Enlightenment was characterised by religious conflicts between the different sects which had sprung up in the wake of the Reformation, and of religious conflicts between Jesuits and anti-Jesuits. There were also conflicts between religious and political movements (Wuthnow, 1989a, p. 169).

By analysing the Enlightenment's cultural development in nine different European countries, Wuthnow concludes that the cultural activities of the Enlightenment were strongest in those countries where the economic growth was strongest and where the bourgeoisie was in the strongest position. Another prerequisite for enabling the cultural activities of the Enlightenment to flourish was that there should be a strong state bureaucracy. There was a strong connection between the elite which created the cultural products of the Enlightenment and the state bureaucracy. It was the state which helped finance the cultural products and sometimes the producers of culture were employed in the state bureaucracy.

A strong centralised bureaucracy was thus a prerequisite for the cultural production of the Enlightenment to have effect. Without a centralised bureaucracy there was a lack of resources for cultural production. Another necessary condition was a separation of powers between Parliament, for example, and the royal executive. Such a division of authority allowed freedom for cultural development. Both these prerequisites were satisfied in France, England and Prussia. Other countries did not satisfy both prerequisites. Holland, Sweden and Austria could not satisfy the first condition, while Russia and Spain could not satisfy the second. A third requirement for Enlightenment activity was the existence of some centrifugal forces, including an independent judiciary, institutionalised channels for resolving religious and ethnic conflicts etc. This requirement was lacking in Russia and Spain. As a consequence, the cultural production of the Enlightenment was strongest in France, England and Prussia.

The cultural producers had an ambivalent relation to the state. On the one hand they were dependent on the support which they could obtain from the state, and on the other hand they had to distance themselves from the same state. This ambivalence gave rise to tensions in their works. On the one hand, they used the rational form which they had learnt through their legal and administrative training, and on the other hand, they were strongly critical of rationalism. This ambivalent attitude towards the state also gave rise to tensions between public and private life, between duty and freedom, and between highly formalised polemic and free fiction (Wuthnow, 1989a, pp. 315-316).

Such tensions were further exacerbated by geographical circumstances. Authors lived in large towns like Paris, London and Berlin, and had the possibility of communicating privately. They could have private exchanges of views which were clearly separated from their public conduct. In their works there was therefore concern for the two separate arenas, the private self and the public roles, and for the relations between these arenas. The more changeable that public life became, the more the self became the subject of reflection. The self was vulnerable and had to be protected. The key to this protection of the self lay in the strength of social relations, and the means for strengthening these relations was discourse.

In this way the discourse of the Enlightenment created a vision that discourse might in itself be valuable. The idea was that the self should be strengthened because, for example, through discursive activity one expresses points of view and adopts attitudes to political questions. In this way discursive activity creates a relationship between the public role and the private self. Where the self is weak, or lacks a public role, it must be defined in relation to other people and base its views on the inclusion of other authorities.

When discourse is important, words and speech are decisive. Words can have several meanings, so there is scope for interpretation; speech acquires the power to construct reality; truth becomes relational; and there is space for creativity. The consequence of this is that discourse can manipulate and redefine categories of reality to the point where new distinctions are created. When words have new relations to each other, they also take on new meanings.

The essence of the thinking of the Enlightenment, according to Wuthnow, was the separation between the private self and the public role which was made on the basis of discourse. When the public role is changeable, this enables authors to create new works. This changeability in public life also leads to a weakening of the self, because the self is dependent on these public roles. When the self does not have any inner authority, it must be defined as a product of social relations and especially as a product of discursive relations. In this way, words are the key to power. And the ability to manipulate words, to objectify them and give them new meanings, is the sign of personal freedom (Wuthnow, 1989a, pp. 321-323).

The discursive field of the Enlightenment was, says Wuthnow, marked by a polarity between traditional institutionalised beliefs and references to nature. On the one side there were the attitudes rooted in the church, educational institutions and the state, and on the other side there were the attitudes rooted in nature. The writers of the Enlightenment were so occupied with nature because of their perception of the split between the public and the private. They found freedom and the opportunity to experiment with lifestyles in nature. It was in nature that they could find the basis for knowledge, morality, feelings for the social etc.

Wuthnow points out that this polarity of cultural products was often based on personal experiences. For example, when Voltaire was at school he recognised that there was an opposition between strict Jesuitical morality and a more tolerant free-thinking morality. This meant that Voltaire could base his thinking both on the highly formalised classical thinking and on the less formal free-thinking. In German thinking, represented by Albrecht von Haller, we see the tension between the evils of urban life and, on the other hand, cultivation and refinement.

Such contradictions could not be allowed to remain unresolved. Rousseau put these contradictions in a chronological perspective in which development moved out of darkness and towards light. At the same time literature created some figural actors who could serve as examples. The citizen, the businessman, was thus a model one could strive to emulate in public life. He was a model for ethical behaviour. Conversely, Enlightenment writers directed their fire against the lifestyles of the landed aristocracy and the court (Wuthnow, 1989a, pp. 330-332).

The separation between public and private life led to the cultivation of specific genres. The first person vanished from literature and fiction prevailed. Personal behaviour could be used in narrow private circles, while public behaviour could be presented in fiction, first and foremost in novels, The writer withdrew and let the characters speak for themselves. Another genre was the historical narrative, in which history was recreated from a personal point of view. In this way it was possible to create a positive line of development in which the negative was replaced by the positive.

Wuthnow emphasises that the writings of the Enlightenment took concrete events as their starting points, but that their aim was to deal with more general topics. It was the universal they were interested in. They gave weight to generalisation, and even abstraction. But this was closely allied to thinking about natural sciences. They built on the idea that nature everywhere gives a basis for the same sorts of abstractions. In the same way the educated elite of Europe created the idea of a cultural zone. The general was emphasised rather than the particular. In this way they ignored the ethnic, national and religious conflicts in Europe (Wuthnow, 1989a, p. 343).

The writers of the Enlightenment created a harmony between text and context by using known genres. They reached their public by using narrative and satire and by expressing themselves briefly. They thus built on the form of communication which had been developed up to the time of the Enlightenment and was known by their readers.

The third ideological movement which Wuthnow focuses on is European socialism from the 1870s up to the First World War. The environmental conditions circumstances for this movement were the growing resources resulting from the growth of industrial production, international trade, the population and colonial relations to the rest of the world. As a result of these developments, a numerically large working class emerged. This was a great challenge to the cultural institutions which had grown up in the Enlightenment: the place of science in the universities, primary education for the wider population, freedom of religious belief, the growing demand for books, etc. (Wuthnow, 1989a, pp. 357-359).

In this connection too, Wuthnow makes a review of the most relevant European countries. He does this by establishing which factors were most significant for the development of socialism. Here again he found that economic growth was significant for the development of ideology, but that it was not in itself sufficient to explain why it was more important in some countries than in others. He thus questions why socialism had greater success in Germany than in France or England. True, Germany had more rapid industrialisation than the other two countries, but urbanisation proceeded just as rapidly in England as in Germany, and the working class grew as quickly in France as in Germany. He also questions why socialism gained equal footholds in Denmark and in Sweden when the two countries were not industrialised in the same tempo.

According to Wuthnow, the answer to these questions is to be found in the political context. In the fight to win the hearts and minds of the proletariat, the socialist movement had to compete with republicans, liberals, state bureaucrats and aristocratic regimes. What was most important for socialist parties was which of these interests held power. Where there was a parliamentary majority dominated by liberal or republican ideas, the bourgeoisie could prevail upon the working class and persuade them away from the socialist movement. This happened in France, England, the Netherlands and to a certain extent in Norway. Where a strongly monarchical state was based on an alliance between the landed aristocracy and the upper ranks of the bourgeoisie, the liberal parties were weak. If the conservative alliance prosecuted and prohibited the socialist parties, as was the case in Germany, for example, a situation arose in which the socialist movement could develop its own identity and aim to win parliamentary influence, set in train activities for legitimising the movement, and develop a true socialist ideology. This is what happened in Germany, Denmark, Sweden and Belgium. There was thus a specific institutional context which was decisive for whether economic growth meant that the socialist movement could develop and take root (Wuthnow, 1989a, pp. 480-481).

According to Wuthnow, the content of socialist discourse was marked by fundamental distinctions between theory and practice and between the existing bourgeois society and the classless society of the future.

The socialist ideology was directed towards practical social reforms, and the legitimacy of the movement depended on its ability to strengthen and improve the conditions of the working class. With the complexity which typified the contemporary institutional context, a desire to strengthen the welfare of the working class had to be accompanied by an effective ideological basis for social practice. The consequence was that different parts of the socialist movement were very much concerned with the question of the relation between theory and practice.

In the socialist discourse a distinction was developed between theory and practice so that the two elements could be developed independently. Theoretical works were written in an obscure and unapproachable style. Their main use was as a frame of reference for the debate between the leading figures of the movement. However, practical ideology was related to the social context. It was in the genre of lists of demands and political platforms (Wuthnow, 1989a, pp. 483-484).

At the same time, the socialist movement aimed at development and change. Thus two opposing poles developed in the discourse. The negative pole was the existing bourgeois society, and in this connection its links with existing religions, dogmas and liberal values came under attack. The bourgeoisie was thus not just a social class, but equally a symbolic construction. The positive pole consisted of a vision of the future, which was a vision of a classless society. But this fundamental polarity was followed by a number of other opposites, as for example between illusion and reality, ideology and science, the past and the future and so on. In this way, the polarity between bourgeois society and the classless society created a discursive space, within which many different debates could be based.

In the light of the distinction between bourgeois society and the classless society, the concept of the proletariat came to play an important role. This concept developed to become a category laden with symbolism, whose content lay somewhere between the workers' institutional experiences on the one hand, and the potentialities the workers would have through the transformation of society, on the other hand. The concept of the proletariat remained very abstract, which Wuthnow believed was due to the existence of highly complex class relations. As a result, many different concepts of the proletariat were developed. The proletariat thus became a symbolic construction that stood both for the negative elements of the bourgeois society and for the possibilities of escaping from these negative elements. Relationally, the proletariat stood for exploitation, alienation and poverty. Functionally, it stood for action, historical progress and the possibility of moving forward to a more humane society. This ideological construction of the proletariat was thus a consequence of the specific discursive field from which it arose, which was the field between bourgeois society and the classless society (Wuthnow, 1989a, pp. 500-501).

The distinction between theory and practice led to focusing on the consciousness of the proletariat. Increased consciousness was necessary for building a bridge between theory and practice. The proletariat had to adopt the discursive vision in order to be able to understand existing conditions and future possibilities. There also had to be a horizon of socialist analysis to replace the bourgeois analysis. By placing himself within this socialist discourse, the worker could have visions. On this basis he was able to make choices about his actions.

The figural actor within the socialist ideology was thus the proletariat. The proletariat constituted the model and served as an example for thinking, acting and changing.

Following the analyses of the developments of the Reformation, the Enlightenment and socialism, Wuthnow puts his results into a wider theoretical context. It is thus his belief that within sociology there are two significant theoretical trends with regard to understanding cultural change. On the one hand there are theories which see cultural development as a result of an ever more complex society. According to this school of thought, cultural development consists of continual adjustment to the increasing level of social complexity. Wuthnow suggests that this school of thought includes Durkheim, Parsons, Luhmann, Bellah and Habermas. On the other hand, there are the theories which see cultural development as legitimising changed class structures. According to this school of thought, as soon as a class becomes sufficiently powerful, ideologies will be developed which will be able to legitimise the dominance of this class. This school of sociological thought includes Marx and Weber.

Wuthnow sees his own findings as a contribution to a third way of understanding cultural change. He believes that an ideology's own internal structures help to ensure an eventual harmonisation between the ideology and its environment.

> "Rather than conceiving of these social conditions as having a purely unidirectional impact on the rise of new ideologies, it has also proven necessary to posit an interactive relation – a process – in which the internal patterns of elements within ideologies play an important role in determining the eventual fit between ideologies and their environments." (Wuthnow, 1989a, p. 537).

When Wuthnow reviews the three historical periods which he is concerned with, he gets an overview of the relationship between capitalism and cultural development. As expressions of capitalism he includes the market, the classes and the state. It is his view that there is no direct reflection from capitalism to cultural development. It is true that the market is the framework for cultural production, but it is not the logic of the market which drives cultural development. The market is itself a result of the social arrangements. It is the same for the classes. Classes consist of a significant element of the social context for cultural development, but ideologies do not reflect these class conditions. They are rather an element of the ideological construction itself. And finally, there is the state. Here Wuthnow points out that, over time, ideology becomes integrated in political power. Nevertheless, it is not political power which lies behind cultural development. It is rather the ideologies which promote the structures of the capitalist state which have prevailed.

It is Wuthnow's view that cultural change grows out of complex historical conditions, but that there is not a necessary connection between these conditions and the actual cultural development. History is made by actors who make choices on the basis of the information available to them, but it is also created by the restrictions of tradition, special interests, economic conditions, and political conditions.

Cultural producers knew about these limitations and were critical of them.

> "Their criticism of these conditions was often extreme and unrelenting. It was sharpened by an alternative vision, a vision constructed discursively, a vision that was pitted authoritatively against the established order, not as its replacement but as a conceptual space in which new modes of behaviour could be considered. The strength of their discourse lay in going beyond negative criticism and beyond idealism to identify working models of individual and social action for the future." (Wuthnow, 1989a, pp. 582-583).

In this major work on three important contributions to the cultural development of Europe, Wuthnow defines culture as being behaviour and the tangible results of this behaviour. More specifically, it consists of the discourse which is accessible in the form of written documents. These can be theological writings, sermons, dramas, novels, philosophical doctrines, political tracts and propaganda. This discourse includes a community of discourse consisting of competing producers, interpreters, critics, audiences, consumers, patrons etc. The concept of ideology is a sub-concept of culture. It is defined as being a constellation of discursive elements which articulate a given social context. Wuthnow thus maintains that culture consists of behaviour, but it is clearly his view that culture is moving more and more in the direction of being discourse. It is the text and the context which is the point of focus in his analyses.

The main purpose of his work is to explain the connection between social conditions and cultural development. To start with, Wuthnow distances himself both from the theory of reflection and from the theory of legitimation. Culture neither reflects nor legitimises social conditions. On the contrary, there is a gradual adjustment between culture and social conditions. Wuthnow emphasises that this process is not automatic. The outcome depends on the choices which human beings make in the light of environmental limitations. It is a basic tenet of Wuthnow's theory that human beings make decisions or selections. The environmental conditions of culture thus consist, not merely of resources and institutional contexts, but also of actions and decisions of producers and consumers. The social process consists not only of the production of cultural products, but also of selection and institutionalisation. The formulation of a given ideology consists not just of articulation but also of disarticulation. On the one hand, certain themes from the social horizon must be included and certain forms of representative behaviour must be developed, and on the other hand these themes and figural actions must be liberated from their concrete circumstances and be put into a more general frame. Space must be made for creative reflection.

Thus, behind this cultural development there lie choices, decisions and creativity. This concerns human activities which unfold within the limitations of environmental conditions. The result of such processes is that the concrete is opposed to the general, so that a discursive space is formed. Within this discursive space there is an adjustment between cultural and social conditions. Thus this adjustment is not automatic. It is a result of human behaviour.

## *Cultural inclusion or exclusion*

In his book *Producing the Sacred*, Wuthnow turns his attention to his own society, America. The question he gets to grips with is how the sacred is produced. It is Wuthnow's opinion that the sacred, the spiritual and the holy are cultural phenomena which must be produced. Therefore, he considers the institutional conditions which can be the basis for such production, including membership of a church, the church hierarchy, special interest groups, academics and public rituals. In his analysis, he reviews these institutions in order to investigate the extent to which they contribute to the production of the sacred.

The starting point for the analysis of how the sacred is produced is a theory of cultural production. Here again we see how Wuthnow emphasises the active role of people. Culture does not merely exist. It is something which people produce intentionally. Wuthnow himself says that the inspiration for this point of view comes from studies of art and literature, where it is evident that culture is produced, so it is relevant to take into account questions about resources and organisations (Wuthnow, 1994a, pp. 24-25).

There must be resources for education, salaries, buildings, etc., and to obtain such resources requires some form of organisation. Since resources are limited, such organisation will often provoke another organisation with competition between the two organisations. Some shared mechanisms will be developed between these organisations. There will be selective adaptation to the surrounding environment, and some organisations will gain in strength while others will disappear. In their search for resources, competing organisations will become more similar to each other in form and content. Finally, the organisations will find niches within their shared field, so that they will appear to be specialised. The consequence of this will be that cultural products will not only be the outcome of a given organisation, but of that organisation's positioning within the wider system. There is thus a long chain of factors which decides which products will prevail and which will not. (Wuthnow, 1994a, pp. 29-33).

> "... cultural production results in both products and by-products, that is, intended and unintended results." (Wuthnow, 1994a, p. 27).

If one looks at the production of the sacred, the intended results will usually be to create openness, inclusiveness, acceptance and love. The problem is that production of the sacred can lead to the opposite, cultural exclusion. In the same way that the increasing emphasis on abstraction can lead to cultural exclusion in the cultural and professional worlds, so too in the religious world products can be developed which contribute to cultural exclusion.

> "... any cultural organisation protects itself by generating products that in turn become the basis for cultural exclusion." (Wuthnow, 1994a, p. 34).

Production of the sacred is linked to questions of correct belief and behaviour. In order to survive in the wider system of organisations, church organisations must aim to attract the most important members of society and the resources which they can bring to the organisation, without opening up for the broad mass of people who want to be associated with these important people. To this end it must identify both its peculiar qualities and its similarities to other organisations. It must practise a belief which differs from that of other organisations. At the same time it must avoid making its beliefs too clear, but rather give them a sprinkling of general wisdom, rooted in historical, philosophical and theological sources. Concrete behaviour is promoted by rewarding people who, because of their social position, want to be included in the church organisation. This is done by giving these people special positions or by having them undertake church activities. The result of this will be that those people who feel uncomfortable with the lack of clarity of content and the absence of reward for their behaviour will leave the church organisation.

According to Wuthnow, church organisations not only produce sacred products. They also need to produce information about themselves. They produce information about their internal administration and planning, about the comings and goings of their leaders, about budgets and accounts etc. Religious organisations often tend to keep these two forms of product separate, but in an open society it is not possible to hide information about organisations. This means that, in addition to the production of the sacred, church organisations also contribute to the production of self-referential knowledge (Wuthnow, 1994a, pp. 38-39).

This distinction between sacred and self-referential knowledge is also reflected in the work of the church. The priest who gives an uplifting sermon must, at other times, take part in planning and budgeting. His work is split between the spiritual, which is necessary for giving a sermon, and the rational, which is necessary for running an organisation in a wider field of organisations (Wuthnow, 1994a, pp. 158-159).

This split is all the more explicit in the case of televangelists, where the pastor speaks of his inner convictions, while the whole arrangement is directed by media professionals. Here too there is a conflict between the rational purpose, to obtain resources for the church organisation through such media performance, and the spiritual purpose, to communicate feelings from the heart about one's belief (Wuthnow, 1994a, p. 165).

This split between the rational and the spiritual will often lead to a reaction. One form of reaction can be a fundamentalism in which a counter-discourse is developed in which God is the absolute who can, at any time, intervene and influence history. Another form of reaction can be a peripheral counter-discourse, characterised by mysticism and demonism (Wuthnow, 1994a, p. 159).

In this work, which Wuthnow describes as an essay, we have a confirmation of the view of culture as being something which is produced intentionally and which requires the use of resources. To some extent this work is an extension of *Communities of Discourse*. The new element which appears here is the distinction between the intended and unintended consequences of this cultural production. Here the explanatory element is the organisational framework for cultural production. When this concerns the production of the sacred, which is included as cultural production, the organisational circumstances, in this case the competition between organisations, can lead to unintended consequences.

Even though, to start with, church organisations aim at openness and inclusion, nevertheless, because of the organisational competition they come to depend on a culturally conditioned exclusion. It is best for them if they can attract the most socially important and economically well funded people without being burdened with the kind of people who would want to join these important people in the congregation. The key to this is the lack of precision of religious content, and rewarding a form of behaviour which few will understand.

Even if church organisations start with the aim of producing spirituality and feelings, because of the competition for resources they put more emphasis on rationality than on spirituality. In order to appear as organisations which are worth supporting, they must appear to be well organised and rational.

In this way the organisational conditions, or as Wuthnow usually expresses it – the institutional framework – is decisive for what comes out of the cultural production on the social level or in terms of content.

## *Channelling through institutions*

In his book, *God and Mammon in America*, Wuthnow investigates the attitudes of the American people to spiritual and material values. The book is based on the results of a nation-wide survey and a series of in-depth interviews.

In this book Wuthnow refers several times to American culture. Both religiosity and the prizing of material goods are part of American culture. Wuthnow considers general culture as being the background to the individual's values and behaviour. His aim is thus to investigate how general culture affects people's values and behaviour.

In the light of the general distinction between the spiritual and the material, Wuthnow investigates the extent to which people who have an active involvement in a church have different material values than people without such an involvement. He thus distinguishes between those who go to church once a week and those who do not. To start with, he shows that there is no distinction between these two groups as regards their position in the labour market. The difference becomes apparent in their attitudes to work and earning money. It appears that people who go to church have a better attitude towards their work than other people. They find their work more fulfilling, they complain less about their pay and they have a better understanding of the purpose of their work. Wuthnow interprets this result as showing that religious feelings have a therapeutic function in relation to economic behaviour in the post-industrial society.

Wuthnow sees this result as an extension of the classical sociological tradition according to which cultural phenomena, which cannot easily be manipulated, have an important influence on the meaning of work.

> "Cultural phenomena that could not so easily be manipulated were examined and shown to have a decisive impact on the meaning of work. Religion was one such phenomenon." (Wuthnow, 1994b, p. 76).

Religion also has a role to play when it comes to work ethic. Wuthnow demonstrates that people who attach importance to religion are more ethical in their behaviour. They are less inclined to bend the rules in their dealings with other people, to be late for work or to use the facilities of their workplace for private purposes.

It is Wuthnow's view that ethics must always be based on some underlying value-orientation. As an example of such value-orientation he refers to the orientation towards personal benefit, orientation towards corporate benefit, altruism, moral absolutism and religiously conditioned morality. Wuthnow demonstrates that these basic value-orientations are significant for basic ethical behaviour in the workplace. It is apparent that people who are oriented towards personal benefit show the lowest ethical standards of conduct in the workplace, while those who are characterised by moral absolutism or religiously conditioned morality have the highest ethical standards of behaviour. And, according to Wuthnow, these two latter value orientations are found first and foremost among people involved in religious groups. Wuthnow therefore sees these religious groups as a kind of counterculture within the broader general culture.

> "Such groups [religious fellowship groups] can serve as a kind of counterculture, helping to combat the more relativistic or utilitarian norms that may prevail in the workplace." (Wuthnow, 1994b, p. 109).

Wuthnow raises the question of how American culture is able to deal with the contradictions and paradoxes which it contains. How does it deal with the conflict between the material and the spiritual and the conflict between individualism and altruism?

> "American culture – perhaps any culture – is built on a foundation of paradox. The paradox of intense individualism being present in the same settings as a deeply altruistic spirit, for example, is one. The simultaneous presence of spirituality and materialism in our society is clearly another." (Wuthnow, 1994b, p. 157).

Wuthnow says that people deal with such paradoxes by drawing symbolic boundaries between the two contradictory elements. For example, the boundary between the spiritual and the material can be a border between the inner and the external lives. This means that it is possible to protect the inner life against the external world. The way in which these symbolic boundaries can be drawn, can vary according to the social circumstances and from individual to individual. (Wuthnow, 1994b, p. 162).

The dualism between the spiritual and the material is thus a general cultural condition in American society. This dualism is a prerequisite for evaluating the material. One must have a sense that something other than the material exists, in other words the spiritual, in order to be able to evaluate the spiritual. Wuthnow's view is that the sense of the spiritual is most apparent in those people for whom religion has the greatest meaning. It is apparent that those who attach the greatest importance to religion are also those who are most concerned about the importance which is attached to materialism and money in American society.

Just as the boundaries between the spiritual and the material are drawn as symbolic borders, so the material is also dealt with as a symbol.

> "... materialism is a symbol. It stands for something else ... To be precise: materialism is a generalized symbol that stands for evil in our culture." (Wuthnow, 1994b, p. 177).

The fact that the boundary between the material and the spiritual is dealt with as a symbolic border does not mean that it has no significance. Wuthnow believes that it is important that such boundaries should be respected. The material sphere will be especially problematic if it transgresses beyond its sphere and invades the spiritual sphere. Here it can influence people to become so involved in the material that they can infringe the normal standards which set a limit to selfishness. The spiritual sphere can be similarly problematic. If it invades the material sphere, it can absorb so much from it that it seems to be infected by materialism (Wuthnow, 1994b, p.183).

Wuthnow thus sees a distinction between the spiritual and the material as a fundamental principle of ordering. This principle establishes some basic categories which influence how other assumptions and ideas are related. Maintaining a special spiritual sphere means that one can evaluate materialism, assign values to it and distance oneself from it. Through the development of such basic distinctions, people adjust to the special social conditions under which they live (Wuthnow, 1994b, p. 188).

In this work, Wuthnow operates with a national culture which consists of some basic distinctions and categories. These basic categories are the result of contemporary social conditions. On the basis of these categories and distinctions, the individual person can develop some general value-orientations and some more specific values and actions. In this way it is possible to generate insight and understanding. How this happens depends on the other aspects of the life of the individual. For example, it can be important whether the person in question is involved in church life. An involvement in church life gives special possibilities for dealing with the contradictions between the material and the spiritual. For example, this is observed in connection with the values and ethics of working life and attitudes to money and materialism. It can thus be said that the general national culture is channelled to individual people through their institutional attachments, and especially through their attachment to or lack of attachment to spiritually based institutions. As a result, people with varying degrees of attachment to spiritual institutions develop differing general value-orientations and thus differing specific values and actions.

## *Cultural constructions*

The last of Wuthnow's works which will be considered in this connection is his book *Poor Richard's Principle*. This book, too, is concerned with American culture. Wuthnow focuses on the American dream. He perceives that this dream has a moral frame. It is his thesis that this moral frame has changed from seeing economics and morality as an integrated whole to seeing these two elements as separate. In the original American dream, hard work and economic progress were linked to personal, family, communal and spiritual values. Towards the end of the 19$^{th}$ century, the American dream was influenced by scientific thinking which made it difficult to integrate personal values with the more formal discussion of economic life. The aim of the book is to investigate the status of the American dream towards the end of the 20$^{th}$ century. Are morality and economics still separate, and if they are, are there sources for the promotion of values which can make it possible to re-integrate morality and economics? And finally, there is the question of whether the original moral discourse can help re-establish a moral framework for American society. Is it possible to re-build the American dream? The methodology on which the book is based is qualitative interviews, and there are also references to survey research.

The problem behind the discussion of morality and economics is the question of the extent to which there are cultural resources which can make it possible to restrict economic behaviour. Where can people find support for limiting work obligations, maintaining ethical standards in working life, and ensuring security for themselves and their loved ones? What resources can people draw on when they set limits to economic life? (Wuthnow, 1996a, p. 9)

The starting point of this discussion is the establishment of the fact that economic life occupies an ever-increasing share of social life. Americans work ever more, have increasingly long working hours, feel that the ethical rules of the game are disregarded, are and feel ever more tired, feel more and more burnt out and so on. Against this background that Wuthnow asks where it is possible to find the resources for restricting economic behaviour.

The question is, what the attitude is of the American people to morality and economics at the end of the 20$^{th}$ century. How are work and money culturally constructed today? Are they constructed in a way which puts limits on economic life? What is the role of morality in setting such limits? Wuthnow pursues such questions in his analysis of the relationship of his respondents to work and money.

The first empirical question is whether the respondents undertake a cultural construction of work by relating it to wider values. Wuthnow investigates this problem by looking at the accounts which these people give for their work.

> "Understanding these accounts will help us recognize how much our commitment to jobs and careers depends on wider cultural understandings rather than monetary pressures alone." (Wuthnow, 1996a, p. 104).

When the respondents were asked to explain why they do their current work, they most frequently referred to the fact that their work is varied, gives them the possibility of making decisions, and gives them a certain pride, even if this may not always be the case. Wuthnow considers such explanations to be cultural constructions, which are more based on ideals than on realities. They are moral in the sense that they emphasise what is regarded as being good in relation to work.

> "These accounts are cultural constructions ... Insofar as they invoke fundamental definitions of reality, insofar as they suggest conceptions of the good, insofar as they tell us how to behave – they are fundamentally moral rather than economic. Yet they have been appropriated and shaped by economic institutions to the point that they seldom show any connection to the larger moral traditions that make up our cultural birthright." (Wuthnow, 1996a, p. 137).

The respondents thus legitimise their work by giving explanations which put their work in a wider moral context. In this way work becomes meaningful to them, and they feel a sense of duty towards their work.

The next empirical question was whether the respondents undertook any cultural construction of money, by relating it to wider values. It is clear that the attitudes of the respondents were characterised by taboos. Money is not something one talks about. Money is thus not only something which is public, it is also something which is highly personal and private. Money is linked to freedom, personal value and security. The lack of money is thus associated with restrictions, low self-esteem and lack of security.

This privatising of money means that it flows more freely than previously in relation to work. Money is linked to consumption which must be legitimised by explanations in the same way as work. Similarly, these explanations do not involve personal values to any great extent. Reference is made to the fact that a given purchase fits a chosen lifestyle, that there should be an appropriate level of comfort in everyday life, that one chooses something which stresses what is unique about oneself. One of the problems which the respondents pointed out is that money affects human relations between, for example, married partners and between parents and children. As a result, it is necessary to draw symbolic boundaries between money and human relations.

The question is, whether there are any institutions which can function as a source of human values and which can relate to work and money and thus make it possible to set limits to economic behaviour. In this respect, Wuthnow points to the family, the local community and religious feelings. The problem is that when these institutions operate as a source of personal values, problems arises in the relationship between these institutions and economic obligations. A family is an emotional haven where it is possible to escape from economic life. It stands as a counterpart to economic life. At the same time, internal relations within the family can be put under strain by economic life. The family is the place where children are influenced by advertisements and therefore where the pressures to consume are increased, where both parents are out at work and therefore away from home a lot, where men cultivate those sides of themselves which are repressed at work, and where women have to try to make daily life cohere. In the case of the local community, there is no longer any natural reciprocity. The individual must find his own balance between his own interests and his obligations towards others. These days, to show concern for others is taken as being to distance oneself from materialism. The problem is that voluntary action becomes a question of feelings, choice, gratitude and greed. It can also be something which is done to obtain a good reputation. Religion emphasises the distinction between the material and the spiritual, but it has always promoted work and the desire to earn money. The problem is that it is not always clear how the material should be limited.

The last question which Wuthnow takes up is whether it is possible to develop a moral framework for understanding economic obligations. For this purpose Wuthnow introduces two traditions, that of ascetic morality and that of expressive morality. Ascetic morality, which comes from the puritan sects, sees morality as a system of rules governing people's rights and duties. One must aim at integrity, beauty, truth, goodness, righteousness and avoid lies, deceit and falsehood. By setting up absolute goals and values, boundaries are set to economic behaviour. Money and work are the means for achieving the goals one sets oneself. Expressive morality, which came to the fore in the 19$^{th}$ century, puts more emphasis on enjoyment and joy. Here, what matters is to cultivate nature, feelings and taste. In this way limits are set to economic behaviour.

By using the interview material, Wuthnow relates these two moral discourses to the present. He investigates whether there are any survivals of this cultural heritage which make it possible to see how morality can be used as a barrier to economic life.

> "I also had another reason for introducing the ascetic and expressive moralist arguments: those are part of our cultural heritage, and, while often neglected in formal discussions of economic life, they probably still have some resonance in popular understandings of work and money. Put differently, we may find residues of these earlier arguments, perhaps modified by late-twentieth-century cultural orientations, that still guide and restrain economic commitments." (Wuthnow, 1996a, p. 335).

Wuthnow's opinion is that it is possible to find traces of the two forms of morality in the values of the American people. He describes two sets of values, each of which illustrate how the two forms of morality make themselves felt today. Today, ascetic morality is built on a looser connection between absolute values and the means that are necessary for putting these values into practice. Expressive morality puts more emphasis on inner experiences. Ascetic morality sees values as being related to objects, while expressive morality sees values in relation to domains of life. This means that they also look differently on the question of roles. Object-related values involve actors who are strong individualists, while domain-related values involve actors who are a part of a system. Ascetic morality is against laziness, lack of ambition etc., while expressive morality is against dependence, an exaggerated sense of duty, indecisiveness etc. Ascetic morality leads to responsibility and guilt, while expressive morality distances itself from guilt feelings. Ascetic morality involves mistrust of feelings, while expressive morality stresses the importance of feelings. Ascetic morality assumes that people know intuitively what is right and wrong, whereas expressive morality emphasises freedom. However, both types of morality emphasise reflection as the background to freedom, responsibility and the right to choose. With ascetic morality this reflection is based on an inner compass bearing, while expressive morality starts from the basis of language and symbols.

As for setting limits to economic behaviour, ascetic morality offers a balance between morality and economics, while expressive morality offers language and argues for differences between people. With ascetic morality people must be allowed to choose their own ways in the world of work, but with expressive morality the emphasis is on people's personal development.

Wuthnow concludes that both types of morality contain arguments which can legitimise restrictions to striving after wealth and material success. They establish opposing positions between concepts and categories. They give the individual the possibility of making choices and underline the need for complex strategies. They do not simply negate the economic world. With the help of a more open framework they bring a new viewpoint to it. Such a new view can make it possible to rescue the American dream.

In this work, Wuthnow operates with the concept of cultural construction. A cultural construction consists of the relation of a given phenomenon to values. More specifically, there is a relation of work and money to values. Through this relation, work and money are culturally constructed. The empirical investigation of such constructions takes place by studying the explanations which people give for their work and their attitudes to money. The values which are necessary for creating a cultural construction must come from somewhere. Here, Wuthnow identifies some social institutions: the family, local communities and religious associations. The problem is that when these institutions function as sources for the development of values, there is a problematic relation between these institutions and economic life. Finally, he points out that cultural heritage is significant to the development of values. Here he is thinking about morality. This morality operates as an open framework, from which opinions and strategies develop, and thus the basis for choice. The values that are necessary for creating cultural constructions can come both from contemporary social institutions and from the cultural heritage.

### *Discussion*

Not much has been written about the writings of Robert Wuthnow. There has been some discussion of his research into religious phenomena, but only very little has been written about his understanding of culture. Of these writings, those of Robertson and Griswold will be considered here.

In his book on globalisation, Robertson discusses, on the basis of the works of Wuthnow and other authors, how far sociology has succeeded in developing a theory of culture (Robertson, 1992). By reference to Wuthnow's preface to *Cultural Analysis*, Robertson refutes the idea that theory and method are especially undeveloped in the field of sociological theory of culture. Robertson believes that the theory of culture has made significant progress in recent years. Here he refers to the works of Parsons, Geertz, Sahlins, Swanson and Bourdieu.

Robertson may well be right in saying that there have been a number of contributions to sociological theory of culture. The problem is that, as there is no clear agreement about the concept of culture, it is difficult to speak of any real theoretical clarification.

In her book, *The Sociology of Culture*, Griswold refers, among other things, to Wuthnow's theory. In her discussion of culture and cultural change she disagrees with Wuthnow's idea that culture should be considered as something tangible. Her view is that culture must be understood on the basis of the choices which the actors make with regard to culture (Griswold, 1992, p. 324). Furthermore, she disagrees with Wuthnow's theory that the connective causes are only such that culture changes as a result of social change. She believes that the opposite can also be the case, that society changes as a result of cultural development (Griswold, 1994, p. 3). Finally, she criticises Wuthnow for his theory that when the moral order breaks down, new ideologies will arise. She believes that the outcome can equally well be that old ideologies are revived (Griswold, 1994, p. 150).

Griswold's criticism of Wuthnow does not express any systematic critique of Wuthnow's scientific work. There is criticism of certain points. It is surprising that she criticises Wuthnow for conceiving culture as being exclusively tangible products, and then goes on to suggest that one ought to consider culture as being expressed through human actions. In fact, the question of actions is central to Wuthnow's understanding of culture. He combined tangible artefacts with actions in his concept of culture. Her other criticisms, that culture can influence social conditions and that old ideas can make a return, are really empirical questions on which a view will not be expressed in this context.

Discussion of Wuthnow's theory of culture is thus sporadic and unsystematic. In what follows I shall try to summarise Wuthnow's understanding of culture and attempt to form a theory of culture. The starting point for this summary will be a statement of the social concerns that must lie behind his theoretical work and the sources of inspiration which he draws on. What do these mean for his methodology and what do they mean for his theory?

Robert Wuthnow's social concerns are most clearly apparent in his later works. He is concerned about the predominant economic behaviour, the growing materialism, about individualism and about rationality. In his works he asks how it is possible to limit and to distance oneself from these phenomena. It concerns him that ethics are disappearing from working life, that there are too few resources for family life, that local community life is becoming less substantial and problematic. He therefore raises questions about the extent to which there are institutions and moral guidelines which can help to set limits to economic life and its associated materialism, and to rationality etc. These concerns are directed towards morality and institutions. When he looks at religious institutions, it concerns him that there is cultural exclusion of people who do not have the right cultural and social background.

While these concerns can be seen most clearly in Wuthnow's more recent works, they can be traced back to his earliest writings. Here there were references to the religious meaning system being in retreat, and of it being replaced with a scientific meaning system and a mysticist meaning system. In his middle phase his concerns were more directed towards sociology than towards social realities. He believed that the sociology of culture had made little progress for many years. This was due to some limiting assumptions in sociology, specifically that culture is a subjective phenomenon, and that culture reflects social reality.

Wuthnow's prime concern is for the cultural development of his own country, and this concern makes him direct his attention to sociology's lack of development within a theory of culture. He requires further development of a theory of culture in order to do research in the area that concerns him most, which is culture.

The desire to develop further a sociological theory of culture leads Wuthnow to study this theory. Specifically, he studies the theories of Berger, Douglas, Habermas and Foucault, but he also follows the threads back to the classical writers. The question is, what these theories mean for Wuthnow's understanding of culture.

Wuthnow points out that the classical writers' concern for whether people could find any meaning in life led them to focus on the question of meaning and on culture's subjective aspects. The question of meaning is there in his earliest writings, and subsequently it is criticised for being inadequate, before turning up again in the more recent works. In the more recent writings the concept of values is introduced. Here Wuthnow defines cultural constructions as relating a given phenomenon to values. The inspiration from Weber is clear.

In the intervening years the classical writers have been banished from Wuthnow's writings. Even the distinction between subject and object is regarded as putting a limit on the development of theory. In this phase Wuthnow was influenced by the four writers whose work is studied in *Cultural Analysis*. With the influence of Habermas, the aspect of action was given prominence; with the influence of Douglas, the aspects of ritual and classification were given prominence; with the influence of Foucault, the aspect of discourse was given prominence; and with the influence of Berger, the aspect of subjectivity continued to be given a role. The result of building on these sources of inspiration was that in this phase culture was defined first as being the symbolic-expressive aspect of human behaviour, and later as being a form of action and the tangible results of these actions.

If we look at the methodological principles in Wuthnow's work, it is clear that the influence of hermeneutics is strongest. It is interpretation and loose-fitting frameworks of concepts which characterise his thinking. Openness and, with it, change characterise his scientific work.

If I am to try, on this basis, to summarise Wuthnow's understanding of culture, it must first be established that this understanding of culture changes throughout his authorship. To start with, culture is defined as being meaning systems, which transcend everyday meanings. In the middle period culture is defined as being the symbolic-expressive aspect of human behaviour, and the tangible results of these actions. And finally, in his most recent works, culture is viewed as fundamental distinctions and categories, and cultural constructions are defined as relating a given phenomenon to its values.

Wuthnow, himself, imposes order on these different definitions of culture by referring to different levels of culture. He distinguishes between the subjective level, where meanings and values belong, the structural level, where categories and patterns belong, the dramaturgical level, where the dramatisation of the moral order belongs, and finally the institutional level, where resources and the channelling of ideas belong. It can be said that the works which have been looked at here start and finish at the subjective level, but that the intervening works run through the other three levels.

The question is whether it is possible to see the outline of a theory of culture in the works studied. With the shifting concepts of culture, the theory of culture in Wuthnow's writing must also be changeable. To start with, the meaning systems are transcendent and enduring, without being unchanging. They create a wholeness for the individual and integration for society. They create a cohesive force because they give the possibility of relating individual phenomena to something larger, and because they set social standards which can regulate people's behaviour. Culture thus creates a wholeness for people and, because it affects behaviour, it helps the integration of society.

Later, emphasis is put on the fact that culture has the ability to dramatise both moral and social orders. It is rituals that communicate the moral order, while ideologies communicate the social order. At the same time, Wuthnow stresses that culture is not a reflection of the social order. Whether a specific ideology gains a foothold, or not, depends on whether the form of the ideology is adapted to the social environment, and whether the ideology is able to communicate something about the social relations in the environment in question. There must also be a social movement which can secure the necessary resources for the dissemination of the ideology. The process through which culture gains a foothold consists of production, selection and institutionalisation. This must not be thought of as an automatic process. The result depends on the choices which people make in the light of the existing limitations. On the one hand, the producer must choose what products to make. On the other hand, patrons and consumers must decide which products they will support or buy. Nor is it sufficient to choose or decide. There must also be space for creativity. This space is created by articulating the general and disarticulating relations to the general. Behind cultural development there thus lie choice, decisions and creativity. The adaptation of the cultural to the social conditions is thus not automatic. It is the result of human behaviour.

In his more recent works, a distinction is made between general national culture and the individual's values and actions. Here, general culture gives the individual some categories and distinctions which can give points of reference for the development of his personal values. How this happens depends on the individual's institutional affiliations. Cultural heritage and social institutions function as sources for the individual's development of values. These values then form the basis for the development of cultural constructions which are, in turn, a prerequisite for people being able to orient themselves and make decisions.

As with the development of the concept of culture, there is a shared view between the earlier and the later works. Here, general culture stands on one side while the individual's values and cultural constructions stand on the other. Culture functions as a source for the development of the values of the individual. This creates wholeness and guidelines for behaviour. The result for society is integration and cohesion. In the middle period emphasis was put on people's choices, decisions and creativity in the formation of culture. Here, it is people who are active in forming their own culture within the allotted guidelines.

Wuthnow's very free form, with the constant construction of concepts, leads him to the situation where concepts and theories undergo changes. The question is, whether the division he makes of culture into different levels, solves this problem. Is it possible to develop a cultural concept and a theory of culture for each level? Has he put himself in the situation where, by basing his ideas on very different sociological traditions, he tries to make theories cohere, even thought they may not be compatible? Can culture be the phenomenon which directs human behaviour, while at the same time people can direct culture through their choices? On the other hand it must be admitted that, by giving weight to the analyses as he has done, he maintains the possibility of analysing culture as a reciprocal relation between people and cultural products. In fact, the whole of his production supports the tradition which he has previously identified as restricting the sociology of culture, and this is the tradition of culture as a subject-object relationship.

# 7

# Pierre Bourdieu: Culture as Classification

Pierre Bourdieu's discussion of, and views on, culture play a very modest role in the literature on Bourdieu. In his treatment of Bourdieu in *Sociologi och epistemologi*, Donald Broady presents three key concepts which he considers are the most important in Bourdieu's work. These are: capital, habitus and field. Culture is not identified here as a key concept. In Broady's view, it is possible to derive a concept of symbolic capital from Bourdieu's concept of capital, and as part of the concept of symbolic capital, it is possible to derive the concept of cultural capital. Thus, culture does not occupy a central role in Broady's view of Bourdieu's theory (Broady, 1990/1991).

In Derek Robbins's book on Bourdieu, *The Work of Pierre Bourdieu*, culture is presented as an element which is linked to the discussion of pedagogy. Robbins particularly concentrates on distinguishing between aristocratic culture, rational culture and popular culture, and the educational challenges to which these distinctions give rise (Robbins, 1991).

One of the few authors who gives a central role to Bourdieu's views on culture, is Bridget Fowler. In her book on Bourdieu, *Pierre Bourdieu and Cultural Theory*, she focuses on Bourdieu's theory of culture. For her, Bourdieu's theory of culture primarily deals with art and literature, and she sees it as being part of a wider discussion of the development from modernism to post-modernism. For her, Bourdieu's theory of culture thus concerns art and literature (Fowler, 1997).

Thus, the literature on Bourdieu's work only deals with his perception of culture to a limited extent. However, Bourdieu himself focused on culture in many of his works. These works will naturally be included in the discussion of how Bourdieu perceived culture, and how he related culture to other social phenomena. Other works are also relevant, because culture is included as part of the theoretical aspects of these works. It is thus necessary to review large parts of Bourdieu's writings in order to obtain a comprehensive view of his perception of culture.

Bourdieu wrote extensively. His works can be divided into four categories. The first category consists of works based on his anthropological studies in Kabyle in Algeria. As a young researcher Bourdieu undertook empirical studies in this area, and in a number of his later works he returned to the interpretation of this material. The most important of these works are *Outline of a Theory of Practice* and *The Logic of Practice*. The second category of works consists of those which deal with education in French society.

Here, too, Bourdieu undertook a number of empirical studies primarily of a quantitative character. These works on education include *The Inheritors* and *Reproduction in Education, Society and Culture*, which were both written together with Jean-Claude Passeron. I will also refer to one of his articles which deals with this topic, "Systems of Education and Systems of Thought", from Young's anthology, *Knowledge and Control*. The third category of works casts light on the question of taste in art and literature. The most important work is *Distinction*, in which he again used his own empirical studies. This category also includes *The Field of Cultural Production*, which is a collection of articles by Bourdieu in which he discussed the production and consumption of art and literature. Finally, the fourth category of works refers to those works in which Bourdieu reflected on his own works. The most important of these is *In Other Words*. Bourdieu wrote numerous other important works, including his book *Homo Academicus*, a collection of articles under the title of *Language and Symbolic Power, An Invitation to Reflexive Sociology*, and a long list of other articles. However, I have chosen to concentrate on those works which I believe are most important for deriving Bourdieu's perception of culture.

## *Symbolic violence*

*Outline of a Theory of Practice*, published in 1972, is based on Bourdieu's studies of agrarian life in Kabyle in Algeria. Bourdieu developed some of his basic concepts in this work; these were the concepts of habitus, practice and capital. In a later work, *The Logic of Practice*, published in 1980, he clarified these concepts and related them to both theoretical and practical logic. *The Logic of Practice* is thus a reflection on the findings in *Outline of a Theory of Practice*.

The most important methodological principle in Bourdieu's thinking was emphasised in the introduction to *The Logic of Practice*; this was the principle of relational thought. According to this principle, each element must be characterised by the relationships which connect it with all the other elements of a system, so that it acquires meaning and function. Using this method of thinking in scientific thinking, one must treat historical facts as systems of understandable relations.

> "The philosophical glosses which, for a time, surrounded structuralism have neglected and concealed what really constituted its essential novelty – the introduction into the social sciences of the structural method or, more simply, of the relational mode of thought which, by breaking with the substantialist mode of thought, leads one to characterize each element by the relationships which unite it with all the others in a system and from which it derives its meaning and function." (Bourdieu, 1980/1995, p. 4).

Bourdieu's approach to anthropological research consisted of mapping the relations of oppositions in the agrarian calendar, in people's relations to their houses, their relations to the day, to their life-cycle, and so on. To this he added the contradictions in symbolic practice between, for example, going in and coming out, opening and closing, filling and emptying, etc. For him, such data operated as intermediate terms which made it possible to reveal new relationships (Bourdieu, 1980/1995, p. 9).

By constructing diagrams of different areas of practice it was possible for Bourdieu to see relations between these areas of practice.

> "... I had constructed diagrams, for the various areas of practice – agrarian rites, cooking, women's activities, periods of the life-cycle, moments of the day, etc. –

> which, … gave visible form to the relations of homology or opposition while restoring the linear order of temporal succession. The 'grouping of factual material' performed by the diagram is in itself an act of construction, indeed an act of interpretation, inasmuch as it brings to light the whole system of relationships …" (Bourdieu, 1980/1995, p. 10).

By forcing himself to relate the identified oppositions to each other, Bourdieu claimed that this eliminated more intuitive interpretations which can arise if one looks at relationships only in isolation.

Such an interpretation cannot use any other evidence of its truth than that which lies in its ability to incorporate the total body of facts entirely coherently. Such an understanding of practical logic requires the researcher to adapt his own dispositions, and surrender everything which would normally be referred to reflection, theory and logic.

However, Bourdieu emphasised that the models of practice which researchers construct should never be confused with the true principles of practice. This is because, as generative principles, practice does not have coherent and independent axioms, but practical patterns which vary according to the situational logic. Practical logic is seldom entirely coherent or entirely incoherent (Bourdieu, 1980/1995, pp. 11-12).

This difference between theoretical logic and practical logic made Bourdieu think about the relationship between the researcher and the object of his research. This brought his relational thinking to the empirical level. He saw that it was necessary to clarify the objective distance between the observer and the observed. According to Bourdieu, this distance is the essential condition for scientific practice in the social sciences. The distance consists of a deep difference between two relations to the world; a theoretical relation and a practical relation (Bourdieu, 1980/1995, pp. 14-15).

The relationship between the observer and the observed is a special instance of the relationship between knowledge and action, interpretation and use, symbolic mastery and practical mastery, and between theoretical logic and practical logic. According to Bourdieu, this difference, which is in-built in intellectual activity and intellectual conditions, is the phenomenon which is the most difficult for intellectual discourse to express with precision.

The relationship between the observer and the observed also involves the fact that, in every external observer there is a native, and thereby a familiarity with ordinary prelogical thinking. This means that the distance between the external observer and the native can only be overcome by creating a distance to the native which has a hidden preexistence in the observer. The way to develop such a distance is by objectifying this inner native. Only in this way can an external observer bring himself closer to the native (Bourdieu, 1980/1995, pp. 19-20).

The consequence of this view is that scientific practice must be subjected to knowledge about the knowing subject of research, and thus to a critical knowledge of the limits to all theoretical knowledge. Theoretical reflection on the limits of theoretical understanding aims to liberate theoretical understanding from the distortion resulting from its epistemological and social basis. The aim of the critique must be to develop the practice theory which theoretical practice implicitly uses, and in this way to make a truly scientific theory of practice and of practical knowledge possible.

If one is to satisfy the most practical requirements of scientific practice, then, according to Bourdieu, one must analyse the specific logic and the social conditions for the social-scientific knowledge (Bourdieu, 1980/1995, pp. 27-29).

Against the background of these general methodological considerations, Bourdieu made a review of the theoretical reasoning which he observed in other anthropological researchers. His criticisms were primarily directed at the schism between objectivism and subjectivism. He thus distanced himself from both pure objectivist thinking and pure subjectivist thinking. He rejected the idea that items of knowledge are passively registered, and instead he insisted that items of knowledge are constructed. Similarly, he rejected idealistic thinking by insisting that the principle behind such construction is a system of inner dispositions, also called 'habitus'. As a researcher, one must descend from the lofty viewpoint of objectivity and enter into practical relations with the world. One must experience the necessities of this world and the things that must be said and done. One must return to practice with its dialectic between structure and habitus.

> "One has to escape from the realism of the structure, to which objectivism, ..., necessarily leads when it hypostatizes these relations by treating them as realities already constituted outside of the history of the group – without falling back into subjectivism, which is quite incapable of giving an account of the necessity of the social world. To do this, one has to return to practice, the site of the dialectic of the *opus operatum* and the *modus operandi*; of the objectified products and the incorporated products of historical practice; of structures and *habitus*." (Bourdieu, 1980/1995, p. 52).

In his dialogue with and his attempt to overcome pure objectivist thinking and pure subjectivist thinking, Bourdieu sought to clarify the dialectical relations between objective conditions and subjective conditions. He thus sought to clarify the dialectical relationship between characteristics of the material universe and the inner dispositions of the individual, between class conditions and feelings of class, between objective conditions and structuring dispositions (Bourdieu, 1980/1995, p. 140). As a step towards clarifying these dialectical relations, Bourdieu developed some fundamental concepts which were relevant to the whole of his theoretical work. These concepts included the most important: habitus, practice and symbolic capital. The empirical basis for these clarifications was his anthropological work in Kabyle.

The concept which was most decisive for Bourdieu's attempt to create dialectical relations between objectivity and subjectivity, was the concept of habitus. Habitus is linked to the individual and functions as the element which links subjectivity and objectivity to each other. Thus, the dialectic consists in the fact that habitus is a product of objective structures, at the same time as facilitating the reproduction of objective structures.

In *The Logic of Practice*, Bourdieu defined habitus as:

> "The conditionings associated with a particular class of conditions of existence produce *habitus*, systems of durable, transposable dispositions, structured structures predisposed to function as structuring structures, that is, as principles which generate and organize practices and representations..." (Bourdieu, 1980/1995, p. 53).

These principles are objectively regulated, without in any way being the result of being subject to rules. They can be put in place collectively, without being the product of organised action.

The most important quality of habitus is that it functions as a generative principle. Habitus is indeed a product of objective conditions, but it is also able to generate new phenomena. Bourdieu saw habitus as being a product of history, but it is also able to produce more history according to the schemes generated by history. Habitus enables the free production of all the ideas, opinions and actions which belong to the conditions which are specific for its production, and only of these. Habitus thus has a tendency to generate all the reasonable, common-sense forms of behaviour which are possible within a given class of objective standards. In all probability, these forms of behaviour will be positively sanctioned because they are objectively in line with the logic which characterises the specific field (Bourdieu, 1980/1995, pp. 55-56).

In explaining the concept of habitus, Bourdieu sought to determine the relationship between the habitus of the individual and the habitus of a class. In this respect he said that, within each class there will be a tendency for a given individual to have a habitus which has a higher degree of similarity to the habitus of other individuals from the same class than to the habitus of individuals from other classes. This is because the habitus within a given class is the outcome of the same objective structures. Nevertheless, the habitus of individuals in the same class will not be identical. It will be characterised by relations of homology, i.e., by variances within the homogeneity which is a consequence of the social conditions.

> "In fact, the singular *habitus* of members of the same class are united in a relationship of homology, that is, of diversity within homogeneity reflecting the diversity within homogeneity characteristic of their social conditions of production. Each individual system of dispositions is a structural variant of the others, expressing the singularity of its position within the class and its trajectory. 'Personal' style, the particular stamp marking all the products of the same *habitus*, whether practices or works, is never more than a deviation in relation to the style of a period or class, so that it relates back to the common style not only by its conformity - ... - but also by the difference that makes the 'manner'." (Bourdieu, 1980/1995, p. 60).

Habitus is decisive for the choices and strategies which lie behind people's behaviour. Bourdieu emphasised that early experiences in life determine how people act later in life. Bourdieu thus stressed that life's early experiences are always dominant in the formation of habitus. This is because habitus will always seek to be constant. Through its systematic choices of information, places, events and people, it will seek to protect itself against crises and critical challenges. Habitus is thus the un-chosen principle which lies behind all choices. As a consequence, the strategies which, on the face of it, could appear to be attempts to achieve certain goals, and thus appear to be determined by the future, are in fact the products of habitus and thus of the past. It is such strategies which enable the individual to meet unexpected and constantly changing situations (Bourdieu, 1980/1995, pp. 60-61).

Thus, we have already been introduced to the second important concept in Bourdieu's theory, the concept of practice. Bourdieu developed this concept as an extension of the concept of habitus. Bourdieu considered practice to be a consequence of habitus, and thus a consequence of objective structures. The dialectical principle is also operative here, in that objective structures form the basis for habitus, and thus for practice, which in turn reproduces the objective structures. However, Bourdieu emphasised that one cannot understand practice by using the same logic that is used for logical thinking. Practice has its own logic.

With the help of a few generative principles, the logic of practice is able to organise thoughts, opinions and actions. These generative principles which lie behind the practical logic are simple and integrated with each other. This is because the logic of practice is based on simplicity and generality. Practice can only operate if it is based on principles which are coherent, relevant and obey economic logic (Bourdieu, 1980/1995, p. 86). No more logic is used than is needed.

When logic is used, it means that coherence is developed within the universe of meaning as well as the universe of practice, but as the logic used is as slight as possible, this means that the coherence becomes loose and opaque. It is as if the two universes close in on themselves.

Within the universe of meaning, coherence arises when pairs of oppositions relate to each other through relations of homology.

> "Because the principle opposing the terms that have been related ... is not defined and usually comes down to a simple contrariety, analogy ... establishes a relation of homology between relations of opposition ... This uncertain abstraction is also a false abstraction which sets up relationships based on ... 'overall resemblance' ... This mode of apprehension never explicitly limits itself to any one aspect of the terms it links, but takes each one, each time, as a whole, exploiting to the full the fact that two 'realities' are never entirely alike in all respects but are always alike in some respect, at least indirectly ..." (Bourdieu, 1980/1995, pp. 87-88).

Within the universe of practice, uniform reactions are developed in relation to different situations with the help of some practical schemes. The coherent force which exists in the universe of practice is due to the fact that a small number of practical schemes can be combined with each other in different ways. The schemes are thus related to each other through their practical interchangeability. The system is thus loose and approximate. This is because the systems only function in relation to practical purposes (Bourdieu, 1980/1995, pp. 92-94).

Objective structures are the basis for the practical systems. Material structures are the foundations for the development such practical operators, so that some given behaviour appears to be a necessity. At the same time, this behaviour, which is the result of the practical schemes, has a tendency to reproduce the objective structures (Bourdieu, 1980/1995, p. 95).

However, Bourdieu emphasised that it is not possible to deduce a given practice from the historical conditions which have produced the habitus, nor from the actual conditions which appear to have promoted it. One can only understand practice by relating the social conditions, which have had constitutive effect for the habitus which has generated the practice, to the social conditions in relation to which the habitus has been implemented. There must be a clarification of the mutual relationship between these two social worlds through scientific work (Bourdieu, 1980/1995, p. 56).

The third concept which Bourdieu developed in *The Logic of Practice*, was the concept of symbolic capital. This concept refers to behaviour which demonstrates the greatest possible credibility. Through their behaviour, people seek to demonstrate the greatest possible amount of symbolic capital in order to secure good alliances and contracts. The background for this behaviour is the habitus which is developed in the earliest years of life and which expresses the objective regulation of economic circumstances. In this way, symbolic capital, practice and habitus are the result of objective structures which they also contribute to reproduce. With all three concepts, it is possible to make a dialectical relationship between objectivity and subjectivity.

Symbolic capital is the basis for all the relationships that express obligations and debts concerning honour, rights and duties. These relationships have been accumulated through generations and can be mobilised under extraordinary circumstances. Economic and symbolic capital are interwoven in such a way that the display of material and symbolic capital can in themselves make a material profit probable. In an economy which is based on trust, as in Kabyle, a good reputation is the best, if not the only, form of economic guarantee. As a consequence, the great families must use every opportunity to demonstrate their symbolic capital. This can consist of the number of family members and allies, of witnesses and guarantors, who can all be mobilised at any time and at any place with a view to affirming the trustworthiness of a transaction or the strength of a contract (Bourdieu, 1980/1995, p. 119).

The display of symbolic capital is one of the only ways to ensure that capital is added to capital. This is because symbolic capital is a credit or an advantage which a group only gives to those who can demonstrate the best symbolic and material guarantees. The group is the ultimate source of credit, and it will be quick to withdraw it if it suspects that a family is not trustworthy. The consequence is that each family has a vital interest in keeping its honour and trustworthiness above suspicion (Bourdieu, 1980/1995, p. 121).

In developing the three concepts of habitus, practice and symbolic capital, Bourdieu's purpose was to explain dominance between people. Linking the three concepts together thus resulted in a theory of dominance. According to Bourdieu, the development of symbolic capital creates relations of dependence which are dressed up under a veil of moral relations, but which in fact have an economic basis (Bourdieu, 1980/1995, p. 123). Bourdieu argued that such dependency relations have the character of symbolic violence.

> "So long as overt violence ... is collectively disapproved of and is liable to provoke either a violent riposte or the flight of the victim ... symbolic violence, gentle, invisible violence, unrecognized as such, chosen as much as undergone, that of trust, obligation, personal loyalty, hospitality, gifts, debts, piety, in a word, of all the virtues honoured by the ethic of honour, presents itself as the most economical mode of domination because it best corresponds to the economy of the system." (Bourdieu, 1980/1995, p. 127).

From the starting point of the concept of habitus, Bourdieu developed his concept of practice. His concept of practice enabled him to develop a concept of symbolic capital, which in turn enabled him to understand symbolic violence as a form of dominance. However, the whole of this development of concepts was based on studies of a pre-capitalist society. The social mechanisms which he analysed within the framework of these concepts thus belong to a pre-capitalist society.

The question which remained for Bourdieu was the degree to which these social mechanisms could be transferred to a society where the social mechanisms are much more institutionalised. In this connection he said that, in a society in which there is a higher level of institutionalisation, there will be a number of independent fields within which forms of dominance can exist, corresponding to the forms which he identified in pre-capitalist societies. These fields include politics, education, legislation, art and culture. In what follows I will investigate how Bourdieu applied his anthropological ideas to a number of fields of modern society. In particular, I will concentrate on those fields which make it possible to study Bourdieu's perception of culture.

## *The relation to culture*

Bourdieu's research into education started in the beginning of the 1960s. The first of his works on education was *The Inheritors*, with the subtitle 'French Students and their Relation to Culture'. This book, first published in 1964, was written jointly with Jean-Claude Passeron. The aim of the book was to link education to culture. As an offshoot from this book a number of articles followed, including "Systems of Education and Systems of Thought". This article was published in 1967 and was later included in Michael Young's anthology, *Knowledge and Control*. The theory of the relation between education and culture was gone into in greater detail in the book, *Reproduction in Education, Society and Culture*, which was also jointly written with Jean-Claude Passeron and published in 1970.

*The Inheritors* is based on empirical data on the connection between choice of education and social background. Bourdieu and Passeron tried to explain this connection by including questions of culture. To start with, Bourdieu and Passeron observed that children from the bourgeoisie were more highly represented at university than children from the working class or the middle class. At the same time, there was a tendency for children of the bourgeoisie to be much freer in their choice of subject of study than children from less privileged backgrounds. For example, they had a greater tendency to study more exotic subjects such as anthropology and mythology.

Bourdieu and Passeron looked for an explanation for these differences by looking at the students' cultural backgrounds. It was assumed that, compared with other students, the students from the bourgeoisie would be privileged with regard to knowledge, taste and insight. This was displayed by differences in their style and manner. Students who only had the cultural ballast given to them in school had to work hard, and this was revealed in their style.

> "For individuals from the most deprived backgrounds, the school remains the one and only path to culture, at every level of education. As such, it would be the royal road to the democratization of culture if it did not consecrate the initial cultural inequalities by ignoring them and if it did not – for example, by denigrating a piece of academic work as too 'academic' – often devalue the culture it transmits, in favor of the inherited culture which does not bear the vulgar mark of effort and so has every appearance of ease and grace." (Bourdieu & Passeron, 1964/1979, p. 21).

Young people who have a general cultural ballast from their home backgrounds will be able to operate easily in the cultural field. There is thus a level of conformity between class-based cultural habits and educational requirements which is essential for the success of young people.

There is a game played by students which further emphasises the importance of their social backgrounds. In this game, students learn the tricks which, together with their class-determined background, give them a good training for their later professional lives. One of the rules of this game is that one should distance oneself from one's class background. It should not be shown off. The demonstration of a controversial political allegiance is a relatively easy way to make a symbolic break with a privileged class background. For example, openly joining a left wing group creates a distance to a bourgeoisie background. This intellectual game, which is based on creating a distance from all kinds of social and occupational restrictions, is in reality a game about differences with a view to maintaining them. In this way, social differences are maintained on the quiet. Students who come from more privileged backgrounds can distance themselves from their studies and only concern themselves with the issues which they themselves choose to put on the agenda, while students from less privileged backgrounds are tied to their university studies, which do not really match their expectations. They therefore become anxious about the future.

> "... the degree of commitment to the intellectual game and to the values it implies is never independent of social origin. The term, seriousness, therefore, covers two distinct ways of living studenthood. One of them is primarily characteristic of students of bourgeois origin who make higher education an experience into which enter no problems more serious than those they put there. The other expresses the anxiety

> about the future characteristic of students who have come from the social strata that are furthest from academic culture and who are condemned to experience that culture as unreal." (Bourdieu & Passeron, 1964/1979, p. 53).

To understand this student game, one must start from an understanding of study as a means of acquiring the ability to create culture or to transfer culture to others. In other words, to study is the same as saying to adopt an interim position. One must work at disappearing as a student. This means that everything happens as if students try to hide the true nature of their work from themselves. They do this by separating their present from their future, and by separating their means from their ends. In this way they are able to forget themselves as students and forget the future. They create the illusion that their time as students is an end in itself. Their student years become endless and autonomous. The students' denial of themselves as students also makes it possible for the teachers to deny themselves as teachers. For teachers, teaching becomes a personal skill (Bourdieu & Passeron, 1964/1979, pp. 55-58).

However, the distance which is created between rational behaviour and magical behaviour depends on the futures which await the students in question. The distance will vary according to class background, the subject studied and gender. The more secure the future, the easier it is to forget about it. Objective chances are decisive as to whether one plays this game of denial of student years as a period of preparation. It is a difficult game to play for women and men from less privileged backgrounds.

For teachers it would be equivalent to abdicating their higher authority, if they decided to teach using the same technique as they use in their intellectual work. For them there is no alternative to maintaining that their teaching is based on charismatic qualities.

This charismatic ideology, which contrasts elegance with work in order to devalue work in the name of elegance, ensures that the privileged classes can legitimise their cultural privileges. In this way these cultural privileges change from being a matter of social inheritance to becoming individual elegance or personal merit.

When there is no methodical formulation of the work of teachers, or of their evaluation of student performances, these evaluations will be based on personal criteria which can vary from teacher to teacher and from situation to situation. Students who come from the cultivated classes are best prepared to adapt to such a system of diffuse and implicit demands, because they implicitly possess the means of satisfying these demands. There is already a high degree of conformity between school culture and the culture of the cultivated classes. Students from these classes can therefore subconsciously satisfy the demands which are made in an exam situation.

In an epilogue to *The Inheritors*, Bourdieu and Passeron identified the problem that, as a result of the increased numbers of people seeking further education, there is increased competition between young people for academic qualifications, and for the chance to turn these qualifications into jobs.

Traditionally, families or individuals from the economically better off classes will seek to ensure their social reproduction by turning their economic capital into educational capital. They will thus follow a reproduction strategy. When there is an increase in the number of people going on to further education, there is an increased risk that the educational capital obtained will not be able to be turned into jobs, and this leads to a compensation strategy. Young people, who are disappointed in their expectations of being able to follow in their parents' footsteps, will seek positions which lie between a student existence and a professional career, for example, within the cultural bureaucracy. Here, they will be able to take advantage of their cultural capital in the form of good taste, good manners and physical charm. In this way they are able to redefine social structures. They seek to distance themselves from those classes which threaten to deprive them of their privileges.

Conversely, young people who come from less privileged backgrounds find that the paper qualifications they have acquired are worthless. The consequence of this will often be protest against the logic of the academic institution and a denial of the whole social order.

> "These young people, whose social identity and self-image have been undermined by a social system and an educational system that have fobbed them off with worthless paper, can find no other way of restoring their personal and social integrity than by a total refusal. It is as if they felt that what is at issue is no longer just a question of personal failure, as the educational system encourages them to believe, but rather the whole logic of the academic institution." (Bourdieu & Passeron, 1964/1979, p. 84).

The overall result of the changes brought about by this increase in the numbers seeking further education is that there has been a redefinition of the social order, but there has simultaneously been a maintenance of the principle of distance in the social order. The underlying principle of the social order is that each social class will seek to distance itself from those who are below them, while seeking to diminish the distance to those who are above. What matters is not positions, but the relationship between positions (Bourdieu & Passeron, 1964/1979, p. 97).

We see the first elements of Bourdieu's perception of culture in this work. The culture which is referred to here has qualities which, to a greater or lesser degree, can be related to individuals and classes. Bourdieu and Passeron spoke about the cultivated classes and about the individual's cultivated behaviour. Cultivation is made apparent through knowledge, taste, insight, style, elegance, ease and good manners. The lack of cultivation is made apparent in toil and hard work, and the vulgar impression which this leaves.

The degree of cultivation varies according to membership of a social class, which means that cultivation is a privilege. Among the truly cultivated there is naturalness and understated understanding which means that the true manner of cultivated behaviour is never formulated. In this way, cultivation becomes a personal characteristic, and, in extreme cases, charisma.

At the same time we see elements of a theory of practice and a strategy which are linked to social background. Those students who come from the bourgeoisie will have a tendency to behave in a way which distances them from that background, while revealing their class origins in the ease with which they view the future. Young people from the working class will have a tendency to worry about the future. The strategic element becomes apparent when the pressure on further education is increased. In this situation, the children of the bourgeoisie will develop a compensation strategy which will lead to a redefinition of the social order, while young people from the working class will have a tendency to protest against the whole logic of the educational system. However, the end result is that the distances between the classes are maintained, so the social order is maintained while it is changed.

In this work we can see parallels with the main concepts which were developed through the anthropological studies. Cultural privileges and charisma have a parallel in symbolic capital. The students' game and strategies have a parallel in practice. And finally, the cultivated individual's ability to demonstrate style and manner has a parallel in habitus. For the time being it seems that culture will be included in both the concept of habitus and the concept of capital.

In the article "Systems of Education and Systems of Thought", which was included in Young's anthology, *Knowledge and Control*, Bourdieu's conceptualisation of culture and the relationship of culture to the family and education was made clearer. By way of introduction, Bourdieu made a link between his anthropological research and his educational research. He saw some analogies in the way that thinking was developed in primitive societies and in school-going societies. He thus raised the question of the extent to which the patterns which shape the thinking of educated people in school-going societies can have the same functions as the patterns which lie behind the myths and rituals of primitive societies.

> "As a social individual, the ethnologist is on terms of intimacy with his culture and therefore finds it difficult to think objectively about the patterns governing his own thought ... He may also be reluctant to admit that, ... the patterns which shape the thinking of educated men in 'school-going' societies may fulfil the same function as the unconscious patterns he discovers, by analysing such cultural creations as rites or myths, among individuals belonging to societies with no educational institutions ..." (Bourdieu, 1967/1971, p. 190).

In this way, Bourdieu created the basis for analogous thinking about, and the development of, concepts for understanding thinking and practice in two very different types of society.

The question which Bourdieu discussed in this article concerned the influence of school on the way in which people think. It was his view that the school system alone is able to establish and develop the patterns which lie behind people's thinking in a given period. This happens through practice, by which the thinking habits are created which are common to a whole generation.

In this context Bourdieu gave a definition of culture.

> "Culture is not merely a common code or even a common catalogue of answers to recurring problems; it is a common set of previously assimilated master patterns from which, by an 'art of invention' similar to that involved in the writing of music, an infinite number of individual patterns directly applicable to specific situations are generated." (Bourdieu, 1967/1971, p. 192).

These patterns can control or regulate mental processes, without being consciously recognised as controlled. It is primarily through this subconscious culture, which the thinker owes to his intellectual training, or more precisely his scholastic training, that the thinker belongs to his time and his society. The only way in which it is possible to be aware of these patterns is by reflexively going back through the operations which one has already carried out. (Bourdieu, 1967/1971, p. 193).

To give an example of this view, Bourdieu referred to Panofsky's analysis of the relationship between gothic art and scholasticism. Panofsky believed that gothic architecture borrowed its special methods from the schoolmen. The principle that logic is an argument had to be presented explicitly, and was clearly transferred to the execution of architecture and sculpture. Panofsky believed that this phenomenon could be explained as the result of mental habits which operated as a principle for the regulation of action. Schools thus create general dispositions or a cultural habitus in those who have been under their influence.

> "... in a society where the handing on of culture is monopolized by a school, the hidden affinities uniting the works of man (and, at the same time, modes of conduct and

thought) derive from the institution of the school, whose function is consciously ... to transmit the unconscious or, to be more precise, to produce individuals equipped with the system of unconscious (or deeply buried) master-patterns that constitute their culture." (Bourdieu, 1967/1971, p. 194).

When Bourdieu explained how a school is able to develop a cultural habitus in its pupils, he sought this explanation in the classifying practice of the school. The school thus unfolded its plans, methods or programmes for thinking. Through its ordered treatment of cultural works, the school passes on the rules which lie behind the orthodox method for approaching these works, and the principles which determine their hierarchies. Therefore, an autodidact can immediately be recognised by an educated man. A school will always classify according to genres and authors, and it will always create hierarchies so that the classic works will stand above the great mass of works.

The problem is that this gradual rationalisation of education can act as a threat to the cultural integration of the educated class. It will lead to specialisation within education, and thus to the production of intellectual clans. What distinguishes these clans from each other is not so much what they have learnt, but the way in which they have learnt it. For example, this can relate to the type of tasks they have been set, the form of examination, the criteria for judgement, and so on. The individual's contact with his culture depends primarily on the conditions under which he has acquired it, including how it has been communicated.

"The formal lecture, for instance, communicates something other, and something more, than its literal content: it furnishes an example of intellectual prowess and thereby indissolvably defines the 'right' culture and the 'right' relation to that culture; vigour and brilliance, ease and elegance are qualities of style peculiar to the act of communication which mark the culture communicated and gain acceptance at the same time as the culture from those receiving it in this form." (Bourdieu, 1967/1971, p. 199).

While these different schools can threaten the integration of the educated classes, the tendency to reserve further education to the economically and culturally privileged classes contributes to the creation of a cultural divide. The dual educational system, with a division between further education for the middle classes and basic schooling for the masses, leads to a cultural split between an academic culture and a popular culture. The most important difference between these two forms of culture is that the popular culture lacks the objectification on which the academic culture is based. (Bourdieu, 1967/1971, pp. 200-201).

In this article we thus get a definition of culture as being a common set of master patterns which can generate individual patterns, which in turn can guide the mental processes. Culture is thus the common patterns which can generate the individual patterns which can generate thinking. When Bourdieu explained these master patterns he introduced schooling as the decisive factor. It is not the content of schooling which determines these patterns, but rather the way in which the content is communicated. The manner of teaching contributes to the division of the cultivated into clans, and the way in which teaching treats groups of pupils helps to divide them between academic culture and popular culture. The ways in which schools communicate and organise culture thus contribute to making divisions between people with regard to their relationships to culture.

The book *Reproduction in Education, Society and Culture* contains a point by point explanation of a theory of symbolic violence, as well as an empirically based theory on the reproduction of the social order. The overarching idea of the book is thus to set out a theory of symbolic violence, and then apply it to empirical material. The result of this is a theory of social reproduction.

The question which concerned Passeron and Bourdieu, in the theory on symbolic violence, was how it was possible to explain culture and the mediation of culture through education. Culture does not appear to be controlled by any principle. It appears to be arbitrary. The same applies to the educational process through which culture is mediated. It, too, appears to be arbitrary. It is this apparent double arbitrariness which they characterise as symbolic violence (Bourdieu & Passeron, 1970/1997, p. xx). However, it was their view that culture is not arbitrary but necessary. This will be apparent if one relates earlier and actual cultures to the social conditions in which they made their appearance and were developed.

> "The 'choices' which constitute a culture ('choices' which no one makes) ... reveal their necessity as soon as they are related to the social conditions of their emergence and perpetuation." (Bourdieu & Passeron, 1970/1996, p. 8).

The same applies to the selection of meaning which is included in educational activities. If one relates these to the social classes, it will be revealed that there is accordance between the educational work and the material and symbolic interests of the different classes. Therefore, educational activities tend to reproduce the divisions of the cultural capital and contribute to the reproduction of the social structures.

> "In reality, because they correspond to the material and symbolic interests of groups or classes differently situated within the power relations, these pedagogic actions always tend to reproduce the structure of the distribution of cultural capital among these groups or classes, thereby contributing to the reproduction of the social structure." (Bourdieu & Passeron, 1970/1996, p. 11).

The pedagogic task, which is to mediate the apparently arbitrary culture, works most effectively when it is based on an implicit pedagogy. On the one hand, it must maintain its apparent arbitrariness, and on the other hand, it must ensure the development of habitus in the students. This starts with the habitus which the pupils have from their families. This means that the habitus which is formed in the family is the basis for the reception of the messages given in the classroom, while the habitus which is formed in the school is the basis for the habitus which enables the individual to receive the messages of the culture industry (Bourdieu & Passeron, 1970/1996, p. 43). The problem is that pupils who do not come to school with a habitus from their families, which must be the starting point for this whole process, will be badly dealt with by the whole of this implicit pedagogy.

The institutional basis for the pedagogic work involves a high level of standardisation, ritualisation and routinisation. The more that pedagogic work is organised to ensure cultural reproduction, the more will school culture become routine. The whole basis for this routinisation is the defence, by the pedagogic agents, of the market value of their diplomas. By defending their own interests, they defend the whole existence of the symbolic market which the system of diplomas consists of. Thus they reproduce themselves. However, the basis for this self-reproduction is the institutionalisation of pedagogic work. Even though the teacher may seem to base his authority on charisma, the dominance of pedagogic work must be explained by the fact that the institution serves the classes whose apparent cultural arbitrariness it reproduces.

> "In any given social formation, the dominant educational system is able to set up the dominant pedagogic work … because … by the mere fact of existing and persisting as an institution, it implies the institutional conditions for misrecognition of the symbolic violence it exerts, i.e. because the institutional means … are predisposed to serve … the groups or classes whose cultural arbitrary it reproduces …" (Bourdieu & Passeron, 1970/1996, p. 67).

Bourdieu and Passeron developed their theory of social reproduction in extension of their theory of symbolic violence. This theoretical development is introduced with a thesis that the productivity of pedagogic work is a function of the distance between the habitus which it is intended to promote, the habitus which is promoted by all prior pedagogic work, and ultimately by the family (Bourdieu & Passeron, 1970/1996, p. 72).

To start with, they presented the results of empirical research which showed that the success of pupils in given subjects must be understood in the light of two concepts: the concept of linguistic capital, and the concept of selection. It was shown that in the social classes where selection is greatest, there will be a tendency to neutralise the advantage of the other social classes by virtue of their linguistic capital. It was shown that, pupils who, because of their social background, would be expected to have the poorest results, in fact had quite good results, and conversely, the results were not so good among those pupils who, because of their social background, would be expected to have the best results. To understand this result, one must take into account the possibilities which the young people had in order to be accepted for different kinds of education. It is thus the probability of the different classes being accepted which explains this possibility of neutralising the original differences with regard to linguistic capital.

If one is to understand the results of pedagogic work, one must construct a system of relations between, on the one hand, the school system which shall reproduce the legitimate culture, and, on the other hand, the social classes which are at varying distances from the academic culture. Only through the construction of such a system of relations is it possible to develop relational concepts on, for example, the probability of permission, disposition to do school work, distance from academic culture, degree of selection etc. In this way it is not only possible to understand the relationship between school and social class, but also to open the way for an understanding of the best hidden aspect of these relationships, which is that a given school system undertakes its function of conserving society through the special way in which it undertakes its communicative function (Bourdieu & Passeron, 1970/1996, p. 102).

It is thus the mode or the manner which are decisive in pedagogic work. Bourdieu and Passeron pointed to a whole range of techniques which emphasise this aspect. One of these techniques is the distancing technique. This concerns the physical and spatial distance in the teaching situation, the use of a special way of speaking, emphasis on the neutrality of the position of the teacher, the stigmatising use of language about the students' mediocrity and their tendency to decry brilliant theories etc. In this way, pedagogic work is set about with a special style. It involves the adoption of a special style, a special relation to language and a special relation to culture by which it serves specific social classes. So, the linguistic capital with which the pupils come to school is the decisive factor for the relationship between class background and educational results. The relationship to language depends on social background.

> "The distinguished distance, prudent ease and contrived naturalness which are the foundations of every code of society manners, are opposed to the expressiveness or expressionism of working class language, which manifests itself in the tendency to move from particular case to particular case, from illustration to parable, or to shun

> the bombast of fine words and the turgidity of grand emotions ..." (Bourdieu & Passeron, 1970/1996, p. 116).

When, rather than its content, the style and manner of the educational system is emphasised, this means that culture is reduced to being a relationship to culture. It ends with a question about the extent to which one makes a vulgar search for culture, or whether one masters a special manner for acquiring culture.

> "... all the ways, declared or tacit, of reducing culture to the relation to culture, in other words, of setting against the vulgarity of what can be acquired or achieved a manner of possessing an acquirement whose whole value derives from the fact that there is but one way of acquiring it." (Bourdieu & Passeron, 1970/1996, p. 130).

In the selection which takes place in the educational system, exams play an vital role. A pre-requisite for exams having such a vital role in selection is, that there should be an institutionalisation of the educational system, so it acquires relative autonomy in relation to its surroundings. The educational system acquires this relative autonomy by incorporating the requirements of the surrounding world in its own traditions (Bourdieu & Passeron, 1970/1996, p. 145). It is the ability to reformulate and re-interpret the requirements of the outside world in the light of inherited norms which is the core of the educational system's relative autonomy.

It is the relative autonomy of the educational system which means that examinations can function as an effective means of selection. The effectiveness of exams is, among other things, that they function according to implicit norms, which are in reality a reformulation of the norms of the dominant classes. Therefore, pupils who do not come from these classes will be handicapped. This inequality will be most marked in those subjects where the norms are most diffuse (Bourdieu & Passeron, 1970/1996, p. 162).

When the selection is made, those who possess the right diplomas will have the possibility of entering into certain positions in society. They do not have this possibility so much by virtue of their technical qualifications, which people without a diploma could equally well have, but just as much by the documentation of their relationship to general culture. In this way the relationship to indefinable culture becomes objectified and monopolised, with the possibility of drawing maximum profit from it. The whole process has the character of transforming social advantages to academic advantages, which in turn are turned to social advantages (Bourdieu & Passeron, 1970/1996, p. 166).

Bourdieu and Passeron believed that if one is to understand the relationship between the educational system and the structure of class relations, it is necessary to introduce the concept of habitus. The concept of habitus must be understood in the light of the objective structures. It is the objective structures which produce the class-determined habitus, and thereby a practice which is in accordance with the structures, so that these are able to function and be reproduced. It is this class habitus which, even if it is produced outside school, is nevertheless the basis for all school performance. The school system helps to maintain existing class relations, while obscuring the fact that school hierarchies reproduce social hierarchies and legitimise them. The problem is that culture, which is determined from birth, makes one blind to the real function of the educational system, which is to ensure the profitability and legitimacy of cultural capital (Bourdieu & Passeron, 1970/1996, pp. 205-210).

We do not get any further understanding of what culture is from this work, but what we get is a relation of culture to pedagogic work and educational institutions. Both the theory of symbolic violence and the theory of social reproduction are present at all three of these levels. The points of departure are arbitrary culture, implicit pedagogic work and routinised institutions. It is the whole of these unspoken understandings and these assumptions which Bourdieu and Passeron tried to penetrate. They did this by relating the three levels to social relations. Culture relates to class structure, pedagogic work relates to class-determined habitus, and the institution relates to class-determined interests. This unveils the class-determined necessity which lies behind arbitrary culture, the class-determined habitus which lies behind implicit pedagogic work, and the class-determined interests which lie behind institutional routinisation.

At the cultural level, one can see the necessity of the culture which appears as legitimate culture in school when one relates it to the relationship of different classes to this culture. It is the distance of the different classes to this legitimate culture which makes it possible to see that culture is not arbitrary. Some classes are closer to school culture than others.

At the pedagogic level, one can see the symbolic violence that lies in the pedagogic work when one relates the implicit pedagogic work to the differences in the pupils' habitus. The way in which culture is mediated is more in accordance with some pupils' dispositions than others'. The pupils are thus divided, depending on whether they can acquire culture easily or with effort. Pupils are divided according to their relation to culture.

At the institutional level, one understands the everyday routinised and ritual actions when one relates the implicit norms of tests and exams to the differentiated norms which pupils have in themselves, depending on their class background. Some of the pupils' norms are closer to the opaque and diffuse examination norms than others'.

The consequence of the whole of this process is that selection is made in relation to the possibility of taking up a position in society. This selection is not based on culture, but on relations to culture. When all else is put to one side, what is left is the contrast between ease and elegance and the vulgar stamp of effort.

## *The profit of distinction*

*Distinction* must be considered as Bourdieu's most important work. The book, which was first published in 1979, contains a comprehensive presentation of a theory on the relations of different classes to culture. Here again, Bourdieu used the concepts of habitus, practice and capital, and we see them applied in interpreting the results of survey research. The research revealed preferences in relation to music, painting and film, moral values in relation to lifestyle, ideals in relation to the establishment of a home, behaviour with regard to visiting museums, going to concerts or reading books, choice with regard to food, sports activities etc. The statistical analysis of the results shows that expressions of cultural preferences and practices are connected to people's social and educational backgrounds. Where the educational background is the same, the social background, including rising and falling in the social scale, can be seen. The more one moves away from the culture which is mediated through school, the more this is so.

In his introduction to the book, Bourdieu acknowledged that the book overstepped some of the intellectual world's most fundamental boundaries. First, he breached a basic taboo against relating intellectual products to the social conditions for their existence. Second, he came close to breaching the academic convention according to which it is a barbarism to expose culture, which is almost a holy phenomenon, to scientific treatment. In order not to breach this convention entirely, he only gave the statistical results a minor role, and instead focussed on the theoretical discussion of the results (Bourdieu, 1979/1984, p. xiii). Already at this point we meet the theme which echoes throughout the book, that culture is something elevated and 'sacred' which, in spite of his introductory comments, Bourdieu tried to reveal by relating culture to the social order.

Bourdieu looked for the origin of the idea of culture's almost sanctified status in Kant's view of aesthetics. Kant's distinction between sensual pleasures and pure pleasures makes it possible to abstain from the low and vulgar and to constitute culture as a good which is pure and elevated above all forms of interest. For Bourdieu it was necessary to remove this sanctified barrier between the pure and the vulgar, between ease and necessity, between form and substance, between the disinterested and the reasonable, in order to be able to reveal the connection between the different types of choices which people make, and their social and educational foundations (Bourdieu, 1979/1984, p. 6).

The problem which confronted Bourdieu was that culture appears to be self-evident, intuitive and silent. In order to overcome this problem, he had to objectify it. Here he met the problem that the cultural game is protected against objectification by all the partial objectifications which the game's actors undertake in relation to each other. Intellectuals and artists each deny the true nature of their own and their opponents' activities. According to Bourdieu, the only solution to this problem was to start from the field of positions and the interests which are associated with a given position. Only thus would it be possible to understand both the shared interests bound up in participation in the cultural game, and the specific interests which are associated with positions and with bringing oneself to such position.

> "Only at the level of the field of positions is it possible to grasp both the generic interests associated with the fact of taking part in the game and the specific interests attached to the different positions, and, through this, the form and content of the self-positionings through which these interests are expressed." (Bourdieu, 1979/1984, p. 12).

Bourdieu started the book by identifying culture's aristocracy, so he made clear from the start his basic view that there is a relation between culture and class. It was his aim to break with the charismatic ideology, according to which taste is a talent, and replace it with a scientific view, according to which taste is a product of upbringing and education. The identification of what is right and what is wrong in the cultural world, which rules apply in the cultural world, and how the 'correct' understanding in the cultural world is justified, therefore takes place in a constant dialogue with the social order.

Bourdieu referred to cultural aristocrats as 'essentialists'. Cultural aristocrats stress the importance of essence and cultivation rather than registration and memory. It is the general culture that counts (Bourdieu, 1979/1984, p. 24). In the field of aesthetics, the emphasis is on form, rather than content or function. It is important to be able to distinguish one particular form by seeing it in relation to other forms. Those who put emphasis on content are regarded as barbaric. The same applies to attempts to apply reason to works of art (Bourdieu, 1979/1984, p. 44).

If one plays along with this cultural game, one must be able to play seriously, but without being consumed by a spirit of seriousness. One must distance oneself from necessity. One must, in a manner of speaking, retain a child's view of the world. The aesthetic disposition is thus a generalised ability to turn a blind eye to necessity and practical purposes. It is an expression of distancing oneself in relation to the world.

The taste which is developed by the cultural aristocracy is regarded as being the most natural taste, while all others are unnatural. Taste is justified through negation, through a distancing from other kinds of taste.

> "In matters of taste, more than anywhere else, all determination is negation; and tastes are perhaps first and foremost distastes, disgust provoked by horror or visceral intolerance ('sick-making') of the tastes of others. 'De gustibus non est disputandum'; not because 'tous les goûts sont dans la nature', but because each taste feels itself to be natural – and so it almost is, being a habitus – which amounts to rejecting others as unnatural and therefore vicious. Aesthetic intolerance can be terribly violent." (Bourdieu, 1979/1984, p. 56).

The problem is that this game of culture is not as innocent as one might, at first, believe. What is at stake in every cultural struggle is the right to establish a particular way of living as being the right way. In such a struggle, an arbitrary lifestyle is proclaimed as being the legitimate lifestyle, so all other lifestyles are dismissed as being arbitrary. However, not all social classes are equally well equipped to enter into this struggle of denial and dismissal. In fact, it is only the members of the dominant class who are able construct a lifestyle out of art. Only they are able to rearrange their own dispositions for lifestyle to a system of aesthetic principles. The petit bourgeoisie is nervous about exposing itself to classification, and the working class sticks to what has already been approved in the aesthetic calendar.

The school system can, of course, help give cultural competence to pupils. However, in order to give such help, there must be a certain rationalisation. This cannot rely on practical schemes of classification, but instead explicit and standardised classification systems must be developed. Visual systems can be developed which can act as typologies for all agents. The problem is that there will always be a difference between true cultural competence and educational qualifications. This difference ensures that authentic culture cannot be reduced to scholastic knowledge.

The difference between authentic culture and scholastic knowledge is reinforced by the ideology of natural taste, which makes differences in acquiring culture a question of natural differences. The most legitimate relation to culture is thus that which is least clear. There ought not to be anything educational or academic about the relation to culture. It ought to be made evident with ease and naturalness as nature's true culture. It is thus made into a new mystery.

> "The ideology of natural taste owes its plausibility and its efficacy to the fact that, like all the ideological strategies generated in the everyday class struggle, it *naturalizes* real differences, converting differences in the mode of acquisition of culture into differences of nature; it only recognizes as legitimate the relation to culture (or language) which least bears the visible marks of its genesis, which has nothing 'academic', 'scholastic', 'bookish', 'affected' or 'studied' about it, but manifests by its ease and naturalness that true culture is nature – a new mystery of immaculate conception." (Bourdieu, 1979/1984, p. 68).

In the struggle over which manner is correct, the dominant groups will always lean towards the least rational and the least transparent methods for acquiring culture.

> "Bourgeois culture and the bourgeois relation to culture owe their inimitable character to the fact that ..., they are acquired pre-verbally, by early immersion in a world of cultivated people, practices and objects." (Bourdieu, 1979/1984, p. 75).

No school attendance can compensate for this acquisition of culture. On the contrary, the educational system will sanction the cultural capital which is inherited in this way. It is this capital which becomes an asset which can be invested and profitably exploited.

On the basis of this analysis, Bourdieu developed his theory of cultural practice. As a starting point for the development of this theory, he considered the methodology.

> "... the dispositions which govern choices between the goods of legitimate culture cannot be fully understood unless they are reintegrated into the system of dispositions, unless 'culture', in the restricted, normative sense of ordinary usage, is reinserted into 'culture' in the broad, anthropological sense and the elaborated taste for the most refined objects is brought back into relation with the elementary taste for the flavours of food." (Bourdieu, 1979/1984, p. 99).

The starting point for the theory of cultural practice is a discussion of the social space and its transformations. It is the positioning and the movement of people within this space which forms the basis for their habitus, dispositions and practice. Therefore, objective classes must be constructed. Bourdieu emphasised that social classes cannot be constructed on the basis of their qualities, but rather on the basis of structures of relations between different qualities (Bourdieu, 1979/1984, p. 106). Bourdieu therefore created a three-dimensional space in which social classes are determined by the resources and power which are derived from the three different forms of capital; economic capital, social capital and cultural capital (Bourdieu, 1979/1984, p. 114). Different classes will have access to these different kinds of capital in varying degrees, and they will therefore develop different strategies for investing in their children's future. Here, Bourdieu included the educational strategies which he had discussed in connection with his works on education. These are not discussed in this context.

However, it is not enough to make a classification within the social space. One must also understand that the people who have been classified will have opinions about the classification. These opinions will depend on the positions which they occupy in the social space. The key to understanding this phenomenon is habitus. Habitus is defined as a generative principle which is the basis both for the practice which can be classified, and the differentiation and evaluation made of the practice and products of others. Habitus is thus not only a basis for action, but also for understanding and developing a point of view. Habitus is also an internalised necessity because practice and the evaluation of practice take on a systematic character. Since different living conditions lead to different types of habitus, practice appears as the systematic expression of different objective living conditions. Practice becomes lifestyle (Bourdieu, 1979/1984, p. 170).

As a result, the basic contradictions of class conditions will become established as basic contradictions in the structuring principles, i.e. in habitus. The necessity and freedom which are built into class conditions will thus be changed into generative principles for behaviour. The contradiction between freedom and necessity will be presented as natural. This classification system continually changes necessities into strategies, limitations into preferences, and it generates the set of choices which constitute a lifestyle. It makes a virtue of necessity by introducing the choice which is adapted to the conditions of which it is a product. It is taste, and not income, which directs the practice which fits the objective conditions.

The consequence of this generative principle, habitus, is that within different areas practices will be developed which are in conformity with one another. There will thus be a homology between different areas of consumption.

> "Bearing in mind all that precedes, in particular the fact that the generative schemes of the habitus are applied, by simple transfer, to the most dissimilar areas of practice, one can immediately understand that the practices or goods associated with the different classes in the different areas of practice are organized in accordance with struc-

> tures of opposition which are homologous to one another because they are all homologous to the structure of objective oppositions between class conditions." (Bourdieu, 1979/1984, p. 175).

This made it possible for Bourdieu to look backwards to the most elementary form of taste, which is the taste for food, and its significance for the development of the class-determined body. Through this, he sought to understand the theory of general taste and cultural practice in greater depth.

In this investigation of taste for food, we meet again the distinction between freedom and necessity. The preferences which Bourdieu explained in the contradiction between rich and poor is the contradiction between light and heavy food, between delicate food and nourishing food. This means that the body also feels this fundamental distinction. On the one hand, there is the refined and cultivated body, and on the other hand, there is the big and strong body. The body thus reproduces the logic of the social structures (Bourdieu, 1979/1984, pp. 190-193).

Even in the meal itself, Bourdieu found the distinction between form and substance. The bourgeois meal is characterised by its form, where the rhythm of the meal is important, including its pauses and waiting. It is style and manners that are important. In the working class, what is important about a meal is its substance, including the quantity of food and the feelings of satiety and strength obtained from the meal (Bourdieu, 1979/1984, p. 197). There is the same distinction in the choice of sporting activities, where there is a difference between physical activities based on style, and physical activities which are aimed at developing and strengthening the body.

It is possible to review different areas and investigate the degree of conformity between the choices which are made within each area. In this way one can build up the formula which lies behind the habitus and determines the lifestyle which appears from finding the homologies between these different areas. (Bourdieu, 1979/1984, p. 208).

Bourdieu regarded such different areas as fields which are subject to dynamic development. Each field acts as a system of differences which allow social differences to be expressed. The field which best expresses such social differences is the cultural field. This is because the distinctional relation is objectively built into this field. A work of art is an objectification of this distinctional relation. As soon as it becomes self-conscious, art is defined through negation, which is itself the basis for the refinement through which simple pleasures are distanced. The same applies to the evaluation of art. Because of its embodiment of the social relation, this is itself a distinctional relation.

When Bourdieu discussed the dynamic in the cultural field, he started by emphasising that objectified cultural capital has its own laws.

> "There is no doubt that the works of art inherited from the past and deposited in museums and private collections and, beyond them, all objectified cultural capital, the product of history accumulated in the form of books, articles, documents, instruments, which are the trace or materialization of theories or critiques of these theories, problematics or conceptual systems, present themselves as an autonomous world which, although it is the product of historical action, has its own laws, transcending individual wills, and remains irreducible to what each agent or even the whole population of agents can appropriate ..." (Bourdieu, 1979/1984, p. 228).

Nevertheless, Bourdieu had to distance himself from theories which operated with the idea of objective knowledge without a knowing subject. In this connection Bourdieu was thinking of Karl Popper, among others.

> "… it has to be pointed out that objectified cultural capital only exists and subsists in and through the struggles of which the fields of cultural production (the artistic field, the scientific field etc.) and, beyond them, the field of the social classes, are the site, struggles in which the agents wield strengths and obtain profits proportionate to their mastery of this objectified capital, in other words, their internalized capital." (Bourdieu, 1979/1984, p. 228).

The profit which the agents can obtain from the cultural struggle is a profit of distinction, which is in proportion to the rarity of the means which are necessary for evaluating the objectified culture, and in addition to this there is a legitimation profit which consists of the confirmation of being what one is and of being right. In this context, Bourdieu brought in the difference between culture's function in a class society and in a society without significant social differences. In a class society, the legitimate culture is a product of dominance, and it is predetermined to express and legitimise dominance. In a non-differentiated society, culture is accessible to all, and can be mastered more or less equally well by all. Therefore it cannot be used for dominance.

The problem for intellectuals and artists is that they are split between, on the one hand, wanting a larger audience and a larger market for their works, while, on the other hand, being concerned for the cultural distinction which is based on their own rarity. When several people acquire a distinctive skill, the profit from distinction is threatened. If the market were not supplied with an endless series of new products and new ways of using them, the profit would disappear entirely (Bourdieu, 1979/1984, p. 230).

Within the cultural field, there is a symbolic struggle over the possibility of acquiring distinctive signs in the form of products or behaviour, and for the possibility of maintaining or changing the principles which are the basis of these distinctive qualities. The dynamic in this struggle lies in the strategies which are the basis of the rarity of the products and the belief in their value. Distinction, and with it social class, can only exist through this struggle for the exclusive ownership of the distinctive sign. They are the basis for the natural distinction.

It was Bourdieu's assessment that the cultural struggle has consequences which may result in one distancing oneself from the struggle. The symbolic struggle cannot be seen, and thus has no possibility of being organised. It is bound to take the form of a competitive struggle, which in itself helps to reproduce the distances which are the whole basis for its being.

> "If the relationship of the different classes with culture can be described indifferently either in the language … of distance from the centres of cultural values or in the language of conflict, this is because the symbolic struggles between the classes have no chance of being seen and organized as such, and are bound to take the form of competitive struggles helping to reproduce the gaps which are the essence of the race." (Bourdieu, 1979/1984, pp. 250-251).

When, in their view of culture, the dominant classes distance themselves from everything which is natural, those who want to get on in the world must change the whole of their nature. For those who want to get on in the world, this means they must distance themselves from everything connected with their previous existence, including language, body and taste, and even social roots, family, friends, and so on.

On the basis of this general theory, Bourdieu presented his analysis of his empirical material on three types of relations to culture and their class background. These concern the sense for distinction, which is associated with the dominant class, cultural goodwill, which is associated with the middle class, and the choice of necessity which is associated with the working class. This comprehensive analysis need not be presented here.

When Bourdieu summarised this major work on the relation of social class to culture, he began with some of the fundamental principles of social science. It was his view that, in constructing the social world, the social sciences must take account of the fact that the agents construct the world through their ordinary practice. It is therefore the task of the social sciences to describe the social genesis for the principles of this construction. One must look to the social world for the basis of these principles (Bourdieu, 1979/1984, p. 467).

The cognitive structures, which the social agents implement in their practical knowledge of the social world, are internalised social structures. When these schemes are a product of the basic social structures, they are common to all agents in society, and they thus enable the production of a shared meaningful world, a common-sense world. All the agents in a given social unit thus share some fundamental schemes of perception, which are capable of receiving a preliminary objectification in pairs of antagonistic adjectives. The whole of this network of oppositions, high/low, spiritual/material, light/heavy, free/forced, unique/common, brilliant/boring, forms a matrix of everything held in common, so it is easily accepted because of the social order which lies behind it. Behind them lie the dominant elite and the dominated masses. This social mythology draws its strength from the fact that it refers back to the most fundamental contradictions in society. This means that these contradictions can be used in different areas in accordance with the principle of homology between fields. Individually, these contradictions are very weak, but precisely because of this, they are good at expressing the indefinable. They work especially in relation to everything which is constantly changing.

> "The same classificatory schemes ... can function, by being specified, in fields organized around polar positions, whether in the field of the dominant class, organized around an opposition homologous to the opposition constituting the field of the social classes, or in the field of cultural production, which is itself organized around oppositions which reproduce the structure of the dominant class and are homologous to it ..." (Bourdieu, 1979/1984, p. 469).

> "... when considered in each of their uses, the pairs of qualifiers, the system of which constitutes the conceptual equipment of the judgement of taste, are extremely poor, almost indefinite, but, precisely for this reason, capable of eliciting or expressing the sense of the indefinable." (Bourdieu, 1979/1984, p. 470).

When these opposing pairs occur in different contexts, there is a further confirmation of them. They therefore appear as the wholly necessary result of two fundamental principles of social division: the division between the dominant and the dominated classes, and the division between the competing factions within a given class.

In this way the objective division is written into the presentation of the social world. Objective limits become a sense for limits, and sense of one's own place, which leads to a person excluding himself from the places, people and products from which that person is himself excluded. A sense of limits means that one forgets the limits. They become a matter of course. Both the real world and the world of thought become self-evident. One comes to act as if one knows the structures of the social world, and one's own place in them. This feeling for social structure has nothing to do with any action based on knowledge. It is a social necessity which is settled in a durable relation to one's own physical being, in one's manner of physical presentation, in the way one moves and so on.

The reality is that the perception of the social world is based on the interests of individuals or groups. The boundaries between classes are due to the strategic interests in letting people in or keeping them out.

> "Here the limits are frontiers to be attacked or defended with all one's strength, and the classificatory systems which fix them are not so much means of knowledge as means of power, harnessed to social functions and overtly or covertly aimed at satisfying the interests of a group." (Bourdieu, 1979/1984, p. 477).

> "In short, what individuals and groups invest in the particular meaning they give to common classificatory systems by the use they make of them is infinitely more than their 'interest' in the usual sense of the term; it is their whole social being, everything which defines their own idea of themselves, the primordial, tacit contract whereby they define 'us' as opposed to 'them', 'other people', and which is the basis of the exclusions ('not for the likes of us') and inclusions they perform among the characteristics produced by the common classificatory system" (Bourdieu, 1979/1984, p. 478).

What is at stake in the struggle for the meaning of the social world is power over the classificatory systems which are the basis of the groups' representation, and thus for their mobilisation and demobilisation. It is only through struggle that the inner limits become barriers which must be moved.

The classificatory system only works because, within a symbolic logic, it reproduces the differences within the established order. But this system gives its own symbolic contribution to the maintenance of the order, because it has its own special symbolic power to make people see and believe.

Classification systems would not be so much a subject of struggle if it were not that they contribute to the existence of classes by strengthening the effects of the objective mechanisms. When one gives a group a name, one gives it a role, a social function. A group exists, or does not exist, depending on its ability to be recognised and win its place in the social order (Bourdieu, 1979/1984, pp. 480-481).

On this basis, the task for the social sciences is to take account of the practical knowledge which the agents develop for themselves, by producing sections and classifications. It must be remembered that the products become converted into distinctive signs, which can be signs of distinction or signs of vulgarity, so it can be understood that representation is an integrated part of the social world. A class is defined just as much by the way it is perceived as by the way it is, just as much by its consumption as by its relation to production. Thus it was Bourdieu's opinion that the individual or collective struggle about classification is a forgotten aspect of the class struggle.

In this comprehensive work it becomes clear that Bourdieu understood culture to be everything which is intuitively understood, self-evident and unspoken, and which it is difficult to objectify. It is everything one has learnt at one's mother's knee, in the preverbal stage. It cannot be explicitly formulated. He also emphasised the need to regress culture to the anthropological concept of culture. Finally, we meet again the idea of a common set of master patterns, which are presented in educational works and to some extent in anthropological works. We find them in the contradictions between freedom and necessity, high and low, free and forced, spiritual and material, and so on. At a more general level, Bourdieu spoke of these oppositions as cognitive structures, as basic systems for understanding, or as classificatory systems. Bourdieu considered such a set of common patterns as social mythology. We thus see three key concepts to illuminate

Bourdieu's perception of culture in *Distinction*, and these are: the intuitively understood, the anthropological, and the mythological.

At the same time, Bourdieu recognised that culture can be objectified. It can exist as works, books, articles, theories, concepts etc. In this form, culture cannot be reduced or made subject to human will. It has its own laws. It exists as cultural capital. However, this objectified capital can only exist through struggle which agents carry on with a view to obtaining profit, understood as distinctional profit or legitimation profit, and the possibility of dominance resulting from this. The possibility of obtaining profit is dependent on the ability of the individual to master the objectified cultural capital, and thus the individual's internalised capital. Objectified culture is a capital which can be internalised and thereby become the basis of profit for the individual.

The relation to culture is also an important theme in this work. Where, in their works on education, Bourdieu and Passeron spoke of the relationship to culture being dependent on educational background, in this work Bourdieu spoke of the relationship to culture being dependent on the combination of social background and educational background. He was primarily interested in the relationship of social class to culture. By illuminating the relationship of social class to culture it becomes possible to understand the possibilities for different classes to obtain profit from cultural capital. It is decisive that the dominant class has a distinctive relation to culture, that the middle class has a pretended relation to culture, and that the working class has a necessary relation to culture.

The fact that culture gives the possibility of profit and dominance means that it becomes the subject of cultural struggle between agents. Here Bourdieu spoke of the symbolic struggle to acquire distinctive products and behaviour. The different agents will develop strategies for ensuring for themselves the exclusiveness of their products and behaviour, or their acquisition of distinctive signs. Furthermore, he spoke of the classificatory struggle. This struggle involves strategies to ensure the maintenance of boundaries and thus to establish who is allowed inside and who is kept out. This cultural struggle has significance beyond the symbolic level. Its result will be decisive for the maintenance of the social order. A social group can only gain a place in the social order if it can win recognition at the symbolic level.

In *Distinction* we thus get some elements for illuminating Bourdieu's perception of culture. At the same time, this understanding is put in relation to material and class conditions. Culture and the different relations to culture are products of these conditions. It also becomes clear that culture is relevant to the maintenance of the social order and to the possibility of changing this order. Therefore, the cultural struggle and the strategies behind this struggle are important.

## *Position-taking*

In the anthology of articles, *The Field of Cultural Production*, edited by Randal Johnson, a number of articles are covered in which Bourdieu clarified his theory of the cultural field. This particularly refers to the articles "The Field of Cultural Production" (1983), "The Production of Belief" (1977), "Principles for a Sociology of Cultural Works" (1986) and finally "Outline of a Sociological Theory of Art Perception" (1968). The other articles in the book help to illustrate the mechanisms which operate in the cultural field. Among others, there are more empirically-oriented articles on Flaubert and Manet. However, these articles will not be discussed here.

In the article "The Field of Cultural Production", Bourdieu emphasised his relational thinking by reference to the German philosopher, Ernst Cassirer. According to Bourdieu, when one undertakes research in the areas of art and literature, it is necessary to break with the substantialist thinking which has a tendency to put the individual in the centre. What one must do instead is to focus on the structural relations between the social positions which have been occupied by the individuals, groups or institutions.

> "Few areas more clearly demonstrate the heuristic efficacy of *relational* thinking than that of art and literature. Constructing an object such as the literary field requires and enables us to make a radical break with the substantialist mode of thought (as Ernst Cassirer calls it) which tends to foreground the individual, or the visible interactions between individuals, at the expense of structural relations – invisible, or visible only through their effects – between social positions that are both occupied and manipulated by social agents which may be isolated individuals, groups or institutions." (Bourdieu, 1968-1989/1993, p. 29).

If one wishes to study artistic and literary fields within a given period, then according to Bourdieu, one should construct two spaces, a space of positions, and another space of position-takings. On the one hand, one must construct the space of positions by looking at each position in relation to other positions within a given field. The structure which one arrives at by this means is in reality a pattern for the distribution of the capital which controls success and profit in the field. Each author or artist must see himself placed within such a space of positions.

> "... the space of literary or artistic positions defined by possession of a determinate quantity of specific capital (recognition) and, at the same time, by occupation of a determinate position in the structure of the distribution of this specific capital." (Bourdieu, 1968-1989/1993, p. 30).

On the other hand, one must construct the space of position-takings by investigating the structures for the manifestations of agents within the fields. The space of position-takings thus consists of the indications produced in the works of the artists or writers.

> "The space of literary or artistic position-takings, i.e. the structured set of the manifestations of the social agents involved in the field – literary or artistic works, of course, but also political acts or pronouncements, manifestos or polemics, etc. ..." (Bourdieu, 1968-1989/1993, p. 30).

These two spaces cannot be separated from each other. Together they form the field within which strategies are developed which are dependant upon the positions, and struggles are fought which can lead to the maintenance or change of the field. Bourdieu said that one must look upon the space of position-takings as a product of permanent conflict. The principle which generates and unites this system is the struggle which is carried on from the starting point of the different positions. It was thus Bourdieu's fundamental belief that the principles behind the position-takings lie in the structures found in the space of positions.

Bourdieu said that the history of a given field is the result of the struggles between established practitioners and young challengers. The ageing of writers does not stem from the mechanical, chronological passing of time. It is the result of the struggle between those who have made their mark, and who struggle to survive, and those who cannot make their mark without outmanoeuvring the agents who have an interest in stopping the clock and extending the present situation into the future.

> "To understand the practices of writers and artists, and not least their products, entails understanding that they are the result of the meeting of two histories: the history of the positions they occupy and the history of their dispositions ... In fact, however great the effect of position ... it never operates mechanically, and the relationship between positions and position-takings is mediated by the dispositions of the agents." (Bourdieu, 1968-89/1993, pp. 61-62).

The field is presented to each agent as a space of possibilities. These possibilities are defined as the relation between, on the one hand, the average chances of gaining access to positions, and on the other hand, the dispositions of each agent. It means that the objective chances in a given field at a given point in time become activated through the schemes of perception, expectations and aspirations which constitute habitus. These schemes, which reproduce the fundamental divisions of the field into pure art/commercial art, bohemian/bourgeois etc., are one of the forms of mediation, through which dispositions become adapted to positions.

A position presents itself to each agent either as a necessary destination which draws to it those who are made for it, or as an impossible destination, or as one which is only temporarily acceptable.

> "This sense of social direction which orients agents, according to their modesty or daring, their disinterestedness or thirst for profit, towards the risky, long-term investments of journalism, serials or the theatre, is the basis of the astonishingly close correspondence that is found between positions and dispositions, between the social characteristics of 'posts' and the social characteristics of the agents who fill them," (Bourdieu, 1968-1989/1993, p. 64).

However, writers and artists with different, or even opposing, dispositions can occupy the same positions, at least for a time. The structural limitations within a given field restrict the freedom of action of dispositions. But there are different ways of acting within these limits. The group which occupies the dominant positions will be strongly homogeneous, while the groups which adopt avant-garde positions will have very different origins. Therefore, sooner or later, they will each go off in their own directions. When their cohesion is no longer supported by their opposition to the dominant groups, they will take up their own positions, as some of them obtain recognition. What divides them is the dispositions which constitute the basis for taking aesthetic or political positions. What affects who wins recognition and who does not, is their level of educational capital and social background (Bourdieu, 1968-1989/1993, p. 67).

Not all agents are inclined to move towards the economically most risky positions. Willingness to take risks seems to depend largely on the possession of substantial economic and social capital. Economic capital gives the necessary indifference to profit, which, together with a sense of the chances of profit, points in the direction of the most exposed avant-garde positions and the riskiest investments. In the longer term these will be the most profitable. This sense for investment seems to be one of the dispositions which is most closely associated with social and geographical origins.

> "... those richest in economic, cultural and social capital are the first to move into the new positions... By contrast, a faulty sense of investment, linked to social distance... or geographical distance... inclines beginners to aim for the dominant positions at a

> time when…, the profits are tending to decline. It may also make them persist in declining or threatened positions when the best-informed agents are abandoning them. Or again, it may lead them to be drawn by the attraction of the dominant sites towards positions incompatible with the dispositions they bring to them, and to discover their 'natural place' only when it is too late, i.e. after wasting much time, through the effect of the forces of the field and in the mode of relegation." (Bourdieu, 1968-1989/1993, pp. 68-69).

Bourdieu ended the article with a question about whether these strategies should be considered as cynical calculation. Is it conscious calculation which ensures compatibility between positions and dispositions? There is no simple answer to this question. It differs from agent to agent and from one time to another. According to Bourdieu, it is questionable whether we are able to cope with the answer to this, and if we cannot, then it is perhaps as well that it is difficult to reveal the truth through a critical explanation.

In this article, Bourdieu was concerned with the question of what determines the content of cultural works, understood as art and literature. The article does not really give any further insight into Bourdieu's perception of culture, but it gives further insight into his understanding of the cultural field. Thus, it contributes to explaining his theory of culture.

When Bourdieu explained what determines the content of cultural works, he included three basic elements: positions, position-takings and dispositions. When an artist finds himself in a given position, either as an established artist or as a newcomer, there will be many possibilities for taking a position for marking distinctiveness of content. The choice of marking will depend both on the actual position and the disposition of the artist.

It is thus the combination of the actual position and an inner feeling of social direction which determines which strategies an artist adopts. Does the newcomer dare to move towards risky marks of distinctiveness, with a chance of a high profit, or should he be more careful and more reticent, with a risk of a low profit or even no profit? The true basis for the feeling of social direction is the social, economic and cultural capital which a person possesses.

According to this article, the true explanation for the content of cultural products is to be found in the combination of the actual position and the social and economic origins. This combination determines strategies and position-takings, and thus the content of works.

In another of the articles in this collection of articles on the cultural field, "The Production of Belief", Bourdieu investigated what determines the value of and belief in a cultural product. He started by stating that dealing in art, which means trading in a good which has no price, is a practice in which the logic of the pre-capitalist economy survives. This practice can only operate if one pretends not to be doing what one is in fact doing. It can only work by suppressing narrow economic interests. One must reject commerce, but when it comes to it, even the most anti-commercial and most visible indifference towards economics has a high degree of economic rationality.

The basis of this economic rationality is the possibility of accumulating symbolic capital within the cultural field. Symbolic capital, said Bourdieu, should be understood as economic or political capital which is denied, unappreciated, and thereby recognised and legitimate. It is a credit which, in the long run and under certain conditions, guarantees economic profit. The economic capital which is necessary for producing cultural products cannot give profit unless it has been converted into symbolic capital. For agents in the cultural field, there is only one legitimate form for accumulation, and that is to create a name which makes it possible to introduce objects or people and thereby attach a value to them (Bourdieu, 1968-1989/1993, p. 75).

The question which interested Bourdieu in this article was, who produces the value of the work? Is it the painter or the dealer, the author or the publisher, the playwright or the theatre? Bourdieu believed that it is the dealer who gives the work value. He is the symbolic bank manager who can offer the security and symbolic capital which he has built up, and which he can lose if he backs a loser. Also, for a dealer, the less visible his investment is, the more productive it will be, symbolically speaking. There is an applicable law that promotion must be understated.

The next question is how the dealer obtains the authority to introduce the author or the artist. What is the source of this authority? The dealer's authority is itself a credit-based value which can only exist in relation to the whole field of cultural production. His authority thus exists through his relations to the artists or writers on his list, and those he does not have on his list. It also exists through his relations with other dealers who either do or do not envy him his list of artists or writers. It exists through his relations with critics who either believe or do not believe in his judgment. And finally, it exists through his relations with clients who either do or do not trust him.

> "... what 'makes reputations' is... the field of production, understood as the system of objective relations between these agents or institutions and as the site of the struggles for the monopoly of the power to consecrate, in which the value of works of art and belief in that value are continuously generated." (Bourdieu, 1968-1989/1993, p. 78).

The value of works is thus generated through countless struggles to establish their value. Such struggles nearly always involve the denial of commercial compromises and calculating manoeuvres. In this way the principle of the denial of economics holds centre stage. It is the principle which comes to control the way it functions and changes.

The principle of the denial of economics is constantly maintained by those who are new to the field, because they have a clear interest in denying selfish interests. At the same time they have an interest in toppling the hierarchy of the field, without upsetting its fundamental principles. Their strategies will therefore frequently tend towards a return to its roots, which will always be the basis for all heretical activity. They will use the weapons which the established artists and writers themselves use to justify their dominance. They will demand respect for the basic principle of the field, which is the denial of economics. Conversely, those who occupy dominant positions will develop defensive strategies. They will try to carry on quietly and discreetly (Bourdieu, 1968-1989/1993, pp. 83-84).

Newcomers must get themselves known, distinguish themselves and ensure that there is recognition of the distance which they have put between themselves and the more established producers. They must create a new position. To create a distance is also to make time. The continuous struggle between newcomers and established artists and writers means that each position is pushed further back in the chronological hierarchy, which is simultaneously a social hierarchy. Thus, the distance between style and lifestyle can be measured in time, both in the artistic space, and in the social space (Bourdieu, 1968-1989/1993, pp. 107-108).

The consequence of this development is that there is no possibility of going back to the styles of previous ages. Because of the game played to acquire distinction, every product in the cultural field must always contain some hint or stylistic reference to contemporary or earlier producers in the field. This excludes amateurs. There is no room for naïve practitioners. Therefore an individual product cannot be reduced to being the artist's own work. In this way artistic work is brought closer to intellectual work. The game played about the belief in the value of a work thus becomes a cultivated game. It is a game for cultural mandarins.

A work is thus not produced just once. It is produced again and again by all those who have an interest in it, and those who can obtain material or symbolic profit from it. This occurs through a continual classification, deciphering, commenting, combating etc. The discourse about a work is thus part of the process of producing its meaning and value (Bourdieu, 1968-1989/1993, pp. 110-111).

However, we do not find any further contribution to an understanding of what culture is in this article either. But we do get a further contribution to the theory of the cultural field and thus to the theory of culture. The importance of this article is in giving an explanation of how the values of cultural products are established. It was Bourdieu's view that the value of a work is due to the authority of the dealer, and this in turn is due to the dealer's relations with other agents in the field. What is important about these relations is that they should be characterised by a denial of economic interest.

This principle of the denial of economic interest is maintained by the practising artists themselves. Newcomers will have an interest in this principle. For them, it is not a matter of earning money, but of distancing themselves from the established practitioners. The result is continuous development and continuous interpretation and thereby a re-creation of works.

The outcome of this theory is that works do not in themselves have any value. The value is produced and reproduced constantly by the agents of the field.

In the third of the selected articles, "Principles for a Sociology of Cultural Works", Bourdieu stated that the fields of cultural production exist as a space with possibilities for the people who are involved in the field. It is the field which defines the universe of problems, references, intellectual assumptions, concepts, and so on. It is this field of possibilities which means that producers within a given period are bound both by their situation and their time, and that they are relatively autonomous in relation to their economic and social surroundings. The space of possibilities is thus a system of common references.

Bourdieu applied this understanding when he discussed the analysis of cultural works. Here too, there was a space of possibilities. On the one hand, there is an internal reading and on the other hand, there is an external reading. Internal reading includes the pure reading of pure literature. In this context, cultural works are considered as a pure form. Bourdieu sketched two traditions of this form of reading: the neo-Kantian, where the works only relate to themselves, and the structuralist where the works relate to a common frame of reference. External reading relates the cultural works to their author's social characteristics. This tradition includes the Marxist-inspired writers (Bourdieu, 1968-1989/1993, p. 180).

It was in opposition to these two traditions that Bourdieu introduced his theory on the cultural field. It was thus his aim to focus on the whole of the microcosm within which the cultural agents operate.

> "... the social microcosm that I call the literary field is a space of objective relationships among positions... and one can only understand what happens there if one locates each agent or each institution in its relationship with all the others. It is this peculiar universe, this 'Republic of Letters', with its relations of power and its struggles for the preservation or the transformation of the established order, that is the basis for the strategies of producers, for the form of art they defend, for the alliances they form,

for the schools they found, in short, for their specific interests." (Bourdieu, 1968-1989/1993, p. 181).

What is the consequence of this on the form of works? To answer this, Bourdieu introduced his concept of homology. He developed a hypothesis of a homology between the space of creative works and the space of positions. In this way, the process which produces works becomes a consequence of the struggle which agents contest from the starting points of their different positions.

The direction of change will depend on the space of possibilities given by historical development, and by the interests which direct the agents as a consequence of their positions.

> "The science of cultural works has as its object the correspondence between two homologous structures, the structure of the works... and the structure of the literary field, a field of forces that is unavoidably a field of struggle. The impetus for change in cultural works – language, art, literature, science etc. – resides in the struggles that take place in the corresponding fields of production." (Bourdieu, 1968-1989/1993, p. 183).

These struggles, which aim to maintain or change power relations within the production field, will apparently lead to maintenance or change within the field of works which are the objects of or tools of the struggle.

The strategies which the agents develop in these struggles depend both on their positions, and thus on their cultural capital, as well as on the space of possibilities which is inherited from previous struggles. It is therefore extremely important to investigate the limits of the theoretical framework one is trapped in.

> "This is why – if I may be permitted a parenthesis and a reflexive look back on what I am trying to do – it is so important, if one is to have a bit of freedom from the constraints of the field, to attempt to explore the limits of the theoretical box in which one is imprisoned. This, in my view, is the principal function of theoretical culture: to provide the means for knowing what one is doing and for freeing oneself from the naïveté associated with the lack of consciousness of one's bounds." (Bourdieu, 1968-1989/1993, p. 184).

If one is to place oneself in relation to the space of possibilities, one must see the space as the result of a long history of struggles between theories and theoreticians, between texts and writers, and between reading and readers.

When a field becomes more and more dependent on its own history, it will simultaneously be less and less dependent on external history. If it is possible to speak of 'pure art' in the field of art, this is due to historical development. It is the relative autonomy of the product fields which makes pure aesthetics possible (Bourdieu, 1968-1989/1993, pp. 188-189).

Bourdieu also emphasised that, to understand the relationships between agents within a production field, it is necessary to take account of their habitus. If one wants to explain a number of positions which a given agent will occupy, one must understand that the practice of the person in question is directed by the dispositions which are the consequence of his social background. These dispositions determine whether an individual agent opts for one possibility or another. This is a subconscious process, a feeling for the game. This is why there is such frequent correspondence between the hierarchy of positions and the hierarchy of social origins.

In this article, Bourdieu was also concerned with the question of how to explain the content of works. What interested him was how to explain the increasing tendency for works to be influenced by their own history, rather than by external forces. Here, the principle of homology is clearly applicable. It was his view that there is a homology between the struggles fought within the cultural field and the works produced in that field. When the struggles start from positions which have been inherited through the history of the field, this means that the works themselves will also be influenced by this history. It is here that one must look for the cause of the field becoming more and more dependent on its own history. However, the actual positions occupied by the agents must be explained on the basis of their habitus.

In the last of the articles from *The Field of Cultural Production* which is considered here, "Outline of a Sociological Theory of Art Perception", Bourdieu discussed the question of what determines the capacity to appreciate cultural products. It was his view that evaluating or deciphering cultural products requires the possession of a cultural code.

> "The work of art considered as a symbolic good... only exists as such for a person who has the means to appropriate it, or in other words, to decipher it... The degree of an agent's art competence is measured by the degree to which he or she masters the set of instruments for the appropriation of the work of art, available at a given time, that is to say, the interpretation schemes which are the prerequisite for the appropriation of art capital or, in other words, the prerequisite for the deciphering of works of art offered to a given society at a given moment." (Bourdieu, 1968-1989/1993, pp. 220-221).

Art competence can thus be understood as knowledge of the possible divisions into complementary categories of representations. One must know the principles of classification. Bourdieu made it clear that this code of art is in reality a social institution.

The disposition to appropriate cultural products is therefore the result of general and specific education. The instruments for appropriating art are not a matter of will or consciousness. The tools which are necessary for understanding artistic works are developed in parallel with the tools which are necessary for producing artistic works. In this way a work is produced twice; it is produced by its creator and by those who behold it, in other words by the producer and by society. The question is, whether those who receive and evaluate a work of art are sufficiently well qualified to understand the complexity of the work. Do the two sets of tools complement one another? This problem will often be most marked during periods of great change in art, rather than in more classical periods. When there is great change in art, the tools for appropriating art will frequently be inadequate. The code for understanding the new art will lie in the new art itself (Bourdieu, 1968-1989/1993, pp. 223-226).

The dispositions which are necessary for appropriating art are the result of the influences of families and schools. If one repeatedly appropriates works within a given artistic style, one will, in time, internalise the rules which guide the production of these works. There is an unconscious acquisition of the rules of art. The knowledge which is obtained through the repeated absorption of works of art is the most privileged form for acquiring the tools for appropriating art. This is because the work of art is presented as an individual work, so that it cannot be reduced to being principles and rules for certain styles. The originality of the work can be noted. Artistic styles are not predetermined. They are created and re-created as a consequence of the artist's habitus. It is the artist's habitus which directs the choice which lies behind the creation of the work, and thus the systematic which is created in the works (Bourdieu, 1968-1989/1993, p. 229).

Even if schools cultivate the ability to admire works, classify works, etc., pre-eminent artistic competence will be possessed by those who have the required ability to liberate themselves from school-taught culture, and develop their own attitudes. Such a genuine culture, or free culture, is only relevant for a small minority of educated people. A genuine artistic education requires the possession of previously acquired competence. This competence is unequally distributed between the social classes.

> "... literary or art education... necessarily presupposes, without ever, or hardly ever, being organized in the light of this principle, that individuals are endowed with a previously acquired competence and with a whole capital of experience unequally distributed among the various social classes (visits to museums or monuments, attending concerts, lectures, etc.)." (Bourdieu, 1968-1989/1993, pp. 231-232).

The problem is that school, which is an institution which could take it upon itself to level the differences in cultural competence, allows these differences to operate as differences in natural talent. This is because teachers are driven by the same culture in their pedagogic work, and because they have been influenced in their own families. In this way, cultural capital is attracted by cultural capital. In this context, Bourdieu defined culture as being a system of schemes of perception, expression and historically constituted and socially conditioned thinking.

> "Thus the intensity and modality of the communication are here again a function of culture (as a system of schemes of perception, expression and historically constituted and socially conditioned thinking) which the receiver owes to his or her family milieu and which is more or less close to scholarly culture..." (Bourdieu, 1968-1989/1993, p. 233).

Bourdieu argued that the ideology of natural talent is the basis for legitimising bourgeois privileges. By denying the relationship between education and culture, it is possible to turn cultural competence into a question of natural talent. The view of cultural competence as a natural talent is the basis for a natural division between the bourgeois class and the other classes. Legitimation occurs through the symbolic shift from economic differences to cultural differences. The spiritual sanctification of culture and art serves a very important function, the maintenance of the social order. As a result, educated people are not only able to distinguish between the civilised and the barbaric, but they are also able to legitimise a specific definition of culture. This means that museums, which preserve the relics of the past, and which are, in principle, open to all, are in truth only accessible to those who possess the capacity to appropriate the works.

> "The museum gives to us all, as a public legacy, the monuments of the splendid past, instruments of the sumptuous glorification of the great figures of bygone ages, but this is false generosity, because free entrance is also optional entrance, reserved for those who, endowed with the ability to appropriate the works, have the privilege of using this freedom and who find themselves consequently legitimized in their privilege, that is, in the possession of the means of appropriating cultural goods or, to borrow an expression of Max Weber, in the monopoly of the handling of cultural goods and of the institutional signs of cultural salvation (awarded by the school)." (Bourdieu, 1968-1989/1993, p. 237).

In this article, Bourdieu gave a definition of culture. Culture is the system of schemes which are used for perception, expression and thinking. At the same time, the article adds a further element to the theory of culture in this collection of articles, which is the recipient's ability to appropriate the cultural product. The article seeks an explanation for this.

Bourdieu's view was that the capacity to appropriate a cultural work is the result of family and educational influences. To be able to decipher a work, one must acquire the codes which are built into the work. Since the works are based on all the previous codes in the field, the decipherment of the work must do the same. Therefore, to decipher a work can never be a natural talent. However, the idea of a natural talent plays a social role, which is to make social differentiations natural. The cultivation of art thus has a decisive role to play in the maintenance of the social order.

The four articles from the anthology on the cultural field which are discussed here, thus give a definition of culture as being a system of schemes of perception. These schemes are exemplified in the discussion through oppositions such as pure art/commercial art, bohemian/ bourgeois etc. They also contribute to the theory of the cultural field and thus to a general theory of culture. They do this by introducing a general understanding of the dynamic of the field as being centred around positions, the positions-takings and dispositions. All the articles treat the cultural field as a microcosm characterised by relations and the struggles between its actors. Furthermore, they help illustrate different elements within the cultural field, particularly the questions of what determines the content of a work, and what determines the ability of the recipient of a cultural work to appropriate the work.

## *Reflections*

In a number of articles, lectures and interviews, Bourdieu reflected on his own research. The book, *In Other Words*, contains such reflections on his works. In these reflections, Bourdieu considered both questions of methodology and of concepts.

On the issue of methodology, in a lecture which he gave at the University of San Diego in 1986, Bourdieu emphasised that one must break away from substantialist thinking. Referring to Cassirer, he emphasised the necessity of using relational thinking about the social world. This relational thinking was essentially developed in the fields of physics and mathematics, but according to Bourdieu, one should also view the social world relationally.

> "In order fully to transcend the artificial opposition that tends to be established between structures and representations, one also has to break away from the mode of thought that Cassirer calls substantialist, and which leads people to recognize no realities except those that are available to direct intuition in ordinary experience, individuals and groups. The major contribution of what one has to call the structuralist revolution consisted in applying to the social world a relational way of thinking, which is that of modern physics and mathematics, and which identifies the real not with substances but with relations.... This relational way of thinking is the point of departure of the construction presented in *Distinction*." (Bourdieu, 1987/1990, p. 126).

In this connection, Bourdieu looked back to his book *Distinction*, and pointed out that it was written on the basis of such relational thinking. He thus stressed that a space of positions should be understood as relations between positions. One should thus understand the different lifestyles laid out in *Distinction* as positions within a space of power positions.

According to Bourdieu, objective relations should be understood as relations between positions achieved in the allocation of resources which can be activated in the competition for scarce goods. Such resources can either be economic capital or cultural capital. The position thus achieved will then be the basis for adjusting to this position. One develops what Bourdieu, with reference to Goffman, called 'a sense of one's own place'. This leads to ordinary people keeping to their ordinary positions and others keeping their distance and avoiding becoming familiar (Bourdieu, 1987/1990, p. 128).

*In Other Words* gives some conceptual guide to Bourdieu's perception of culture. The book starts with an interview with Bourdieu by Honneth, Kocyba and Scwibs in 1985. In this interview, Bourdieu looked back at his educational research, including his article, "Systems of Education and Systems of Thought." It was originally his intention to carry out a social criticism of culture. Therefore, in the article he sought to show that mental structures are built into the school system so that divisions in the educational system are the basis for forms of classification. Such forms of classification are also forms of dominance (Bourdieu, 1987/1990, pp. 23-24).

Later in the same interview, Bourdieu referred to culture as being a source of inspiration.

> "It's the role of culture to point out those authors in whom you have some hope of finding help… Culture is that sort of freely available and all-purpose knowledge that you acquire in general at an age when you don't yet have any questions to ask. You can spend your life increasing it, cultivating it for its own sake. Or else, you can use it as a sort of more or less inexhaustible toolbox." (Bourdieu, 1987/1990, p. 29).

It was Bourdieu's view that, as a consequence of the logic of their education, intellectuals treat the works which they have inherited from the past as culture, as a treasure which they can cultivate and thereby obtain for themselves prestige and symbolic dividends, rather than treating them as productive capital which can be invested in research. He himself said that, in order to promote a pragmatic point of view, one must have a barbaric attitude to culture, especially philosophy, which is culture *par excellence*.

In a paper written in 1983, Bourdieu said that in order to master culture, one has to master forms. Such a mastering of culture cannot be developed in one day. It requires the learning of rules which make it possible to play the game to its limits and thus present excellence (Bourdieu, 1987/1990, p. 78).

In another paper from 1981, Bourdieu discussed the question of the dialogue between different academic disciplines. On this issue he spoke of different cultures. If one is a member of one academic discipline, one must decipher what is said in another discipline in accordance with its own codes and its own culture (Bourdieu, 1987/1990, p. 87).

Finally, in a paper dating from 1987, which contains answers to a number of critical points, there are some thoughts relating to culture. Here, Bourdieu argued that culture is a specific capital (Bourdieu, 1987/1990, p. 107). He said that such capital is symbolic and exercises a specific form of domination which he called symbolic power or symbolic violence, when it is known and acknowledged, i.e. when it becomes an object of knowledge and recognition.

> "Culture is our specific capital and…, we tend to forget the true foundation of our specific power, of the particular form of domination we exercise." (Bourdieu, 1987/1990, p. 107).

> "I contend that a power or capital becomes symbolic, and exerts a specific effect of domination, which I call symbolic power or symbolic violence, when it is known and

recognized…, that is, when it is the object of an act of knowledge and recognition." (Bourdieu, 1987/1990, p. 111).

Bit by bit, the different parts of the book, *In Other Words*, add to the picture of Bourdieu's perception of culture. Culture is thus considered as forms of classification, as a treasure which can be used for its own cultivation with a view to obtaining further dividends, or as a tool for solving problems, or it can be viewed as a form, as a code or finally as a form of capital which can be the basis of domination.

At the same time, culture is presented as being, on the one hand, a treasure one can benefit from when solving scientific problems, and on the other hand, a means for securing one's own interests, and a means for exercising dominance, violence and repression.

## *Discussion*

In his thesis on Pierre Bourdieu, Donald Broady puts forward the argument that Bourdieu was inspired by the historical epistemology represented by Gaston Bachelard, among others. It is Broady's view that Bourdieu's theory is primarily a theory of knowledge. Some of the scientific principles which Broady finds in Bachelard and then finds again as fundamental principles in Bourdieu's sociology, are an adapted rationality, relational thinking and science as a construction.

Apart from this epistemologically oriented argument, Broady argues that Bourdieu was also influenced by classical sociological thinking. This argument is supported by a discussion of the three concepts which Broady considers are the most fundamental in Bourdieu's theory: capital, habitus and field. Broady argues that these three concepts were inspired by Marx, Husserl and Weber, respectively (Broady, 1990/1991, p. 297). Broady thus places Bourdieu between Marxism, phenomenology and classical sociology.

Broady believes that classical sociology in particular was significant to Bourdieu's studies of symbolic and cultural phenomena. He believes that on this issue, Bourdieu was strongly influenced by the studies of religion made by Weber and the disciples of Durkheim (Broady, 1990/1991, pp. 198-199).

It is especially in connection with the discussion of the concept of capital that Broady deals with Bourdieu's perception of culture. He considers cultural capital to be a subcategory of symbolic capital, which in turn is a sub-category of the concept of capital. However, Broady points out that Bourdieu's concept of culture developed from being a relatively vague and general concept of culture to become a narrower concept. In his earlier works Bourdieu used a broad anthropological concept of culture, covering any form of human form of life and system of symbols, but, towards the end of the 1960s, he began to refer to culture as the legitimate, authorising and dominant culture. According to Broady, this is what, in the Swedish context, is called high culture. In Broady's view, popular culture cannot be covered by Bourdieu's concept of culture. Consequently, says Broady, Bourdieu's concept of culture can be used to study high culture as one part of culture in a wider anthropological context (Broady, 1990/1991, pp. 222-224).

Broady's treatment of Pierre Bourdieu is one of the most thorough studies of Bourdieu. In order to judge his argument that Bourdieu was inspired by historical epistemology it is necessary to have a closer acquaintance with French philosophy. I will therefore not pursue this argument here, but instead concentrate on his argument that Bourdieu's sociology was characterised by relational thinking. I think this argument is right. Likewise, I think it is right to regard Bourdieu's theory as having been influenced by both Durkheim and Weber. On the other hand, I am not convinced that Bourdieu's theory of culture developed from being a broad anthropological concept to a narrow concept of high culture. Bourdieu's concept of culture remained broad and anthropological throughout his work, but he did use studies of art and literature, among other things.

In the anthology, *Bourdieu: Critical Perspectives*, edited by Craig Calhoun, Edward LiPuma and Moishe Postone, there are a number of articles which are relevant to the question of Bourdieu's perception of culture (Calhoun et al., 1993).

In his article, Edward LiPuma writes that Bourdieu's theory of culture involved a kind of functionalism. If culture becomes an instrument of power, it will have practical functions and thus it will be practical logic which creates the cohesive force in culture. The consequence of seeing knowledge and understanding as a product of positions and the positions-takings is, according to LiPuma, that one must question what such a theory says about society (LiPuma, 1993, pp. 20-23).

Nicholas Garnham addresses the same problem. He, too, points out that if cultural production is reduced to being a power struggle, then cultural content will disappear. He therefore asks whether it is adequate to explain cultural practice on the basis of a struggle for scarce resources (Garnham, 1993, p. 185).

Finally, the anthology contains an article by Scott Lash in which Bourdieu's theory of culture is considered as a theory on the economy behind symbolic practice. Lash focuses on Bourdieu's understanding of cultural economy. As his starting point he argues that Bourdieu's theory is not merely the best, but the only theory on the subject. It is Lash's opinion that neither Marx, Weber nor Durkheim gave even the elements of a theory of culture. It is also his opinion that modern theory is either concerned solely with cultural production, or exclusively with perception. In contrast to these limited approaches, Lash states that Bourdieu's theory of the economy behind symbolic practice provides the tools for analysing cultural production, texts, cultural consumption, the roles of institutions and the media, and the social and historical changes which lie behind cultural practice. Lash sees Bourdieu's model as being primarily a theory on the cultural market. It contains supply, goods and demand, and habitus functions both on the supply and the demand side (Lash, 1993, pp. 193-196). Lash argues that the essential advantage of Bourdieu's theory on the cultural economy is that it gives us a theory for action, in which the action itself is fully structured. With its classificatory capability, habitus is, on the one hand, the basis for understanding specific types of cultural goods, and on the other hand, it is the basis for the production of cultural goods.

When Lash asserts that the classical sociologists did not give so much as the elements of a theory of culture, I must naturally declare my disagreement with this view. The classical sociologists have indeed given us the elements of a theory of culture. Lash reduces Bourdieu's theory of culture to an economic theory on commodities, supply and demand. There is no doubt that the objective aspects were very important to Bourdieu, but I cannot agree with a view that wholly disregards the interpretive and constructional element of Bourdieu. For Bourdieu, culture was not just a commodity.

In this anthology there are thus two opposing views about Bourdieu's ideas on culture. On the one hand, we have LiPuma and Garnham, who criticise Bourdieu for suggesting that culture is determined by struggles for power and the position-takings, so that the content of culture disappears. And on the other hand there is Lash, who considers that Bourdieu's theory is the only theory which can give a cohesive understanding of cultural phenomena. According to Lash, this view is arrived at by seeing the cultural economy as a market for supply, demand and commodities.

In her book, *Pierre Bourdieu and Cultural Theory*, Bridget Fowler concentrates on Bourdieu's cultural sociology with special reference to his analyses of literature and painting. She believes that Bourdieu saw modernism as a period in which the acquisition of culture was reserved for a small elite. The masses were deprived of their culture in the same way that farmers were deprived of their land. This is a process, the terror of which it is difficult to understand in its full consequences. Fowler's aim with her book on Bourdieu is to refute this view (Fowler, 1997, p. 11).

It is Fowler's view that Bourdieu based his theory particularly on a combination of Marx and Weber, as has been seen earlier with Lukacs. According to Fowler, Bourdieu's ideas contain a development of the materialist thinking which is contained in the writings of Marx. The criticism which Marx makes of production is used by Bourdieu in relation to the sphere of cultural goods (Fowler, 1997, pp. 29, 43 and 85).

Fowler's criticism is in many ways linked to the criticisms already noted in the writings of LiPuma and Garnham; it is a criticism more related to substance. It is her view that in his theories, Bourdieu excluded the art which is produced by members of the dominated classes, and he thus undervalued both mass produced and folk art. It is also her view that Bourdieu's theories see artists as involved in a constant search for dominance. Fowler believes that this means that Bourdieu overlooked the fact that artists can very well seek dominance at the same time as acting as prophets. She believes that certain artistic movements can be compared with the poor peoples' church. They can act as prophets, promote new aspects and criticise when others are silent. She thus criticises Bourdieu for having a passive perception of authors. She believes one should develop a more active view of authors. One should understand that, through the practice of their art, they show an ability to interpret and develop the discourse for their time. Fowler thus criticises Bourdieu for undervaluing the subjective aspect (Fowler, 1997, pp. 64-65 and 176-179).

It is relevant to ask to what extent Bourdieu undervalued the substance of culture. Do writers and artists really have no substantive intentions in the works they create? On the other hand, I do not believe one can interpret Bourdieu's theory in a way which deprives the masses of their culture. Popular culture still exists in Bourdieu's theory. It is just not objectified. For Bourdieu, the essential problem was the dominance which exists in the cultural field.

In his book on Bourdieu, Richard Jenkins reviews and discusses a number of important questions about Bourdieu's ideas. To start with he discusses Bourdieu's sources of influence. His view is that Bourdieu based his concept of practice on Marx, his theory of classification on Durkheim, and his theory on lifestyle and status on Weber. As well as these, he names Levi-Strauss, Sartre, Wittgenstein, Goffman, Husserl and Nietzsche as sources of influence.

Jenkins argues that a key aspect of Bourdieu's work was to understand the relationship between subjectivity and the objective world. However, he believes that Bourdieu lacked the ability to deal with the issue of subjectivity. Jenkins believes that this meant that Bourdieu undervalued the actors' knowledge of the social world. In the same way, Bourdieu also undervalued rationality. According to Jenkins, this resulted in a deterministic theory. In Jenkins's opinion, Bourdieu was a prisoner of objectivity. Bourdieu objectified what he studied, and then objectified his objectification. Jenkins's main criticism of Bourdieu is thus that he said that he would overcome the dualism between subject and object, while all the time being rooted in objectivism, and that he rejected determinism while developing deterministic models (Jenkins, 1992/1996, pp. 25, 91, 97 and 175).

Jenkins also criticises Bourdieu for having an unclear concept of culture. He believes that, on the one hand, Bourdieu presented culture as being material artefacts, and, on the other hand, he presented it as a concept to encompass the unconscious. Jenkins says that habitus acts as an analogy for culture in Bourdieu's explanation of human behaviour. Jenkins suggests that this raises questions about how habitus should be related to the concept of culture (Jenkins, 1992/1996, p. 92).

According to Jenkins, the habitus concept should involve the embodiment of culture. This means that culture is not merely a matter of ideas. Jenkins thinks this is an original and challenging idea. However, he also points out that the consequence of this idea is that thinking becomes reduced to being an appendix or an effect of the body (Jenkins, 1992/1996, pp. 93 and 98).

Jenkins focuses on the fact that the cultural unconscious, habitus, is developed in school as categories for cultural consumption. This means, says Jenkins, that Bourdieu's theory does not cover the question of cultural production. Bourdieu solved this problem, says Jenkins, by insisting that the same principles apply to cultural production as to cultural consumption (Jenkins, 1992/1996, p. 136).

Finally, Jenkins argues that, in Bourdieu's work, high culture is subsumed in anthropological cultural perceptions. High culture becomes absorbed in general culture. Jenkins hints at his criticism of this approach when he says that Bourdieu ought to have put anthropology to one side and go out and meet the people he wrote about (Jenkins, 1992/1996, pp. 128 and 149).

Jenkins thus makes a number of criticisms of Bourdieu's theory. At the general level these criticisms concern determinism and the absence of scope for knowledge and rationality in human action. On the aspect of culture, the criticisms concern the lack of care in dealing with the concept of culture. In many ways, Jenkins has identified some important questions about Bourdieu's theory.

The last work which is discussed here is Derek Robbins's book, *The Work of Pierre Bourdieu*. This book is a general introduction to Bourdieu's work, and an attempt to reconstruct Bourdieu's mental approach. Towards the end of the book, Robbins makes a comparison between Bourdieu and the English romantics. Robbins believes that the English romantics had a concept of habit which corresponded to Bourdieu's perception of habitus. In both cases the result was a weak determinism.

Robbins believes that Bourdieu considered it was his task to give sociological form to Kant's view of pure and practical reason and aesthetic evaluation. This sociological form avoids any form of psychological interpretation. It is pre-Freudian (Robbins, 1991, p. 170).

According to Robbins, Bourdieu believed that it was necessary to regard both culture and social relations as internally coherent systems. However, this breaks with classical rationalism which distinguishes between the eternal truths of formal logic and historically conditioned empirical truth. Instead, one must acknowledge that social reality must be understood as a system with in-built necessity (Robbins, 1991, p. 75).

As for his perception of culture, Robbins believes that in the 1960s Bourdieu was faced with a dilemma with three types of culture: aristocratic culture, rational culture and popular culture. Aristocratic culture creates a social hierarchy. The purpose of museums and galleries is to transform this aristocratic culture. Rational culture should harmonise society and get it to function on a democratic basis. It is rational pedagogy which undertakes this task. Popular culture should be included in and used by the other two forms of culture. For example, it is expressed in photography (Robbins, 1991, p. 53). Robbins believes that, at the start of the 1960s, Bourdieu argued for a rational culture, but that towards the end of the 1960s he recognised that the educational system performed a necessary logical function in society (Robbins, 1991, p. 62).

Robbins thus believes that there was a development of Bourdieu's ideas on culture, which was especially linked to the pedagogic question. However, this argument seems somewhat random and unsystematic. He does not otherwise add anything new and significant to the discussion on Bourdieu's cultural ideas.

On the basis of this review of the secondary literature, a number of significant points of discussion of Bourdieu's theory have been highlighted. As for the intellectual background to Bourdieu's theory, there appears to be an argument about how far he built it up by drawing on a wide range of sources in the intellectual universe, or whether it is possible to discover a more coherent principle to explain his theory. As for culture, there appears to be an argument about the extent to which this should be understood solely as the result of power struggles and the position-taking, or whether culture should be understood more substantively as an expression of human ideas, ideals and desires. And finally there is the question of the relationship of social class to culture. Is culture exclusively for the elite, or does popular culture also exist?

In what follows, I shall give my interpretation of Bourdieu's ideas on culture and of culture's relationship to other social phenomena. As a starting point for this presentation of Bourdieu's perception of culture, I will discuss the background to it. What was the societal background to his theory? What problems concerned him? What were his major influences, and what was the significance of these influences for his theory of culture?

Bourdieu's theory was founded in the 1960s and it bears the marks of the contemporary concerns for repression. The war in Algeria focussed his interest on the Algerian people and on understanding their way of life. The massive increase in the numbers going on to further education attracted his attention to educational work. And finally, differences in the acceptance of different forms of cultural expression directed his attention towards art and literature. It is thus repression and dominance in the Third World, in education and in culture that were the background to the development of Bourdieu's thinking. Bourdieu's theory is not concerned with revealing raw or direct forms of repression. It is concerned with revealing symbolic repression. It is symbolic violence and the mechanisms of repression which operate at the symbolic level which concern him. This form of dominance is hard to recognise and difficult to organise against. The problem is that symbolic dominance is accompanied by material advantages.

On an intellectual level, Bourdieu's theory is characterised by the schism between objectivist thinking and subjectivist thinking which was prevalent among intellectuals in France in the1960s. The representatives of objectivism included the structuralist oriented anthropologist Levi-Strauss and the structuralist oriented linguist Saussure. The representatives of subjectivism included the phenomenology oriented anthropologist Mauss and the existentialist philosopher, Sartre. The essential question is whether human behaviour is conditioned by objective structures, or whether human beings can act of their own free will. Bourdieu could not avoid taking a position on this question in the intellectual arena of France in the1960s. His solution was to try to build a bridge between objectivism and subjectivism. He wanted to create a relationship between objective structures and the human subject.

In order to do this, Bourdieu borrowed ideas from philosophy. He referred frequently to the German philosopher, Ernst Cassirer, whose fundamental idea was that scientific thinking leads us from substantive thinking to relational thinking. It was thus Cassirer's belief that mythological thinking is substantive, while modern science, including mathematics and natural sciences, is relational (Cassirer, 1910/1953 and 1921-1929/1955). It is this basis of relational thinking which creates a coherence in Bour-

Bourdieu's works and has constitutive effect for his theory. It is this relational thinking which makes it possible for him to relate the subject to objective structures.

In addition to this, Bourdieu operated with the principle of including the best products of the thinking of his predecessors. He believed that their ideas should be used as tools for further thinking. In this way, access to their thinking becomes truly productive. He explained this approach in, among other things, the article "The Genesis of the Concepts of Habitus and Field" (1985).

When Bourdieu had to solve the theoretical problems he encountered, he thus drew on different kinds of thinking from philosophy, sociology, art history and so on.

He used this principle when, for example, he had to bridge objective and subjective thinking. In this context, habitus was an important concept, and he developed it in order to break with structuralism without having to fall back on the individualism of economic thinking. His aim in developing the concept of habitus was thus to reintroduce the individual who actively takes action, the creative agent. In the article "The Genesis of the Concepts of Habitus and Field", he explained that the habitus concept goes all the way back to Aristotle and his use of the concept of *hexis*, but that he was primarily influenced by the art historian, Panofsky (Bourdieu, 1985, p. 13). In his book, *Gothic Architecture and Scholasticism*, Panofsky developed a theory that there is a parallel between these two forms of cultural expression. According to Panofsky, both scholastic thinking and gothic architecture are characterised by a wholeness, a systematic, division into parts, clarity and explicitness. In this connection, Panofsky used the concept of mental custom, and defined it as a principle for regulating action. Such mental customs exist in all civilisations and can, in this instance, explain the parallels between gothic architecture and scholastic thinking (Panofsky, 1951/1976, pp. 20-21).

Also, when Bourdieu had to bridge external reading and internal reading he had to develop a new concept, the concept of field. The aim of developing this concept was to be able to understand a given work both in the light of its inner necessity and its external necessity. A work does not merely follow the rules of reason or beauty. It also follows the rules which lie in the field and the relations between its positions. The source for this concept came primarily from Weber's studies of religion, and in particular his chapter on religion in *Economy and Society*. In this chapter, Weber analysed the different kinds of agent in the religious world, at the same time as analysing different kinds of religious ideas. It was in this chapter that he introduced the distinction between priests and prophets, between the learned and the charismatic, between rationality and revivalism (Weber, 1956/1968, p. 425). Where, according to Bourdieu, Weber adopted a perspective of interaction in relation to the agents in the religious world, he himself was of the view that the religious field is constructed of objective relations. Bourdieu thereafter saw it as his task to transfer the principles which he had identified in the religious field to other fields, under the principle of homology (Bourdieu, 1985, pp. 17-18). The principle of homology is thus a principle of his scientific thinking.

Bourdieu did not himself identify Weber as the origin of the distinction between economic capital and cultural capital. However, I suggest that Weber's distinction between class and status was a possible source of Bourdieu's idea of the distinction between the two forms of capital.

In summarising this discussion of Bourdieu's intellectual background, two principles are apparent. The first principle is relational thinking. The second is the principle that problems in current thinking can be solved by using the ideas of previous thinkers as problem solving tools. As a consequence, Bourdieu had both some basic principles for his thinking, and a tendency to draw inspiration from numerous other sources. He had a productive relationship with existing culture.

In the course of his different works, Bourdieu gave explanations of some of his methodological principles. It is characteristic that he used the same principles for both practical logic and theoretical logic. He thus used the same principles for understanding empirical phenomena and scientific phenomena. These principles include relating, constructing and objectifying.

The principle of relating is both a scientific and an empirical principle. Bourdieu distinguished between theoretical relating and practical relating. Bourdieu considered relational thinking, understood as thinking which emphasises relations rather than substance, to be a scientific principle. At the same time, he studied how humans struggle to develop certain kinds of relations between each other and to culture.

The principle of constructing is likewise both a scientific and an empirical principle. Here, Bourdieu distinguished between theoretical logic and practical logic. In theoretical logic the researcher must construct and interpret on the basis of the material which the person in question has available. The researcher must investigate whether there is homology or contradiction between different kinds of empirical phenomena, between different fields. The only test of the truth of such constructions is the cohesion of the constructions. Bourdieu considered practical logic to be built up on the same principles as for construction. Everyday understanding of the world around us is based on principles of homology or contradiction. If oppositions exist in one area, they will be transferred to another area.

Finally, there is the principle of objectification. Here Bourdieu distinguished between objectifying the researcher's relations to phenomena and objectifying phenomena. The principle of objectification applies equally to empirical phenomena and to the researcher's relations to empirical phenomena. The researcher is thus required to objectify his own relations to his research, and to objectify the phenomena which are the subjects of his research.

The methodological principle which was most significant for Bourdieu's perception of culture was the principle of construction, or the principle of homology. In all of Bourdieu's works we see opposing pairs as an expression of social mythology. This is the case, regardless of whether these relate to anthropological studies in Kabyle, or educational or cultural research in France. Everywhere he saw these pairs of oppositions which, together, formed what he called the common sets of master patterns or basic schemes of perception. In several places Bourdieu defined these common sets of master patterns as culture. Culture is thus the common schemes of perception, common forms of classification, common codes etc., which, according to the principle of homology can be transferred from one domain to another. For Bourdieu, culture was common.

This does not mean that Bourdieu denied the existence of objective culture. In several places he refers to objective culture, understood as works, treasures, accessible knowledge, theories, sources of inspiration and so on.

Bourdieu's concept of culture can thus be considered as including, on the one hand, common schemes for perceiving the world around us, and, on the other hand, objective culture as a source of inspiration for the individual's further development of culture.

The principle of relating is essential for the theory of culture derived from Bourdieu's works. Bourdieu's theory of culture is in reality a theory about the relations of individuals and social classes to culture. At the level of the individual, which we find in his educational research, Bourdieu distinguished between the relation to culture which is characterised by ease, elegance, mastery, style and taste, and the relation to culture which is characterised by worry, toil and vulgarity. At the level of class, which is especially prominent in the book *Distinction*, Bourdieu distinguished between the dominant

dominant class's distinctive relation to culture, the middle class's pretended relation to culture, and the dominated class's relation of necessity to culture.

The principle of objectification becomes apparent when Bourdieu had to explain these relations to culture. In his educational research he objectified culture, pedagogic work and even educational institutions by relating them to the objective structures which lie behind them. Culture thus relates to class, or more correctly to a specific class, the dominant class. Pedagogic work relates to habitus, or more correctly to a specific habitus, which is the habitus which is developed when growing up in the families of the dominant class. Institutions are related to class interests, or more correctly to the interests of the dominant class.

In his analyses of art and literature, the principle of objectification becomes prominent when Bourdieu had to explain how one form of culture becomes more legitimate than another. Here, too, he made a relation between culture and class. The social space forms the background for determining which cultural expression becomes the most legitimate. At the same time, Bourdieu objectified the relations within the cultural field. He related the position-takings, through the production of individual works, to the objective positions which the artists or writers already occupied. In this way there is an objectification of the products which are created within the cultural field. Cultural products take on the character of position-takings, and they are the result of the interplay between the position which the artists and writers adopt, and the dispositions which they have developed through their upbringing.

If, on this basis, one tries to summarise Bourdieu's theory of culture on a more substantive level, one must say that it is primarily a theory of cultural dominance, or more precisely, of symbolic violence. In classless societies symbolic violence is evidenced by the showing of trust, obligations, loyalty, hospitality, gifts, in other words, in everything that is part of an ethic of honour. This symbolic violence creates dependency between people. The result of this is dominance, not merely symbolically, but also materially.

In societies which have class divisions, symbolic violence is evidenced by making an apparently arbitrary culture natural and legitimate, and thus creating a distance between it and other forms of culture. A key means for ensuring this naturalisation of an arbitrary culture is the pedagogic work of the educational system. This work itself appears to be arbitrary. However, this double arbitrariness is not in itself arbitrary, but necessary. Therefore the arbitrariness is itself symbolic violence. Naturalness and arbitrariness are both the basis for symbolic and material dominance.

The dominance in pedagogic work occurs by its being related in its complete form to the habitus which is most widespread among the pupils of the dominant class. This thus legitimises the culture which they bring with them. Pupils from other classes find that the culture which they bring with them from their families is not legitimate. These pupils from the dominated classes not only find that the culture which they have acquired in their families is not accepted, they also find that the culture which they acquire in school is not the authentic culture. School learning, with its classification of materials, is merely a vulgar version of authentic culture, which is based on the correct habitus. There is therefore no purpose in acquiring this school-based culture. It is only a pale imitation of the real thing. In any case, authentic culture cannot be learnt; one must grow up with it. In this way it obtains an aura of mysticism and inscrutability. Through the legitimisation of this authentic culture, there is a legitimisation of the class which is the bearer of the culture. The consequence of legitimising the culture of the dominant class is the legitimising of the classification which is in the interests of the dominant class. There is a natural drawing of boundaries between classes, and between those who are on the inside and those who are outside. Symbolic violence thus provides the basis, not only for symbolic dominance, but also for material dominance.

Class background is also important for those who want to be agents within the cultural field. New producers will develop a strategy for succeeding in the field, but this strategy will only be effective if it fits in with the class habitus. There is no purpose in wanting to be an avant-garde artist if one does not have the ability to master the objectified cultural capital and if one does not have a natural sense for where to invest. The foundation for this natural sense for culture and for cultural investment must be laid while growing up. The consequence of this view is that both the ability to produce and the ability to receive cultural products are dependent on class determined habitus. Symbolic violence is also apparent here. It is not really possible to be a cultural agent unless one has the right class background. One will be dropped, but unfortunately one will not find this out until it is too late.

If Bourdieu's theory is a theory of symbolic violence, it has to be said that the symbolic violence is not without its clashes and armed exchanges. Students who find that their schemes of understanding are not accepted in educational institutions will distance themselves from the whole way the institutions operate. Members of the dominated classes who find that their way of interpreting the world is not legitimate, will try to make a virtue of necessity and will distance themselves from those who do not do the same. Artists who do not possess the right sense for cultural investment will take up the fight against the established field and develop strategies for occupying a dominant position. Here, too, there is a principle of distancing from those who already occupy leading positions. And finally, there is all the classification which takes place on the basis of a general view of the world through opposing pairs. If this classification means that one is put in a class with a disadvantaged position, there will be conflict over the classification. One must distance oneself from the existing classification, and try a more advantageous classification. Symbolic violence has its limits.

One of the questions one can ask about Bourdieu's theory is, how far he succeeded in bridging objective and subjective thinking. Did he succeed in creating a theory with room for the subject dealt with, the agent? The link should be habitus, which is a result of the objective structures and at the same time a generative principle for the actions of the agent. However, Bourdieu's methodological principle of objectifying means that all phenomena are referred back to the objective structures. Habitus refers back to class, culture refers back to the social space, institutions refer back to class interests, cultural products refer back to habitus and objective positions and so on. How many different possibilities for action do the agents really have? The strategies they develop work best if they are in conformity with their habitus. The choices they make are a consequence of habitus. The products they create are a consequence of habitus and positions. Habitus is a consequence of the objective structures. Is habitus a concept which makes it possible to see the agent as a subject who has the possibility of taking action and influencing his surroundings, or is habitus a concept which makes us see the agent as a subject who contributes to the reproduction of his surroundings? How important are the struggles about positions, about classification and about symbols, if the strategies which lie behind the struggles are controlled by habitus, and thus by objective structures? Will they change anything in everyday life, or will they first become significant when the objective structures are put under so much strain that the system cannot function any more, as was, for example, the case with the educational structures in France in the 1960s, or with French rule in Algeria?

Another question which can be asked of Bourdieu's theory is, how far he succeeded in bridging internal and external reading. Is field a concept which makes it possible to see cultural products in the light of previous products and of external influences? Is the struggle for positions within a given field decisive for which products are produced? Have writers and artists no message they want to give? Is it merely a question of distancing oneself from those who are on top of the heap in order to gain a position for oneself? Must we admit that objectifying is so all-embracing that the subject, with its ideas and ideals, totally disappears?

A third question which can be asked of Bourdieu's theory is, how far he succeeded in creating a theory which applies both to empirical phenomena and to scientific phenomena. If we consider the principle of construction through homology, this principle was developed through the studies of farmers in Kabyle. These primitive people developed their understanding of the world using the principle of homology. They transfer the principles from nature to humans, to the house, to the relationship between the sexes, etc. In this way they establish a coherence in their understanding of the world through opposing pairs. The basis for this homology in their thinking, is their own habitus. However, the question is whether it is possible to transfer this principle to scientific thinking. Can scientific thinking also be developed by using the principle of homology? Is it possible to imagine that, because a principle applies in one field, it will also apply in another? Is it plausible that it is possible to explain developments in the field of cultural production according to the same principles which apply in the field for cultural consumption? Is it plausible that the principles which apply in the cultural field also apply in other kinds of fields? What is the basis for this homology? Is it the habitus of the artists, the consumers or of the dealers which makes this possible? With Bourdieu, the principle of homology was extended so far that it could cover how farmers in Kabyle think and how French scientists think. Is it plausible that, with the principle of homology, mythological thinking and scientific thinking can be controlled by the same principle of homology? What is the basis of this similarity? Is it the habitus of the researcher? If so, what does this say about the factual circumstances? Do we know anything about the empirical circumstances, or do we know something about the researcher's habitus?

This raises the more general question of how far it is possible to develop a sociological theory on the basis of studies of classless societies and then transfer it to studies of societies which have different classes. Is it reasonable to imagine that such widely differing social units as farmers in Kabyle and the cultural aristocracy in Paris should operate under the same principles? Did such a concordance exist only within Bourdieu's mind, as a result of his habitus, or does it exist in the empirical conditions which result from the similarities between the habitus of the agents studied?

# Part III
# Conclusion

# 8

# Conclusion: From Concern to Distance

Sociology originated as criticism. When one reads the writings of Durkheim, Weber and Simmel, it is clear that their shared point of departure was criticism of the German historical school. In his biography of Durkheim, Lukes writes that he was strongly influenced by the German historical school, but that he also sought to distance himself from it, because historians had a tendency to describe rather than explain. Weber wanted to reform the historical school by distancing himself from its highly objectivist approach. On the one hand he wanted to retain its ideas of value-freedom and neutrality, and on the other hand he wanted to open the way for a more interpretative approach. Simmel, too, developed his theory in a dialogue with the German historical school and its belief that it is possible to make a photographic image of reality.

It is thus clear that the founders of sociology were both inspired by the German historical school and wished to distance themselves from it. They were interested in the problems of history, but were critical of the methodological principles which the German historical school used. They did not believe in the highly objectivist and 'photographic' approach. What they wanted, instead, were explanations, interpretations and coherence.

The starting point for sociology was thus the dilemma between wanting to keep hold on the scientific premises of value-freedom and objectivity, and wanting to establish the freedom to be able to explain and interpret the wider developmental trends of society. This methodological dilemma is the basis for an important tension in sociology.

## *Classical theory of culture: Concern and criticism as the driving forces*

For Durkheim, taking his point of departure in the German historical school meant that, on the one hand, he was concerned to be able to generalise and to conceptualise social phenomena, and, on the other hand, he wanted to be able to explain their development. The whole of his methodological principle of social facts had the aim of ensuring the development of valid concepts for understanding actions which were of fundamental importance for society. At the same time he wanted to establish the relations between cause and effect in the behaviour of the past and to develop rules for future behaviour. Durkheim himself emphasised that his approach to sociology was rationalist.

The question is why the issue of methodology was so important for Durkheim. Why was it important to develop concepts and to explain? It was so because explanation, and especially scientific explanation, are parts of his theory of how social development can be influenced, and it was his concern for social development which was the thread which ran through his work.

Concern for social development can become tangible in a concern that economic life, which is without moral rules, will predominate. The consequence would be a crisis for European society. The question of morality greatly concerned Durkheim. He characterised morality as mediocre, and if it was to be improved, explanations had to be found. Explanations can affect individuals, so explanations are important.

Durkheim found inspiration for his development of explanations in biology. It was the concepts of biology, such as cells, germs and systems, which he transferred to the social sciences. One must go back to the original cell or germ in order to be able to explain later developments, and increasing complexity and systematisation. This was why he called his method the genetic method.

The bases for Durkheim's beliefs about culture were, on the one hand, a dispute with the traditional historical method, and the consequent search for an explanatory method, and on the other hand a concern for societal development. It is against this background that we must understand his proposals for a concept of culture and a theory of culture.

For Durkheim culture was a subject/object relation. There is an external culture of treasures which are preserved by society, and an internal culture of personal characteristics which are linked to the individual. Durkheim created a relation between the external and the internal culture by opposing the system and the individual to each other. Culture is considered as a system of rules for living, a system of rituals and a system of categories. These systems can be transferred to people, where they become systems of habits, emotions and ideas. The fact that culture is transferred to people means that systems are developed in these people. Their behaviour and thinking will be regular and predictable. In contrast to these very general expressions there are the more concrete expressions which, on an objective level, are the cultural treasures consisting of works of art, writings, buildings etc., and which, on a subjective level, are linguistic capability, the ability to think, the ability to acquire knowledge and insight etc. Culture is thus both general and specific. It is both systematised and concrete. It is both scientific and historical.

If we look at Durkheim's texts in more detail, there are two types of relations which he develops explanations for. On the one hand he tries to answer the question about how society affects culture, and on the other hand he tries to answer the question of how objective culture influences subjective culture.

On the question of how society affects culture, Durkheim developed no fewer than four different explanations. There is the reflection explanation, according to which the collective creates the categories which it already knows from its social organisation. There is the constitutive explanation, according to which society needs the categories which are instituted through rituals and the emotions to which these rituals give rise. There is the resource explanation, according to which increased welfare and social integration provide a peaceful environment for intellectual work and thus a basis for cultural development. And finally, there is the conflict explanation, according to which culture's development is determined by conflicts between different social groups.

Durkheim also developed a series of explanations for how objective culture affects subjective culture. The most important of these are the emotion-based explanation and the explanation based explanation. The emotion-based transfer of culture is linked to rituals. Rituals are able to transfer culture to individuals because, through rituals, a feeling is created for the symbols of society. It is thus the emotions of the individual which ensure the continued existence of the symbols and society. The explanation based transfer of culture is linked to education. Education can transfer culture to the individual because of the capacity for exploiting a child's natural disposition to develop emotions of duty and ideals and the possibility of linking these duties and ideals to empirical circumstances. The duties and ideals can thus be explained.

It is here that the significance of the explanation comes into the picture. The explanation, and with it the scientific explanation, has a special significance. Sociology, as a science of cultural phenomena, can create explanations, and these explanations can form the basis for the development of morality, thinking and knowledge in the individual. One must understand cultural phenomena and be able to explain them. It is in this way that one can influence them.

Thus, Durkheim ascribes to sociology and its explanations of cultural phenomena great significance for the development of culture and thus for the development of society. That is why it was important for Durkheim to give explanations rather than descriptions.

When one reads the writings of Durkheim, one gets a clear impression that the tension between historical thinking and systems thinking lives on in his analytical work. Some of his works seek explanations for historical changes, while others seek explanations for systematisation. In some of his works human beings appear as dynamic actors in the struggle between different ideas. In others the categories of ideas are laid down in primitive societies, and are then reinforced through history, despite increasing complexity. The question I have raised is what this tension, or contradiction as Durkheim would have called it, means for the further development of sociology.

For Weber, the fact that his point of departure was the German historical school, meant that he was particularly concerned with the problem of values. On the one hand he retained the historical school's requirement of value-neutrality in relation to the results obtained. The researcher must not take a view about the phenomena studied. The results must speak for themselves. On the other hand, in his choice of research topic and in the development of his concepts, the researcher must be guided by his own values. A researcher cannot develop concepts without such value-relations. Without values there would be no research. Thus the researcher's own values make the whole difference between the historical school's descriptive research and Weber's sociological research. Therefore, all kinds of research must also be analysed for their value-content. One must reveal the values which have guided the researcher's treatment of a given topic. One must find the vulnerable points in a given text. When the value-content has been clarified, one can try to explain how the text came into being. One can study the circumstances which prompted the researcher to produce the text.

Here, too, one may ask why it was important to make this methodological argument. Why was it important to replace descriptive with value-related research? It was because Weber wanted to study particular historical phenomena. It was the spirit of capitalism, the Protestant ethic, the Chinese mandarin culture, western rationalism etc. which interested him. One cannot describe such phenomena. They are too wide-ranging and complex to be described. They must be understood. The tools for understanding them are general concepts, or ideal types, as Weber called them.

Weber chose to study these high-level phenomena because of his concern for the general development of society and for cultural development. It was capitalism, rationalism, social fragmentation, specialisation and the breaking down of man as a whole which concerned him. He believed that it was increasingly impossible to maintain the cultivation of man as a whole. His concerns were thus directed at the increasing degree of complexity of culture and its increasingly ruinous lack of meaning.

Even though Weber was critical of the German historical school and worried about cultural development, he remained faithful to German cultural tradition. He did not add new forms of thinking to the existing forms. He was neither convinced by historical materialism nor by positivism. In truth, he upheld German cultural thinking and made it into a scientific principle.

The starting points for Weber were thus, on the one hand, a dispute with the German historical school's descriptive methods and its consequent reliance on the development of a value-based cultural science, and, on the other hand, a concern for the continued development of culture and its consequent loss of meaning. It was against this background that he developed his ideas of culture and his proposals for a theory of culture.

For Weber, culture is that part of the world which people relate to their values and thus give them meaning and significance. Culture consists of those phenomena which have been ascribed meaning. It is those phenomena which are significant for people. Among the values which contribute to constituting culture, and thus creating meaning, are ethics, aims, emotions, beliefs and aesthetics.

When one reviews Weber's writings, several theoretical perspectives stand out, including society's influence on culture, culture's influence on society, culture's influence on culture, culture's influence on people and culture as an excluding phenomenon.

It was Weber's view that culture is influenced by a multiplicity of forces, which include socio-economic structures, interest groups, institutions and ideas.

Culture's influence on culture consists of one idea's development being inspired by another. When an idea is generated, it will have been inspired by other ideas, but it will also be the basis for the development of new ideas. It was this continuous process which Weber regarded so pessimistically. It leads to increasing complexity and confusion within culture.

Culture's influence on people includes aspects both of cultivation and of behavioural rules. There is a transfer of culture to people. The problem is that, with the increasing degree of complexity and confusion, it is difficult for any individual to absorb culture as a whole. If the aim is perfect cultivation, it becomes impossible. No single person can acquire the whole of culture. One must be selective and be satisfied with acquiring parts of it. Another aspect of the influence of culture on the individual is culture as a regulator of behaviour. A particular idea leads to a particular kind of behaviour. In this way culture can be transferred to the individual and create a particular social order.

Finally there is culture's excluding function. In his basic explanation of social structures, Weber distinguished between classes and status groups. Classes are economically determined, while status groups are determined by lifestyle and culture. Status groups involve a community within which certain cultures can thrive. The individual must acquire these cultures. This takes place through education, for example. The outcome is that only those people who have acquired an education can have access to the culture and have the possibility of acquiring the relevant values. The acquisition of culture and values is a question of the selection of the right status groups. In this way culture has an excluding function.

Weber developed his value-based cultural science with a view to being able to analyse the phenomena which concerned him. In this way, sociology as a cultural science becomes a tool for developing concepts and being able to understand the phenomena which cause concern.

The problem was that Weber thereby added to the problem which concerned him. His research into culture contributed to culture's further progress towards complexity.

His contribution led to culture becoming even more complex and confusing. It can be said that Weber was confronted by a dilemma in relation to culture as a topic of study. He was critical of cultural development, but nevertheless he made cultural values a decisive element of his methodology. He was critical of culture's excluding function. Nevertheless he made cultural values a pre-condition for being able to understand developments in culture and society.

Finally, there was the problem that the researcher must retain value-freedom in relation to his results, while values form the basis for the choice of topic of study and for the development of concepts about the phenomena studied. The question is whether this leaves tensions in sociology. Can there be value-freedom in relation to results obtained through a value-based research process?

For Simmel, taking his point of departure in the German historical school meant that he was very interested in the question of *a priori* categories and personality as preconditions for research into both historical phenomena and philosophical texts. On the one hand he retained an interest in historical phenomena. On the other hand he determined to develop an alternative to the belief in historical research as a photographic image of empirical reality. This alternative was based on his view that it is only possible to analyse empirical phenomena by using *a priori* categories, and by being guided by one's own personality. Categories can create order in the empirical world, while personality can create coherence. As a result, one must adopt a personal point of view in research.

The question is, why did Simmel feel he had to have this methodological disagreement with the German historical school? Why was it important for research to be guided by personality and *a priori* categories? Simmel's interest in these methodological aspects was due to his interest in the development of forms. In order to understand the constant change of forms, Simmel had to develop a method which would make it possible to understand these forms in all their changeability.

For Simmel, the constant development of forms was a matter of great concern. Forms change because life changes. There are more forms because forms produce forms. This means that there is an ever increasing differentiation between forms. At the same time the distance between forms and people becomes ever greater, because the forms increasingly obtain an independent function. What worried Simmel was that people would no longer be able to adopt forms, let alone direct their development. People would, instead, be subjected to forms.

Simmel used German philosophy and psychology as sources for developing concepts to understand these problems. Even he did not see any scope for positivism or historical materialism. He used Kant's concept of *a priori* categories. However, he did not accept them as being eternally valid. He saw them as empirical, and thus as subject to change. From psychology he took the concept of personality, which was the phenomenon to create coherence in the interpretation of phenomena.

Simmel's starting point was thus, on the one hand, a dispute with the German historical school and its requirement for making a photographic image of empirical reality – with its consequent pursuit of categories and personalities as the basis for the interpretation of phenomena – and, on the other hand, a concern about the rapid development of forms and the consequent distance between people and forms. It is against this background that we should understand his concept of culture and his proposals for a theory of cultural phenomena.

For Simmel, culture was synonymous with form. One can say that what concerned him was the development of culture. Form is a concept which runs through many of Simmel's works. It was his most basic epistemological concept, and a central feature of his understanding of art, science, literature, religion and economics, and it was also a central feature of his understanding of society and its organisation.

There are two particularly prominent theoretical perspectives in the Simmel texts which have been studied, and these are the relation between form and life and the relation between form and personality.

The relation between form and life concerns how life's continual development creates new forms. This means that, in due course, forms become obsolete and come into conflict with life. The consequence is a conflict between form and life.

The relation between form and personality concerns how increased distance is created between forms and people. The starting point for this process is the relation between form and life. As a consequence of life's development, forms undergo a differentiation of values, so they contain both a substantive value and a cultural value. When these two forms of value are separated from each other, the substantive value can be developed according to its own rules, without regard to whether it has value for the people who are to be cultivated. In this way a distance is created between forms and people which makes the cultivation of the individual more difficult. As a result, the individual must develop his own personal relation to the forms. On the one hand the individual must learn to recognise the forms in order to be able to acquire culture. On the other hand, he must add his own personal viewpoint to these forms.

It can be said that the relation between form and life creates the basis for the relation between form and personality. It is the continual development of life which creates the basis for forms which are independent of people. This means that people must take possession of forms, but this must be on their own terms. This means that the individual becomes active in taking possession of forms. Personality is decisive for how individuals take possession of forms.

Simmel emphasised the introduction of personality into his methodology and his theory of culture because personality was seen as being a phenomenon with great cohesive power. Personality is the phenomenon which creates coherence in research and in other cultural phenomena. It is personality which gives coherence in literature, art, science etc.

The question I have raised is whether this idea can succeed. If each personality creates its own form of coherence, this must lead to the creation of distances between different products. Personalities are not the same, so that diversity rather than coherence will result. The attempt to create wholeness may result in novel forms of differentiation.

If one looks at these three classical contributions to sociology's understanding of culture together, it will be seen that there are ideas which are common to all three and ideas which diverge.

The shared starting point for Durkheim, Weber and Simmel is the methodological dispute with the German historical school. This dispute both brings inspiration from historians and a distancing from their ideal of making a photographic image of reality and an objective description. This inspiration means that all three continued to be interested in historical analysis. Their criticisms resulted in new thinking about methodological problems. However, here there were differing key concepts in each of the three writers. For Durkheim, the key element were the formation of concepts and explanation. For Weber, the key element was the value-relation of research. And for Simmel, the key elements were *a priori* concepts and personality. Durkheim's source of inspiration was biology, Weber's was the German cultural tradition, and Simmel was influenced by German philosophy and psychology. They were in agreement in their criticism, but their sources of inspiration and their theoretical solutions differed.

Another shared starting point for these classical sociologists was their concern about social and cultural developments. However, their substantive concerns were not entirely identical. Durkheim was worried about the prominence of the anomic economy, and thus for how morality could be strengthened. Weber was worried about the continual development of culture and differentiation, and thus the difficulties in ensuring the cultivation of man as a whole. Simmel was worried about the continuous development of forms and the difficulties for people to take possession of and control forms. What was common to all three was their concern about contemporary developments which prompted the methodological debate. They chose to apply their new methods to research which would clarify developments and perhaps help influence these developments.

If we look at the cultural understanding which results from these new methodologies, it will be apparent that there are differences here too. With Durkheim, culture was something which is made into a system. For Weber, culture was that to which meaning was ascribed. Simmel was concerned with culture as form. The key words are thus, system, meaning and form. Nevertheless, there are some common characteristics in their general understanding of cultural phenomena. Common to them was the view of culture as a subject/object relation. With Durkheim, this can be seen in his distinction between objective culture and subjective culture. Objective culture can be acquired by individuals. With Weber, this is apparent in a corresponding distinction between objective culture and subjective culture. He identified the problem for the individual in acquiring objective culture. With Simmel, this distinction is seen in the separation between form and personality. Forms have their own lives, and it becomes increasingly difficult for people to possess objective culture. People become subjected to forms.

However, this agreement about the fundamental relation to culture does not lead to agreement about how culture's other relations should be understood. Durkheim had an optimistic view of culture. He delighted in cultural treasures and wished people to take possession of these treasures. He believed that culture would form the basis for a strengthening of morality and thus for systematisation and predictability of behaviour. Science has a role in this process because it can explain the phenomena which the individual is confronted with. This means that there is an increased possibility for improving morality through educational work. Weber had a pessimistic view of culture. He observed, with concern, how culture became more and more complex and thus more difficult for the individual to acquire. He also pointed out the excluding function of culture, as it is only people from certain status groups who have access to objective culture through education. Simmel also regarded cultural development with pessimism. The development of life, the development of forms, and the fragmentation of forms into substantive forms and functional forms make it increasingly difficult to ensure that people can acquire objective culture. The distance between forms and people becomes ever greater.

The solutions to the problems they were concerned with depended on the methodological developments which they made. With Durkheim, sociology had to be able to give an explanation in order to contribute to an improvement of morality. With Weber, sociology had to be able to develop new concepts for significant social phenomena so as to bring clarity and understanding to the phenomena which caused concern. And with Simmel, personality had to be able to bring coherence to research and the acquisition of objective culture.

However, the methodological solutions chosen introduced new tensions into sociology. In Durkheim we see the tension between history and system. On the one hand, he wanted to explain historical development, and on the other hand he wanted to clarify the systematisation of culture and social forms. In Weber we see the tension between value-freedom and value-neutrality. On the one hand he wanted to maintain the researcher's distance from his own results, and on the other hand he emphasised that research must be directed by the researcher's own values. Another tension in Weber's work consisted in his pessimistic opinion of culture and his use of culture as a fundamental methodological approach. In Simmel we see tension between form and personality. On the one hand, research must start from *a priori* categories, and on the other hand, it must start from personality. Categories should create order, but they were considered as being confusing. Personality should give coherence, but at the same time it differs from person to person.

In this way, three of the most important founders of sociology created a sociology based on shared concerns for social and cultural development, and a common acknowledgement of the necessity for creating new methodological principles. Their views of culture were characterised both by shared ideas and by differing conceptual definitions. What was common to them all was that their methodological dispute with the German historical school created a number of tensions in sociology. What has this meant for the subsequent development of sociology? What has happened to the basic methodological principles, the underlying concerns, the development of concepts and theories, and what have these tensions meant for further theoretical development? Questions such as these will be considered in the ensuing discussion of the contributions by Archer, Wuthnow and Bourdieu.

## *Contemporary theory of culture: Pursuit of unicity and distance*

Archer's theory has been developed under the influence of Anglo-Saxon sociology and philosophy. Through her reading of English sociologist, David Lockwood's article on social integration and system integration, she has developed a new methodological principle, which is the principle of analytical dualism. The principle of analytical dualism is thus inspired by Lockwood's combination of conflict theory and general functionalism.

With her principle of analytical dualism, Archer distances herself from the whole of sociology. She has criticised sociologists for not having used this principle. As a consequence, some of them, notably Parsons, Sorokin and Lévi-Strauss have committed the error of downwards conflation, others, notably Miliband, Marcuse and Habermas, have committed upwards conflation, and finally a group, notably Bauman and Giddens, have committed central conflation.

The question is, what is the driving force behind this methodological dispute with much of sociology? Why is it so important to follow the route of analytical dualism? It is because it gives Archer the possibility of distinguishing between structure and action. On the basis of this fundamental distinction she can develop a theory both for culture and for structural change. She can focus on both cultural and structural rules. Dualism makes it possible for her to distinguish between culture and structure, and between the cultural system and socio-cultural interaction, and between social structures and social interaction. She can develop a theory on the mutual influences of these pairs of concepts, without conflating them. Furthermore, it gives Archer a basis for creating a theory which no other person has advanced before. She can, on the one hand, distance herself from all previous theories and, on the other hand, advance a unique theory.

Archer has two good reasons for advancing her methodological principle of analytical dualism. First, she has created a theory which can analyse change in both the cultural sphere and in the structural sphere. Second, she has distanced herself from large parts of sociology, so that her theory appears as a unique theory.

To her methodological principle of analytical dualism Archer adds her theoretical understanding of change as a morphogenetic cycle. The process of change has three phases: the starting point, which can be called the existing structure; a middle phase, where there is interaction between people; and the final phase, in which new structures are developed. Archer's thinking on this is influenced by the systems theoretician, Walter Buckley.

In her more recent works Archer has also been influenced by the theory on change of the philosopher Roy Bhaskar. With his critical realist philosophy, Bhaskar has developed further concepts for understanding the processes of cultural and structural change. The concept of emergence is important here. Within the concept of the emergence of new phenomena there lies the view that new phenomena arise on the basis of earlier phenomena, without being able to be reduced to those earlier phenomena. The new phenomena have an independent existence.

When Archer's thinking relates more specifically to the cultural sphere, the philosophers Karl Popper and Imre Lakatos, are more important sources of inspiration. When Archer developed her concept of culture, she turned to Popper's idea of the third world. Culture is thus everything which is accessible to man's understanding. When she developed her theory on the potential for ideas to generate cultural change, she turned to Lakatos's idea of consistency as being the decisive criterion for the validity of a theory. The internal consistency of ideas is decisive for whether cultural agents are pushed to cultural change or not.

It is on the basis of these many sources of inspiration that Archer has developed her theory of cultural phenomena. In her theory, culture becomes everything which can be made subject to understanding. On the basis of this concept of culture, she develops her concept of the cultural system as logical propositions which can be either true or false. In opposition to the cultural system she sets up socio-cultural interaction which she defines as being the influence which people exercise on each other in relation to culture. Under the principle of analytical dualism, the relation between the cultural system and socio-cultural interaction will be decisive for whether there will be morphogenesis or morphostasis.

The starting point for cultural morphogenesis is cultural conditions. What matters is whether the relations between the logical propositions are contradictory or complementary. Contradictions will give the cultural actors problems, while complementarities need not give rise to problems. Here, Archer brings in examples from classical sociology. Durkheim's analyses of the development of educational ideas in France is an example of situational logic characterised by constraining contradictions, while Weber's analyses of ancient China and India are examples of situational logic characterised by concomitant complementarities.

However, Archer emphasises that cultural situational logic is not in itself decisive for whether there will be cultural change. Change requires socio-cultural interaction, and this interaction will be characterised by the attempt to maintain or to expand vested interests. Socio-cultural interaction is governed by material interests.

The decisive question, therefore, is how the cultural system and socio-cultural interaction fit together. It is of no avail if the cultural system is full of inconsistencies crying out for change, if the power relations are such that any attempt at change can be repressed. Nor is it of any avail if the cultural system is full of complementarities, giving good possibilities for adding new elements to the existing cultural system, if those in power use all means to stop it. Thus, the second phase in the morphogenetic cycle, so-

socio-cultural interaction and its use of power or withholding of power, are decisive for whether the outcome will be morphogenesis or morphostasis.

It is Archer's view that it is possible to suppress change, under highly ordered socio-cultural conditions, for months, years or even centuries, but it is impossible to do so in the long run. Sooner or later a situation will arise when even the cultural elite will see that it is in its interest to accede to the demand for a revision of culture so that inconsistencies are diminished, or where it will be forced to open up to new cultural elements if it is to retain its position. Sooner or later, the third phase of the morphogenetic cycle will become a reality.

All the while this cultural morphogenesis is taking place, there will be another morphogenesis. The cultural morphogenesis will lead to a morphogenesis of action. When culture changes, there will also be socio-cultural interaction around the cultural change. Relations between agents within the cultural sphere will be affected by the cultural change. Here, too, power relations can prevent restructuring among the corporate agents for some time. As long as the elite can distance itself from the primary agents, there will not be change. The problem is that the primary agents will, in time, join together and become corporate agents. The consequence will be a re-grouping. The morphogenesis of action will then become a reality, so there will be a double morphogenesis.

The morphogenesis of action will lead to yet another morphogenesis, that of the actors. When there is a re-grouping of the agents, new roles will emerge. The number of roles to be allocated will be greater. Here, too, a morphogenetic process will be set in motion. There will be a triple morphogenesis.

However, Archer emphasises that both agents and actors are rooted in people. People have the ability to reflect and be creative and the ability to have authentic inner experiences. This means that a person can make a decision. Therefore there is nothing automatic about the morphogenesis either of the action or the actors. The processes are rooted in people who can evaluate and choose.

In Archer's thinking, structural morphogenesis takes place under the same principles as cultural morphogenesis. They are identical processes. The question is, how are these two processes related to each other? There are also questions about how socio-cultural interaction can affect structural development, and how social interaction can affect cultural development. Archer points out that these mechanisms are really very simple.

If a structural interest group needs to draw attention to itself and legitimise itself, it will seek a doctrine which it can use to promote its interests. The problem is that, as soon as it has done this, it will find that it has placed itself in the middle of the cultural situational logic. But it is not only this group which has to adopt a position in relation to the advanced cultural struggle. This also applies to other structural interest groups which it is allied with or opposed to. These, too, must seek to make their mark or legitimise themselves, but they must do this in the light of the choice which the first group makes. In this way, socio-cultural interaction intrudes into the structural domain.

If a socio-cultural interest group forms an alliance with a structural interest group in order to secure resources for its work, it will surrender part of its universality. It must subordinate itself to the particular interests of the structural interest group in question. Finding a sponsor for cultural activities does have its price. The problem is that when one socio-cultural group has secured resources through such an alliance, then other socio-cultural interest groups have to do the same. If other socio-cultural interest groups want to avoid falling behind the first group, they must also find themselves sponsors among the structural interest groups. In this way socio-cultural interest groups are drawn into the power struggle which takes place between structural interest groups. Thus, structural interaction intrudes into the cultural domain.

On the basis of this comprehensive theoretical construction, Archer raises the question of how it is possible to understand the relations between theory and empirical materials. She characterises the morphogenetic approach to cultural analysis and the structural analysis as a format. To this format, one should add analytical histories about the developments which do in fact take place. An example of such an analytical history in the structural domain is her own analysis of the development of educational systems.

Archer's theory prompts a number of questions. The linking together of analytical dualism and the morphogenetic principle means that, over time, system thinking will take over and displace the conflict thinking which was originally the basis for the distinction between system integration and social integration. Furthermore, as pointed out, the link between analytical dualism and Popper's three worlds means that the idea about the mental processes, as the element which links objective thinking with the physical world, disappears. It is not so easy to link analytical dualism with other kinds of theories.

Wuthnow's theory has been developed through criticism of classical sociology. Wuthnow interprets the classical theory, which for him means Marx, Weber and Durkheim, so that it is based on the distinction between, on the one hand, culture as a subjective phenomenon and, on the other hand, the social structures as objective phenomena. Wuthnow mistakenly ascribes to the classical sociologists the view that culture is a subjective phenomenon. Wuthnow disputes this view by drawing in some of the more recent sociologists who emphasise the importance of studying patterns, rituals and institutions in culture. He refers in particular to Douglas, Habermas and Foucault. Wuthnow develops a number of sequences of concepts in order to study patterns, rituals and institutions in a number of examples of ideological change.

Methodologically, Wuthnow distances himself from the difficulties of studying culture as a subjective phenomenon, and concentrates instead on developing methods for studying the elements of culture which are observable, in other words, actions and cultural products. Having identified the observable aspects of culture, he then looks at how these should be interpreted. He uses the principle of openness and the continual development of new concepts.

What is the importance for Wuthnow of this possibility for open interpretation of observable cultural phenomena? It is important because it gives him the freedom to pursue new interpretations of both theoretical and empirical phenomena. In the world of theories he can give these theories his own interpretation. In the world of empirical phenomena he can also give them his own interpretation. And Wuthnow has a great need to be able to interpret empirical phenomena. He is very concerned about some of the fundamental trends in American society, including individualism, materialism and rationalism. A significant part of his research is focused on the impact of economic life, at the cost of local community, family life, business ethics etc.

For Wuthnow, the benefit of the interpretative approach is that it gives the possibility of developing concepts for interpreting the phenomena that cause him concern. At the same time, he has the opportunity to develop unique interpretations. He has the opportunity to make his own contribution to sociology's understanding of culture.

Wuthnow's mistaken interpretation of the classical sociologists has meant that throughout his writings he has been strongly interested in the question of what significance subjectivity and meaning should be ascribed in the understanding of culture. It can be said that he alternates between giving subjectivity and meaning key positions in his understanding of culture, and allowing subjectivity and meaning to disappear out of the picture, to be replaced by action and artefacts.

The questions of subjectivity and meaning are included in that part of Wuthnow's research which relates to those aspects of American society which cause him concern. The questions of subjectivity and meaning are omitted from that part of Wuthnow's research which relates to ideologies and wider cultural changes, and replaced by studies of the symbolic expressive aspects of actions and of the cultural products which are created through these actions.

Thus, Wuthnow's research tends to be split into two parts. On the one hand there is the research in which subjectivity and meaning are decisive, and on the other hand there is the research in which actions and artefacts are decisive. It is always possible to observe two kinds of sources of inspiration. On the one hand, there is the influence of the classical sociologists, and on the other hand, there is the influence of more recent sociology. Among the classical sociologists, the phenomenological ideas, particularly of Berger, to a certain extent influence Wuthnow's studies involving subjectivity and meaning. In his studies concerning actions and artefacts, Wuthnow is influenced by a group of sociologists which he refers to as post-structuralists, including Habermas, Foucault and Douglas.

On the basis of the ideas of the classical sociologists and from Berger, Wuthnow is able to maintain the subjective aspect of culture. And, with the influence of Habermas, Foucault and Douglas, Wuthnow is able to focus on the observable aspects of culture. Under the influence of Habermas, the aspect of action is prominent. Under the influence of Foucault, the aspect of discourse is prominent. And under the influence of Douglas, the aspects of classification and ritual are prominent.

Under these twin influences, Wuthnow develops two kinds of cultural research. One kind is found in his earlier writings, and is taken up again in his most recent writings. The other kind is found in his middle period. This results in two kinds of understanding of culture and two kinds of theoretical contribution in relation to culture.

If we look first at the concept of culture, then in the early and most recent parts of his writings it is defined as being meanings systems and as the relating of meaning to a given phenomenon. In his middle period, culture is considered as symbolic-expressive aspects of actions and as the tangible results of such actions. So, on the one hand there is meaning-related culture, and on the other hand there are observable actions and artefacts. In the former case there is subjectively based culture, and in the latter case there are observable aspects of culture.

In order to accommodate these very different views of culture, Wuthnow has introduced different levels of cultural analysis. He distinguishes between the subjective level, to which categories and patterns belong, the dramaturgical level, to which the dramatising of the moral order belongs, and the institutional level, where resources and the channelling of ideas belong. This makes it possible for Wuthnow to accommodate different views of culture within a common overriding categorisation. Meaning-related culture is placed at the subjective level, while action-related and product-related culture are placed at the other three levels. However, the question remains whether this splitting into different levels solves the problem that Wuthnow in fact operates with two sets of concepts and, as we shall see, two sets of theories.

When we come to the question of how Wuthnow analyses contributions to the development of the theory of culture, we can also see two main trends. From his earlier and more recent work it is possible to derive the view that culture consists of enduring meanings systems or a general national culture which gives wholeness and values to the individual. In this way, individual phenomena are related to the greater whole, and social standards and behavioural guidelines are created. This leads to integration and coherence in society. The one of the main themes of Wuthnow's analyses, which originates from his concerns for society, is to see culture as a higher, value-related phenomenon which can influence people's outlook on life and behaviour, and thus influence social integration.

From the works of Wuthnow's middle period it is possible to derive the view that culture has the capacity to dramatise the social and moral order. Rituals communicate the social order, while ideologies communicate the moral order. Wuthnow emphasises again and again that culture is not a mirror of the social order. Whether a given ideology gains acceptance or not depends on whether the form of the ideology is suited to the social environment, and whether the ideologies are able to communicate anything about the social movements in the environment in question. At the same time, there must be a social movement which can secure the necessary resources for spreading the ideology. Wuthnow thus operates with a cultural process in three phases: production, selection and institutionalisation. However, he emphasises that this process does not take place automatically. The outcome depends on the choices which people make in the light of the circumstances. Producers must choose which products they will create, and consumers must choose which products they will buy. But there must also be space for creativity. Such a space is created through the articulation of the concrete and the disarticulation of the concrete through relation to the general. In this way the cultural processes become the result of human behaviour and of human choices and creativity.

Even though Wuthnow makes a division into different levels, he does not avoid his work being split into two parts. In one part he is influenced by the classical sociologists. In the other part he is influenced by the tradition which he calls post-structuralist. In the one part he studies culture as meaning, and in the other part he studies actions and products. Can culture simultaneously be a phenomenon which is controlled by general values and a phenomenon which is controlled by choices and creativity? It can be said that Wuthnow has put himself in between two distinct forms of theories of action, between the idea of action being controlled by values and the idea of action being controlled by free choice.

Bourdieu's theory was developed through his criticism of two major intellectual schools of thought among his contemporaries; these were pure objectivist thought and pure subjectivist thought. On the basis of this dispute he developed some new methodological principles, which were the principle of relational thinking, the principle of construction and the principle of objectification.

One may ask, what prompted this methodological dispute? Why was it important to be able to construct a theory based on these particular methodological principles? It was because, on the one hand, he wanted to build a bridge between objectivism and subjectivism, which necessitated relational thinking, and because, on the other hand, he wanted to construct and explain a new insight which necessitated construction and objectification. But why did Bourdieu need a new insight? He needed it because he wanted to uncover some absolutely fundamental mechanisms in French society. His theory is nothing less than a withering criticism of the cultural aristocracy which he had encountered on his way up through the French educational system. But it also quickly became clear that he was himself able to exploit the mechanisms which he uncovered most elegantly. He identified the distancing technique as an important mechanism of the cultural aristocracy, while he himself established a clear distance in relation to other intellectual schools. He identified naturalness and understated understanding as being the most effective forms of symbolic dominance, while he himself used naturalness and understated understanding in his analysis of cultural phenomena. He identified institutionalisation as the most effective form of naturalisation of interests, while he himself built up institutions.

Bourdieu thus had two good reasons for developing new methodological principles. First, they gave him the tools to carry out a critical analysis of the symbolic repression which he had witnessed in the elitist French educational system. Second, it bought him up to the top of the cultural aristocracy. His ability to reveal mechanisms and to use these same mechanisms for his own purposes was remarkable.

His methodological distancing was particularly notable in relation to pure objectivist thinking and pure subjectivist thinking. Bourdieu distanced himself from structuralist-oriented anthropology represented by Lévi-Strauss, from phenomenology-oriented anthropology represented by Mauss, and from existentialism represented by Sartre. He disagreed with the idea that people's behaviour is conditioned by objective structures, and with the idea that human beings have free will to decide. What he did instead was to set himself the aim of developing a new idea that could create a relation between objective structures and the human subject.

Bourdieu's decisive new methodological development was the introduction of relational thinking. In developing his relational thinking Bourdieu found inspiration in the work of the German philosopher Ernst Cassirer. In Cassirer's work, relational thinking was the decisive basis for scientific thinking. Bourdieu was also influenced by the American art historian Panofsky. It was from Panofsky that he took the concept of habitus. The relation between subject and objective structures is created by the introduction of the concept of habitus. Habitus is the mental habit which is created by objective structures and laid down in the individual. When it is laid down in the individual it forms the basis for the individual's actions, and thereby for the further formation of objective structures. Bourdieu wanted to use the concept of habitus to re-introduce the active individual, the creative agent.

The second of Bourdieu's new methodological developments was the principle of construction. It was Bourdieu's opinion that the researcher must construct and interpret on the basis of his material, and thereafter investigate whether the construction so developed can be transferred from one field to another under the principle of homology. In order to evaluate such constructions there is only one validation criterion, and this is the coherence of the construction. Bourdieu himself pointed out that the source of this principle of the construction of fields was Weber's analyses of religion, in which a distinction was made between the ideas and the agents of the field.

Bourdieu's third new methodological development was the principle of objectification. According to this principle, the researcher must objectify both his own relations to the research and to the phenomena which are the object of the research. Bourdieu did not himself refer to any sources of influence for this principle.

On the basis of these methodological principles, Bourdieu created his concept of culture and the elements for his theory of culture.

The principle of construction leads to the development of an understanding of culture as common patterns of understanding. Through construction and homology between fields, Bourdieu saw pairs of opposites which could fit into many different contexts. These pairs of opposites operate as patterns of understanding.

The principle of relational thinking leads to a theory of culture which puts into focus the relationship of people and of social classes to culture. The individual's relations to culture are decisive for his understanding of cultural and social reproduction through education. The relations of social classes to culture are decisive for understanding how some classes are able to maintain their dominance over other classes.

The principle of objectification leads to a theory of culture in which culture relates to classes, where pedagogy relates to habitus, and where institutions relate to interests.

The consequence of the development of these methodological principles was a concept of culture in which culture is understood as patterns of understanding. This does not mean that Bourdieu disregarded objective culture. He saw it as a source of inspiration for productive work with the development of new cultural expressions. However, this aspect does not play a leading role in his work.

For Bourdieu, culture concerned cultural dominance and symbolic violence. In non-differentiated societies, this symbolic violence is revealed through the showing of trust, hospitality, obligations, loyalty etc. It is everything which can be contained within the concept of an ethic of honour. All the elements referred to create dependence between people. The result of this is not only symbolic dominance, but also material dominance.

In societies with class structures, symbolic violence is evidenced by making apparently arbitrary culture the natural and legitimate culture. This creates a distance between it and other forms of culture. Naturalness and arbitrariness thus form the basis for both symbolic and material dominance.

In the educational system, pedagogic work is related to a particular habitus, which is the habitus of the dominant classes. This means that pupils who come from a different background find that their cultural background is not accepted. They also find that the culture which they acquire in school is not accepted as an authentic culture.

In the areas of art and literature, one must have a particular habitus in order to have a feeling for where it is right to invest one's efforts and to be able to develop the strategies which mean that one can distance oneself from others in the field, to obtain profit and acknowledgement.

Meanwhile, the whole of this symbolic repression does not take place without a clash of arms. Those groups of students or artists who find that their style and expression is not accepted as legitimate will take up the fight against those who occupy the leading positions, distance themselves from them and will try to occupy those positions themselves. In this struggle they will dispute the existing classifications and the common patterns of understanding with a view to introducing classifications which are more advantageous to themselves. There will be a dispute about classification.

There are a number of questions to be asked about Bourdieu's theory. The most important of these is whether Bourdieu did in fact succeed in building a bridge between objectivist thinking and subjectivist thinking. The means for creating this should be habitus. The problem is that habitus is determined and controlled by objective structures. The question is, what happens to the active agent?

Another question concerns his principle of construction and its homologous application. This principle was developed through his studies of Algerian farmers, applied to the French cultural aristocracy, and then turned into a scientific principle. One may well ask whether a principle which is of a more or less mythological character can be transferred first to French society, and from there to French science, without the whole thing appearing to have a certain tinge of mythology.

If we now look at the three representatives of contemporary sociology together, and their thinking about culture, their differences are more apparent than their similarities.

Something which is common to Archer, Wuthnow and Bourdieu is their tendency to distance themselves from other theories and to develop their own theory. Unicity is clearly a matter of great importance to all three of them. One gets the impression that distancing oneself from the others and creating a new and distinct theory is an end in itself.

Another common feature is that they distance themselves through some fundamental methodological argument and new creation. These methodological creations differ widely, however, laying down the basis for very different theories.

With Archer, the new methodological creation consists of the development of analytical dualism. With Wuthnow, it consist of a dispute with subjectivity, with a view to interpreting the observable aspects of culture. And with Bourdieu, it consists of a dispute with both objectivism and subjectivism, with a view to building a bridge between these two forms of thinking. The result of these methodological principles is that Archer develops controlling principles for her research, Wuthnow is very open in relation to his research, and Bourdieu had the possibility of, on the one hand, being open and, on the other hand, developing fixed principles for his research. One can say that Archer and Wuthnow each pull in diametrically opposed directions, methodologically speaking, while Bourdieu placed himself in between.

If we look at the concepts of culture used by the three contemporary sociologists, it appears that Archer looks at culture with logical principles, Wuthnow approaches culture in all its aspects, and Bourdieu regarded culture as a tool for understanding. Archer considers the cultural system to be logical propositions; Wuthnow switches between seeing culture as meaning-related phenomena and observable actions and artefacts; while Bourdieu saw culture as being common classification schemes. The key words are thus, for Archer – logic, for Wuthnow – meaning and discourse, and for Bourdieu – habitus.

Also, when we come to consider their contributions to a theory of culture, we see clear differences. Archer's theory is a theory of cultural change. It is the relations between logical propositions which determine whether there is any basis for agents and actors to change culture, and it is their mutual power relations which determine whether they do in fact change culture. Actions are thus influenced by logic, material interests and power. Wuthnow's theory is, on the one hand, a theory about morality and, on the other hand, a theory about how people affect cultural development. In the former case there are meanings systems which give the individual wholeness and guidance for action. In the latter case, we see actions and artefacts which are created through people's choice and creativity. We thus see actions which are influenced by culture and cultivation and actions which are influenced by choice and creativity. Bourdieu's theory is a theory of symbolic dominance. Some people have the positions and power to make their culture the legitimate culture. By creating a distance to other forms of culture, they make other people's culture less legitimate. The key to legitimising the dominant culture is naturalness and understated understanding. Symbolic violence is developed through such naturalness and understated understanding, the consequence of which is both symbolic and material dominance. Against this symbolic violence there is not only a struggle to regroup, but also to redefine. This means that there is not only a struggle between classes, but a struggle about classification.

If we compare the three theories with each other, we must again place Archer and Wuthnow at either extreme, and put Bourdieu somewhere in the middle. In Archer's theory, people are not at all influenced by cultivation. They are exclusively influenced by logical relations and by power and material interests. Human beings are not marked by their culture; it is entirely external. In Wuthnow's theory, people are, on the one hand, marked by their culture, but they also make choices in relation to a cultural field. Culture creates figurative actions, in other words, moral examples. In Bourdieu's theory, people are influenced by patterns of understanding, which are laid down in their formative years, and they are also influenced by the interests which are associated with participation in cultural life. They seek their own cultural profit. One can say that, in

Archer's thinking, people do not act on the basis of cultivation, but on the basis of material interests; in Wuthnow's thinking, people act primarily on the basis of cultivation, but also to a lesser extent on the basis of choice and creativity; while in Bourdieu's thinking, people act both on the basis of their cultivation and their interests.

For all three of these sociologists there are some problematic aspects to their theories. For Archer the main problem is that she can in fact only maintain analytical dualism by violating her other sources of inspiration, including Buckley's thinking on morphogenesis and Popper's division into the three worlds. With Wuthnow there is a clash between his highly meaning-oriented understanding of culture and his action-oriented understanding of culture. There is a clash between his ideas of free choice and cultivation. Bourdieu had problems in bridging between the subjective and the objective approaches because, when it came to it, he let everything be objectified. There was not truly a place for free will. In addition to this, he applied the principle of homology both to mythological and to scientific thinking. This means that his scientific thinking contains a touch of mythology.

These three contributors to contemporary sociological ideas about culture leave the impression that distancing and new developments are the ruling principles. This has led to great differences both in methodology and in the developments of concepts and theories. This differentiation makes a pattern where Archer and Wuthnow are at opposite ends of a scale, and Bourdieu is in the middle. In Archer's view, people act on the basis of material interests. In Wuthnow's view, people act primarily on the basis of their cultivation. While in Bourdieu's view, people act on the basis of their cultivation, but with a clear view to material advantages.

## *The synthesis between natural scientific and cultural scientific thought*

The question which now remains concerns the extent to which it is possible to understand the selected theories as a distinction between natural scientific and cultural scientific thought, and whether there is an attempt to overcome this contradiction in these theories.

It is my opinion that, among the classical writers, Durkheim and Weber were inspired by natural scientific and cultural scientific thought, respectively, and that this is reflected in important differences between their concepts and theories of culture.

Durkheim sought to develop a scientific method characterised by natural scientific thought. His approach to sociology was rationalist. He tried to identify the relations between cause and effect in past behaviour with a view to being able to understand the rules for future behaviour. The central concept in Durkheim's methodology was the concept of social facts, by which he meant the actions which are able to impose limits in relation to the individual. In explaining social facts one should, according to Durkheim, use the genetic method. One should look back to a given social phenomenon's originating cells and germ, and from there follow its development forward towards complexity. Durkheim's analyses were thus characterised by the conceptual apparatus of biology. He analysed social phenomena by using concepts such as genetics, cells and germs. To these he added the concepts of evolution, periodicity, categorisation and system.

Natural science thinking influenced Durkheim's understanding of culture. Natural science thinking means that a system-oriented and evolutionary perspective is imposed on culture. Culture is a system which can influence people to behave in a regulated and predictable fashion. At the same time, culture develops in such a way that the best ideas survive. The natural scientific approach also meant that Durkheim sought an explanation for culture. He explained culture by means of society. On the one hand, society is the source of the representations of the world which people create, and on the other hand it is the organiser of culture.

As against this there is Max Weber's view of social science as a part of cultural science. This view meant that the question of values came to play a central role in his methodology. In his view, in order to be able to study or practice social science, it was necessary to take account of questions about values. Weber explicitly distanced himself from the natural scientific pursuit of explanations. Instead, he emphasised that social sciences must interpret and understand. One must discover the value content of a phenomenon, and then seek to understand it by uncovering its background. Finally, Weber emphasised the importance of not following the natural sciences in trying to discover laws. What one should do instead is to try to understand unique historical events.

On the basis of this cultural scientific thinking, Weber considered culture to be those parts of the world to which people have related values and thereby given them meaning and significance. In Weber's thinking, culture was primarily understood through the concept of meaning. To this were added concepts such as belief, ethics and human nature.

It is my opinion that, in contemporary sociology, Archer is inspired by natural scientific thinking, while Wuthnow is inspired by cultural scientific thinking. This is decisively important for their thinking about culture.

Archer seeks to transfer the rational approach of natural scientific thinking to the social sciences. She refers to Karl Popper and other philosophers who have been inspired by the natural sciences, as sources of inspiration. She emphasises that social phenomena should be studied as objective phenomena which are capable of explanation. Furthermore, she bases her theory on logical and causal relations.

What does this natural science-oriented thinking mean for Archer's understanding of cultural phenomena? The consequence of this is that Archer considers culture to be a system and she defines this system as consisting of logical propositions which can either be contradictory or complementary. Culture is thus subjected to the rules of logic. It also means that people are regarded as actors who, in relation to culture, pursue their material interests. In this way, culture becomes a matter of logic and power.

Wuthnow's methodology and theoretical thinking about culture stands opposed to this view. Wuthnow works with a hermeneutic approach. Thus, he believes that sociological work consists of interpretation rather than revealing objective facts. He argues that one should put forward a loose-fitting framework rather than a fixed system of concepts. Such loose-fitting frameworks of concepts can give a structure to empirical investigations, without casting them in concrete. It will then be possible to make changes in the light of empirical results.

This very open and interpretative approach to sociology means that Wuthnow does not have a clear and unambiguous view of culture, nor of how cultural analysis should be carried out. During his career there have been changes and inconsistencies in his writings on the understanding of culture. These changes and inconsistencies are centred on Wuthnow's relation to the concept of meaning. In his earlier writings the concept of meaning played a decisive role in his understanding of culture, in his middle period he disputed the concept, and in his most recent writings the concept has been reintroduced. Wuthnow's concept of culture thus switches between meaning and symbolic-expressive actions, including primarily discursive expression.

Thus, it is clear that Durkheim worked on the basis of natural scientific thought, while Weber worked in the basis of cultural scientific thought. It is equally clear that Archer works on the basis of natural scientific thought, while Wuthnow works on the basis of cultural scientific thought. It therefore makes sense to understand the sociological theory of culture through the distinction between natural scientific and cultural scientific thought. Furthermore, it appears that this distinction is relevant both to classical and to contemporary sociology.

The question that remains is, how are we to interpret Simmel and Bourdieu? Is Simmel's theory an expression of a synthesis between the two modes of thought in classical sociology? And is Bourdieu's theory an expression of a synthesis between the two modes of thought in contemporary sociology?

Simmel's thinking was primarily based on Kant's philosophy, and so he was in the same tradition as the later Cassirer. What was common to Simmel and Cassirer was their search for general concepts for the understanding of many different forms of expression. In Simmel's work, the general concept which he used in many different contexts was the concept of form. For Simmel, form was a general category which expressed the most general within religion, art, science, law, production, metaphysics, etc. Form means the same as *a priori* categories, and as such it is constantly changing.

This search for the most general concept, and its use in many different areas, makes it possible to see Simmel's theory as a theory which tries to achieve such a high degree of general applicability that it can build a bridge between natural scientific and cultural scientific thought.

If we look more specifically at this question, it appears that it is indeed the concept of form which is the fundamental concept in his understanding of culture. For Simmel, culture was synonymous with form. The consequence was that culture became the general phenomenon which should combine natural scientific with cultural scientific thought.

It is especially in the two areas of methodology in relation to historical science and the philosophy of money that we see Simmel linking together natural scientific and cultural scientific thought.

In these methodological discussions, Simmel distinguished between the treatment of facts and the mental processes which occur in the understanding of these facts. On the one hand there must be a registration of facts, a scientific simplification, and a selection of data. On the other hand, there must be a process of mental reconstruction, in which the historian's personal point of view determines what understanding the research leads to.

In the philosophy of money there is a link between the dynamic of the objects themselves and people's lifestyles. On the one hand there are some objective forms which have their own inner relations and their own ability to generate new forms. On the other hand there is a lifestyle through which people seek to express the meaning they have found in life. The relation between these two elements is culture, and its inner relation between objective culture and subjective culture. When the distance between objective culture and subjective culture is increased, the distances between objective forms of money and the division of labour, and subjective forms of lifestyle are also increased. According to Simmel, this results in continual conflict between form and life.

Simmel thus tried to develop a theory with broad applicability. In this theory the concept of form was so general that it could be used in all fields. At the same time, the concept of form becomes the concept which connects natural scientific and cultural scientific thought.

The problem which Simmel left for his successors was that he did not create any coherence between the different kinds of cultural expression. As life unfolds, so new forms are created, and by virtue of the inner logic of these forms, yet further forms are created. The concept of form is thus general, but the forms themselves become ever more complex and intransparent. People are unable to maintain an overview and see the coherence in the increasing degree of complexity.

Perhaps these problems have been too complicated for succeeding sociologists. Whatever the reason, Simmel has not had any great influence on the contemporary theories of culture which have been selected, here, for closer analysis. They restrict themselves to Durkheim and Weber, as sources of inspiration.

Is it, then, possible to understand Bourdieu's theory as an attempt to develop a synthesis between natural scientific and cultural scientific thought, within contemporary sociological theory of culture?

Bourdieu's linking together of natural scientific and cultural scientific thought was most explicit in his methodological considerations. The three principles of relational thinking, construction and objectification represent an exchange between the two forms of scientific thought. His relational thinking was inspired by Cassirer's studies of modern natural science, where the relations are more important than the substantial elements which are related to each other. With his principle of construction, Bourdieu emphasised the need for openness in the interpretation of any given material. On the basis of his material, the researcher must undertake a construction, whose only criterion for validity is its inner coherence. However, such a construction must be subjected to objectification, in other words its ability to relate to objective circumstances.

At the methodological level, Bourdieu also made a link between natural scientific and cultural scientific thought. In particular, he attached importance to the use of both statistical methods and interpretative discussion.

At the theoretical level, Bourdieu linked together cultural expression and objective conditions. On the one hand we see perceptive pedagogy, natural taste and the legitimate lifestyle as cultural elements. On the other hand we see the social space which these cultural elements must relate to, if we are to understand them. It is precisely this relation between culture and the social space which is so important, so the theory is more focused on the relation to culture than on culture itself.

How does Bourdieu carry this thinking over the divide between natural scientific and cultural scientific thought? In this connection, the most important concept is the concept of habitus. What he meant by habitus was the classification scheme which is established in the individual at the pre-verbal stage of development.

The concept of habitus is also the fundamental concept in Bourdieu's understanding of culture. For him, culture was common classification schemes. Thus, for Bourdieu, too, culture was the link between natural scientific and cultural scientific thought.

Bourdieu also left a number of unresolved problems. First, the concept of habitus and its relation to objective structures cannot give the individual subjectivity. The individual becomes a reflection of objective structures. As a result of this, the content of Bourdieu's theory emphasises social reproduction. It seems almost impossible to explain change on the basis of this theory.

Another problem is that, through his thinking about relations, Bourdieu allowed the substantive content of culture to disappear. Everything concerns relations to culture. Culture itself has no message.

It is my opinion that both Simmel and Bourdieu have provided two attempts at syntheses between natural scientific and cultural scientific thought within a sociological theory of culture, but that while these attempts are full of perspectives, they are not without problems. They have left behind them some problems, but they also give good possibilities for interpreting and explaining empirical phenomena within the cultural world.

# References




Archer, M. S. and Giner S. (eds.) (1971) *Contemporary Europe. Class, Status and Power.* London: Weidenfeld and Nicolson.

Archer, M.S. (1979) *Social Origins of Educational Systems.* London: Sage Publications Ltd.

Archer, M.S. (1982) "Morphogenesis versus structuration: on combining structure and action" in *The British Journal of Sociology,* 33:4, pp. 455-483.

Archer, M.S. (1985) "The Myth of Cultural Integration" in *The British Journal of Sociology,* 36:3, pp. 333-53.

Archer, M.S. (1988/1996) *Culture and agency. The place of culture in social theory.* Revised Edition. Cambridge: Cambridge University Press.

Archer, M.S. (1995) *Realist social theory: the morphogenetic approach.* Cambridge: Cambridge University Press.

Bhaskar, R. (1993) *Dialectic. The Pulse of Freedom.* London: Verso.

Blegvad, M. (1996) "Max Webers sociologi i teorihistorisk lys" in *Dansk Sociologi,* 7:4, pp. 19-30.

Bourdieu, P. & Passeron, J. (1964/1979) *The Inheritors. French Students and their Relation to Culture.* Chicago: The University of Chicago Press.

Bourdieu, P. & Passeron, J. (1970/1996) *Reproduction in Education, Society and Culture.* London: Sage Publications.

Bourdieu, P. & Wacquant, L. (1992) *An Invitation to Reflexive Sociology.* Cambridge: Polity Press.

Bourdieu, P. (1967/1971) "Systems of Education and Systems of Thought" in Young M.: *Knowledge and Control. New Directions for the Sociology of Education.* London: Collier-Macmillan Publishers.

Bourdieu, P. (1968-1989/1993) *The Field of Cultural Production. Essays on Art and Literature.* Edited and Introduced by Randal Johnson. Cambridge: Polity Press.

Bourdieu, P. (1972/1995) *Outline of a Theory of Practice.* Cambridge: Cambridge University Press.

Bourdieu, P. (1977-1984/1992) *Language and Symbolic Power.* Edited and introduced by John B. Thompson. Cambridge: Polity Press.

Bourdieu, P. (1979/1984) *Distinction. A Social Critique of the Judgement of Taste.* London: Routledge & Kegan Paul.

Bourdieu, P. (1980/1995) *The Logic of Practice.* Cambridge: Polity Press.

Bourdieu, P. (1984/1988) *Homo Academicus.* Cambridge: Polity Press.

Bourdieu, P. (1985) "The Genesis of the Concepts of Habitus and of Field" in *Sociocriticism* no. 2: 11-24.

Bourdieu, P. (1987/1990) *In Other Words. Essays Towards a Reflexive Sociology.* Cambridge: Polity Press.

Broady, D. (1990/1991) *Sociologi och epistemologi. Om Pierre Bourdieus författerskap och den historiska epistemologin.* Stockholm, HLS Förlag.

Bruun, H.H. (1972) *Science, Values and Politics in Max Weber's Methodology.* Copenhagen: Munksgaard

Buckley, W. (1967) *Sociology and Modern Systems Theory.* Englewood Cliffs, New Jersey: Prentice-Hall, INC.

Calhoun, C, LiPuma, E. & Postone M. (eds.) (1993) *Bourdieu: Critical Perspectives.* Cambridge: Polity Press.

Cassirer, E. (1910/1953) *Substance and Function and Einstein's Theory of Relativity.* New York: Dover Publications, Inc.

Cassirer, E. (1921-1929/1955) *The Philosophy of Symbolic Forms.* Vol. 1.: *Language.* Vol.2: *Mythical Thought.* Vol.3: *The Philosophy of Knowledge.* New Haven: Yale University Press.

Collin, F. (1996) "Værdi og idealtype hos Max Weber" in *Dansk Sociologi,* 7:4, pp. 53-70.

Crone, M. (1996) "Max Weber mellem etik og nihilisme - Leo Strauss om Webers dobbelte værdibegreb" in *Dansk Sociologi,* 7:4, pp. 71-78.

Durkheim, E (1912/1995) *The Elementary Forms of Religious Life.* New York: The Free Press.

Durkheim, E. (1893/1997) *The Division of Labor in Society.* New York: The Free Press.

Durkheim, E. (1895/1966) *The Rules of Sociological Method.* New York: The Free Press.

Durkheim, E. (1925/1968) *Moral Education. A study in the theory and application of the sociology of education.* New York: The Free Press.

Durkheim, E. (1938/1977) *The Evolution of Educational Thought. Lectures on the formation and development of secondary education in France.* London: Routledge and Kegan Paul.

Durkheim, E. (1950/1992) *Professional Ethics and Civic Morals.* London: Routledge.

Fowler, B. (1997) *Pierre Bourdieu and Cultural Theory. Critical Investigations.* London: Sage Publications

Frisby, D. (1981) *Sociological Impressionism. A Reassessment of Georg Simmel's Social Theory.* London: Heinemann.

Gadamer, H. (1960/1993) *Truth and Method.* Second, Revised edition. London: Sheed and Ward.

Garnham, N. (1993) "Bourdieu, The Cultural Arbitrary, and Television" in Calhoun, C, LiPuma, E. & Postone M. (eds.): *Bourdieu: Critical Perspectives.* Cambridge: Polity Press.

Gellner, E. (1968) "Holism Versus Individualism" in M. Brodbeck (ed): *Readings in the Philosophy of the Social Sciences.* London: The Macmillan Company.

Giddens, A. (1979) *Central Problems in Social Theory.* London: Macmillan.

Giner, S. and Archer, M. S. (eds.) (1978) *Contemporary Europe: Social Structures and Cultural Patterns.* London: Routledge & Kegan Paul.

Gramsci, A. (1932/1975) *Letters from Prison: Antonio Gramsci.* Edited by Lynne Lawner. New York: Harper Colophon.

Griswold, W. (1992) The Sociology of Culture: Four Good Arguments (and One Bad One). *Acta Sociologica,* 35: 323-328.

Griswold, W. (1994) *Cultures and Societies in a Changing World.* Thousand Oaks, California: Pine Forge Press.

Gunder Hansen N. (1991) *Sansernes Sociologi. Om Georg Simmel og det moderne.* Copenhagen: Tiderne Skifter.

Habermas, J. (1967/1988) *On the Logic of the Social Sciences.* Cambridge: Polity Press.

Habermas, J. (1971) *Towards a Rational Society.* London: Heinemann.

Hayek, F. A. (1973) "From Scientism and the Study of Society" in J. O'Neill (ed): *Modes of Individualism and Collectivism.* London: Heinemann.

Jenkins, R. (1992/1996) *Pierre Bourdieu.* London: Routledge.

Lash, S. (1993) "Pierre Bourdieu: Cultural Economy and Social Change" in Calhoun, C, LiPuma, E. & Postone M. (eds.): *Bourdieu: Critical Perspectives.* Cambridge: Polity Press.

Lévi-Strauss, C. (1958/1969) *Structural Anthropology.* London: Allen Lane. The Penguin Press.

LiPuma E. (1993) "Culture and the Concept of Culture in a Theory of Practice" in Calhoun, C, LiPuma, E. & Postone M. (eds.): *Bourdieu: Critical Perspectives.* Cambridge: Polity Press.

Lockwood, D. (1964) "Social Integration and System Integration" in G. K. Zollschan and W. Hirsch (eds): *Explorations in Social Change.* London: Routledge & Kegan Paul.

Luhmann, N. (1984/1995) *Social systems.* Stanford, CA: Stanford University Press.

Lukács, G. (1918/1991) "Georg Simmel" in *Theory, Culture and Society.* 8:3, August 1991. A Special Issue on Georg Simmel. No 3: pp. 145-150

Lukes, S. (1973) *Émile Durkheim - His Life and Work. A historical and critical study.* London: Allen Lane The Penguin Press.

Mandelbaum M. (1973) "Societal Facts" in J. O'Neill (ed): *Modes of Individualism and Collectivism.* London: Heinemann.

Marcuse, H. (1964) *One-Dimensional Man.* London: Routledge & Kegan Paul.

Miliband, R. (1969) *The State in Capitalist Society.* London: Allen and Unwin.

Nedelmann, B. (1991) "Individualization, Exaggeration and Paralysation: Simmel's Three Problems of Culture" in *Theory, Culture and Society.* 8:3, August 1991. A Special Issue on Georg Simmel. No 3: 169-193

Panofsky, E. (1951/1976) *Gothic Architecture and Scholasticism. An inquiry into the analogy of the arts, philosophy, and religion in the Middle Ages.* New York: New American Library.

Parsons, T. (1951) *The Social System.* London: Routledge & Kegan Paul.

Popper, K. R. (1972/1992) *Objective Knowledge. An Evolutionary Approach.* Revised Edition. Oxford: Clarendon Press.

Ringer, F. K. (1969) *The Decline of the German Mandarins. The German Academic Community, 1890-1933.* Cambridge, Massachussetts: Harvard University Press.

Ringer, F. K. (1992) *Fields of Knowledge. French academic culture in comparative perspective, 1890-1920.* Cambridge: Cambridge University Press.

Ringer, F. K. (1997) *Max Weber's Methodology. The Unification of the Cultural and Social Sciences.* Cambridge, Massachussetts: Harvard University Press.

Ritzer, G. (1992) *Sociological Theory.* New York: McGraw-Hill.

Robbins, D. (1991) *The Work of Pierre Bourdieu.* Milton Keynes: Open University Press.

Robertson, R. (1992) *Globalization. Social Theory and Global Culture.* London: Sage.

Schroeder, R. (1992) *Max Weber and the Sociology of Culture.* London: Sage Publications.

Simmel, G. (1905/1977) *The Problems of the Philosophy of History. An Epistemological Essay.* Translated and Edited, with an Introduction, by Guy Oakes. New York: The Free Press.

Simmel, G. (1907/1978) *The Philosophy of Money.* London: Routledge and Kegan Paul.

Simmel, G. (1907/1986) *Schopenhauer and Nietzsche.* Chicago: University of Illinois Press.

Simmel, G. (1950/1964) *The Sociology of Georg Simmel.* Translated, edited, and with an introduction by Kurt H. Wolff. New York: The Free Press. London: Collier-Macmillan

Simmel, G. (1959) *Georg Simmel, 1858-1918.* A Collection of Essays, with Translations and a Bibliography. Edited by Kurt H. Wolff. Columbus: The Ohio State University Press.

Simmel, G. (1968) *Georg Simmel: The Conflict in Modern Culture and Other Essays.* Translated, with an introduction by K. Peter Etzkorn. New York: Teachers College Press.

Simmel, G. (1971) *Georg Simmel: On Individuality and Social Forms. Selected Writings.* Edited and with an Introduction by Donald N. Levine. Chicago: The University of Chicago Press.

Simmel, G. (1976) *Georg Simmel: Sociologist and European.* Edited by P. A. Lawrence. Nairobi: Nelson.

Simmel, G. (1984) *Georg Simmel: On Women, Sexuality, and Love.* Translated and with an Introduction by Guy Oakes. New Haven: Yale University Press.

Sorokin, P. (1957) *Social and Cultural Dynamics.* London: Peter Owen.

Spykman, N. J. (1925/1992) *The Social Theory of Georg Simmel.* Aldershot, Hampshire: Gregg Revivals.

Vaughan M. and Archer M.S. (1971) *Social Conflict and Educational Change in England and France: 1789-1848.* Cambridge: Cambridge University Press.

Watkins, J.W.N. (1968) "Methodological Individualism and Social Tendencies" in M. Brodbeck (ed): *Readings in the Philosophy of the Social Sciences.* London: The Macmillan Company.

Weber, M. (1904-05/1970) *The Protestant Ethic and the Spirit of Capitalism.* London: Unwin University Books.

Weber, M. (1904-17/1949) *The Methodology of the Social Sciences.* Translated end Edited by E. A. Shils and H.A. Finch. New York: The Free Press.

Weber, M. (1926/1995) *Max Weber, A Biography.* New Brunswick: Transaction Publishers.

Weber, M. (1948/1970) *From Max Weber: Essays in sociology.* Translated, Edited and with an Introduction by H. H. Gerth and C. Wright Mills. London: Routledge & Kegan Paul.

Weber, M. (1956/1968) *Economy and Society. An outline of Interpretive Sociology.* Edited by G. Roth and C. Wittich. New York: Bedminster Press.

Weingartner R. H. (1960) *Experience and Culture. The Philosophy of Georg Simmel.* Middletown, Connecticut: Wesleyan University Press.

Wuthnow, R. (1976) *The Consciousness Reformation.* Berkeley: University of California Press.

Wuthnow, R. (1978) *Experimentation in American Religion. The New Mysticisms and Their Implications for the Churches.* Berkeley: University of California Press.

Wuthnow, R. (1987) *Meaning and Moral Order. Explorations in Cultural Analysis.* Berkeley: University of California Press.

Wuthnow, R. (1988) *The Restructuring of American Religion. Society and Faith Since World War II.* Princeton: Princeton University Press.

Wuthnow, R. (1989a) *Communities of Discourse. Ideology and Social Structure in the Reformation, the Enlightenment, and European Socialism.* Cambridge, Massachussetts: Harvard University Press.

Wuthnow, R. (1989b) *The Struggle for America's Soul. Evangelicals, Liberals and Secularism.* Grand Rapids, Michigan: W. B. Eerdmans Publishing Company.

Wuthnow, R. (1991) *Acts of Compassion. Caring for Others and Helping Ourselves.* Princeton: Princeton University Press.

Wuthnow, R. (1992) *Rediscovering the Sacred. Perspectives on Religion in Contemporary Society.* Grand Rapids, Michigan: W. B. Eerdmans Publishing Company.

Wuthnow, R. (1993) *Christianity in the 21'st Century. Reflections on the Challenges Ahead.* New York: Oxford University Press.

Wuthnow, R. (1994a *Producing the Sacred. An Essay on Public Religion.* Urbana and Chicago: University of Illinois Press.

Wuthnow, R. (1994b) *God and Mammon in America.* New York: The Free Press.

Wuthnow, R. (1994c) *Sharing the Journey. Support Groups and America's New Quest for Community.* New York: The Free Press.

Wuthnow, R. (1995) *Learning to Care. Elementary Kindness in an Age of Indifference.* New York: Oxford University Press.

Wuthnow, R. (1996a) *Poor Richard's Principle. Recovering the American Dream through the Moral Dimension of Work, Business, and Money.* Princeton: Princeton University Press.

Wuthnow, R. (1996b) *Christianity and Civil Society. The Contemporary Debate.* Valley Forge, Pennsylvania: Trinity Press International.

Wuthnow, R. (1997) *The Crisis in the Churches. Spiritual Malaise, Fiscal Woe.* New York: Oxford University Press.

Wuthnow, R. (1998) *After Heaven. Spirituality in America since the 1950s.* Berkeley: University of California Press.

Wuthnow, R., Hunter, J.D., Bergesen, A., Kurzweil E. (1984) *Cultural Analysis. The Work of Peter L. Berger, Mary Douglas, Michel Foucault, and Jürgen Habermas.* London: Routledge & Kegan Paul.

Zeuner, L. (1999) "Margaret Archer on Structural and Cultural Morphogenesis" in *Acta Sociologica,* 42:1, pp. 79-86.

Zeuner, L. (2001) "Theory of Culture. Margaret Archer versis Classical Sociology" in *Cultural Dynamics,* 13:1, pp. 92-116.

Østerberg, D. (1988) *Metasociology. An Inquiry into the Origins and Validity of Social Thought.* Oslo: Norwegian University Press.

UNITAR

# THE CENTENNIAL OF THE FIRST INTERNATIONAL PEACE CONFERENCE

## REPORTS & CONCLUSIONS

*edited and introduced*
*by*

Frits Kalshoven



KLUWER LAW INTERNATIONAL
THE HAGUE / LONDON / BOSTON

A C.I.P. Catalogue record for this book is available from the Library of Congress



ISBN 90-411-1463-7 (HB)
ISBN 90-411-1464-5 (PB; available through UNITAR)

---

Published by Kluwer Law International,
P.O. Box 85889, 2508 CN The Hague, The Netherlands.

Sold and distributed in North, Central and South America
by Kluwer Law International,
675 Massachusetts Avenue, Cambridge, MA 02139, U.S.A.

In all other countries, sold and distributed
by Kluwer Law International, Distribution Centre,
P.O. Box 322, 3300 AH Dordrecht, The Netherlands.



*Printed on acid-free paper*



Printed in the Netherlands.

# Contents

## Abbreviations

| | |
|---|---|
| ABM | Anti-ballistic missile |
| ADR | Alternative dispute resolution |
| AJIL | *American Journal of International Law* |
| *Ann Dig* | *Annual Digest of Public International Law Cases* |
| *Annuaire* | *Annuaire de l'Institut de droit international* |
| ASEAN | Association of South East Asian Nations |
| BC weapons | Bacteriological (biological) weapons |
| BYIL | *British Yearbook of International Law* |
| CFE | Treaty on Conventional Armed Froces in Europe (1990) |
| CTBT | Comprehensive Nuclear Test Ban Treaty (1996) |
| CTBTO | Comprehensive Nuclear Test Ban Organization |
| CWC | Convention of the Prohibition of the Development, Production, Stockpiling and Use of Chemical Weapons and on Their Destruction (1993) |
| *Documents* | A. Roberts and R. Guelff, *Documents on the Laws of War*, 3rd ed. (2000) |
| DSB | Dispute Settlement Body |
| DPKR | Democratic People's Republic of Korea |
| ENMOD Convention | Convention on the Prohibition of Military or Any Other Hostile Use of Environmental Modification Techniques (1977) |
| EHRR | *European Human Rights Reports* |
| GATT | General Agreement on Tariffs and Trade |
| IAEA | International Atomic Energy Agency |
| ICAO | International Civil Aviation Organization |
| ICBM | Intercontinental ballistic missile |
| ICC | International Criminal Court |
| ICJ | International Court of Justice |
| ICLQ | *International and Comparative Law Quarterly* |
| ICRC | International Committee of the Red Cross |

| | |
|---|---|
| ICSID | International Centre for the Settlement of Investment Disputes |
| ICTR | International Criminal Tribunal for Rwanda |
| ICTY | International Tribunal for the Former Yugoslavia |
| ILC | International Law Commission |
| ILM | *International Legal Materials* |
| ILO | International Labour Organization |
| ILR | *International Law Reports* |
| INF | Intermediate-range nuclear forces |
| Merrills | J.G. Merrills, *International Dispute Settlement* (1991) |
| NAFTA | North American Free Trade Agreement |
| NATO | North Atlantic Treaty Organization |
| NGO | Non-governmental organization |
| NPT | Non-Proliferation Treaty (1968) |
| OAS | Organization of American States |
| OAU | Organization of African Unity |
| OSCE | Organization for Security and Co-operation in Europe |
| PCA | Permanent Court of Arbitration |
| PTBT | Partial Test Ban Treaty (1963) |
| RdC | *Recueil des Cours* (of the Hague Academy of International Law |
| SC | Security Council |
| SG | Secretary-General |
| START | US-USSR/Russia strategic arms reduction talks |
| START I | US-USSR Treaty on Reduction and Limitation of Strategic Offensive Arms (1991) |
| START II | US-Russia Treaty on Further Reduction and Limitation of Strategic Offensive Arms (1993) |
| START III | ongoing US-Russia discussions about further reductions |

| | |
|---|---|
| UN | United Nations |
| UNCITRAL | United Nations Commission on International Trade Law |
| UNCLOS | UN Convention on the Law of the Sea |
| UNGA | UN General Assembly |
| UN Handbook | *United Nations Handbook on the Peaceful Settlement of Disputes between States* (1992) |
| UNSCOM | UN Special Commission on Iraq |
| UNTS | UN Treaty Series |
| WHO | World Health Organization |
| WTO | World Trade Organization |
| YBIHL | *Yearbook of International Humanitarian Law* |

# INTRODUCTION

by Frits KALSHOVEN[1]

1. The First Hague Peace Conference of 1899 (or, with its official name, the International Peace Conference) stands out as a landmark in the history of mankind, and rightly so. Not because it achieved the impossible – peace, or significant cuts in the armaments of States: far from it. But this was the first time a diplomatic conference had been convened to discuss these and suchlike issues outside any direct connection with topical events such as a war actually being waged or a peace that had to be concluded, and then not just for the sake of discussion but with the set aim to work towards tangible results. While there shall be more to say about the Conference and its results below, I may now simply note that it doubtless belongs in the class of international events worthy of being commemorated on the occasion of their one-hundredth anniversary.[2]

2. This is precisely what was done with the Centennial of 1999, organized by the Governments of the Kingdom of the Netherlands and the Russian Federation under the aegis of the United Nations and within the framework of the UN Decade of International Law.

1. Professor emeritus of international and humanitarian law, University of Leiden; member and acting president of the International Fact-finding Commission established pursuant to Article 90 of Protocol I (1977) Additional to the Geneva Conventions of 1949. -Having been invited by the Netherlands Minister of Foreign Affairs to act as editor in chief of the compilation of papers and documents relating to the Centennial Conference that appear in the present volume, I take this opportunity to express my gratitude to him for entrusting me with this honourable function.

2. For a critical appraisal of the Conference and its aftermath, see: G. Best, "Peace conferences and the century of total war: the 1899 Hague Conference and what came after", 75 *International Affairs* (1999) No.3, pp. 619-634. See also: G.A. Aldrich and C.M. Chinkin (eds.), "Symposium: The Hague Peace Conferences", 94 AJIL (2000) pp. 1-98. For a general historical overview of the Conference, see also: A. Eyffinger, *The 1899 Hague Peace Conference: The Parliament of Man, the Federation of the World* (1999).



*F. Kalshoven (ed.),*
***The Centennial of the First International Peace Conference,* 1–39.**

Measured against its illustrious precedent of 1899, the 1999 Centennial stands out as the "bigger" event in every respect. It lasted longer: from the early initiatives[3] to the present publication of the main reports and conclusions, a period of six years. It involved more actors: representatives of countless States[4] as compared to the 26 of 1899; and, apart from States, the actors included international governmental and non-governmental organizations as well as local groups and individual persons – "civil society" at work! And this multitude of actors engaged in a great variety of activities, ranging from free-style discussions on the Internet and individual papers to more structured seminars and (regional and other) conferences.[5]

3. All this activity centred around the three themes that had also been the main items on the agenda of the 1899 Conference. These were, in the order of the commissions that dealt with them: the reduction of armaments, the laws of war on land, and the peaceful settlement of disputes. To stimulate and structure the debate, the organizers at an early stage had invited experts to prepare reports on each of these themes: Dr. Hans BLIX on disarmament and arms control, Professor Christopher GREENWOOD on the laws of war, and Professor Francisco ORREGO VICUÑA and Dr. Christopher PINTO on dispute settlement.[6] Their initial reports were distributed over all the known participants to the various activities and were also made available on the Internet, as were reports of preparatory seminars and conferences held in different parts of the world as they became available.

4. Thus prepared, the stage was set for the "grande finale" of 1999, in two phases. One, in May at The Hague, consisted of two events: 12-15 May, the tumult of the non-governmental Hague Appeal for Peace; and 18-19 May, first session of the more sedate, governmental

3. The idea was first publicly expressed by President Yeltsin in his 1995 address to the UN General Assembly.

4. "Countless" because their numbers fluctuated by the day and were moreover different for the meetings in The Hague and St. Petersburg, respectively.

5. All these contributions are included on the CD-ROM accompanying this book.

6. Of the six rapporteurs originally invited (two for each topic) two weren not in a position to finalize their reports.

Centennial Conference convened at the level of Legal Advisers. The other, from 22 to 25 June at St. Petersburg, was the second session of the Centennial. Both the Hague Appeal and the Centennial Conference produced a document at the end of their activities: the "Hague Appeal for Peace and Justice in the 21st Century," and the "Outcome of the Celebrations of the Centennial of the First International Peace Conference: Report on the Conclusions". The Hague Appeal in its final shape is the product of a core group and may not even have been seen by a majority of the participants.[7] And the Centennial Report is not a true "report" either: although promulgated among the participants, it was drawn up under the authority of the chairmen of the two meetings and does not attempt to provide an official, complete report of the discussions; rather, it aims to reflect the main views and trends of opinion that emerged from the debate.[8] Both texts are included in this volume immediately after the reports of the Rapporteurs.

5. After the above events, the Rapporteurs were given the opportunity to complete and adapt their reports so as to take into account, as appropriate, comments at the various stages of the celebrations. The present volume provides the final versions of the reports. It should be noted that these texts too, are not "reports" in the sense of reflections of proceedings: they are the product of their authors, who therefore are entitled to all the praise their writings deserve, while at the same time remaining alone responsible for the end result of their labours.

6. The reports are included in this book in the order of 1899: (1) the law relating to disarmament and arms control; (2) the laws of armed conflict; (3) dispute settlement.

7. The "Hague Appeal for Peace and Justice for the 21st Century" was transmitted to the UN by a letter dated 17 May 1999 from the Permanent Representative of Bangladesh to the Secretary-General, and published as UN Doc. A/54/98.

8. The Chairmen's Report on the Conclusions of the Centennial likewise was transmitted to the UN by a letter dated 10 September 1999 from the Permanent Representatives of the Netherlands and the Russian Federation to the Secretary-General, and published as UN Doc. A/54/381.

7. As noted above, the Centennial measures as a "bigger" event than the Peace Conference had been. The difference in size accurately reflects societal changes that took place over the last century. It does not, of course, imply that the Centennial will go down in history as the more significant event as well: even by its aim, it was a far more modest affair than the Peace Conference had been. Even so, the comparison at least provides an excuse to ask ourselves for a moment: what, indeed, has made the Conference of 1899 qualify as an important event? This question obviously was also dealt with by the Rapporteurs, each in their own fields. Yet there is room for some brief remarks on my part too. And I should state immediately that while perhaps a failure in the eyes of the public at the time, it is precisely through its after-effects that the Peace Conference has earned its place on the list of really outstanding international events.

8. "Peace," the goal that figured in its title, the Conference did not achieve, nor any system of compulsory dispute settlement; yet the modest steps realized in that area with the adoption of the Convention for the Pacific Settlement of International Disputes and the ensuing establishment of the Permanent Court of International Arbitration (PCA),[9] have acted as the catalyst that set in motion further developments, up to and including the creation of the International Court of Justice (ICJ). A similar remark may be made about "disarmament," or, more properly, rigorous reduction of armaments: nothing of the kind was realized, and one has to look very closely to find any result that even remotely resembled a disarmament measure.[10] Yet here again, the idea had been firmly implanted that arsenals cannot be permitted unlimited growth both in a quantitative and qualitative sense, and also this idea would bear – always modest – fruit in the century that followed.

9. The Conference scored its greatest instant success with the adoption of the Convention and Regulations Respecting the Laws

9. On this, see the Report by Orrego Vicuña and Pinto, paras. 14 et seq.

10. On this, see the Report by Blix, paras. 37 et seq.

and Customs of War on Land[11] – rules on the conduct of warfare precisely in the type of situation it had vainly tried to preclude or bring under control in the first place. Disappointing though this may have been at the time, it has since become evident that this result too must be positively appreciated, marking as it does an important step on the road to what much later, in the 1970s, would come to be termed the "reaffirmation and development of the international humanitarian law applicable in armed conflict".[12]

10. "Reaffirmation and development": the phrase aptly describes the struggle throughout the 20th century to preserve or restore the spirit of 1899 and, often against all odds, construct on that basis, systems and processes that might make for a better and safer world. It is not here the place, nor my competence, to sketch the history of that century. Rather, I merely wish to note a few points of particular relevance in the context of the Centennial, including some that follow from developments that have occurred in the period since the authors concluded work on their reports.

11. First, then, war, and the law relating thereto. Throughout the 20th century, wars were being waged in all shapes and sizes, from the two World Wars to the 1980-88 war between Iraq and Iran; to the wars of national liberation that brought an end to so-called "salt-water colonialism"; down to the odd short-lived border incident with "prisoners of war" at least on one side; to the strictly local, rapid secession of Slovenia from Yugoslavia – even all the way down to the construct of a "30-hours armed conflict" waged on 23 and 24

11. On this, see the Report by Greenwood, paras. 2.6 et seq.

12. From 1974 to 1977, a diplomatic conference with that title was held in Geneva, to elaborate and ultimately adopt two Protocols Additional to the Geneva Conventions of 12 August 1949; texts in A. Roberts and R. Guelff, *Documents on the Laws of War*, 3rd ed. (2000) (hereinafter: *Documents*) at pp. 419, 481.

January 1989 at La Tablada, Argentina.[13] In retrospect, it seems permissible to split the century into two periods, with the wars in its first half belonging mostly in the class of international armed conflicts (with the Spanish Civil War as a striking exception) and the majority of those in the second half falling under the heading of non-international armed conflicts. (The "wars of national liberation" of this period were regarded as internal affairs by the colonial Powers, although other actors, including the UN General Assembly, increasingly preferred to regard them as international armed conflicts.)[14]

12. Ironically, this division of the century into two almost equal halves finds its parallel in a coincidental split in the development of the law of armed conflicts. Up to and including the Second World War, the relevant treaty law formally applied only in "wars" between States and could at best be made applicable in "civil wars" through the device of recognition of belligerency. Then, in 1949, the Diplomatic Conference that negotiated and adopted the Geneva Conventions for the protection of war victims,[15] introduced into these instruments a common Article 3 that for the first time provided a short list of fundamental principles for the protection of persons not, or no longer, taking part in an internal armed conflict, and to be respected by all the parties to such a conflict whenever it occurred.[16]

13. The capture by members of the *Movimiento Todos por la Patria* of a military barracks located at La Tablada, followed by the recapture of the place by the army, which altogether had taken some 30 hours, was construed by the Inter-American Commission on Human Rights as an armed conflict in the sense of Art. 3 common to the Geneva Conventions of 1949; Report No. 55/97, Case No. 11.137, Argentina; OEA/Ser/L/V/I.97, Doc.38, 18 Nov. 1997. See also Greenwood, Report paras. 3.31, 5.32 and 6.29.

14. At the 1974-77 conference mentioned in note 12, pressure in this direction resulted in the insertion into Protocol I (applicable in international armed conflicts) of Art. 1 (4) classifying defined liberation wars as international armed conflicts.

15. Reprinted in *Documents* pp. 195 (Convention I), 221 (Convention II), 243 (Convention III) and 299 (Convention IV).

16. Emulating this example, the 1954 Hague Convention for the Protection of Cultural Property in the Event of Armed Conflict (*Documents* p. 371) was likewise

(continued...)

Another closely related and equally important event occurred on 10 December 1948, when the UN General Assembly adopted the Universal Declaration of Human Rights: like the long list of human rights treaties that were to follow, this too set norms to be respected by States in all situations including those of armed conflict, unless expressly excepted.

13. Another noticeable innovation, already implicit in the foregoing, was the introduction in the Geneva Conventions of 1949 of the term "armed conflict." This was not just a semantic device to get away from the odious "war" (as in the Charter Preamble's "scourge of war"), nor from its politico-legal connotations (the "declared war", perhaps even without any actual fighting yet with all its consequences for treaties, third parties etc.). Rather, "armed conflict" was expected to provide an objective description of given situations and thus determining the application of the Conventions (in their entirety, in a situation of international armed conflict; only common Article 3, in an internal armed conflict). Even though the new terminology is less immune from politization than may have been hoped, it is now in current use to indicate the law applicable in armed conflict, or international humanitarian law (IHL).[17] Obviously, the

16. (...continued)
equipped with a provision on respect for cultural property in "conflicts not of an international character" (Art. 19).

17. The existing IHL treaties do not make provision for an authoritative determination, as-it-were over the heads of the party or parties concerned, that a situation is one of armed conflict. The ICRC, for its part, usually prefers not to rely on qualification of situations but rather goes for the protection of victims regardless. Among international political organs, the Security Council acting under Chapter VII of the Charter may "decide", in circumstances with binding force, that a given situation represents an armed conflict. Again acting under Chapter VII, the Security Council in 1993 established ICTY (see below, para. 24). As a judicial organ, this has from its inception been determining, with legal effect, whether situations objectively qualified as (international or internal) armed conflicts. The point is made explicit in the recent Blaškić Judgement, where the Trial Chamber states that "the parties to the conflict may not agree between themselves to change the nature of the conflict, which *is established by the facts whose interpretation, where applicable, falls to the Judge*." (emphasis added); *The Prosecutor* v. *Tihomir Blaskic*, Judgement, 3 March 2000, Case No. IT-95-14-T, p. 29: para. 82.

word "war" has also remained in use. Thus, in a political context: "The Vietnam War was a war of national liberation." (It also was an (internal, or international, or internal-yet-internationalized) armed conflict.) Or as a simple alternative to the longer phrase "armed conflict". And of course, frequently nowadays, in the phrase "crime of war".

14. This brings me to the last feature marking the start of the second half of the 20th century I want to mention here: i.e., the post-World War Two trials at Nuremberg and Tokyo[18] and the acceptance of the universality principle for "grave breaches" as defined in the Geneva Conventions,[19] as first steps on the road to international regulation of individual criminal liability for violations of the law of armed conflict, or war crimes.[20]

15. With all this, international society appeared well prepared to cope with the wave of internal armed conflicts that swept over the world in the period under review. A last important feature, detailed rules elaborating the principle of protection of civilian populations against the effects of hostilities, was added in 1977 with the adoption of two Protocols Additional to the Geneva Conventions of 1949, one (Protocol I) for international armed conflicts and the other (Proto-

18. Besides war crimes, these trials also involved crimes against peace and crimes against humanity.

19. Arts. 49 (Convention I), 50 (Convention II), 129 (Convention III), 146 (Convention IV).

20. Much earlier, in 1919, the "Commission on the Responsibility of the Authors of the War and on Enforcement of Penalties" submitted its plan for an international war crimes tribunal to the Preliminary Peace Conference at Versailles. The tribunal would have jurisdiction over actual perpetrators, those who ordered the crimes, as well as "all authorities, civil or military, belonging to enemy countries, however high their position may have been, without distinction of rank, including the heads of states," who ordered or failed to prevent or repress violations of the laws or customs of war. And the applicable law would be "the principles of the laws of nations as they result from the usages established among civilized peoples, from the laws of humanity and from the dictates of the public conscience" – the Martens clause! Extracts in: L. Friedman, *The Law of War, a Documentary History* (1972) pp. 842 et seq.

col II) for internal armed conflicts,[21] followed a little while later by the 1980 UN Conventional Weapons Convention[22] with annexed Protocols, which in large part serve to protect civilians from the adverse effects of weapons such as land mines and incendiary weapons.

16. Yet, the more complete and elaborate the law of armed conflict, the less it was respected, to the point where, in the closing decade of the century, persons and objects protected under the law such as civilians and civilian objects, or Red Cross workers and their means of transport appeared to have become the targets of choice, and this not merely in so-called "failed States". Reactions to this alarming state of affairs were numerous and continue to this day. A few of these may be mentioned here.

17. At the instigation of the International Committee of the Red Cross (ICRC) the Swiss Government convened a first International Conference for the Protection of War Victims, Geneva, 30 August – 1 September 1993. In the opening paragraph of the Final Declaration of the Conference, the participants "solemnly declare" that they:

> … refuse to accept that war, violence and hatred spread throughout the world, and fundamental rights of persons are violated in an increasingly grave and systematic fashion. We refuse to accept that wounded are shown no mercy, children massacred, women raped, prisoners tortured, victims denied elementary humanitarian assistance, civilians starved as a method of warfare, obligations under international humanitarian law in territories under foreign occupation not respected, families of missing

21. Protocol I, Part IV – Civilian Population; Protocol II, Part IV – Civilian Population.

22. The full title is "UN Convention on Prohibitions or Restrictions on the Use of Certain Conventional Weapons Which May be Deemed to be Excessively Injurious or to Have Indiscriminate Effects." The three original Protocols are on: weapons the primary effect of which is to enjury by fragments which in the human body escape detection by X-rays (I); the use of mines, booby-traps and other devices (II), and the use of incendiary weapons (III); 19 ILM (1980) p. 1523; *Documents* p. 515.

> persons denied information about the fate of their relatives, populations illegally displaced, and countries laid to waste.[23]

18. Similar expressions of dismay may be found in other declarations made in the course of the closing decade of the century. Particularly striking were the statements delivered on the occasion of the 50th anniversary of the Geneva Conventions, on 12 August 1999 in Geneva. Thus, Kofi ANNAN, Secretary-General-General of the United Nations, focussing on the fate of civilians, noted that "the ethnic wars of the 1990s have been characterized by the abominable practice of making civilians the very targets of warfare, in campaigns of genocide and 'ethnic cleansing'." And he continued:

> It is not, therefore, merely a question of protecting civilians *in* armed conflict, but protecting them *from* armed conflict. These flagrant violations of international humanitarian law – the wholesale expulsion of an entire people from their native land, summary and arbitrary executions, mutilation, rape, forced displacement, denial of the right to food and medicines – have taken place not as the effect of war, but as the essence of warfare.
> [...]
> As the United Nations enters a new century, our commitment to ensuring respect for international humanitarian law and ending the culture of impunity will be at the heart of our efforts to promote peace and security. As we do so, we will continue to find guidance, inspiration and courage in the principles of the Geneva Conventions.

19. One way the Secretary-General could give expression to this commitment was by announcing that on that very day, his Bulletin on "Observance by United Nations forces of international humanitarian law," dated 6 August 1999, had entered into force, thus (at least temporarily) putting an end to a discussion about application of IHL to UN forces that had been going on for a very long time.[24]

23. The Final Declaration was published by the ICRC in 75 *International Review of the Red Cross* (1993) pp. 337 et seq.

24. ST/SGB/1999/13, reprinted in *Documents* p. 721. See Greenwood, Report paras. 3.48 to 3.57; and, by the same author, "International Humanitarian Law and United (continued...)

20. The celebration of the 50th anniversary of the Geneva Conventions was marked by the signing of a "Solemn Appeal," by which the signatories "[called] on the world:"

> to reject the idea that war is inevitable and to work tirelessly to eradicate its underlying causes;
> to demand of those involved in armed conflicts and all who are in a position to influence the course of such conflicts that they respect the essential humanitarian principles and the rules of international humanitarian law;
> to spare civilians the agony of war;
> to foster relations between individuals, peoples and nations on the basis of the principles that inspired the Geneva Conventions, namely:
> respect for human dignity in all circumstances;
> compassion for those who suffer;
> solidarity.

21. The 27th International Conference of the Red Cross and Red Crescent, Geneva, 31 October – 6 November 1999, took note of this appeal, fully endorsed it and "[undertook] to contribute towards the achievement of its aims." It should be noted that the Conference was as much a matter of the participating States parties to the Conventions as of the components of the Red Cross and Red Crescent Movement (the national societies, their International Federation, and the ICRC). The Conference, which had as its motto "the *power* of **humanity**", also adopted a Plan of Action for the years 2000-2003 (i.e. up to the next regular International Conference). The first chapter lists five "final goals" to be achieved for the "protection of victims of armed conflict through respect of international humanitarian law,"[25] and elaborates these into a number of concrete under

24. (...continued)
Nations Military Operations", 1 Yb IHL (1998) pp. 3-34.

25. The goals listed are the following:
(1) full compliance by all the parties to an armed conflict with their obligations under IHL to protect and assist the civilian population and other victims of the conflict and to respect protected objects;
(2) an effective barrier against impunity through the combination of relevant international treaties and national laws concerning the repression of violations of IHL, and
(continued...)

takings.[26]

22. At the United Nations, too, the alarming level of disrespect for civilians and other victims of armed conflict caused much concern. On 17 September 1999, after a two-day debate on a report of the Secretary-General on the protection of civilians in armed conflict,[27] the Security Council adopted a resolution by which it "strongly [condemned] the deliberate targeting of civilians in situations of armed conflict as well as attacks on objects protected under international

25. (...continued)
the examination of an equitable system of reparations;
(3) universal acceptance of IHL and the adoption of all necessary measures by States at the national level to ensure the implementation of their obligations under international law;
(4) integration, by States, of their obligations under IHL in relevant procedures and training; promotion of this law among relevant persons and bodies;
(5) conformity of weapons with IHL, the establishment of effective controls on the availability of arms and ammunition, and an end to the human tragedy caused by anti-personnel landmines.

26. Given the frequency of internal armed conflicts and the difficulty of having basic precepts of humanity respected in those situations, particular interest attaches to the 3rd para. elaborating goal 1.1:

> Organised armed groups in non-international armed conflict are urged to respect international humanitarian law. They are called upon to *declare their intention to respect that law* and teach it to their forces. (emphasis added)

While such an expression of intention to respect IHL may be a useful device to clarify the stance of "organised armed groups" in that regard, the problem remains that the government of a country involved in the conflict may be unhappy with such a declaration on the part of a party they do not wish to recognize, or see recognized, as a "party to the conflict".

27. Report of 8 September 1999, S/1999/957. Reiterating his concern expressed on the occasion of the 50th anniversary of the Geneva Conventions, the Secretary-General writes (para. 8) that:

> In many of today's armed conflicts, civilian casualties and the destruction of civilian infrastructure are not simply byproducts of war, but the consequence of the deliberate targeting of non-combatants. The violence is frequently perpetrated by non-state actors, including irregular forces and privately financed militias. In many conflicts, belligerents target civilians in order to expel or eradicate segments of the population, or for the purpose of hastening military surrender.

In the next paragraph, he recognizes the difficulty in respecting civilians that nowadays, "the dividing line between civilians and combatants is frequently blurred."

law, and [called] on all parties to put an end to such practices."[28]

23. Again, in the General Assembly debate on the end of the UN Decade of International Law and the report on the Centennial,[29] a message of the Secretary-General stated that:

> Notwithstanding the achievements of the Decade, there is little reason for euphoria when we look at the current state of international affairs. International and national conflicts are still a part of our life today. Loss of life, untold suffering, hunger, dangerous diseases and denial of the basic rights of hundreds of thousands of human beings is a sad reality.

24. Among the "achievements of the Decade" the Secretary-General mentioned in his message, I single out two that strike me as particularly significant, so to speak, for the preservation of human dignity in that all too bleak closing decade of the 20th century. The first was the establishment by the Security Council of the International Tribunal for the former Yugoslavia[30] (ICTY, 1993) and of a similar Tribunal for Rwanda[31] (ICTR, 1994). These measures, in themselves already a quantum leap in international society's reaction to situations of blatant, gross and systematic violations of IHL including crimes against humanity and genocide, were completed in 1998 with the adoption of the Rome Statute of the International Criminal Court[32] (ICC). Once established, the ICC will be permanently available to deal with "the most serious crimes of

28. S/RES/1265 (1999). The Resolution sets forth a number of suggestions and recommendations for the improvement of the lamentable situation.

29. Meeting of 17 November 1999, A/54/PV.54.

30. S/RES/827 (1993), approving the Report of the Secretary-General pursuant to para. 2 of its earlier Res. 808 (1993) [S/25704 & Add. 1 (1993)] with annexed Statute of the International Tribunal (para. 1), and establishing the Tribunal (para. 2); extracts of the Statute in *Documents* p. 565.

31. S/RES/995 (1994), with annexed Statute of the International Tribunal for Rwanda; extracts of the Statute in *Documents* p. 615.

32. Adopted on 17 July 1998 by the UN Diplomatic Conference of Plenipotentiaries on the Establishment of an International Criminal Court, A/Conf. 183/9*, extracts in *Documents* p. 667.

concern to the international community as a whole",[33] as opposed to the ad-hoc Tribunals which have their basis in political decisions of the Security Council. As with the Tribunals,[34] the jurisdiction of the ICC will encompass defined violations of IHL committed in internal armed conflicts as well.[35]

25. The other "achievement" I mention here consists in the adoption of an impressive series of treaties or protocols to existing treaties: 1993, the Convention on the Prohibition of the Development, Pro-

33. Art. 5 (1) of the Statute.

34. Writing in his Report about the jurisdiction of ICTY over the deliberate targeting of civilians, Greenwood refers in a footnote (101) to the case pending before the Tribunal of the Croatian General Blaškić "which involved allegations of unlawful bombardment." In its recent Judgement (supra, note 15) the Trial Chamber finds the accused guilty, first, of "having ordered a crime against humanity," inter alia, for "attacks on towns and villages". It also finds that "by these same acts, in particular, as regards an international armed conflict, General Blaškić committed: a violation of the laws or customs of war under Article 3 of the Statute and recognised by Article 51(2) of Additional Protocol I: unlawful attacks on civilians (count 3)", and another similar violation "recognised by Article 52(1) of Additional Protocol I: unlawful attacks on civilian objects (count 4)" (etc.). -The Chamber's argument on the latter point runs as follows. On the one hand (para. 170) "it should not be necessary to rule on the applicability of Protocol I. The specific provisions of Article 3 of the Statute satisfactorily cover the provision of the said Protocol relating to unlawful attacks upon civilian targets. The specific provisions of Common Article 3 [of the Geneva Conventions] also satisfactorily cover the prohibition on attacks against civilians as provided for by Protocols I and II." While this suggested the possibility of a finding of guilt for a violation of *customs* of war, the Chamber, having found earlier (paras. 75 et seq.) that the conflict was international, went on to point out (para. 172) that both parties had ratified the Protocols and moreover had signed an agreement in 1992 that they would be bound by Arts. 51 and 52 of Protocol I dealing with attacks on civilians and civilian objects. Protocol I thus applying as written *law* of war, the application of Protocol II was excluded – hence, the express phrase in the Disposition "as regards an armed conflict."

35. In parallel with these developments on the political and diplomatic front, another noticeable development is the remarkable increase in public attention, not just for the events of war but for the punishment of perpetrators and their bosses. As a particularly interesting example, reference may be made here to R. Gutman and D. Rieff (eds.), *Crimes of War: What the Public Should Know* (1999).

duction, Stockpiling and Use of Chemical Weapons;[36] 1994, the Convention on the Safety of UN and Associated Personnel;[37] in 1995, a new Protocol IV on Blinding Laser Weapons[38] and in 1996, an amended Protocol II on Prohibitions or Restrictions on the Use of Mines, Booby-Traps and Other Devices,[39] both to the Conventional Weapons Convention of 1980; 1997, the Ottawa Convention on the Prohibition of the Use, Stockpiling, Production and Transfer of Anti-personnel Mines and on Their Destruction;[40] and finally, by a diplomatic conference which convened at The Hague from 15 to 26 March 1999, a Second Protocol to the Hague Convention of 1954 for the Protection of Cultural Property in the Event of Armed Conflict[41] (opened for signature at The Hague on 17 May, the day before the start of the official Centennial celebrations, and vastly improving the system of protection provided by the Convention).[42]

26. The Secretary-General's report is silent on one feature that yet appears to be of increasing importance in the application and interpretation of IHL. It is the inclination to rely on customary law, or what is held for it, occasionally on grounds of actual practice of belligerent parties but where that is lacking (or may be regarded as unsatisfactory) on the basis of expressions of opinion or intuition as found, e.g., in UN General Assembly or Security Council resolutions. While the ICJ has cautiously ventured onto this path in the

36. 32 ILM (1993) p. 800.

37. 34 ILM (1995) p. 484.

38. 35 ILM (1996) p. 1218; *Documents* p. 535.

39. 35 ILM (1996) p. 1206; *Documents* p. 536.

40. 36 ILM (1997) p. 1507; *Documents* p. 645.

41. *Documents* p. 699.

42. It may be noted here that work is in progress on a solution of yet another problem: that of the protective emblem (with the Israeli Magen David Adom as the greatest stumbling bloc). If all goes according to expectations, the end result might be a third Protocol to the Geneva Conventions of 1949, coupled with the requisite amendments to the Statutes of the International Red Cross and Red Crescent Movement. This might then be a first, welcome result in this new century.

*Nicaragua* case[43] and in its *Nuclear Weapons* Advisory Opinion,[44] ICTY is the real trend setter here.[45] That Tribunal obviously finds itself in the unique, and uniquely difficult, position of having to adjudge complex cases of individual criminal liability on the basis of a set of rules that were not drafted for that purpose, were not earlier tested in the context of criminal procedure, and especially in so far as applicable in internal armed conflicts, leave many substantive

43. *Military and Paramilitary Activities in and against Nicaragua (Nicaragua* v. *United States of America), Merits*, Judgment, ICJ Reports 1986, p. 14, at pp. 103-104: paras. 217-219.

44. *Legality of the Threat or Use of Nuclear Weapons*, Advisory Opinion, ICJ Reports 1996, p. 226, at pp. 35-36: paras. 78-82, setting great store by the Martens Clause in the Preamble to the 1899 Hague Convention on Land Warfare, repeated in a modernized version in Art. 1 (2) of Additional Protocol I, 1977.

45. Thus, in the Judgement of Trial Chamber II (Judge Antonio Cassese, Presiding) in *Prosecutor* v. *Zoran Kupreskic et al.*, 14 January 2000, Case No. IT-95-16-T, the Tribunal raises the question whether the conventional prohibitions of reprisals against the civilian population and civilian objects (Arts. 51 (6) and 52 (1) of Additional Protocol I, 1977), "assuming that they were not declaratory of customary international law, have subsequently been transformed into general rules of international law." In the lengthy and complicated argument by which it arrives at a positive answer, a striking feature is the juxtaposition of its admission that "there does not seem to have emerged recently a body of State practice consistently supporting the proposition that one of the elements of custom, namely *usus* or *diuturnitas* has taken shape" with the statement that "This is however an area where *opinio iuris sive necessitatis* plays a much greater role than *usus*, as a result of the aforementioned Martens Clause." Ibid., p. 205: para. 527. See, in this connection, Greenwood, Report para. 5.26, wondering (with Sir Hersch Lauterpacht) whether "criminal trials are the best forum in which to resolve difficult questions about the content of the law regarding weapons, targets and the conduct of hostilities." And see L. Zegveld, *Armed Opposition Groups in International Law: The Quest for Accountability*, thesis Rotterdam (2000) Part 2, paras. 15-19, noting in the closing sentence of para. 19 that "the primary role international bodies play in articulating *opinio iuris* fits in the current trend that the practice of international bodies is becoming increasingly important at the expense of the actual practice of states."
On the Martens Clause see: A. Cassese, "The Martens Clause: Half a Loaf or Simply Pie in the Sky?", in 12 *European Journal of International Law* (2000) pp. 187-216; on its historical origin (not a masterpiece composed by Martens to save the Conference but a compromise formula written in Brussels and, in slightly modified form, dictated by Auguste Beernaert, Head of the Belgian delegation, to Frédéric de Martens as Head of the Russian delegation, "*qui le présenta comme émanant de lui-même*" – emphasis added) see R. Coolsaet, "La Belgique et la première Conférence de la Paix de La Haye (1899)", essay written for the Centennial (on CD-ROM).

questions wide open. ICTY moreover is performing its functions in an increasingly "humanitarian" climate of public opinion – with the actual events, in contrast, continuing to deviate markedly from "desirable" conduct.

27. In these circumstances, the temptation for judges to "find" customary law on the basis of civilized opinion rather than crass conduct must be strong indeed. Even so, and with all due respect, judges might be suggested to pay somewhat more marked attention to the actual behaviour of non-State parties (and, indeed, of the States themselves),[46] thus reducing the risk of creating over-optimistic expectations, especially when the point at issue is, for instance, whether an IHL treaty provision accepted after long and acrimonious debate for international armed conflict only, may now be transplanted as customary law to situations of internal armed conflict as well.

28. In this whole matter, we are eagerly awaiting the study on "customary rules of IHL applicable in international and non-international armed conflicts" the ICRC has been invited to carry out and which, we are informed, may be expected to appear in print in 2001. Both the amount of time that has passed since the original request was made[47] and the quality of the persons involved in the study give us every reason to look forward to a most valuable, thoroughly researched and well-documented end result.

46. As for reprisals against the civilian population, both Italy (in somewhat oblique terms) and the UK (in crystal-clear language) have reserved the right to resort to such reprisals as an *ultimum remedium* and subject to a number of conditions that bring such planned actions in line with the classical rules on recourse to reprisals. See, by this author, "Reprisal", in Gutman and Rieff, op. cit. note 33, p. 309; *Belligerent Reprisals* (1971).

47. The invitation to undertake the study came from the 26th International Conference of the Red Cross and Red Crescent, Geneva, November 1995, endorsing a suggestion to that effect of an Intergovernmental Group of Experts for the Protection of War Victims which had met in January 1995 on the invitation of the Swiss Government as a follow-up to the International Conference for the Protection of War Victims, Geneva, 30 August – 1 September 1993 (see above, para. 17).

29. Turning next to the matter of arms reduction, it may be noticed that in spite of the two "big bangs" over Japanese cities that, putting a final end to the Second World War, marked the transition to the second half of the 20th century, the UN Charter does not single out the "atom bomb" as a feature of special concern. Indeed, disarmament and the regulation of armaments figure in the Charter in the broadest possible terms, as a matter the General Assembly "may consider"[48] and the Security Council is responsible for formulating plans about.[49] These rather vague terms bring to mind the somewhat more precise formulation in the Covenant of the League of Nations, which set the goal as the "reduction of national armaments to the lowest point consistent with national safety."[50] That goal may have been more precise, but at the end of the road the result was nil.[51]

30. In this respect, the post-World War Two record, although better, is decidedly mixed. As is evident from Dr. BLIX' Report, attention for a long time concentrated almost exclusively on the issue of

48. Art. 11 (1): "The General Assembly may consider the general principles of co-operation in the maintenance of international peace and security, including the principles governing disarmament and the regulation of armaments, and may make recommendations with regard to such principles to the Members or to the Security Council or to both."

49. Art. 26: "In order to promote the establishment and maintenance of international peace and security with the least diversion for armaments of the world's human and economic resources, the Security Council shall be responsible, with the assistance of the Military Staff Committee referred to in Article 47, plans to be submitted to the Members of the United Nations for the establishment of a system for the regulation of armaments."

50. Covenant, Art. 8.

51. The League made two major attempts to give effect to this provision. The first was the 1925 International Conference on the Control of the International Trade in Arms, Munitions and Implements of War (which drafted a never-ratified convention on supervision of the private arms trade, and which as a by-product, produced the Gas Protocol: the 1925 Geneva Protocol for the Prohibition of the Use in War of Asphyxiating, Poisonous or Other Gases, and of Bacteriological Methods of Warfare; *Documents* p. 155). The other was the Disarmament Conference, 1932-34, which strove to bring about a complex set of agreements both on quantitative and qualitative disarmament among the participating States, but succumbed in the end to the political forces that were undermining the League. On this whole episode, see, by this author, "Arms, Armaments and International Law," 191 RdC (1985-II) p. 187, at pp. 307-309.

nuclear weapons, sometimes together with the other so-called "weapons of mass destruction": bacteriological (biological) and chemical weapons. His Report also shows that on these issues a good deal has been achieved. B and C weapons are now categorically banned, by treaties of 1972 and 1993, respectively; and a long list of bilateral and multilateral treaties deal more or less effectively with various aspects of the existence and the ensuing threat of nuclear weapons. That this threat remains a matter of grave international concern is evidenced, for instance, by the fact that half of the 22 resolutions the General Assembly adopted on 1 December 1999 under the heading "general and complete disarmament" deal with nuclear weapons.[52] One, entitled "Towards a nuclear-weapon-free world: The need for a new agenda," expresses the Assembly's concern "at the prospect of the indefinite possession of nuclear weapons, believing that the contention that nuclear weapons can be retained in perpetuity and never used is not supported by the history of human experience", and then sets forth a 22-points plan of action towards further reduction of nuclear weapons.[53] It may be noted in passing that in terms of the Charter provisions, such a "plan of action" might rather have been expected from the Security Council.

31. Always on the matter of nuclear weapons, a positive point is that in April 2000, the Russian Duma ratified the bilateral (US-Russia) START II nuclear arms reduction treaty and endorsed the multilateral Comprehensive Test Ban Treaty (CTBT). In either case, the United States has yet to follow suit. The Russian steps were accompanied with some qualifying statements, though. One was the announcement of a new policy on use of nuclear weapons, reserving the option of first use even in the face of an attack with conventional weapons.[54] The other point concerned the American desire to develop weapon systems against long-range missile attacks from

52. A/RES/54/54 A-F, K, L, P, Q.

53. A/RES/54/54G.

54. This may be a sign of a loss of confidence in the deterrent effects of the Russian conventional armed forces. An interesting question is how the Russian authorities would explain this shift in their position in the light of the ICJ Advisory Opinion on nuclear weapons (see above, note 44).

"rogue" countries or terrorist groups: if the US were to go ahead with this plan (which Russia felt would be in contravention of the 1972 Treaty on the Limitation of Anti-Ballistic Missile Systems, or ABM Treaty) it would feel free to reconsider its position in relation to START II.

32. When it comes to so-called "conventional weapons" (the weapons that are actually used in armed conflicts) the record of the post-World War Two period is hardly any better than that of the League period. The single treaty qualifying as a disarmament instrument in this category of weapon is the 1997 Ottawa Convention banning anti-personnel mines.[55] Reference may also be made of the 1980 Conventional Weapons Convention,[56] which, although setting limits to use rather than possession of certain weapons and thus mentioned under the heading of IHL treaties, in its Preamble pays ample lip service to the issue of disarmament.[57] Then, on the level of concrete measures, mention must of course be made of the arms embargoes the Security Council has occasionally (rather than systematically) imposed in respect of countries or regions in conflict.[58]

33. As for public debate at the General Assembly, the discussions in its regular and special sessions on conventional weapons for a long

55. See above, para. 25 and note 40.

56. See above, para. 15 and note 22.

57. The 6th, 7th and 9th paragraphs of the Preamble read as follows:
*Desiring* to contribute to international détente, the ending of the arms race and the building of confidence among States, and hence to the realization of the aspiration of all peoples to live in peace,
*Recognizing* the importance of pursuing every effort which may contribute to progress towards general and complete disarmament under strict and effective international control, (...)
*Wishing* to prohibit or restrict further the use of certain conventional weapons and believing that the positive results achieved in this area may facilitate the main talks on disarmament with a view to putting an end to the production, stockpiling and proliferation of such weapons, (...).

58. On the day of writing this part of the Introduction, the 17th of May 2000, the Security Council unanimously imposed an arms embargo on Ethiopia and Eritrea.

time were no more than repetitive statements for the record (and the home front), showing a clear lack of political will seriously to tackle the matter.[59]

34. The dramatic events of the last decade may now finally have made international society acutely aware that the issue of small arms, and of conventional weapons generally, is indeed an urgent matter. A number of recent statements and declarations demonstrating this awareness deserve to be mentioned here, and first of all, the Report on the Conclusions of the Centennial Conference[60] and the Plan of Action adopted by the 27th International Conference of the Red Cross and Red Crescent.[61]

59. See the Report by Dr. Blix, paras. 71 et seq. See also, by the present author, op. cit. note 49, pp. 319, 322.

60. Para. 57, recognizing that "small arms ... had been responsible for most casualties in recent conflicts" and recommending that "an international code of conduct might be developed, including, *inter alia*, criteria for export of small arms, in addition to existing regional arrangements."

61. Final goal 1.5 requires, inter alia, "the establishment of effective controls on the availability of arms and ammunition". This goal is elaborated as follows:

> States enhance the protection of civilians in armed conflict and post-conflict situations by seeking to strengthen controls on the availability of arms, in particular small arms and ammunition, at the national, regional and international levels, including by improving export regulations. States examine the establishment of means to integrate the consideration of respect for international humanitarian law into national decision-making on transfers of arms and ammunition, and, where relevant, examine ways of integrating such considerations into "codes of conduct".
>
> The Movement [of the Red Cross and Red Crescent] will promote public awareness of the human costs of unregulated arms transfers and widespread arms availability and continue to promote the ratification, and faithful implementation, of the relevant norms of international humanitarian law governing weapons.

35. The UN Secretary-General, taking up the issue in his report to the Security Council on the protection of civilians in armed conflicts,[62] "recommend[s] that the Security Council:"

> 26. Impose arms embargoes in situations where civilians and protected persons are targeted by the parties to the conflict, or where the parties are known to commit systematic and widespread violations of international humanitarian and human rights law, including the recruitment of child soldiers; and urge Member States to enforce these embargoes in their own national jurisdictions.

Introducing his report to the Council, he emphasizes that: "To ensure that these crises are brought to an end, *the United Nations must be ready to respond with more than meetings, speeches and reports. It must take action* in the name of the principles of the Charter and the values of humanity."[63] The response of the Security Council, although more cautious, at all events acknowledges the existence of

62. S/1999/957, 8 September 1999, para. 23:
> The widespread use of small arms, light weapons and anti-personnel landmines has had a significant impact on the scope and level of the violence that affects civilian populations in armed conflict. The absence of effective controls on the transfer of small arms along with their low cost make them popular weapons in today's conflicts. These light and easy-to-use weapons have made it much easier to turn children into soldiers. Their easy availability to untrained combatants has also greatly increased the risks of delivering humanitarian assistance in affected areas.

Para. 55:
> The proliferation and abuse of light weapons and small arms fuel conflicts, exacerbate the suffering of civilian victims and contribute to the breakdown of societies. A number of international and regional initiatives are seeking to address this difficult problem. I fully endorse these initiatives. Controlling the availability of arms is an essential prerequisite for a successful peace-building process. It requires a multi-dimensional approach involving demobilization, rehabilitation of combatants, law enforcement, measures to stop illegal trafficking and regulations for the legal registration and use of arms.

63. Press Release SG/SM/7134 SC/6729, 16 September 1999; emphasis added.

an "excessive accumulation and destabilizing effect of small arms and light weapons."[64]

36. One week later, on 24 September 1999, the Council had the same matter on its agenda again. The Presidential Statement issued after the debate inter alia makes the following points: recognition of the "destabilizing accumulation" of small arms; emphasis that "the challenge posed by small arms is multifaceted and involves security, humanitarian and development dimensions," and emphasis on "the importance of regional cooperation in tackling the issue of illicit trafficking in small arms." The Council also welcomes the idea of "an international conference on the illicit arms trade in all its aspects no later than 2001," encouraging Member States "to participate actively and constructively" in the preparations for this conference, "with a view to ensuring that the conference makes a meaningful and lasting contribution to reducing the incidence of illicit arms trafficking."[65] Members participating in the discussion may have cast their minds back to the conference held in 1925 under auspices of the League of Nations, which ended with a still-born convention on the arms trade.[66] That should not happen a second time.

37. Broaching the matter in the General Assembly on the occasion of the closure of the UN Decade of International Law, Mr. Hans VAN MIERLO, Minister of State and representative of the Netherlands Government, but speaking first and foremost as Chairman of the Dutch National Committee for the celebrations of the Centennial in The Hague in May 1999, had the following to say:

64. S/RES/1265 (1999), 17 September 1999, para. 17:
*Notes* that the excessive accumulation and destabilizing effect of small arms and light weapons pose a considerable impediment to the provision of humanitarian assistance and have a potential to exacerbate and prolong conflicts, endanger the lives of civilians and undermine security and the confidence required for a return to peace and stability.

65. S/PRST/1999/28.

66. See above, note 51.

> In the St. Petersburg sessions of the centennial celebrations, I took up the issue of small arms as one of the remaining gaps in international law today. The Norwegian Minister for Foreign Affairs had done likewise even earlier, about a year ago, in his famous Fridtjof Nansen memorial lecture. Last February, at a preparatory meeting of the centennial celebrations in New Delhi, some speakers even identified small arms proliferation as a greater threat to humanity than nuclear weapons. An estimated 500 million to 1 billion small arms are in circulation world-wide. They cause untold suffering, destabilize societies and prolong conflicts, and when conflicts end, they stand in the way of reconstruction and sustainable development. In 46 out of the 49 conflicts that have taken place during the Decade of International Law, small arms were the only weapons used. (...) Regulation of the small arms issue should be dealt with as a matter of priority.[67]

38. The resolution adopted after the debate on the results of the Centennial (and on the report of the Sixth Committee)[68] does not specifically mention the small-arms issue. Yet the item may be regarded as incorporated, together with all other specific items, in the "invitation" extended to "States, organs of the United Nations, international organizations and other relevant international forums to take note of the outcome of the centennial of the first International Peace Conference and to consider, where appropriate:

> (a) Giving attention to the outcome of the thematic discussions within the sphere of their respective competencies or mandates;" (etc.).

39. Back again at the Security Council, the matter crops up once again on 30 November 1999 in a one-day debate on the role of the Council in the prevention of armed conflicts. The Presidential Statement issued after the debate notes in a paragraph devoted to "preventive measures such as the establishment of demilitarized zones and preventive disarmament" that "progress in preventing and combatting the excessive and destabilizing accumulation of and illicit

67. A/54/PV.54, 17 November 1999.

68. A/RES/54/27, 17 November 1999.

trafficking in small arms and light weapons is of vital importance to the prevention of armed conflict."[69]

40. The issue was under discussion at the same time in the General Assembly as well, this time on the report of the First Committee and under the item "general and complete disarmament." As mentioned before, half of the resolutions adopted at the end of the debate, on 1 December 1999, dealt with the nuclear issue and the other half therefore with general matters, including conventional weapons and small arms in particular. Two of these (A/RES/54/54 I and O) have an identical title ("transparency in armaments"), use largely identical language and decide in identical terms "to include in the provisional agenda of its fifty-fifth session the item entitled 'Transparency in armaments'." This seems wasteful and may not be the best manner to promote the cause of transparency in armaments.

41. Three resolutions deal with the problems posed by the accumulation of small arms: "Small arms" (V), "Illicit traffic in small arms" (R) and "Assistance to States for curbing the illicit traffic in small arms and collecting them" (J), illustrating the complexity of the issue. Worth noting is the decision "to convene the United Nations Conference on the Illicit Trade in Small Arms and Lights Weapons in All Its Aspects in June/July 2001."[70]

69. S/PRST/1999/34, 30 November 1999.

70. A/RES/54/54/V, operative para. 1; the Conference will be hosted by the Swiss Government at Geneva. – In an address to the "Millennium Forum" (an NGO meeting preceding the September 2000 events, see next note), New York, 22 May 2000, the Secretary-General expressed the hope that "civil society organizations will be invited to participate fully" in the planned Conference.
From among the remaining resolutions under this item I single out A/RES/54/54/U on "Convening of the fourth special session of the General Assembly devoted to disarmament." Recalling the special sessions on that topic of 1978, 1982 and 1988 and reiterating "its conviction that a special session of the General Assembly devoted to disarmament can set the future course of action in the field of disarmament, arms control and related international security matters," but noting with regret the lack of a consensus on the purposes of a 4th special session, it effectively postpones the convening of that session under the wondrously deceptive formula: 'Decides, subject to the emergence of a consensus on its objectives and agenda, to convene the fourth
(continued...)

42. The issue of small arms and other conventional weapons came up again recently in a report of the Secretary-General to the Security Council on the role of UN peacekeeping in disarmament, demobilization and reintegration. Shifting the issue from the theoretical to a concrete and starkly realistic level, the report defines disarmament as:

> the collection of small arms and light and heavy weapons within a conflict zone. It frequently entails the assembly and cantonment of combatants; it should also comprise the development of arms management programmes, including their safe storage and their final disposition, which may entail their destruction. Demining may also be part of this process.[71]

Through this brief paragraph, one glimpses the case histories of disarmament and peace making efforts in theatres such as Northern Ireland, Angola, Cambodia, Bosnia and Kosovo – to mention just a few.

43. As a last item under the heading of disarmament and arms control in general and the small arms issue in particular, I mention the report produced by the Secretary-General for the forthcoming Millennium Summit[72] and presented to the General Assembly on 3 April 2000 under the title "WE the PEOPLES " – The Role of the United Nations in the 21st Century.[73] In this extremely rich report, the last two sections of the Chapter on the "Freedom from Fear" deal with "small arms" and "nuclear weapons", respectively. Rather than quoting at length from the text of these sections, which eloquently elaborate the points made in his earlier writings, I may just cite here the proposals by which the Secretary-General concludes his observations (with bold as in the original). On the matter of small arms:

70. (...continued)
special session'."

71. S/2000/101, 11 February 2000, para. 6 (a).

72. To be held at New York from 6 to 8 September 2000; A/RES/54/254, 23 March 2000.

73. A/54/2000.

**I urge Member States to take advantage of this conference to start taking serious actions that will curtail the illicit traffic in small arms.**
The many recent expressions of concern about small arms proliferation are a welcome sign that the importance of the issue is being recognized, but words alone do nothing to prevent the ongoing slaughter of innocent people. Dialogue is critical, but we must match the rhetoric of concern with the substance of practical action.

On nuclear weapons:

**To help focus attention on the risks we confront and on the opportunities we have to reduce them, I propose that consideration be given to convening a major international conference that would help to identify ways of eliminating nuclear dangers.**

One can only add the wish that these proposals may lead to the result they deserve: that is, effective, practical action on the part of Member States and, indeed, of international society as a whole, including its "civil society" component.

44. The Security Council debates on "the prevention of armed conflict" and "the role of UN peacekeeping in disarmament, demobilization and reintegration" and the Secretary-General's report relating thereto, obviously were not limited to "disarmament and arms control" alone. Indeed, the discussions fitted at least equally well under the heading of "peaceful settlement of disputes": not perhaps as that phrase was understood by the participants at the 1899 Hague Peace Conference but certainly in the broad sense it has meanwhile assumed.

45. The broad connotation the phrase has acquired is well illustrated by the various chapters in the Report of Messrs. ORREGO VICUÑA and PINTO, and consequently, in chapter II.3 of the Report on the Conclusions drafted on the basis of the discussions at the Hague and

St. Petersburg sessions of the Centennial Conference.[74] Then, in Geneva, the Solemn Appeal launched on the 12th of August 1999 on the occasion of the 50th anniversary of the Geneva Conventions, implicitly emphasizes the need of peaceful settlement of disputes, when it "calls on the world to reject the idea that war is inevitable and to work tirelessly to eradicate its underlying causes."[75]

46. Peaceful settlement of disputes in the sense of conflict prevention was the topic of the aforementioned Security Council debate of 29 and 30 November 1999 on "the prevention of armed conflict."[76] With the Secretary-General urging the Council "to examine how it could make prevention a tangible part of its day-to-day work," speakers for 38 countries, among them the five permanent members, "expressed a diverse array of views ranging from the need to address the roots of conflict, such as poverty, to the relationship between the principles of maintaining international peace and security and that of States' sovereignty." The inconclusive character of the debate is apparent when one compares the heading of the press release for the first day ("Security Council Told Key is Effective Deterrent Action") with that for the second day: "Some Speakers Urge More Decisive Action, Others Caution on Need to Respect National Sovereignty". The debate, in other words, had not brought any radical changes to the stance of the Council, nor of the UN Members. Positive points are, of course, that many speakers at least expressed dissatisfaction with the poor record of the Council in matters of conflict

74. The reader is referred to that chapter (where he may notice that not all of the forward-looking suggestions of the Rapporteurs were equally enthusiastically received).

75. See above, paras. 20-21; see also the chapter on "Root causes of war / culture of peace" in the Hague Agenda for Peace, in this volume.

76. Press Releases, SC/6759, 29 November 1999; SC/6761, 30 November 1999. The quotations are from these documents.

prevention,[77] and that they recognized the need to continue to work for an improvement of this situation.

47. Neither the forthcoming three-day "Millennium Summit" nor the ensuing Millennium Assembly will be able to solve all the outstanding problems of this world. Yet they may be hoped, nay, demanded, to set in motion processes that help overcome the tremendous difficulties that prevent large segments of the world population to enjoy "freedom from want" and "freedom from fear".

48. Even the world leaders in 1899 were already expected to bring about such miracles. They did not, but perhaps unwittingly have started processes that have brought us to where we are now, with a United Nations that even in its present shape is capable of much more than its Members permit it to achieve. Pending proposals for restructuring could only improve those capacities. The tools are there: they should be used.

49. The Millennium Report of the Secretary-General may be hoped to contribute to activating our present world leaders to set their shoulders under the immense task ahead. I may quote the Report again (adding bold for emphasis):

> **Let the Millennium Summit signal the renewed commitment of Member States to their United Nations, by agreeing on our common vision. Let the world's leaders prove their commitment by acting on it as soon as they return home.**

50. The "immense task ahead" falls apart into innumerable detailed ones, each probably equally daunting. One of these I wish to mention in particular, that has to do as much with the peaceful settlement of disputes as with the implementation of international humanitarian

77. Speaking for Japan towards the end of the first day, Mr Yukio Satoh said, as rendered in the press release: "Timely action was key to the Council's role in conflict prevention, but in that area the record of the Council's recent actions was not one of total success." This statement surely deserves the "Understatement of the Year Award".

and human rights law. It is, in briefest terms, the issue of "peace vs. justice". While particularly agonizing in (the aftermath of) internal armed conflicts, it may play an equally important role in relation to international armed conflicts; and, in both cases, even long after the hostilities have been terminated.

51. Armed conflicts of either variety more often than not have international repercussions: they are a "matter of international concern", even to the point of involving some sort of activity on the part of the Security Council. One particular manifestation of such Security Council activity has been the establishment, in the last decade of the 20th century, of ICTY and ICTR, as measures taken under Chapter VII of the Charter and hence designed to help restore the peace in the areas involved, i.e., the former Yugoslavia and Rwanda. The "peace" meant here obviously is not just the absence of "war": it must be understood to imply the peace of mind that comes with justice done, and seen to be done. The same idea must underlie the creation of the ICC which, once established, will have its seat at The Hague, as the "legal/judical capital of the world".

52. As with the ICJ, which is not given all the legal/political inter-State disputes to settle, the ICC will get to adjudge a mere fraction of the crimes of war, crimes against humanity, and acts of genocide (as well as, when the time comes, acts of aggression). And for the present, it is even more evident that the two "ICTs" were random reactions, leaving most scenes of equally ugly contravention of the basic precepts of humanity without an international criminal forum. We have to live with that, as we have been doing for a long time now.

53. There is however the capacity – not so much of "the world's leaders" but of the national judicial systems – to deal with this peace-disturbing and conflict-aggravating criminality. In theory, it is a capacity of each and every State: first, and as a matter of course, for such acts as are done within its borders or elsewhere by its agents; and second, on the basis of the universality principle, for crimes committed no matter where, in respect of those delicts that are

recognized to fall under the scope of that principle. This includes serious violations of IHL committed in international armed conflicts as well as, according to a current trend of opinion, the most serious of those crimes committed in the course of an internal armed conflict.

54. This is the theory. In practice, by far the greater part of all such armed conflict-related criminality, of which we have witnessed such a depressingly awful amount over the past years, is never brought to trial. In Latin America, in the context of the internal conflicts that long ravaged that continent, this has turned "impunidad" into a household word. On other continents and in other situations of armed conflict, the practice of impunity is equally widespread.

55. Impunity during the conflict, whether as a consequence of sheer impossibility to cope or as a conscious policy, is one thing. Another thing is the continuation of impunity once the hostilities are terminated and "peace building" becomes the task in hand. Here, a difficulty arises: on the one hand, justice should finally be done; on the other, yesterday's adversaries may have to be today's and tomorrow's colleagues. In the internal order, this may lead to a desire for an amnesty: internationally, the same feeling may be shared. At the same time, voices clamouring for the prosecution of particular crimes may continue to be heard.

56. Both national States and the international community have wrestled with this dilemma more than once, and a variety of solutions have been applied, from the international "no amnesty" solution of ICTY and ICTR (best liked by international criminal lawyers) to the total amnesty laws in countries like Chile and Peru (much preferred, nay, demanded by the military in those countries). Somewhere in between, and with a term aptly describing the dilemma, we find the various "truth and reconciliation" commissions, as applied for instance in El Salvador and South Africa. While the South African case may be the most successful one and, at all events, appears to be least open to criticism, the point to note is that virtually every specific solution involves its own imperfections.

57. Thus, on 27 May 1999, ICTY announced the indictment of Slobodan MILOŠEVIĆ, President of the Federal Republic of Yugoslavia, together with four others, for their role in the conflict in Kosovo (an internal conflict).[78] Earlier on in the 1990s, when such a step was frequently speculated about in relation to the events in Bosnia, i.e., in relation to what more closely resembled a situation of international armed conflict, the question was occasionally raised whether his indictment might not impede the conclusion of a peace accord, an act for which he was deemed to be indispensable. And today, the media wonder: will he ever actually appear before the Tribunal – and if not, will this not damage its credibility? No matter how one might wish to answer these questions, the fact of the matter is that they were posed at all and thus bring out two particular features of the Yugoslav situation: one, the possible political drawbacks attending the attempted prosecution of a powerful actor in an ongoing armed conflict; two, the practical difficulty of laying one's hands on that selfsame actor as long as he is staying in unoccupied territory. It may be emphasized, though, that the indictment of Milošević, a functioning Head of State, demonstrates that this can be done without the step leading to violent repercussions, for instance, in the Security Council.[79]

58. At about the same time, another high official who had been the Head of State in his country, General PINOCHET, was even closer to being put on trial following his arrest in London on 24 March 1999. As with MILOŠEVIĆ, the individual criminal liability of PINOCHET for the past events in Chile may not be overly difficult to establish. For the rest, the cases are as different as can be. The only point of interest to me here is that the acts and omissions attributable to PINOCHET appeared to be covered in his own country by an amnesty, in effect,

78. *The Prosecutor* v. *Milosevic et al.*, Indictment of 22 May 1999, Decision on review and application of consequential orders by Judge David Hunt, 24 May 1999; IT-99-37.

79. It may be recalled that the 1919 Commission on the Responsibility of the Authors of the War and on Enforcement of Penalties, almost as a matter of course had included the Heads of States among the authorities over whom the proposed Tribunal would have jurisdiction. See note 20.

one he himself had proclaimed while still in power. Could that really be true: can a country so simply throw overboard elementary considerations of justice, in favour of – what: Peace?

59. Not only "impunidad" is a Latin American household work: so is "amnistía", as an almost self-evident measure to smooth over the after-effects of a situation of violent conflict. No matter how self-evident, the question of the acceptability remains, not least in the light of the appalling viciousness of some of the acts allegedly committed in various Latin American countries in the last half-century. This question has come up time and time again in cases brought before the two organs established by the American Convention on Human Rights, the Inter-American Commission on Human Rights (IACHR) and the Inter-American Court of Human Rights (IACtHR).

60. Quite a few of these cases have to do with El Salvador. After a 12-year internal armed conflict (1980-1991, the last three years running parallel with peace negotiations) the two parties, the Government and the FMLN ("Frente Farabundo Martí para la Liberación Nacional") on 16 January 1992 concluded a peace accord at Chapultepec, Mexico. As one important element in the peace accord, the parties recognized:

> the need to clarify and avoid any special treatment for officers of the Armed Forces, especially in cases relating to respect for human rights. To this end, the Parties will leave consideration and resolution of this point to the Truth Commission.[80]

The mandate of the Truth Commission was to investigate "the serious acts of violence that have occurred since 1980, whose *impact on society urgently requires that the truth about them be made*

80. Section 5, "preventing impunity", of the peace accord; quoted here from an English version of the "Report on the Massacre of the Jesuits in El Salvador", IACHR, No. 136/99, Case 10.488, *Ignacio Ellacuría, S.J., y otros.*, 22 December 1999, para. 59 and note 22.

*known to the public.*"[81] Composed of three non-Salvadorans appointed by the UN Secretary-General in agreement with the parties,[82] the Commission set to work and eventually, on 15 March 1993 released its Report titled "From Madness to Hope, the Twelve-Year War in El Salvador." The Report sets forth in great detail a series of events, specifying the victims, the actual perpetrators and those intellectually responsible for the crimes. The question was: would it stop the madness; would justice be done – and how would this relate to peace?

61. To illustrate this point, no case seems better suited than that of Monsignor ROMERO, Archbishop of San Salvador, assassinated on 24 March 1980, at the very outset of the conflict, while he was celebrating mass in the chapel of the "Hospital de la Divina Providencia". In the final phase of the procedure before the IACHR, decided by its Report of 13 April 2000, the only real point of controversy was that of amnesty.[83]

81. Ibid., para. 59 and note 23; emphasis added.

82. Ibid., para. 60. The members of the Commission were: Belisario Betancur, former President of Colombia; Reinaldo Figueredo Planchart, former Minister of Foreign Affairs of Venezuela, and Thomas Buergenthal, former President of the Inter-American Court of Human Rights (and, we are pleased to note, since January 2000, Judge in the ICJ).

83. IACHR, Informe N° 37/00, Caso 11.481, *Monseñor Oscar Arnulfo Romero y Galdámez*, El Salvador, 13 April 2000 (an English version is not yet available). The Report notes the grave impact "moral, espiritual y psicológico" the assassination had exerted on the Salvadoran society; para. 35. In a text quoted in para. 38, Dr. Pedro Nikken, Past President of the IACtHR and one-time Special Rapporteur of the UN Commission on Human Rights for El Salvador, qualifies the assassination of Monsignor Romero, together with the massacre of the Jesuit priests (above, note 81), as the two cases that had particularly shocked the world.
I confine myself in this Introduction to this one case, as a classic example of a serious treatment by all parties of the difficult question of amnesty as a means to overcome the after-effects of internal armed conflict. I see no reason, in particular, to go into an amnesty accord as scandalous and surrealistic as the one included in the Lomé Peace Agreement of 7 July 1999; on this, see: A. J. M. McDonald, "Sierra Leone's Uneasy Peace: The Amnesties Granted in the Lomé Peace Agreement and the United Nations' Dilemma," in *Humanitäres Völkerrecht* (2000) pp. 11 et seq.

62. The facts of the case, a cold-blooded murder carried out by one Héctor Antonio REGALADO on the orders of Major Roberto D'AUBUISSON and Captain Alvaro SARAVIA, have been public knowledge at least from the time they were unravelled by the Truth Commission. It is also evident that up to the date of publication of its Report, 15 March 1993, no serious efforts had been made by the authorities to bring the authors to trial. Then, five days after the release of the Report, the Legislative Assembly of El Salvador approved a General Amnesty Law that granted "full, absolute and unconditional amnesty to all those who participated in any way in the commission, prior to 1 January, 1992, of political crimes or common crimes linked to political crimes or common crimes in which the number of persons involved is no less than twenty."[84] In application of the Amnesty Law, the ROMERO case was completely dropped.[85]

63. The Report of the IACHR, having set forth the positions of the claimants[86] and the Government[87] and after an exhaustive analysis of the events in the light of the applicable provisions of the American Convention,[88] once again (not, for sure, for the first time) explains its

84. Ibid., para. 133; Decree 486, Art. 1.

85. Ibid., para. 18. On 31 March 1993, the case against Alvaro Saravia was formally dropped. The magistrate saw no need to take a similar decision with regard to Roberto D'Aubuisson: that person had never been officially accused, and moreover, he was now dead. The case against Regalado had been effectively shelved already at an earlier stage; para. 15.

86. Ibid., para. 19; their position, relying on Arts. 4, 8, 25, 1 (1) and 2 of the Convention was that application of the Amnesty Law had rendered the Government responsible for a violation of the American Convention on Human Rights.

87. Ibid., para. 20; the Government did not contest the allegations of fact and law of the claimants (except, obviously, for their conclusion on responsibility); instead, it asked the Commission to shelve the case, on the argument that the Amnesty Law adopted after the publication of the Report of the Truth Commission had served to ensure peace and preserve human rights.

88. Ibid., paras. 30-55. I note two points: (1) the assassination of Monsignor Romero had not only violated the right to life, recognized in Art. 4 of the Convention, but also "constituye una grave transgresión de principios básicos del derecho internacional humanitario" and in particular of Art. 3 common to the 1949 Geneva Conventions and Art. 13 of Protocol II of 1977 (paras. 66-67); (2) irrespective of direct participation by
(continued...)

doctrine on the (in-)compatibility of the Amnesty Law with that Convention. Its central point is that application of amnesty laws that impede access to justice in cases of serious violations of human rights, renders ineffective the obligation of States Parties to the Convention to respect the rights and freedoms recognized therein, and to guarantee to every person subject to its jurisdiction the free and full exercise of his rights without discrimination.[89]

64. Applying its doctrine to the case in hand, the IACHR finds, first, that the application given to the General Amnesty Law of 1993 is incompatible with the international obligations of El Salvador in that it renders ineffective the right to judicial guarantees and judicial protection established in the Convention, as well as with its general obligation to respect and ensure respect for the rights established in that instrument.[90]

65. To this, it adds another argument: by application of the Amnesty Law, the State has violated the "right to the truth"; a right not just for the victim's relatives, but for the community as a whole.[91] This is not limited to a right to know the facts but is part of the right to reparation for human rights violations, both by way of satisfaction

88. (...continued)
State agents, the latter "es en todo caso internacionalmente responsible por actos violatorios de los derechos humanos perpetrados por individuos o grupos de individuos organizados, tales como los escuadrones de la muerte, que actuán con el beneplácito, acquiescencia, tolerancia o incluso colaboración de sus fuerzas de siguridad." On the latter point, see also Zegveld, op. cit. note 45, pp. 61 et seq.

89. Ibid., paras. 126-130. The IACHR finds support for its "doctrine and practice" both in the conclusions on impunity arrived at by Louis Joinet in a report produced as Special Rapporteur of the UN Commission on Human Rights (E/CN/4/Sub.2/1997/20/Rev.1, 2 October 1997), and in a Judgement of the IACtHR holding that a State cannot invoke dispositions of its internal legal order in order to divest itself of its international obligations (Caso Loayza Tamayo, Reparaciones, 27 November 1998; text quoted by the Commission: para. 168).

90. Ibid., para. 131; the State hence is deemed to have violated Articles 2, 8 and 25 of the Convention, in conjunction with Article 1, paragraph 1.

91. Ibid., paras. 142 et seq.

and as a guarantee that the same will not happen again.[92] Seen under this light, the "right to the truth" cannot be regarded as having already been fulfilled by the work, no matter how important, of the Truth Commission: its functions were no substitute for the judicial process as a method to arrive at the truth.[93]

66. The conclusion of the IACHR follows logically: by applying the Amnesty Law to the case of Monsignor ROMERO, the State has violated the right to justice as well as its procedural obligations under the Convention. It accordingly recommends that the State stages a complete, impartial and effective judicial procedure to identify, adjudge and punish all the material and intellectual actors of the violations established in the Report; sets right all the consequences of these violations, and adjust its internal legislation to the American Convention, so that the Amnesty Law is put out of effect.[94]

67. On the latter point, the Government replies that the IACHR does not appear to understand fully the grounds that underlay the Amnesty Law, which was to carry on with the peace process and attain national reconciliation, in a society badly traumatized by the violence of the conflict. Viewed thus, the Amnesty Law was not merely based in law but had been a necessary response on the part of the national conglomerate.[95]

92. Ibid., para. 148. The IACHR writes: "El derecho de una sociedad a conocer íntegramente su pasado no sólo se erige como un modo de reparación y esclarecimiento de los hechos ocurridos, sino que tiene el objeto de prevenir futuras violaciones."

93. Ibid., para. 149: "La CIDH considera que, pesa a la importancia que tuvo la Comisión de la Verdad para establecer los hechos relacionados con las violaciones más graves *y para promover la reconciliación nacional*, las funciones desempeñadas por ella no sustituyen el proceso judicial como método para llegar a la verdad. *El valor de las Comisiones de la Verdad es que su creación no está basada en la premisa de que no habrá juicios, sino en que constituyen un paso en el sentido de la restauración de la verdad y, oportunamente, de la justicia.*" (Emphasis added)

94. Ibid., paras. 157-159.

95. Ibid., para. 161. The last sentence reads: "... la Ley de Amnistía de 1993, no sólo está basada en Derecho, sino que se dio como respuesta necesitada por parte del
(continued...)

68. Again, therefore the question: what is to prevail: peace, or justice? The IACHR restates its case one last time: peace is of the utmost importance in a country like El Salvador that has suffered the effects of armed violence. Yet, the peace of society as a whole cannot stand in the way of justice, which includes the investigation and punishment of individual human rights violations.[96]

69. Peace, thus, concerns the situation in a country as a whole: justice is a matter of the individual cases which need to be set right – in the interests of society as well. Neither one should prevail, both should be honoured fully. That peace without justice can leave wounds which refuse to heal, may be demonstrated by means of a totally different episode, dating back to the Second World War. During the Japanese occupation of the Philippines, local women and girls were often used by the occupying forces as "comfort women". Many of them have needed years, if not decades, to learn to cope with this traumatic experience. Cases are now pending before the Japanese courts that aim to get "satisfaction" for still surviving victims of these reprehensible acts. For the women, money is not the primary goal of their complaints: it is the moral satisfaction of finally seeing a judicial procedure handling their misery.

70. Nor is "victory" the goal of the Japanese lawyers who are pleading the women's cases: their focus is on keeping the population conscious of what has been done half a century ago, that it was not

95. (...continued)
conglomerado nacional."

96. Ibid., para. 162, referring back to para. 155, where the IACHR emphasizes that "Las consideraciones de carácter general sobre la situación en un Estado no pueden de manera alguna ser utilizadas para impedir *una decisión de la Comisión* a un caso individual." (emphasis added). – It may be noted that in this whole discussion no role was played by Art. 6 (5) of Protocol II: the famous provision prescribing that at the end of hostilities, "the authorities in power shall endeavour to grant the broadest possible amnesty to persons who have participated in the armed conflict…" (etc.); this while the IACHR had explicitly qualified the assassination as a violation of Art. 3 common to the Geneva Conventions and Art. 13 of Protocol II (see note 86). It may therefore be clear that the Romero case was not just a matter of any odd human rights violation, in respect of which the statement of the IACHR might be regarded as a bit too bland.

right, and that society should openly and officially recognize this blemish on its historical record.[97] They may not win the cases: they simply have wanted to make their point, in a society that is at peace but may find it difficult to reconcile this situation with the needs of justice that arise out of its past.

71. Even these few examples of the difficulties inherent in the struggle of "peace vs. justice", or impunity and amnesty, suffice to show that it is an issue of daunting proportions, apt to haunt society long after a conflict, international or internal, is ostensibly over. And it is just one issue out of the many that may be gleaned from the reports of the three Rapporteurs and the other documents in this volume, and that are implied as well in the Millennium appeal of the Secretary-General.[98] The participants at the Hague Peace Conference of 1899 can at best have been dimly aware of the immense difficulties that lay ahead. A century later, those who celebrated the Peace Conference's Centennial and who now are preparing for the Millennium Summit, both authorities and civil society, cannot fail to realize the magnitude of the challenges they are facing. May they assume their responsibilities, with wisdom and courage.

97. See: H. Fujita, I. Suzuki and K. Nagano (eds.), *War and the Rights of Individuals* (1999).

98. See above, para. 51.

# INTERNATIONAL LAW RELATING TO DISARMAMENT AND ARMS CONTROL
## with special focus on verification and compliance

Revised report prepared for the Centennial of the First International Peace Conference
by Hans BLIX*

## PREFACE

1. The subject of this report, the development of international law relating to disarmament and arms control since the First International Peace Conference of 1899, is vast. Indeed, one hundred years after the Conference one may marvel that legal rules on arms control and disarmament, non-existent at the time except for some prohibitions of use of specific weapons and restrictions on the use of all weapons, have expanded to such an extent that they now constitute a separate *body of law* next to other new bodies of international law, like the law of the environment or space law.

2. A survey of this vast body of international law of disarmament and arms control and its development might perhaps be best pursued through the collective effort of a group of experts at an institute for peace research or international law. The size appropriate for this report does not permit such a comprehensive and systematic treatment of the subject. Rather, the rapporteur has felt that he could best contribute to the subject and stimulate discussion and further practical action by highlighting material, discussing problems and advancing ideas in some of the areas which are central and in which he has had a good deal of first-hand experience as a representative of his country or as an international official.

*. Director-General Emeritus of the International Atomic Energy Agency



*F. Kalshoven (ed.),*
***The Centennial of the First International Peace Conference,*** 41–159.

3. For a number of years from 1962 he provided legal advice to the Swedish delegation to the successive multilateral disarmament bodies negotiating in Geneva, and he headed the Swedish teams to the various conferences on international humanitarian law which took place in the 1970's, including those which dealt with the prohibition or restriction of use of specific weapons. Most recently, as Director-General of the International Atomic Energy Agency 1981-1997, he had rich experience of the problem of non-proliferation of nuclear weapons, including the problems of verification and compliance which were raised by the cases of Iraq and North Korea.

4. The rapporteur is aware that the approach taken is somewhat selective even though he has tried not to neglect important agreements and developments. Within the approach taken the focus has been further narrowed by the consistent highlighting of two questions which were not much on the minds at the time of the 1899 Hague Peace Conference but which are now central and likely to remain relevant for the foreseeable future, namely *verification* and *compliance*.

5. Other limitations in the scope of the report flow from the subject which the rapporteur has been asked to deal with, namely, international law. That means existing law - *lex lata*. Although the report sometimes points to problems in various existing rules and practices and concludes with some personal suggestions regarding possible pathways forward, it is restrained in advancing ideas for new rules - *lex ferenda* - and in examining proposals which have not been adopted.

6. The rapporteur is not aware of any rules of *customary law* in the field of disarmament proper. However, it is generally recognized that some proscriptions of use of weapons - notably in the Hague Conventions - have hardened into customary law. By contrast, although reference is often made to the *nuclear non-proliferation regime* and a *norm of non-proliferation*, the International Court of Justice (ICJ) did not accept the contention that this regime has developed into a

customary international law prohibition of the threat or use of nuclear weapons.

7. One must be aware that, while a good many measures and actions are taken by States in the area of arms control and disarmament without constituting a performance of legally binding treaty obligations, *unilateral* but *parallel* measures may sometimes be the performance of implied agreements. The so-called "agreed framework" drawn up by the United States and the Democratic People's Republic of Korea (or DPRK) in 1994 concerning, *inter alia,* the freezing of the indigenous DPRK nuclear programme and the facilitation of a new programme based on relatively proliferation-resistant nuclear power reactor technology, might be such a case. Although the two States avoided stating that they had agreed on anything - except to make the statement - and the document simply spells out what each State *would do*, these predictions certainly look like commitments assumed by each State in consideration of what the other does.

8. In other cases no contractual commitment may be discernible. The highly significant declarations by President BUSH and President GORBACHEV in September and October 1991 concerning the withdrawal of tactical nuclear weapons from theatres of deployment and from ships were clearly related but they were made unilaterally and can hardly be said to constitute legally binding commitments - however desirable that would be. Another example of a very important - but political rather than legal - engagement may be seen in the "Founding Act" drawn up in Paris 27 May 1997 between NATO States and the Russian Federation.

9. *Confidence-building measures* have played an increasingly important role in East-West relations, for instance "hot lines" to be used to defuse critical situations that might arise as a result of accidents or misunderstandings. Other examples may be schemes under which parties oblige themselves to notify each other about their military manoeuvres or, indeed, invite representatives to be present at such manoeuvres to see for themselves that they are not preludes to armed attacks. Openness and transparency generally

promote confidence about the absence of aggressive intentions or plans to act by surprise, and about compliance with arms control and disarmament agreements.

10. Important as they are and developed successfully especially within the framework of the Organization for Security and Co-operation in Europe (OSCE), confidence and security building measures do not generally regulate the strength of armed forces or impose reductions. Although some of them may fall within the - rather elastic - concept of "arms control", only a few cases will be referred to in this report.

11. Although export control regimes present themselves chiefly as informal mechanisms for consultation about and harmonization of national rules and decisions on restrictions of export of sensitive equipment and material, this report will devote some discussion to them as they are a significant - and at times controversial - part of the arms control.

12. The Rapporteur would like to thank the Government of the Netherlands for inviting him to prepare this report, and the many experts on international law and on disarmament who have taken the trouble to read a first draft and to suggest many corrections, modifications and additions.

# THE REPORT

## I. Aims of the First Hague Peace Conference

13. Looking back at the very end of the 20th century on the aims that animated the First Hague Peace Conference in 1899 one may feel some optimism as to their further progressive and perhaps eventually full realization - an optimism for which there would not have been much justification even in the mid-1980s. The end of the Cold War between the Communist-ruled countries and the market economy

countries stands out as the closing of a long and perilous period during which State conduct radically different from that sought at the Conference was a distinct possibility, namely, "mutually assured destruction" (MAD) through nuclear weapons. After the close of this period a door may now be ajar to another era in which armed force is no longer used on a global scale, although it may still not be avoided at the regional and national levels.

14. While the world of 1999 is thus vastly different from that of 1899 and could even raise hopes about the eradication of war between great powers and blocks, it is of interest to note that many of the sentiments and considerations which motivated the governments in 1899 remain alive, relevant - and more likely to bear fruit today.

15. The fundamental aim of the First Hague Peace Conference was to seek "the most effective means of ensuring to all peoples the benefits of a real and lasting peace."[1]

16. Considering that countless armed conflicts and two world wars have been fought since the Conference took place, it cannot be said to have been more successful in this lofty aspiration than many statesmen and thinkers before it - and after it. However, it stood for fresh approaches in several respects and presented substantial innovations. Moreover, it did not choose a comprehensive approach to realize its overall lofty aspiration but preferred a selective one in actually focussing on three more precise - though not much less difficult - aims, namely:

- to promote the peaceful settlement of disputes,
- to limit the cruelty of warfare on humanitarian grounds, and
- to limit the burden of armaments.

17. There are, of course, links between these three aims and the overall aspiration of the Conference. In particular, if peaceful settlement of disputes becomes the practice and norm, cruelty in warfare is avoided and governments may be more inclined to arms control and

1. Russian note of 30 Dec. 1898.

disarmament. However, we also find that the wish to limit the cruelty of warfare, which resulted at The Hague in "humanitarian law", e.g. restrictions in the *use* of weapons and the complete prohibition of the use of certain weapons, at the turn of the 20th century is leading, not only to the maintenance of old and the adoption of new rules on use, but to rules of "disarmament law", requiring the destruction and banning the production, acquisition and possession of certain weapons.

18. This report deals with the third - and least successful - aim of the conference: to limit the burden of armaments. Nevertheless, the links between that aim and the two other topics and the overall aspiration of the Conference suggest some brief introductory comments on all three aims before the report focusses on the international law relating to disarmament and arms control. It is evident, for instance, that the best boost for global or regional disarmament is a climate in which there are no serious contradictory territorial or other claims and in which peaceful (non-armed) means of settlement are perceived as offering acceptable solutions. Conversely, reductions in armaments to reach a verified balance and/or a deliberately accepted vulnerability, enabling potential adversaries mutually to inflict intolerable injury, are incentives to resort to peaceful settlements - or no settlements.

## I.1 The peaceful settlement of disputes

19. The search for ways and means of peacefully settling disputes between States that are sovereign and equal was not new in 1899 and is still on today. Nevertheless, it should be acknowledged that the result of the Conference marked considerable progress, in particular in creating permanent machinery for the judicial settlement of disputes.

20. Today we note that the "classical" methods of conciliation, mediation, arbitration and judicial settlement have not changed drastically in the last 100 years. However, the number of differences

which are handled through such "classical" methods has grown considerably and the number of institutions applying these methods is much greater and so is their level of development.

21. If the "classical" methods have not changed much, several other factors of great importance for the peaceful settlement of disputes have changed considerably. A large number of universal and regional intergovernmental institutions for co-operation and mutual adjustment are now active, which did not exist 100 years ago. The United Nations is the all-embracing organization in terms of membership and functions, including the aim of saving the world from "the scourge of war". Then, regional organizations like the OSCE for Europe, the OAS for the Americas, the OAU for Africa, and ASEAN for South East Asia, or sectoral ones, like WTO for international trade and ICAO for aviation, have conflict-preventing or conflict-settling roles too.

22. Also new at this time is the increased mutual dependence of States - e.g. in terms of communications, finance and trade, giving rise to leverages which can be used in the efforts to help prevent the use of force and to settle disputes. This development does imply a new and greater equality between States, but it does mean, for instance, that economic power may often be more relevant for influence than military power. Germany and Japan are influential States not because of their military but their economic capacity.

23. In the last resort the Security Council is given the authority under the Charter[2] in any case of threat to the peace, breach of the peace or act of aggression to resort to or authorize the threat or use of force on behalf of the State community. In the climate of great power détente which prevailed until recently, and which hopefully will be restored, the required concurrence of the five permanent members to

2. Arts. 24 (1), 39, 42.

decisions[3] is no longer a condition that renders the ability of the Council to act in large measure hypothetical. Even though the Council, created some 50 years ago, no longer well represents the economic, military and political power in today's world and the informal G 7/8 group in some respects could wield more power, effective measures and action by the Security Council acting under the legal authority of the UN Charter, is now a more distinct possibility than it used to be in the bi-polarized world of the first 45 years of the United Nations. This general comment is not negated by the fact that in several cases agreement has not been attainable authorizing interventions by armed force and that Members may feel reluctance to allow the organization to be drawn into non-international conflicts.

24. Thus, the institutional conditions are far more favourable to-day than they were 100 years ago for preventing or stopping armed conflicts between States. With the end of the Cold War there is also no nation ready to use force in crusading for a particular social or economic organization. Although fundamentalist doctrines are preached or pursued here and there, and rabid nationalism and fanaticism still lead to horrible persecution and armed conflict in several regions and countries, pragmatism is by and large dominating at the global level.

25. Another favourable factor of great practical importance today to reduce the risk of armed conflicts between States - as distinct from non-international armed conflicts - is that territorial controversies between great powers and blocks have largely disappeared or lost relevance.

26. In the Helsinki Declaration of 1975 the participating States - East and West - declared that they "regard as inviolable all one another's frontiers as well as the frontiers of all States in Europe". Although the principle was balanced by another provision to the effect that "frontiers can be changed, in accordance with international law, by

3. Art. 27 (3).

peaceful means and by agreement..." the net result was that the borders in Europe, as they resulted from the Second World War - including the long disputed Oder-Neisse line - were confirmed as inviolable, though not immutable. Already today we can see how many of these borders will become lines of less significance among partners of the European Union.

27. It has to be noted, of course, that territorial controversies of lesser magnitude continue to simmer here and there. Between Greece and Turkey such a controversy is - barely - kept under a lid with the help of a common institutional framework: NATO. It is perhaps remarkable that the dissolution of the Soviet Union could take place without significant territorial controversies remaining today. Moreover, the formerly disputed long border between China and Russia is no longer a subject of controversy. In Asia, the unsolved controversy between Japan and Russia about the South Kurile islands seems unlikely to lead to the use of force. The various claims made to the Spratley islands and Paracels have so far not led to shooting incidents, but they are a potential source of serious conflict and could test the declared determination of the States in the region to limit their actions to peaceful means.

28. Territorial disputes also seem to have faded in South America, while Africa remains an area where disputes about territory and borders inherited from colonial times still easily erupt and call for regional or international efforts of settlement.

29. Yet another factor that will be discussed below[4] is that the existence of nuclear weapons and the risk that they could be used in an armed conflict might have a restraining influence on pressures to initiate the use of armed force.

4. Para. 44.

## I.2 Humanitarian grounds for restrictions on means and methods of warfare

30. A second powerful sentiment behind the efforts at the First Hague Peace Conference had strong humanitarian roots. While it was realized that armed conflicts were inevitably cruel, it was felt that the business of war was not to give vent to hatred, but to prevail over an adversary to achieve a specific objective, e.g. to capture territory. As the purpose was not to inflict pain and suffering, acts which had such effect and which were not necessary to attain the objective of the armed conflict could not be justified and should be excluded on humanitarian grounds.

31. Further, as civilians were seen to have only marginal importance to the armed contest, no necessity of war should prevent their protection - so long as they did not take part in the armed actions and thus became of importance to that contest. They could be affected by attacks on military targets but were not themselves legitimate targets. A conclusion was that indiscriminate means and methods of warfare, which would make them targets, would be impermissible.

32. Also, the necessity of war did not call for the maiming of the enemy. It was considered *enough to* disable armed enemy soldiers to prevent them from taking further part in the armed contest. The well-known formulations of the St. Petersburg declaration of 1868 stated:

> That the only legitimate object which States should endeavour to accomplish during war is to weaken the military forces of the enemy;
> That for this purpose it is sufficient to disable the greatest possible number of men;
> That this object would be exceeded by the employment of arms which uselessly aggravate the sufferings of disabled men, or render their death inevitable.

33. The preamble of the Second Hague Convention of 1899 succinctly stated that the parties were inspired by "the desire to diminish the evils of war so far as military necessities permit", and

the attached Regulations accordingly held that "the right of belligerents to adopt means of injuring the enemy is not unlimited."[5]

34. This line of thinking logically resulted in general restrictions on the use of weapons (means) and the complete prohibition of use of some weapons. As we shall see in this report the philosophy has remained alive and provides the rationale for many modern rules.

*a. Non-discrimination and the protection of civilians*

35. The "launching of projectiles and explosives from balloons or by other similar new methods" would put non-armed civilians at risk and was not perceived as a necessity of war. Hence the humanitarian consideration could and should prevail and a ban on such methods could be adopted. It was done in 1899 for a period of five years.[6]

36. We are bound to note that the philosophy reflected in the declaration has not stood in the way of modern air warfare, not even prevented area bombardment.[7]

*b. "Excessively" cruel weapons. The ban on dum-dum bullets*

37. The 1899 Hague Peace Conference banned the use of "bullets which expand or flatten easily in the human body" - the so-called dum-dum bullet.[8] The necessity of war was not deemed to require more than piercing a hole to disable a man. Bullets which did not have hard envelopes and which mushroomed on impact and tore their way, mutilating the soldier, were not needed. Hence humanitarian considerations demanded that the use of them should be dispensed

5. Art. 22.

6. Declaration IV, 1.

7. See, by this author, "Area Bombardment: Rules and Reasons", 31 BYIL (1978).

8. Declaration IV, 3.

with. As we shall see the ban has not prevented the modern use of small calibre, high velocity bullets, fragmentation bombs etc.

## c. *Terror weapons*

38. At the Conference the use of "projectiles, the sole object of which is the diffusion of asphyxiating or deleterious gases" was prohibited.[9]

39. The rationale here appears to have been that the projectiles were perceived to be of an "unnecessarily cruel" nature. Later bacteriological weapons, gas and other chemical weapons generally, as well as weapons relying for their effect chiefly on radiation have been seen as particularly odious - "terror weapons". As such weapons have been used only relatively rarely (exception being made for gas in the First World War) or not at all, the abhorrence of them may have been strong enough in the past to prevail over whatever arguments might have been advanced about their military effectiveness.

40. The post-World War II discussions about the legality of use of nuclear weapons illustrate that the rationales invoked for prohibition of specific weapons have not changed very much since the 1899 Hague Peace Conference. Their use is protested both on the ground that their effects allegedly cannot be limited to legitimate military targets and that they are thus by nature indiscriminate, and on the ground of excessive cruelty (heat and radiation).[10]

## d. *Public opinion*

41. One element of influence that should be discerned is public opinion, which was often active, both at the end of the last century and later in support of prohibitions of specific weapons. Nevertheless

9. Declaration IV, 2.

10. The point is extensively discussed infra, e.g. in para. 132.

it is hard to avoid the impression that in the last resort it has been up to the military experts to judge whether a particular weapon's usefulness to the armed contest is so great that the suffering it brings must be seen as a "necessity of war".

42. As for nuclear weapons, the widespread and intense engagement shared by fairly large segments of public opinion in many countries, and by a number of governments as well, has not led to an agreement even on a no-first-use proposition. Uncertainty about their possible use has evidently been seen as a great military value and has led several governments to consider such use as a potential "necessity of war".

43. Not until we get to the 1997 Ottawa Convention on Anti-Personnel Mines do we find a case where the public's assessment of what is a "necessity of war" prevails. However, it remains to be seen whether that Convention, which is to enter into force when 40 signatories have ratified it, will also be accepted by all great military powers.

*e. Do nuclear weapons deter from the use of arms?*

44. The point is sometimes made that precisely the fact that modern warfare and modern weapons - especially nuclear weapons - have become so cruel and tend to affect civilian populations so widely, could now constitute incentives to achieve non-violent settlement of disputes. It is a proposition that is hard to prove and one that might be more plausible regarding some actors than others. We may note that despite several critical moments in the relations between nuclear-weapon States, there has not been any direct armed confrontation among them. On the other hand, it is known that in some

other tense relations the use of nuclear weapons has been discussed internally - and rejected.[11]

45. It should be added that raising the possibility that the huge arsenals of weapons of mass destruction might have had a restraining influence is not the same as welcoming these weapons. In the Non-Proliferation Treaty (NPT) of 1968 there are both expressions which reflect recognition that the existence of these weapons demand political restraint and a commitment to nuclear disarmament.

## I.3 The burden of armaments

46. A third rationale behind the efforts at the First Hague Peace Conference in 1899 was one that has had strong echoes in modern times. It was expressed in the consideration - to quote the Final Act of 1899:

> that the restriction of military charges, which are at present a heavy burden on the world, is extremely desirable for the increase of the material and moral welfare of mankind.

47. The Conference advanced the specific wish that governments might "examine the possibility of an agreement as to the limitation of armed forces by land and sea, and of war budgets". Regrettably, it can be safely observed that the wish has had less impact on the size of armaments than has the global or regional security climate prevailing at any given time.

48. It might be added that although the only explicit rationale adduced at The Hague in 1899 for what today is called "arms control and disarmament" was that of economy, another, implicit, rationale lay in the wish to reduce the horrors of war through some restrictions in the use of weapons and, even more so, in the prohibition of use of some specific categories of weapons. As we shall see, some bans of

11. See infra, para. 138.

use established at the Hague on account of their cruelty - gas, poison - have been transformed in the last few decades into prohibitions of acquisition and possession - disarmament.

## II. Focus on the time after the First Hague Peace Conference

49. It has not been the purpose of the preceding discussion to pass facile judgement on the relative successes and failures of the ambitions articulated at the First Hague Peace Conference. Rather, the idea was to show that several of the ambitions and rationales which inspired the actors of 1899 have remained valid during the following 100 years. During this period the world to which the ambitions have applied, has changed in ways that no one (except perhaps Jules Verne) could have imagined in 1899. The means of warfare and the resources for war have expanded many times over. Two world wars have brought mega-killings, mega-destruction, mega-horrors and ever increasing suffering for the civilian populations, *inter alia* through air bombardment. The armament budgets did not shrink in this period. Rather, with more economic resources available, they skyrocketed when security concerns were high. And while conventions, e.g. regarding prisoners of war, had great humanitarian importance during armed conflicts, the holocaust was more cruel and inhumane than anything previously witnessed.

50 It would certainly be of interest to trace and analyse the many legal instruments which were drawn up prior to the end of the Second World War and which relate to subjects treated at the First Hague Peace Conference.[12]

12. See, e.g., J. Goldblat, *Agreements for Arms Control* (1982) and id., *Arms Control* , (1994); Schindler and Toman, *The Laws of Armed Conflicts* (1981, 3rd ed. 1988); G. Best, *Humanity in Warfare: The Modern History of International Law of Armed Conflicts* (1980, paperback 1983).

51. There are the clauses on limitations of armaments imposed on vanquished States after the world wars, the Covenant of the League of Nations as the first full-scale world organization devoted to the settlement of disputes and the prevention of war, the very significant Washington Treaty on limitations in naval armaments of 1922 and the Geneva Protocol of 1925 prohibiting the use of gas and other chemical weapons and bacteriological weapons. An analysis of these and other inter-war documents would no doubt help us better to understand some questions we face today and certainly show that many of these, for instance, regarding verification and enforcement were intensely examined and discussed long ago.

52. Yet, considering the colossal changes which have been brought about by such developments as the process of decolonization and the global exercise of self-determination, the end of the Cold War, and the accelerated integration of the States of the world into a "global village", it might be permissible to embark directly on a discussion of some of the results of - and some of the issues which are central in - today's efforts to realize the aims and visions of the First Hague Peace Conference. Some considerations of this kind have already been advanced above in direct connection with the description of three central aims of the conference.

53. While this report seeks to give a factual overview of important arms control and disarmament measures which are in force or maybe expected to enter into force, there is no aim to examine *all* agreements reached and provide a detailed assessment of their impact. The examination will zero in on some problems and possibilities which exist in arms control and disarmament today, notably those that are connected with verification of compliance - which appear central to progress.

## II.1 Realization of the aims of the Peace Conference regarding disarmament and arms control in today's world

54. As noted at the opening of this report,[13] the climate for agreements on arms control and disarmament improved radically with the end of the Cold War, the geopolitical changes in Europe and the growing awareness of the catastrophic consequences of a war involving weapons of mass destruction between great powers. Indeed, a greater readiness to agree on measures to prevent crises and to reduce the risk of armed conflict arose already before the end of the Cold War, in the wake of the Cuban missile crisis in 1962, but after the end of the Cold War the evolution accelerated. Regrettably, there is a risk at the present time that frictions which have arisen in the relations between several of the great military powers as a result of a variety of decisions and actions, may put a break on the remarkable successes of recent years.[14]

## II.2 The rationales of arms control and disarmament today

55. Before proceeding to an overview of important modern arms control and disarmament measures it may be appropriate to consider whether these efforts have been driven by other or additional rationales than those which inspired the First Hague Peace Conference.

56. A first point to be noted is that sincere talks about arms control a precondition for measures appear to require the existence of at least a measure of mutual confidence that the other side gives high priority to avoiding an armed conflict. One does not discuss disarmament - at least not sincerely - with a potential adversary when the risk of armed action is perceived as imminent.

13. Para. 13.

14. See comments infra, paras. 89 and 199.

*a. Economy*

57. The principal rationale which the Hague Peace Conference gave for limiting armaments, that of saving resources for the welfare of mankind, has clearly retained its full relevance. Indeed, with the immeasurably greater human, economic, and material resources devoted to military purposes in the modern world, the potential savings are correspondingly higher. The argument has sometimes been made that moving upward in the arms spiral only results in the same insecurity at higher cost. While constituting an incentive to arms control that argument is only persuasive, however, if the goal of parity is accepted and there are reliable means of checking that parity.

*b. Abhorrence of specific weapons*

58. A feeling of abhorrence led the First Hague Peace Conference to prohibit the use of some weapons which were deemed to cause "unnecessary suffering", like asphyxiating gases, poison, and dum-dum bullets.

59. Similar feelings have come to be an important factor behind the demands for bans on *use* and the prohibition of development, testing, acquisition and possession of some modern weapons. Indeed, it would have been surprising if public opinion had remained passive, for instance, in the face of reports that a nuclear war could have resulted in the end of human civilization. The START I Treaty (1991), which stipulated important limitations on US and Soviet strategic offensive arms, cited the familiar sentence that "nuclear war would have such devastating consequences for all humanity, that it cannot be won and must never be fought."

60. And already the over 20 years older NPT (of 1968) committed the parties:

> to pursue negotiations in good faith on effective measures relating to cessation of the nuclear arms race at an early date and to nuclear disarmament, and to a treaty on general and complete disarmament under strict and effective international control.[15]

### c. *Reliability of restrictions*

61. In the interest of greater reliability a strengthening has been sought of the early bans on the use of some specific weapons of mass destruction - biological and chemical - into disarmament conventions prohibiting production and possession of these weapons.

62. This aim is also present and active in the case of some conventional weapons. A preambular paragraph of the 1981 Convention on Prohibitions or Restrictions on the Use of Certain Conventional Weapons which may be deemed to be Excessively Injurious or to have Indiscriminate Effects records the belief of the parties:

> that the positive results in this area may facilitate the main talks on disarmament with a view to putting an end to the production, stockpiling and proliferation of such weapons.

63. Strikingly, while the early bans on use of weapons never required ready procedures or mechanisms for investigation of violations or for verification of compliance, this is today a common condition based on the need for reliability.

### d. *Strategic stability*

64. It is clear that governments in East-West relations have come to believe that a reasonably equal balance of military power between great powers and blocks and a preserved second-strike capacity is

15. Art. VI.

likely to suffice to deter from any adventures. The 1979 Treaty between the United States and the Soviet Union on the Limitation of Strategic Offensive Arms (SALT II) recorded that the parties were "guided by the principle of equality and equal security".

65. Hence agreements have been sought which aim at balance and openness - later, an openness including on-site verification - which will enable the parties to measure their respective strength with a degree of confidence.

66. If these conditions are fulfilled, the military planning becomes mutually more predictable which, in turn, may allow a desired greater stability.

67. In the Treaty of 1990 on Conventional Armed Forces in Europe (CFE) the rationale of balance and strategic stability is well articulated:

> Committed to the objectives of establishing a secure and stable balance of conventional armed forces in Europe at lower levels than heretofore, of eliminating disparities prejudicial to stability and security and of eliminating, as a matter of high priority, the capability for launching surprise attack and for initiating large scale offensive action in Europe.

## e. *Protecting the environment*

68. A relatively new rationale for arms control is found in the wish to avoid catastrophic environmental effects of the use of specific means or methods of warfare. This rationale is strongly pronounced in the 1963 Partial Test Ban Treaty.[16] However, environmental consider-

16. See infra, para. 148.

ations figured already in the Antarctic Treaty of 1959 and turns up in a number of other treaties, e.g. the Outer Space Treaty of 1967.[17]

*f. Limiting the military capacity of aggressor States*

69. It is understandable that at the end of armed conflicts victor States impose - as a condition of peace - limitations on the weapons the vanquished State can have in the future, thereby seeking to prevent new threats arising from the State in question. Arms limitations were imposed on the losers both after the First and the Second World War. A more recent case of restrictions imposed upon a vanquished State can be seen in the key resolution of the Security Council of the United Nations establishing the conditions for a cease-fire with Iraq at the end of the Gulf War.[18]

## II.3 Categories of arms control and disarmament treaties

70. An overview of the vast body of arms control and disarmament agreements reached after the Second World War can be subdivided along different lines: those that relate to weapons of mass destruction and those relating to conventional weapons; or those that are bilateral between the Soviet Union/Russia and the USA and those that are regional or universal etc. However one slices the big cake there will be pieces that do not quite fit the pattern. In the following sections, agreements are discussed under four headings:

- Limitations on the level of armaments;
- Prohibitions or restrictions of use of specific weapons;
- Prohibition of testing, deployment and on attacks on the environment;
- Prohibition of development and acquisition of specific weapons.

17. See infra, para. 161.
18. SC/RES/687 (1991).

## *a. Limitations on the level of armaments*

### *1. Conventional weapons*

### *i General and Complete Disarmament*

71. For many years during the 1950s and 1960s general and complete disarmament was discussed at the Geneva Conference on Disarmament and its successors. Although no agreement was reached it is mentioned here because the subject had such high visibility for a long time. However, the discussion was mainly an exercise in public relations, one that took place to the music of an armament race, both in the field of conventional weapons and weapons of mass destruction. An evident ambition on the Communist side was to appeal to various public peace movements in the hope that they would work for reductions in the armed capacities of the Western States.

72. One major touch-stone was the issue of verification. From the Soviet side it was suggested that the "effective verification", which all agreed was necessary, should consist of full inspection of the destruction of weapons which was to take place - but no verification of the arsenals that remained. This "bonfire" concept was rejected by the West and was seen as evidence that the whole Soviet campaign was a propaganda gimmick. On the Soviet side the Western emphasis on verification was criticized as "control without disarmament", as efforts to pry open a society the closed character of which was felt to be - and perhaps was - a military advantage.

### *ii The 1990 Treaty on Conventional Armed Forces in Europe*

73. If general and complete disarmament was not a very plausible item for successful negotiation in Geneva, years of discussions in Vienna between the Warsaw Pact and NATO countries during the last decade of the Cold War, in the 1980s, resulted in success in the Treaty of 19 November 1990 on Conventional Armed Forces in Europe (CFE). Negotiated between the group of States which at the time belonged to the Warsaw Pact and the group of States which at the time belonged to NATO, the Treaty now falls under the auspices of the OSCE, which has developed an extensive regime of con-

fidence and security building measures for all the members of the organization.

74. The central idea of the CFE was to reduce the total amount of conventional war material which had been assembled during the Cold War in the area between the Atlantic and the Ural mountains, to provide for military balance between the two alliances, and to lessen the concentration of armed forces in Central Europe. Each group of States was obliged to ensure that within 40 months after the entry into force of the treaty the number of battle tanks, armoured combat vehicles, artillery pieces, combat aircraft, and attack helicopters did not exceed the ceilings set.[19]

75. The CFE entered into force in 1992. It comprises extensive arrangements for mutual verification and confidence building measures, notably regarding on-site inspections;[20] on the use of national technical means for information, e.g. satellites;[21] on the duty not to interfere with such means;[22] on the duty not to conceal relevant objects;[23] on the creation of a joint group for consultation on implementation;[24] and on the right of withdrawal if a Party "decides that extraordinary events related to the subject matter of this Treaty have jeopardized its supreme interests."[25]

76. The implementation of the treaty has led to drastic reductions in and redistribution of conventional armaments in the area. By the end of the period the 30 States parties had destroyed or converted to other uses more than 50.000 pieces of the items for which ceilings had been set and some 2.300 intrusive on-site inspections had taken place.

19. Art. IV.
20. Art. XIV.
21. Art. XV (1).
22. Art. XV (2).
23. Art. XV (3).
24. Art. XVI.
25. Art. XIX (1); and see discussion infra, para. 317.

77. With the end of the Cold War and the dissolution of the Warsaw pact the treaty became outdated almost as soon as it had entered into force and a summit of OSCE States in Lisbon in 1996 decided on negotiations to modify the treaty to fit the new geopolitical situation. These negotiations appear now[26] to have led to agreement on a new instrument to replace the original treaty and to be signed in November 1999 at a summit meeting in Istanbul. While the original treaty was based on parity of strength between the groups of States in the two alliances, the new instrument appears to treat every participating country individually and to ensure that no single country can have military forces at levels which could give it a dominating position in the area.

*iii. UN Register of Conventional Arms (1992)*

78. Mention might be made of this register which is operated by the United Nations.[27] It might conceivably help to dispel some misunderstandings and impede some destabilizing accumulations of conventional weapons. However, its importance is more likely to be in the field of confidence building than arms control. Since 1992 a total of 138 UN Member States have provided very substantial amounts of information on their import and export and holdings of seven categories of conventional arms.

79. The register does not cover small arms, a category of weapons on which there is increasing interest, as they are very easily available and result in many casualties, not least in non-international conflicts.

*2. Nuclear weapons*

*i SALT (1972)*

80. The Strategic Arms Limitations Talks (SALT) which began between the United States and the Soviet Union in 1969 resulted in 1972 in two agreements:

26. i.e. the spring of 1999.

27. General Assembly resolution A/RES/46/36.

- the Interim Agreement on certain measures with respect to the limitation of strategic offensive arms (SALT I), and
- the Treaty on the limitation of anti-ballistic missile systems (ABM Treaty).

81. Neither of these agreements which deal with long-range ballistic missiles laid down any limitations on the number of nuclear weapons or the quantity of fissionable material that each party could have, but indirectly they have had a profound importance on the strategies, the nuclear weapons capacity and the further arms control efforts of the two States.

82. SALT I, concluded for five years, created a freeze on the further construction of fixed land-based ICBM launchers and ballistic missile launchers on modern submarines.

*ii. The ABM Treaty (1972)*

83. Under the ABM Treaty each party undertook not to deploy anti-ballistic missile systems for the defence of its territory or of an individual region, with the exception that such defence would be permitted as specified for an area centred on each country's capital and another area containing ICBM silo launchers. The treaty was to be of unlimited duration but there is a right to withdraw from it with six months' notice "if a party decides that extraordinary events related to the subject matter of this treaty have jeopardized it supreme interests." Under a Protocol signed in 1974[28] the two parties agreed that only one area in each country would be allowed to be protected by an ABM system.

84. Both agreements relied on "national technical means of verification" to be used "in a manner consistent with generally recognized principles of international law." The parties agreed not to interfere with these means of verification and also not to use deliberate concealment measures to impede the verification. In addition a Standing Consultative Commission was established with broad competence to

28. entering into force in 1976.

consider inter alia questions of compliance, proposals for furthering the viability of the treaty.

85. The ABM Treaty has been and remains of fundamental importance because so long as each party refrains from protecting itself against the risk of ballistic missiles being launched by the other party, there remains a mutual second strike capacity, which should deter any incentive to a first strike: the mutually assured destruction (MAD) is preserved. Of equal importance is that neither party is prompted to increase its stock of missiles to improve the chance of penetrating the other party's defence against missiles. Through the ABM treaty a vital basis was thus created for later agreements limiting stocks of missiles and warheads (the strategic arms reductions treaties, START).

*iii. SALT II (1979)*

86. The SALT II agreement reached in 1979 set ceilings for certain launchers and missiles and sought to establish quantitative parity. It required the dismantling of a certain number of nuclear-weapon delivery vehicles both in the US and in the Soviet Union. The provisions regarding verification and compliance were the same as in the SALT I and the ABM treaties. The treaty never entered into force but was in the main respected by both parties for a number of years.

*iv. Star Wars (1983) and TMD (1998)*

87. The ABM Treaty was in jeopardy when the United States in 1983 launched the Strategic Defence Initiative (SDI) - often called "Star Wars" as it was designed to be space-based. While this grand initiative to create a defensive shield against incoming ballistic missiles subsided for technical and economic reasons, new schemes have been presented which are said to aim at protection not against great powers but against possible less powerful but more reckless adversaries. Thus, in 1992 a project named Global Protection against Limited Strikes (GPALS) was discussed and, again, in the past year the project Theatre Missile Defence (TMD).

88. Questions arise whether systems of limited defence, intended for use against missiles from "low-capacity" State adversaries or terrorists can offer a protection that stands in any reasonable relation to the costs; whether, indeed, in the modern world of easy travel and transport 100 % protection is attainable against the threat posed by the possible existence of small quantities of weapons of mass destruction clandestinely in the hands of such adversaries, who may choose much more primitive means of delivery than ballistic missiles; and, whether this gain in protection, such as it would be, would outweigh the likely negative consequences for arms control among the eight States which are identified today as having nuclear weapons.

89. Currently the discussion of the TMD seems to impede a formal adoption of START II. It does not seem unlikely, moreover, that it could be very difficult to get general agreement on limitations on nuclear arsenals and on a cut-off of production of highly enriched uranium and plutonium for weapons purposes, if limited shields were created against reckless missile attacks, say, in the Far East. Lastly, it would seem that a limited missile defence could only be a part - albeit a very expensive part - of the answers to the problems posed by reckless regimes or sub-national groups. The matter will be somewhat further discussed below.

*v. The INF Treaty (1987)*

90. The INF (intermediate-range nuclear forces) Treaty of 1987 marks a new generation of US-Soviet Union arms control agreements and was of signal importance, not least to Europan countries, which were the most directly affected by this category of nuclear armaments. Although only a small part of the total stock of US and Soviet nuclear delivery vehicles was eliminated and warheads could be returned to stockpiles, it did away with the whole class of intermediate-range and shorter range missiles, resulting in the destruction of a total of 2695 missiles.

### *vi. Verification, compliance and withdrawal under SALT, ABM, INF*

91. The INF treaty, which was concluded after Gorbachev had taken over the leadership in the Soviet Union, contained elaborate provisions concerning verification. It repeated the provisions in the SALT and ABM treaties about the use of "national technical means of verification" (notably meaning satellites) and the duty of the parties not to interfere with them or to use concealment measures impeding their effectiveness.

92. The great innovation on the verification side in the INF Treaty lay in the introduction of mutual on-site inspection and on-site long-term monitoring.[29] Although on-site inspection was foreseen - and had actually taken place as early as 1963 on Soviet Antarctic installations - under the Antarctic Treaty of 1959,[30] the INF Treaty marked a first full-scale introduction of such verification at home in the two superpowers. In addition, special agreements were made to allow Soviet inspection of US missile sites in some NATO countries and US inspection in Soviet sites in two Warsaw Pact countries. The Treaty also established "Nuclear Risk Reduction Centers" for continuous technical communication and a "Special Verification Commission" to deal with questions of compliance and effectiveness of the treaty.[31]

93. The INF Treaty was accompanied by an extremely detailed separate Protocol, which seems to have left few questions unanswered regarding the procedures to follow, appointment of inspectors, visa, right to access, immunities etc.

94. Like the ABM Treaty the INF Treaty prescribed that it was of unlimited duration, but withdrawal was possible - with six months notice - if a Party "decides that extraordinary events related to the

29. Art XI.

30. Arts. V and VII.

31. Art. XIII.

subject matter of this Treaty have jeopardized its supreme interests".[32]

*vii. START I (1991)*

95. The Treaty on the Reduction and Limitation of Strategic Offensive Arms (START I), signed by the United States and the Soviet Union on 31 July 1991, was the first treaty to bring very substantial cuts in their respective stocks of strategic delivery vehicles and warheads. With regard to verification, it contains in Article IX provisions similar to those found in the SALT on the use of "national technical means" but also arrangements for extensive and intrusive on-site inspection. A separate protocol lays down very detailed rules on inspections and continuous monitoring activities. An idea of the extent of the activities may be gained from its stipulation that the list of inspectors "shall not contain at any one time more than 400 individuals, and the list of monitors shall not contain at any time more than 300 individuals." For comparison it may be mentioned that the IAEA has some 200-300 inspectors to inspect all nuclear installations submitted to safeguards under the NPT and other agreements. Another protocol establishes a Joint Compliance and Inspection Commission, somewhat like the Special Verification Commission for the INF.[33]

96. START I, which entered into force 5 December 1994, was made for a period of fifteen years and contained the traditional withdrawal clause concerning "extraordinary events".[34] That the continued mutual vulnerability which is assured by the ABM Treaty was a vital premise for Soviet acceptance of START I can be seen in a recorded statement that:

> the extraordinary events ... also include events related to withdrawal by one of the Parties from the Treaty on the Limitation of Anti-Ballistic Missile Systems, or related to its material breach.

32. Art. XV (2).
33. See supra, para. 92.
34. Art. XVII.

97. It should finally be noticed that while START I was signed by the Soviet Union in July 1991, the dissolution of the Soviet Union occurred in December of the same year and Belarus, Kazakhstan and Ukraine became independent States, with a great deal of the strategic nuclear weapons and launchers on their territory. Through a Protocol signed in Lisbon on 23 May 1992 the three States were recognized as successor States of the Soviet Union in relation to the START I Treaty and, thus, became individually bound by its provisions. Subsequently all nuclear weapons were transferred from the three States to Russia. All three States adhered to the NPT and submitted their (peaceful) nuclear installations to IAEA safeguards.

*viii. START II (1993)*

98. The Treaty on Further Reductions and Limitations of Strategic Offensive Arms (START II) which was signed by the US and Russia on 3 January 1993,[35] requires parity in the numbers of strategic nuclear weapons on each side and stipulates reductions in two stages. At the end of the second stage, which is to be attained by 1 January 2003[36] each side shall have no more than between 3000 and 3500 deployed strategic warheads and only ICBMs carrying a single warhead shall be allowed.

99. Inspections under START II are to be conducted in accordance with the provisions laid down in START I.[37] In addition, a Bilateral Implementation Commission is established to resolve questions relating to compliance and to agree on measures to improve the viability and effectiveness of the treaty.[38]

35. The Treaty has not yet entered into force.

36. The date was later postponed to 2007.

37. Art. II (7) and Art. V.

38. Art. V.

100. The START II Treaty is to remain in force so long as START I is in force and it is subject to the traditional right of withdrawal in the case of "extraordinary events".[39]

*ix. START III (199?)*

101. At a US-Russian summit meeting in Helsinki a Joint Statement of 21 March 1997 envisaged the negotiation of a START III which would reduce the number of strategic nuclear weapons on each side to the level of 2000-2500. However, due to current frictions between the two States, not even START II has come into force.

*x. Sub-strategic Nuclear Weapons (1991)*

102. In 1991 the United States and the Soviet Union made unilateral - but clearly co-ordinated - important declarations about the withdrawal of sub-strategic nuclear weapons from theatres of deployment and ships and discarding of such weapons.

103. The United States announced[40] that it would eliminate its entire world-wide inventory of ground-launched short-range nuclear weapons. All nuclear artillery shells and short-range ballistic missile warheads would be taken home and destroyed. Furthermore, steps would be taken that normally no US ships would carry tactical nuclear weapons. Weapons that would not be destroyed would be secured in central areas.

104. The Soviet Union announced[41] that it was taking similar steps "leading to the elimination of tactical nuclear weapons". It called on other nuclear-weapon States to join in these efforts.

105. Responses came in June 1992, when France declared that production of the tactical nuclear missile Hades would be cancelled, and the United Kingdom announced that deployment of tactical nuclear

39. Art. VI.

40. On 27 September 1991.

41. On 5 October 1991.

weapons by the navy and air force would be curtailed and the weapons withdrawn would be destroyed.

106. All announcements were made unilaterally and might not be legally binding. The form might have been dictated by the urgency to ensure that the imminent dissolution of the Soviet Union would not make a number of Soviet republics nuclear-weapon States through the presence of tactical nuclear weapons on their territory. There was no procedure or mechanism for verification. A legally binding confirmation of the undertakings would be desirable.

*xi. Disposition of weapon-origin fissile material (1998)*

107. At a US-Russia summit meeting on 2 September 1998 a "Joint Statement of Principles for Management and Disposition of Plutonium Designated as No Longer Required for Defence Purposes" was adopted. Under this Statement each party committed itself to irrevocably remove 50 tons of plutonium from dismantled nuclear weapons and military stocks. Much discussion has taken place as to the further management of fissile material which is no longer needed for defence purposes. Such material must be handled in ways which guarantee that it does not go back into new weapons or other military use. Highly enriched (weapons grade) uranium is least problematic: diluted with natural uranium it becomes low enriched uranium and can be used as fuel in power reactors. In a major transaction originally made in 1993[42] the US has bought 500 metric tons of HEU from Russia to be delivered after dilution.

108. Plutonium raises greater problems, but can either be transformed into a mixed oxide fuel (MOX) which can be burnt in power reactors or mixed with nuclear waste for disposal as waste. Both methods are envisaged.

109. Owing to the large quantities which will arise a good deal of material will have to await transformation and use as fuel, and interim storage will be necessary. Both for the storage and for the

42. The transaction was confirmed in 1999.

fabrication and burning of the fuel based on this material international verification through the IAEA is contemplated to give confidence that no material goes back to military use or disappears. Since 1996 discussions have taken place between the US, Russia and the IAEA on technical, legal and financial issues related to such IAEA verification.

110. The joint US-Russian statement and the trilateral discussions which have taken place demonstrate that nuclear disarmament cannot be limited just to a dismantling of warheads. The fissile material is the most essential part of the weapon and until it has been rendered unsuitable for weapons use it needs to be under verification.

### *b. Prohibition or restriction of use of specific weapons*

111. This category of regulations has not changed dramatically since the time of the First Hague Peace Conference in 1899, when the use of asphyxiating and deleterious gases and poison and dum-dum bullets was banned.[43] These rules have doubtless hardened into customary law but, as noted earlier, there may be different views as to how far the rules go. The large-scale use of gas by belligerents during the First World War caused abhorrence which in the 1919 Versailles Peace Treaty led to a strict prohibition for Germany to produce, stock or import the prohibited chemical weapons,[44] and in 1925 to a new multilateral regulation in the Geneva Gas Protocol.

#### *i. The Geneva Protocol of 1925*

112. The 1925 Geneva Protocol for the Prohibition of the Use in War of Asphyxiating, Poisonous or Other Gases and of Bacteriological Methods of Warfare confirmed and re-codified the existing rules regarding gas, included "analogous liquids, materials or devices" in the ban and extended the ban to cover the use to "bacteriological

43. Hague Declarations IV, 2 and IV, 3.

44. Art. 171.

methods of warfare". This regulation, too, is deemed to have subsequently become customary law.

113. It has been questioned whether the ban in the Geneva Protocol covered the use in armed conflicts[45] of tear gas and herbicides. A resolution adopted by the UN General Assembly in 1969 answered this question in a positive sense.[46] It may be noted here that the 1993 Convention on Chemical Weapons,[47] the main thrust of which is to prohibit development, production and stockpiling of chemical weapons, actually also explicitly prohibits the use of chemical weapons.[48] As the preamble of the Convention recognizes the prohibition of the use of herbicides "as a method of warfare" and the parties undertake not to use riot control agents "as a method of warfare",[49] the matter which caused this controversy at the end of the 1960s seems to have been settled.

114. The value of the Geneva Protocol has been considered undermined by many reservations which, in effect, reduced it to a prohibition of first use for the reserving parties.

115. Like the 1899 bans on the use of gases and dum-dum bullets, the regulation of 1925 contains no verification mechanism. It was assumed that any violations would be evident or could be established through *ad hoc* means of verification. Compliance would be induced, partly by the universal abhorrence of these weapons, partly by the awareness that a violation (at least regarding the use of gas) could bring retaliation in kind.

116. The ban on the use of gas has been violated several times since the First World War and the adoption of the Geneva Protocol, e.g, in the 1930's by Japan in Manchuria and Italy during the war in

45. As distinguished from use in the domestic sphere.

46. RES 2603 A XXIV.

47. See infra, para. 186.

48. Art. I (1)(b).

49. Art. I (5).

Ethiopia. After the Second World War, during which gas was not used, the prohibition was violated in Yemen (1967) and in the 1980s in the war between Iraq and Iran and by Iraq against Kurds on its own territory.

117. A resolution by the UN General Assembly of 1982[50] authorized the Secretary-General to use expert groups to examine reports about possible violations of the Geneva ban. In March 1984 and March 1986, the Secretary-General did send such groups to examine the charges that Iraq had used C-weapons, which was affirmed in 1986.

118. In line with the thinking, developed first with regard to nuclear weapons, that prohibitions of use do not give enough reassurance and bans on production and acquisition are necessary, work began at the Geneva disarmament conference on a convention containing such bans as regards chemical weapons. After many years of negotiations this resulted in the Convention of 1993, which will be discussed below.[51]

119. There do not seem to be any well-documented modern cases of battlefield uses of bacteriological (biological) weapons. However, a readiness to use such weapons[52] seems to have been wide-spread. A convention which prohibits the development, production and acquisition of biological weapons - but does not contain any machinery for verification - was concluded already in 1972. It will be discussed below.

### *ii. The 1977 Protocols Additional to the Geneva Conventions and the Convention of 1981*

120. During the 1970s a number of conferences convened either by the ICRC or the Swiss government dealt with, what they called, the "Reaffirmation and Development of International Humanitarian Law Applicable in Armed Conflicts", and in UN terminology: "Human

50. 37/98 D.

51. Para. 186.

52. E.g. anthrax.

Rights in Armed Conflicts". In plainer language, the work dealt with the modernization of the rules applicable in armed conflicts, including restrictions in the use of specific conventional weapons. The whole of this work was guided by the humanitarian concept on which the First Hague Peace Conference and the instruments adopted at it was based. The military input in the negotiations was strong, ensuring that the "military necessity" aspect was fully considered in the context of all proposed restrictions. While this reduced the humanitarian effect of many proposals it hopefully led to provisions which stand a better chance of being applied in action.

121. In 1977 the conferences resulted in two Protocols Additional to the Geneva Conventions of 1949, one (Protocol I) dealing with international armed conflicts, the other (Protocol II) with non-international armed conflicts.

122. Article 35 of Protocol I confirms the general principle of the Hague Conference that it is prohibited to use weapons and methods of warfare "of a nature to cause superfluous injury or unnecessary suffering", but it adds a prohibition of "methods or means of warfare which are intended, or may be expected, to cause widespread, long-term and severe damage to the natural environment."[53]

123. Article 36 of Protocol I enjoins parties developing or acquiring new weapons to determine whether the employment of such weapons "would, in some or all circumstances, be prohibited". We do not know, of course, what horror weapons might have been stopped on the drawing boards as a result of this duty.

124. Protocol II (applicable in non-international armed conflicts) contains no provisions in the area of weapons.[54]

53. See infra, para. 163.

54. But see para. 127 on anti-personnel mines.

### *iii. 1981 Convention on Excessively Injurious or Indiscriminate Conventional Weapons and Protocols attached to it*

125. An additional result of the effort to modernize the laws of war is a framework Convention on Prohibitions or Restrictions on the Use of Certain Conventional Weapons which may be Deemed to be Excessively Injurious or to have Indiscriminate Effects. It is sometimes referred to as the "inhumane weapons convention." This seems entirely inappropriate as all weapons are inhumane. It was opened for signature in 1981 and contained three annexed Protocols. A fourth Protocol prohibiting the use *and transfer* of blinding lasers was added in 1985.[55]

126. The Convention and the three Protocols originally attached to it are of some interest in this context. Protocol I prohibits the use of weapons the primary effect of which is achieved by fragments which in the human body cannot be detected by X-rays.

127. Another Protocol (II) contains restrictions on the use of mines, booby-traps and other devices. It requires, *inter alia*, that maps be made of preplanned mine-fields, and introduces a duty on belligerents to exchange maps at the end of hostilities to facilitate the clearing of mines. It further establishes certain rules to reduce the risk of indiscriminate effects of mines laid by remote means and prohibits the booby-trapping of various types of objects, like toys and food. This Protocol was amended and strengthened in 1996, *inter alia* extending its application to non-international conflicts. The amended Protocol and the Ottawa Convention on anti-personnel landmines which was adopted two years later[56] appear to be poorly harmonized.

128. Protocol III contains a ban on the use from the air of napalm and other incendiary weapons against cities, villages or other areas where there are concentrations of civilians.

55. On the Convention and the three protocols, see F. Kalshoven, "Arms, Armaments and International Law", 191 RdC (1985-II).

56. See infra, para. 187.

129. It is evident that all three Protocols are directly based on the concepts of "unnecessary suffering" and/or indiscriminate effects. It is also clear that their scope was rather limited. The military assessment of "necessity" weighed heavily and prevailed in large measure over the public revulsion against the extensive use, particularly during the Viet Nam war, of incendiary weapons with very cruel effects, extremely injurious high-velocity small-caliber projectiles and remotely delivered anti-personnel mines with inherent risks of indiscriminate effects.

130. None of the restrictions introduced in the Protocols on the use of specific weapons were subject to any mechanism of verification. They were thus akin to older restrictions or prohibitions of use of specific weapons, like the 1925 Geneva Protocol on BC weapons.

*iv. Prohibition of use of nuclear weapons ? Advisory Opinion of the International Court of Justice (1996)*

131. As noted above[57] the legality of *use* of nuclear weapons has been challenged by individuals, citizens' movements and many governments. Through a resolution adopted in 1994 by the UN General Assembly the controversial question was placed before the ICJ It may be appropriate to examine what the Court answered. It was asked to give an advisory opinion on the question: "Is the threat or use of nuclear weapons in any circumstances permitted under international law?"

132. The Court rendered its opinion on 8 July 1996.[58] By 11 votes to 3 it concluded that [t]here is in neither customary nor conventional international law any comprehensive and universal prohibition of the threat or use of nuclear weapons as such."

57. Para. 40.

58. *Legality of the Threat or Use of Nuclear Weapons*, Advisory Opinion, ICJ Reports, 1996 p. 226.

133. However, the Court further concluded - by unanimity - that:

> A threat or use of nuclear weapons should also be compatible with the requirements of international law applicable in armed conflict, particularly those of the principles and rules of international humanitarian law, as well as with specific obligations under treaties and other undertakings which expressly deal with nuclear weapons.

134. From that premise it concluded, by 7 votes to 7, the President's vote deciding, that: "the threat or use of nuclear weapons would generally be contrary to the rules of international law applicable in armed conflict, and in particular the principles and rules of humanitarian law."

135. It added, however, that it could not conclude definitively "whether the threat or use of nuclear weapons would be lawful in an extreme circumstance of self-defence, in which the very survival of a State would be at stake."

136. In a final paragraph it concluded, unanimously, that "there exists an obligation to pursue in good faith and bring to a conclusion negotiations leading to nuclear disarmament in all its aspects under strict and effective international control."

137. The rules of international law which the whole Court seems to have found relevant to the question were those which emanated from the Hague Conferences and which require that means and methods employed in warfare to be lawful must be capable of distinguishing between civilian and military targets, and must not inflict unnecessary suffering on combatants.[59] In addition, the Court seems to have been agreed on the validity and relevance of the principle of proportionality in the degree of force applied (in response to attacks).

138. While in the view of the majority of the Court the use of nuclear weapons seemed "scarcely reconcilable" with these requirements, its dissenting Vice-President (Stephen SCHWEBEL) noted that many

59. See supra, paras. 30 et seq.

different situations could be imagined. In his view, for instance, "the use of a nuclear depth charge to destroy a nuclear sub-marine that is about to fire nuclear missiles ... might well be lawful". He also cited a conversation in Geneva on 9 January 1990 in which the American Secretary of State, James BAKER, purposely left the then Foreign Minister of Iraq, Tarek AZIZ, "the impression that the use of chemical or biological agents by Iraq could invite tactical nuclear retaliation". Iraq, which had both chemical and biological weapons, used neither in the Gulf war; and Judge SCHWEBEL cites evidence suggesting that the US warnings had been relevant, although President BUSH is reported in fact to have decided (unbeknownst to Iraq) that the US would not use nuclear weapons in retaliation against an Iraqi use of chemical weapons. The dissenting Judge concluded that:

> in some circumstances, the threat of the use of nuclear weapons - as long as they remain weapons unproscribed by international law - may be both lawful and rational.[60]

139. It is of interest to note that when the ICJ concluded - in reply to no question by the General Assembly - that there was an obligation to "pursue in good faith and bring to a conclusion negotiations leading to nuclear disarmament .."[61] it did so against the background of observations that "the pattern until now has been for weapons of mass destruction to be declared illegal by specific instruments."[62] It did not find any corresponding general treaty regarding nuclear weapons but rightly noted that there were a large number of treaties designed to limit:

- the acquisition, manufacture and possession of nuclear weapons;
- the deployment of nuclear weapons; and
- the testing of nuclear weapons.

60. ICJ Report, 1996, pp. 323-328.

61. Under Art. VI of the NPT.

62. Biological Weapons Convention and Chemical Weapons Convention.

140. The Court also noted that two treaties establishing nuclear weapon-free zones[63] have protocols attached to them under which nuclear-weapon States may commit themselves not to use nuclear weapons against parties to the treaties and that the nuclear-weapon States have done so to varying degrees and with various declarations.

141. It may seem surprising that the NPT does not contain any express clause prohibiting the use of nuclear weapons. However, if it had, the difference in obligations between the nuclear weapon and non-nuclear-weapon States parties would have been even more striking. Nevertheless, as the Court observed, nuclear-weapon States have given both positive and negative security guarantees in connection with the NPT, most recently on the occasion of the unlimited extension of the treaty in 1995.

142. While the positive security guarantee is simply a commitment to refer to the Security Council any case of a threat or use of nuclear weapons against a non-nuclear-weapon State party, and to act within the Council in accordance with the Charter to bring assistance to the State victim of the aggression, the negative security guarantees given by four nuclear-weapon States commit them to refraining from the use of nuclear weapons against a non-nuclear-weapon State party to the treaty, unless that State in association with a nuclear-weapon State has attacked them, their allies or their forces.

143. In conclusion, the ICJ stopped short of declaring the use of nuclear weapons unlawful in all circumstances and stressed the duty of the States parties to the NPT to negotiate and to reach agreement on nuclear disarmament. In so doing it seems to have felt - rightly - that the world community was not yet attacking the issue head on but was as it were trying to encircle and to reduce the threat that the continued existence of nuclear weapons poses to the world, by concluding a host of treaties on the deployment, testing and acquisition of nuclear weapons and by creating some other legal commitments.

63. Treaty of Tlatelolco for Latin America, Treaty of Rarotonga for the South Pacific.

The Court observed that these treaties "could be seen as foreshadowing a future general prohibition" of the use of nuclear weapons. The Court did not refer in this context, as it might have done, to the important nuclear arms control and disarmament treaties concluded between the US and the Soviet Union.

c. *Prohibitions of testing, deployment and attacks on the environment*

144. Efforts within the sphere of "arms control and disarmament" are only part of a more comprehensive objective of preventing or limiting the use of injurious and destructive means and methods in conflicts. As noted above,[64] Article 22 of the 1899 Convention (II) with respect to the Laws and Customs of War on Land stipulates that "The right of belligerents to adopt means of injuring the enemy is not unlimited." This rule was repeated with minor changes in Article 35, paragraph 1, of the 1977 Protocol I Additional to the Geneva Conventions of 1949:

> In any armed conflict, the right of the Parties to the conflict to choose methods or means of warfare is not unlimited.

145. Arms may indeed be the most common "means" to inflict injury and destruction and so bring pressure on an adversary, but they are not the only way to create such pressure. Methods like blockades and sieges to cut off food and other provisions have the same objective and have - logically - also been subjected to restrictions or bans. While this report is mainly dealing with the prevention of the use of arms, the current section will also take up some provisions which may or may not have regard to arms, namely, rules prohibiting destruction of the environment.

146. Furthermore, it will be shown that although a prohibition of use of specific weapons - such as nuclear, biological and chemical

64. See supra, para. 33.

weapons - is obviously the most straight-forward way to seek the non-use of the weapon in question, there are other, partial and supplementary approaches, such as the prohibition of testing and deployment.

147. In several treaties more than one approach to prevent, impede or limit the use of means and methods of warfare is found. In the discussion below the apparent main objective of a treaty will determine in which section it will be mainly examined.

*i. Prohibition of the testing of certain weapons*

148. The prohibition of *testing* of weapons may have several rationales. In some cases concern about the environment may be the dominant motive. This was certainly true for the 1963 Partial Test Ban Treaty, a preambular paragraph of which expresses the wish of the parties "to put an end to the contamination of man's environment by radioactive substances."

149. The 1996 Comprehensive Nuclear Test Ban Treaty may have been desired also with a view, if possible, to curtail a further qualitative development of nuclear weapons.

150. The prohibition of testing of "any type of weapons" in the Antarctic Treaty of 1959[65] and a similar prohibition in the 1967 Outer Space Treaty[66] were further probably motivated mainly by environmental concerns.

151. The bans on testing in the treaties establishing nuclear weapon-free zones[67] might have had environmental as well as security-related

65. Art. I.

66. Art. IV.

67. E.g. Art. 6 of the 1985 Rarotonga South Pacific Nuclear Weapon Free Zone Treaty.

grounds, while provisions on testing in some other treaties[68] must be assumed to have security-related objectives. The Biological Weapons Convention of 1972 and the Chemical Weapons Convention of 1993 contain no specific provisions on testing.

*ii. The Partial Test Ban Treaty (1963)*

152. The Partial Test Ban Treaty (PTBT) of 1963 prohibited the testing of nuclear weapons and other nuclear explosions except underground. It responded to strong concerns about radioactive fall-out, especially cesium, strontium 90 and iodine 131.

153. The treaty did not have any verification mechanism. It was felt that national technical means, in particular for measuring radioactive fall-out, would suffice to give evidence of any nuclear explosion that did not take place underground. It was the first treaty of many which contain the clause, mentioned above, that explicitly allows a Party "exercising its national sovereignty" to withdraw from the treaty "if it decides that extraordinary events, related to the subject matter of this Treaty, have jeopardized the supreme interests of its country."[69]

154. For many years a number of States resisted the proposal of a complete test ban, often contending that underground tests below a certain yield could not be detected and asserting that they could not take the risk of committing themselves to an unverified ban.

*iii. The Threshold Test Ban Treaty (1974)*

155. In 1974, the United States and the Soviet Union concluded a Threshold Test Ban Treaty (TTBT) committing the parties not to carry out any underground nuclear weapon test having a yield exceeding 150 kilotons and to limit the number of their underground tests to a minimum. The limitation was the result of the position that tests of lower yield could not be reliably detected as well as the wish to retain the freedom to carry out some tests. This treaty referred

68. Such as Art. IV in the 1972 ABM Treaty, Art. IV in the 1979 SALT Treaty and Art. V in the 1991 START I Treaty.

69. Art. IV.

expressly to the parties relying on national technical means of verification at their disposal.[70] However, under a Protocol of 1990, the parties agreed to mutual on-site inspections.

*iv. The Comprehensive Nuclear Test Ban Treaty (1996)*

156. After many years of underground testing by the five declared nuclear-weapon States the widespread demand for a complete test ban was met and the Comprehensive Nuclear Test Ban Treaty (CTBT) was concluded in September 1996.[71] Its purpose may be said to be broader than the preceding two treaties, as it aims not only at guaranteeing that no further radioactive contamination will occur as a result of nuclear testing, but also, if possible, to impede the further qualitative development of nuclear weapons.

157. After the adoption of this treaty India and Pakistan, which have neither signed the PTBT nor the CTBT, have tested nuclear explosives in 1998, while until the spring of 1999 all other States, including the five declared nuclear-weapon States, have refrained from any testing after its conclusion. Following their tests India and Pakistan have observed moratoria on further testing and appear to have declared that they will sign the CTBT.

158. If by 24 September 1999[72] the treaty has not been signed and ratified by 44 States which have been listed as having nuclear power plants or research reactors, the UN Secretary-General may have to convene a conference of the States that have ratified it to examine what measures may be taken to accelerate the ratification process.

159. The CTBT contains an elaborate system of verification which is based on seismological, radio-nuclide, hydro-acoustic and infra-sound monitoring. It is to rely on several hundred monitoring stations and some 170 primary and auxiliary seismic stations all over the world as well as an International Data Centre in Vienna, where the

70. Art. II (1).

71. At the time of writing (May 1999) the CTBT had not yet entered into force.

72. Three years after the date of its opening for signature.

organization of the treaty (CTBTO) is located. The Secretariat (236 posts foreseen in the 1999 budget) does not analyze and evaluate the data which the monitoring system obtains, but transmits them to member States, which have to judge whether they consider that particular data suggest a nuclear test. The member States, but not the secretariat, can ask for consultation and clarification and on-site inspections. In an urgent case of non-compliance, the Executive Council may bring the issue to the attention of the United Nations.[73]

160. As all the non-nuclear-weapon States parties to the NPT are prohibited already by that treaty to test any nuclear explosive device, a complete test ban treaty could theoretically have been restricted in its membership to the five declared nuclear-weapon States and non-parties to the NPT.[74] However, the global interest in the complete ban was such that there does not seem to have been any suggestion that the treaty could have been of less than universal membership.

### v. *Prohibition of attacks on the environment*

161. Mention has already been made of the relevance of the 1963 PTBT for the protection of the environment against radioactive fall-out.[75] Environmentally motivated bans on the testing of weapons are included in the 1959 Antarctic Treaty and the 1967 Outer Space Treaty.[76] The Antarctic Treaty goes beyond a ban on testing in providing that "any nuclear explosions in Antarctica and the disposal there of radioactive waste material shall be prohibited."[77]

### vi. *The ENMOD Convention (1977)*

162. Reference must be made also to the 1977 Convention on the Prohibition of Military or Any Other Hostile Use of Environmental Modification Techniques, (the ENMOD Convention). This treaty did not aim at any particular weapon but rather at preventing States from

73. Art. V (4).
74. Notably India, Pakistan and Israel.
75. See supra, para. 152.
76. See supra, para. 150.
77. Art. V.

engaging in "military or any other hostile use of environmental modification techniques having widespread, long-lasting or severe effects as the means of destruction, damage or injury to any other State Party."[78]

163. It should perhaps be noted that this formulation is much broader than a similar provision in Article 55, paragraph 1, in Additional Protocol I, which refers to "widespread, long-term and severe damage".[79]

164. The background of the ENMOD convention of 1977 was the use during the Viet Nam war of artificial rainmaking through the seeding of clouds with silver iodide to cause difficulties for the enemy by muddying roads and flooding lines of communication. The convention was much broader in scope, however, and covered "any techniques for changing - through the deliberate manipulation of natural processes - the dynamics, composition or structure of the Earth, including its biota, lithosphere, hydrosphere and atmosphere, or of outer space." During the negotiations examples were mentioned, such as changes in ocean currents, the triggering of earth quakes, cyclones, tornadic storms etc.

165. Without specifically saying so the Convention relies for verification on national technical means. In addition it enjoins the parties to "consult one another in solving any problems which may arise"[80] and refers a party that suspects a breach to complain in the Security Council and to submit all relevant information and possible evidence.[81] It does not contain the Test Ban Treaty-type of withdrawal clause in case of an "extraordinary event" jeopardizing the "supreme interests" of a State party.

78. Art. 1 (1).

79. See infra, para. 166.

80. Art. V ( 1).

81. Art. V (3).

### *vii. Additional Protocol I to the Geneva Conventions of 1949*

166. It should finally be mentioned in this context that Article 55 of Additional Protocol I contains a general provision that:

> Care shall be taken in warfare to protect the natural environment against widespread, long-term and severe damage. This protection includes a prohibition of the use of methods or means of warfare which are intended or may be expected to cause such damage to the natural environment and thereby to prejudice the health or survival of the population.[82]

167. It also lays down a principle under which:

> works or installations containing dangerous forces, namely dams, dykes and nuclear electrical generating stations, shall not be made the object of attack ... if such attack may cause the release of dangerous forces and consequent severe losses among the civilian population ....[83]

168. It is significant that the provision just quoted is included in identical terms in Article 15 of Protocol II relating to non-international armed conflicts.

169. Armed attacks on nuclear installations are a concern as they might lead to releases of radioactive material. The Israeli attack on the Iraqi research reactor OSIRAK in 1981 occurred before that reactor had been loaded and the Iraqi attack on Busher in Iran occurred while the two power reactors had no nuclear equipment. It is to be regretted that the provisions are limited to "nuclear electrical generating stations", as installations for the storage of nuclear waste and for the reprocessing of such waste would be susceptible of more serious releases of radioactive material than those protected. The reason for this limitation might be that spent nuclear fuel and reprocessing plants could contribute to the production of plutonium for weapons production.

82. See supra para. 162 regarding the formulation in the ENMOD Convention.
83. Art. 56 (1).

*viii. Prohibition of the deployment of weapons*

170. Treaties prohibiting the deployment of nuclear or other weapons of mass destruction in a given area or environment seek to reduce the risk that the weapons will be put to use in that area or environment.

171. Treaties establishing nuclear weapon-free zones have the primary aim of committing the States in the zone not to acquire nuclear weapons. However, in addition, some of the treaties also explicitly prohibit the deployment of nuclear weapons in the territory of the zonal States. This emerges from the Tlatelolco and Rarotonga Treaties.[84] Each of these treaties also has a protocol attached to it, under which outside powers may commit themselves not to introduce nuclear weapons into territories for which they are *de facto* or *de jure* responsible within the respective zone. A net effect of these provisions is to preclude the arrangement which was followed within NATO, where some non-nuclear weapons member States which were also parties to the NPT were hosts of nuclear weapons under US control. The protocols have been signed with a variety of reservations and declarations by the States concerned.

*ix. The Antarctic Treaty of 1959*

172. The Antarctic Treaty stipulates that:

> Antarctica shall be used for peaceful purposes only. There shall be prohibited, inter alia, any measures of a military nature, such as the establishment of military bases and fortifications, the carrying out of military manoeuvres, as well as the testing of any type of weapons.[85]

173. The treaty is sometimes characterized as establishing the world's first nuclear weapon-free zone, which is not wrong. However, the article cited evidently goes further and prohibits the deployment of any military weapons. The treaty has detailed provisions permitting aerial observation and obliging the parties to keep all their

84. Art. 1 (1)(b) of the 1967 Tlatelolco Treaty (for Latin America) and Art. 5 of the Rarotonga Treaty (for the South Pacific).

85. Art. I (1).

stations and installations mutually open to inspection by "observers".[86]

*x. The Outer Space Treaty of 1967*

174. The Outer Space Treaty requires that:

> States Parties to the Treaty undertake not to place in orbit around the earth any objects carrying nuclear weapons or any other kinds of weapons of mass destruction, install such weapons on celestial bodies, or station such weapons in outer space in any other manner.[87]

175. Similarly to the Antarctic Treaty, the Outer Space Treaty contains provisions requiring mutual openness[88] and the possibility for "visits".[89]

*xi. The Seabed Treaty (1971)*

176. While in the Antarctic Treaty and in the Outer Space Treaty the non-deployment of weapons is only one objective among several others, the Seabed Treaty of 1971 has the non-deployment of weapons of mass destruction and facilities related to the storing, testing or using such weapons as its sole objective.[90] It contains explicit provisions about the right mutually to verify compliance through observation.[91] Where doubts about compliance remain the parties shall co-operate to find procedures for verification, including appropriate inspection.[92] In the last resort a party may refer the matter to the Security Council,[93] a provision which has no parallel in the less security-related treaties about the Antarctic and Outer Space.

86. Art. VII.

87. Art. IV.

88. Art. X.

89. Not inspections, Article XII.

90. Art. I (1).

91. Art. III (1).

92. Art. III (2).

93. Art. III (4).

## d. *Prohibition of development and acquisition of specific weapons*

177. The prohibition of development and acquisition of specific weapons obviously represents a more ambitious approach than a prohibition of use or a restriction in use or numbers. If a State has no nuclear, chemical or biological weapons, it can use none. So great has been the concern for the dangers of a world loaded with nuclear, chemical and biological weapons that as regards these types of weapons it has been considered desirable to go beyond mere prohibitions of use and seek bans on the very possession of the weapons. A number of treaties have this purpose.

### i. *The Non-Proliferation Treaty (1968)*

178. The NPT may be seen as a dual bargain to attain a nuclear weapon-free world. The treaty obliges non-nuclear-weapon States parties to refrain from acquiring nuclear weapons[94] and nuclear-weapon States parties (as well as other parties) to negotiate in good faith toward nuclear disarmament and general and complete disarmament.[95] It entered into force in 1970 and was extended without time limit in 1995. It is the most adhered to of all arms control agreements, having some 180 parties.

179. The NPT is supplemented by a number of treaties committing States within specific regions to non-nuclear weapon status. In addition to the basic obligation these treaties contain provisions of special interest to the specific regions. Even before the NPT was concluded, the Tlatelolco Treaty for the Prohibition of Nuclear Weapons in Latin America was signed in 1967. It was the first agreement after the Antarctic Treaty of 1961 to establish a nuclear weapon-free area. Several other regional instruments of similar thrust have been concluded later, notably:

- the 1985 Treaty of Rarotonga for the South Pacific,
- the 1995 Treaty of Bangkok for Southeast Asia, and
- the 1996 Treaty of Pelindaba for Africa.

94. Art. II.

95. Art. VI.

180. The philosophy of the NPT might be said to seek commitments by all States which had not already at the time of the conclusion of the treaty, by carrying out test explosions manifested themselves as nuclear-weapon States, to remain without such weapons, and to seek a commitment of the five declared nuclear-weapon States to negotiate toward an elimination of those weapons. The difference between the two types of commitment must be noted. In the case of non-nuclear-weapon States the commitment not to acquire nuclear weapons is absolute. In the case of the nuclear-weapon States there is only an obligation to negotiate toward nuclear disarmament[96] and, for that matter, toward general and complete disarmament.[97]

181. During the nuclear armament race in the long years of the Cold War, the failure of the nuclear-weapon States to pursue effective negotiations on nuclear disarmament made the latter obligation look cosmetic. In the view of many it concealed a permanent non-recognized, yet real, difference between the two categories of States. This criticism was stressed at the conference in 1995 at which the NPT was extended for an indefinite period of time. However, with the INF Treaty (1987), START I (1991) and II (1993), the withdrawal by the United States and the Soviet Union of tactical nuclear weapons from foreign territory and from ships (1991) and the incipient discussions about a total elimination of nuclear weapons, it would seem that both declared aims of the NPT have become credible.

182. The NPT as well as the various nuclear weapon-free zones contain provisions which require that the States committing themselves to non-proliferation shall accept verification that their various programmes and projects for the peaceful use of nuclear energy are not misused to develop or prepare for the development of nuclear weapons. In all cases such verification is effected through comprehensive IAEA safeguards. India, Israel and Pakistan, which have not adhered to the NPT, have submitted some specific nuclear instal-

96. Art. VI.

97. The ICJ in 1996 stressed the obligation of the parties not only to negotiate but also to bring such negotiations to a conclusion, see supra, paras. 136 and 143.

lations to IAEA safeguards. In these cases the safeguards verification has only the objective of verifying that the specific installations are not used in support of weapons-related programmes. The five nuclear-weapon States parties to the NPT have also on a voluntary basis accepted IAEA safeguards on some or all of their peaceful nuclear installations.

183. Questions relating to safeguards and nuclear verification will be discussed in some detail below.[98]

*ii. Biological Weapons Convention (1972)*

184. A Convention on the Prohibition of the Development, Production and Stockpiling of Bacteriological (biological) and Toxin Weapons and on their Destruction was concluded in 1972. Unlike the NPT discussed above, the Chemical Weapons Convention discussed below and the Complete Test Ban Treaty, the Convention does not (yet) have an institutional mechanism for verification. Like the ENMOD Convention[99] it enjoins the parties to "consult one another and to co-operate in solving any problems which may arise in relation to the objective of ... the Convention."[100] A party that finds that another party is acting in breach may complain to the Security Council, presenting "all possible evidence." Parties are obliged to co-operate in carrying out any investigation intiated by the Council.[101] A Test Ban Treaty-type withdrawal clause is also provided.[102] Efforts are at present underway to negotiate a specific verification agreement supplementing the prohibitions contained in the biological weapons Convention.

185. It should perhaps be noted that while in the first half of the 20th century biological weapons were considered as somewhat exotic and were long believed to be practically difficult to use in a militarily

98. See paras. 216 et seq.

99. See supra, para. 162.

100. Art. V.

101. Art. VI (1, 2).

102. Art. XIII (2).

effective way, there has been a more recent concern that these weapons - as well as chemical weapons - might be seen and developed as the "poor man's" weapons of mass destruction and that the practical problems in using them might be overcome. The revelations during inspections in Iraq, especially in 1998, have confirmed these fears and contributed to the determination to add a verification mechanism to the prohibition of the production and acquisition of the weapons.

*iii. The Chemical Weapons Convention (1993)*

186. After many years of negotiations the Convention on the Prohibition of the Development, Production, Stockpiling and Use of Chemical Weapons and on their Destruction, the Chemical Weapons Convention (CWC), was signed on 13 January 1993 in Paris. As its official title shows, it contains comprehensive prohibitions regarding chemical weapons, including the confirmation of the prohibition of their use.[103] It also provides an extensive regime of verification, which in many respects is inspired by the safeguards system of the IAEA but also improves on that system. An international "technical" secretariat, including staff for on-site inspections, has been established at The Hague[104] and elaborate rules concerning clarification, consultation and challenge inspections are laid down.[105] In cases of particular gravity a Conference of the parties shall bring the issue to the attention of the UN General Assembly and Security Council.[106] The Convention contains a Test Ban Treaty-type clause allowing a party to withdraw "if it decides that extraordinary events related to the subject-matter of this Convention, have jeopardized the supreme interests of its country".[107]

103. See supra, para. 112, on the 1925 Geneva Protocol.

104. Art. VIII (D).

105. Art. IX. See further infra, para. 275.

106. Art. XII (4).

107. Art. XVI (2).

*iv. The Ottawa Convention on Anti-personnel Mines (1997)*

187. The Ottawa Convention on Anti-personnel Mines was signed on 18 September 1997. It contains provisions on the prohibition of use, stockpiling, production and transfer of anti-personnel mines and on their destruction. This arms control agreement is unusual in that action by non-governmental organizations was instrumental in inducing its negotiation and adoption. The motivations were the same as those which animated the weapons restrictions reached at the turn of the century, above all the tragic and cruel effects upon civilians of the many millions of anti-personnel mines which have been used, many of which remain active decades after the end of hostilities.

188. In providing for the total elimination and destruction of anti-personnel mines[108] the Ottawa Convention goes far beyond the 1981 Protocol on prohibitions and restrictions on the use of mines, booby-traps and other devices.[109] The treaty obliges the parties to report to the Secretary-General within 180 days of entry into force on specific implementation measures which are to be taken.[110]

189. No ongoing or periodic verification is foreseen, but annual meetings of the parties are foreseen to consider application and implementation. Furthermore, a party wishing clarification of questions relating to compliance can set in motion procedures under which, in the last resort, a special meeting of the parties may be called, which may decide by simple majority on the dispatch of a fact-finding mission of experts to collect additional information on the spot or in other places directly related to the alleged compliance issue.[111] Such a mission must be received, may bring equipment necessary for its task, be "given the opportunity to speak to all relevant persons" and be granted access "to all areas and installations ... where facts relevant to the compliance issue could be expected to be collected." The mission shall report through the Secretary-General to the

108. Art. 1 (1-2).

109. See supra, para. 127.

110. Art. 7.

111. Art. 8 (1-10).

meeting of the parties.[112] Provisions on certain restrictions on access, e.g. regarding "sensitive equipment, information and areas"[113] may have been inspired partly by formulas in the recent IAEA protocol on strengthened safeguards.[114]

190. The Convention obviously creates a very intrusive verification regime. Considering that a number of important countries taking part in its negotiation strongly objected to the idea of verification, especially of production and stockpiling, there will remain a risk of non-adherence or, at any rate, a risk of resistance to putting this regime into operation in concrete cases.

### II.4 Actual arms control and disarmament achieved compared to stated aims

191. It was noted at the beginning of this report[115] that the aspiration of the First Hague Peace Conference to reduce the burden of armaments was not successful. The Conference was followed by an arms race and the First World War. During the interwar period extensive - and not very successful - efforts were made to achieve disarmament, only to be followed by the Second World War. What of the efforts made during the second half of the 20th century: how should they be assessed?

192. As pointed out earlier,[116] the aspirations of the Conference to save resources through disarmament and to reduce the horrors of war through general restrictions on the use of arms and prohibitions of specific arms, have remained fully relevant. A number of further rationales or aims were identified, which seem to have inspired

112. Art. 8 (11-17).

113. Art. 8 (14 b).

114. See Art. 7 of IAEA INFCIRC / 540 of 1997.

115. Para. 47.

116. Paras. 57-58.

modern arms control and disarmament measures.[117] After our overview of a great many arms control and disarmament measures which have been accomplished, it might be appropriate at this point to assess - briefly - to what extent the post-World War II generations have been able to realize their aspirations in this area.

### a. *Economy. Saving of resources*

193. For a number of years during the 1970s and 1980s the economic rationale was highlighted under the item "Disarmament and Development", which figured prominently on the international agenda, notably at the United Nations. Extensive studies were undertaken and ample evidence was provided about the enormous resources - in terms of men, money and material - that could be saved if less were spent on armaments and how they could be transferred to productive development. In the chilly security climate that prevailed at the time between the great military powers these studies and exhortations had little or no impact. "General and complete disarmament" was invoked in every possible context for long periods, but was scarcely taken seriously and is not discussed today.

194. What we have seen in the post-World War Two era as a whole is a tremendous development in expensive high-technology military equipment sought by practically all countries and, in addition, a spread of armaments to many developing countries which can afford them even less than the richer countries.

195. This dismaying assessment must not, however, cloud the fact that in the favourable global security climate which arose as the Cold War petered out and gave place to détente among the great powers, very significant cuts were made in military resources which were burdensome and excessive. Thus, the CFE achieved substantial

117. Paras. 61-69.

reductions in conventional armaments in Europe, and START I[118] and START II[119] enable and oblige the United States and Russia to dismantle vast numbers of nuclear warheads.

196. In view of what appeared like a wave of disarmament there was a good deal of discussion about a "peace dividend", part of which many hoped would result in more aid to developing countries. However, although reductions in military budgets have been a common - but by no means universal - feature resulting from the détente, whatever dividends there were in industrialized countries did not increase public assistance to developing countries. And while in some regions of developing countries, like Latin America, the security climate has generally been favourable for arms restraint, some other regions where tensions remain high, notably the Middle East, have continued to carry very heavy military expenditures.

197. A point that should perhaps also be noted here is that disarmament does not always bring an immediate economic gain. For instance, the dismantling of nuclear weapons that is taking place at an accelerated pace in the United States and Russia is a complicated and expensive process, and safely storing the huge quantities of highly enriched uranium and plutonium and refashioning them into fuel for power reactors or disposing of them also draw costs. Enormous costs are also incurred by the extensive satellite and other surveillance and intelligence systems used by the great powers to give mutual confidence that arms control and disarmament commitments are respected.

198. Yet, not building more intercontinental missiles and warheads saves resources. Perhaps not so many swords will be made into ploughshares but generating electricity by burning plutonium from dismantled warheads is also an attractive proposition. Moreover, while the economic motive of disarmament remains valid, today the security and stability sought are even more important.

118. 1991.

119. 1993, but not yet in force.

199. In the spring of 1999, unfortunately, there are not only military tensions and even armed conflicts in several regions, but détente between the great powers has come under some strain. A continued reduction of military budgets still remains a common feature but cannot be taken for granted unless confidence is restored that global détente resumes.

*b. Abhorrence of specific weapons*

200. The abhorrence of weapons of mass destruction and of the massing of weapons and techniques of warfare which are liable to cause great losses of in life and mass destruction of property and environment have remained a central ground for the modern demands for arms control and disarmament.

201. There have been some recent successes in this area. The ban of the Geneva Protocol of 1925 on the use of chemical and bacteriological weapons has been confirmed and transformed into bans on production and possession. Such bans have also been adopted regarding antipersonnel landmines, although it is yet uncertain how effective the new Convention will be. Some other minor restrictions have been adopted, e.g. relating to the use of blinding lasers as an antipersonnel weapon.

202. The major debate has concerned the demands for a universal ban on the use, first use, production and possession of nuclear weapons. On the whole these demands have not been successful and, although their numbers recently have gone down somewhat, they still hang as a sword of Damocles over the world. During the long years of the Cold War considerations of security easily prevailed over demands by important segments of public opinion.

203. Nevertheless, although the nuclear-weapon States have recognized only very qualified - and uncertain - restrictions on their

latitude to use these weapons,[120] we can register the successful adoption of some rules to limit the testing and deployment of nuclear weapons, and to limit possession of them to a few States. Moreover, as the Cold War has subsided, drastic reductions are on the way in the huge stockpiles of nuclear weapons; the whole category of intermediate range nuclear missiles has been discarded, and tactical nuclear weapons such as nuclear artillery shells and mines have been destroyed or withdrawn. Certainly, we must note that with détente the great military powers have been moving decisively in the direction of nuclear disarmament, as is in their own and everybody's interest.[121] Yet, enough remains to pose horrible dangers to the world for many years. The complete elimination of nuclear weapons, although now broached as a serious subject, is not around the corner.

204. Further, it is clear that although the 1977 Additional Protocols have modernized the laws of war and maintained the principle that civilians must not be the object of attack, modern wars cause ever greater numbers of civilian casualties. The old concept of "unnecessary suffering" remains valid and recognized, but so many more means and methods of warfare have been developed which the States - the potential parties to armed conflict - find "necessary". Fragmentation bombs, incendiary weapons and many others remain in use. The dum-dum bullet was banned in 1899, but the small-calibre high-velocity bullet is in use today. And although for the first time Additional Protocol II seeks to introduce some restraints in non-international conflicts, the actual practices of armed forces and "para-military forces" in Yugoslavia, Sierra Leone or Zaire have been horrifying. Armed conflicts have not become less inhumane.

120. Negative security guarantees, commitments under nuclear weapon free zone treaties.

121. And as is required under Art. VI of the NPT.

*c. Reliability of prohibitions and restrictions*

205. The strongest guarantee against the use of a weapon is its non-existence. It was the arrival of nuclear weapons that convinced governments that prohibitions of use, mutual deterrence[122] and the right of retaliation are not good enough, and that led them to make agreements under which bans on production and possession are accepted by all but eight States of the world. How to bring these eight States to zero nuclear weapons is now a problem on which serious discussion has started,[123] but which will be with us for a long time.

206. Meanwhile the philosophy which developed for nuclear weapons rubbed off on two other categories of "weapons of mass destruction", namely, the chemical and the biological, and here the efforts to agree on bans on production and possession have been successful. The same is true for antipersonnel landmines.

207. While bans on the use of weapons which it was not illegal to produce or possess,[124] were never coupled with ready procedures for verification of possible violations, confidence in the reliability of commitments to non-production and non-possession requires elaborate systems of verification, including on-site verification. Such systems - global,[125] regional[126] and bilateral[127] - are well established for nuclear weapons. For chemical weapons a global system of verification is developing and for biological weapons it is under negotiation.

208. In addition, extensive systems of verification have been created bilaterally between the United States and Russia to verify reductions

122. As in the case of gas.

123. E.g., Report of the Canberra Commission on the Elimination of Nuclear Weapons, August 1996.

124. Like the bans in the 1925 Geneva Protocol.

125. IAEA.

126. Euratom.

127. Argentina/Brazil.

in the nuclear and missile capacities of these two States, and multilaterally to verify reductions in conventional armaments in Europe. The most recent multilateral verification system is that which is being set up monitor the 1996 Comprehensive Test Ban Treaty.

209. The development of effective systems and institutions for verification of arms control and disarmament agreements is of great importance as such systems may allow parties to have confidence that neighbours and other parties respect their commitments. This development as well as a greater general readiness to accept openness and practise greater transparency constitutes major progress compared to earlier periods. An example is the 1992 Treaty on Open Skies. However, this remarkable new development is by no means without problems and the subject of verification will therefore be discussed in a subsequent separate section.

### *d. Strategic stability*

210. Without strategic stability through arms control agreements or otherwise there is a greater risk that competitors will race as fast as they can afford to avoid falling behind the feared "progress" of the competitor.

211. The ABM Treaty would appear to be a major success, under which the parties made themselves mutually vulnerable to a second strike and thereby reduced the need for great stocks of strategic missiles and weapons. True, the more actors on the globe may acquire an important missile capacity and some weapons of mass destruction capacity, the riskier such a deliberate vulnerability may be. It is a serious question, however, whether the response to the hypothetical threat of some lesser actors should be sought in measures which might undermine strategic stability between the larger actors.

*e. Protecting the environment*

212. Concern for the environment is increasing generally in the world and the devastation brought by area bombardment, the lasting dangers caused in large areas by land-mines and the risk of catastrophes resulting from destruction of various huge installations, like hydro-dams, have led to agreements demanding restraint.[128]

213. In practical terms the 1963 PTBT probably did more than any other arms control treaty to spare the environment from negative impacts.

*f. Limiting the military capacity of aggressor States*

214. Such limitations may be required in certain situations and may for a period of time be of significance to put a lid on a difficult actor. We have also seen how after World War II the prohibitions in Peace Treaties on the development of nuclear weapons helped the vanquished States to transform to a nuclear weapon-free status under the NPT.

215. Nevertheless, commitments which are accepted only because a vanquished State wishes to avoid the consequences of further conflict are, as experience has shown, less dependable than those that are reached without duress.

128. See supra, paras. 161 et seq. In a booklet entitled "War and the Environment" (Stockholm 1981) the rapporteur has written an article on the subject "Arms control treaties aimed at reducing the military impact on the environment".

## III. The issue of verification

216. It may be taken for granted that the First Hague Peace Conference was as anxious as any diplomatic conference to see full compliance with the rules it adopted, for instance the ban on the use of gas. Yet, no step was taken to create any machinery or mechanism which could help to establish authoritatively whether violations had occurred. It was probably assumed that such violations, occurring in war, would be manifest and the consequent risk of retaliation in kind - or not in kind - would act as a deterrent against violations. The first assumption worked in the First World War - the use of gas was manifest - and after that war it has been possible in most cases to establish some *ad hoc* inquiry, when needed. The second assumption failed in the First World War, when gas was used by belligerents on both sides, but it worked in the Second World War when all parties refrained from using gas - as it is believed - for fear of retaliation.

217. The demand for compliance in peace-time with rules requiring reductions in the numbers of particular weapons or the non-possession of some types of weapons which might be easily concealed, raises the issue of verification in a serious way. The storage of, say, canisters of gas, especially in closed societies, will not be manifest as the use of the gas might be in war. Yet, if a State is to destroy its stock of chemical weapons pursuant to an agreement, it will want to be confident that potential adversaries parties to the agreement do the same. If a State is to reduce its number of some type of missile under an agreement that is believed to establish parity with another party, it will want to be confident that the other party respects its part of the bargain. In such cases States may seek that confidence - or early warning about violations - through different means: the scanning of media, intelligence, satellite surveillance, or an agreed mechanism of verification that may include on-site inspection in other countries. Indeed, we have found that such verification now has become a central issue and an indispensable element in practically all bans or limitations on specific weapons. As we look forward to further regulations in the arms control and dis-

armament field, we therefore have reason to analyse problems and possibilities which exist in the field of verification and on-site inspection. An extensive practice already exists, as has been shown in earlier sections of this report. Much has, of course been written and published about the issue of verification.[129]

218. The establishment of procedures, mechanisms and machinery for effective verification, including on-site inspection, in the fields of arms control and disarmament encounters the difficulty that States traditionally are very jealous about exercising exclusive control over their territories. It would in all likelihood have been difficult to get acceptance of any such verification before the Second World War. Even during the discussions of the question of general and complete disarmament in the 1960s it was held by the Soviet Union - at that time a closed State - that inspection, except for witnessing the actual destruction of weapons, would be tantamount to espionage.

219. The world has come a long way since such attitudes dominated our thinking. It is now generally realized that in a world moving toward fewer weapons, notably fewer weapons of mass destruction, extensive verification and on-site inspection are indispensable. Indeed, the more far-reaching the restrictions contemplated, the stronger verification will be demanded to give confidence against undetected violations. For instance, if an agreement were reached setting a ceiling at 1000 for some weapon, non-detection of 10 or even 100 over that number might perhaps not matter much in terms of security,[130] but if the commitment were to have been to zero weapons, non-detection of even one could be a more dramatic matter.

129. Reference may be made here to two UN studies, in UN Doc. A/45/372 of 28 August 1990 and UN Doc. A/50/377 of 22 September 1995.

130. Depending upon the kind of weapon the restriction applied to.

220. Part of the reason for the long delay in the achievement of the CTBT[131] was the position taken by several States that it could not be adequately verified, given the control techniques existing at the time. In the discussion of proposals for a complete elimination of nuclear weapons the verification issue will be prominent, as can be seen from the Canberra Report.[132]

221. With détente and growing international integration, governments have generally become much more accommodating as regards the acceptance of verification, the provision of information on items subject to verification and on-site inspection. The notion that "sovereignty" somehow conceptually makes it impossible for a government to accept that functionaries of a foreign State or an international organization perform some official activities within its jurisdiction is giving way to a more pragmatic - but still restrictive - attitude which accepts some verification activities, when they are deemed to be in the interest of the State and take place on the basis of agreed rules. Indeed, one might turn the arguments about unwelcome intrusions around and suggest that at least impartial international verification and on-site inspection constitute a service to a State! After all, the State has a direct interest in convincing neighbours and the world that it is abiding by its arms control or disarmament obligations or else face the consequences of suspicions which could arise in the absence of impartial credible control. To draw a prosaic parallel: inspections by municipal authorities that the sanitary conditions in restaurants are satisfactory give customers confidence to go to them.

222. It is another matter that any inspection - into any sphere - should be made as little intrusive, expensive and cumbersome as is compatible with the need to achieve confidence. As will be discussed below, some modern techniques have proved helpful by being very effective without being very intrusive.

131. See supra, para. 156.

132. Op. cit. note 123.

## III.1 Procedures, mechanisms and institutions for verification

223. There is a wide spectrum of procedures, mechanisms and institutions that can be employed for verification and on-site inspection.

224. Even below the level of prepared procedures, mechanisms and institutions importance is rightly attached to general openness and transparency. Open, democratically organized States with a free inquisitive press and citizens who do not fear to express themselves, naturally raise less difficulties in terms of credible verification than closed authoritarian societies, where the possibility of concealing violations of arms control commitments is greater.

225. At the lower end of the spectrum we find arrangements and ready procedures for the creation of fact finding expert groups. Thus,[133] a resolution of the UN General Assembly allowed the Secretary-General to appoint such groups to investigate possible violations of the 1925 Geneva Protocol prohibiting the use of gas in armed conflicts. Another example is found in Article VI of the 1972 Biological Weapons Convention,[134] which stipulates that the Security Council is the appropriate organ to which complaints can be directed and obliges parties to the Convention to co-operate with the Council in investigations. To sum up, the creation of *ad hoc* groups for verification is rarely likely to pose insuperable problems. Getting co-operation from the State on whose territory the verification is to take place, may prove the difficult part.

226. We also find at the lower end of the spectrum treaties which diplomatically refer to "visits" rather than "inspections."[135]

133. As noted supra, para. 117.

134. The Convention still does not have a special institution set up for verification.

135. See supra, paras. 173 and 174 for the 1967 Outer Space Treaty, and for the 1959 Antarctic Treaty, which refers to "inspection" by "observers."

### *a. Inspection in bilateral relations*

227. In the early days of nuclear exports, agreements between the United States and importing countries stipulated visits by US inspectors to verify that the imported material or equipment was used only for peaceful purposes, as required by the agreements. Later, such inspection rights were transferred to the IAEA.

228. The acceptance of inspectors representing a global organization in which the inspected country is a member is usually less difficult for such country than bilateral inspection. However, this report has cited several US-Russian agreements in the field of nuclear arms control and disarmament, which establish large-scale bilateral verification schemes, including extensive on-site inspection.[136]

229. Doubtless, in instances like these the two major nuclear-weapon States would not accept outside inspection. For one thing, out of non-proliferation concerns they might want to have inspectors only from States which themselves have nuclear weapons. For another, they might wish to be able themselves to press directly for the clarification of any questions arising rather than relying on an independent outside inspectorate. A third reason might be cost. If the parties themselves have to foot the bill for inspection, why not carry it out themselves? Yet, in another context, where nuclear material is moved from the military to the peaceful sector in Russia and the United States, the thinking in the two States moves in the direction of asking the IAEA to verify the exclusively peaceful use or storage of the material.[137] In this case the interest of the outside world to be ensured that the two States are actually doing away with their weapons-usable material needs to be taken into account.

136. See supra, para. 92 for the INF Treaty and para. 96 for START I.

137. See supra, para. 109.

### b. *Verification on regional basis*

230. There are a few regional verification mechanisms. The oldest is that of Euratom for the countries of the European Union. It predates the IAEA safeguards system. When safeguards verification was to be established for the non-nuclear-weapon States of the European Community in pursuance of their adherence to the 1968 NPT, agreement could only be reached on the use of IAEA safeguards, as European verification was seen by some as "self-inspection". The result was a rather costly duplication which has been alleviated only a few years ago. The lesson, however, is probably that regional verification may not have full credibility unless the relations between the parties in the region appear to ensure sufficient vigilance.

231. The 1990 Treaty on Conventional Armed Forces in Europe (CFE) which regulates very significant disarmament in the larger European space has an elaborate system of verification of its own, including on-site inspection.[138]

### c. *Verification by global organizations*

232. Global organizations responsible for verification and on-site inspection are the IAEA,[139] the Organization for the Prohibition of Chemical Weapons (OPCW),[140] the CTBTO,[141] and the UN Special Commission on Iraq (UNSCOM).[142]

138. See supra, para. 75.

139. For inspection by the Agency under the NPT, see supra, para. 182 and infra in this section.

140. See supra, para. 186 and infra in this section.

141. See supra, para. 159 and infra in this section.

142. See infra in this section.

### *d. Bilateral vs. regional and global verification*

233. Although this section focusses on questions raised in verification by globally based institutions, some comments may be warranted on the choice between bilateral, regional or global arrangements or combinations thereof. Reference has already been made to the historical reasons why there is a European Union based nuclear verification system overlapping with the globally based one. Some reasons why the large nuclear-weapon States have chosen bilateral verification systems for fundamentally important arms control agreements have also been noted, a basic one being that they consider the verification of these agreements so vital to their security that they trust only themselves to administer it.

234. There may be some justification for the concern that authorities of an inspected State may feel less inhibited to try to "push around" an international inspectorate than an inspector from a great Power with which the State has delicate relations and whose government is able and likely to react quickly and strongly to any attempt to interpret their inspection rights narrowly. However, if the States members of the international organizations are sufficiently supportive of the international verification and inspection system (without meddling in the management) and the secretariats of the organizations are ready to make use of that support without dangerous delay, the risk of too great tolerance and patience on their part should be.

235. It is of interest to note the view sometimes expressed that UNSCOM, being a "subsidiary organ" of the Security Council[143] very frequently reporting to it and obtaining its support in the efforts to inspect Iraq and eradicate weapons of mass destruction, was a desirable model. However, too close an embrace by supportive, forceful member States may also have its risk, as some problems surrounding UNSCOM have shown. In a report by a panel established by the Council in 1999 it is stated that:

143. Under Art. 29 of the Charter.

> As a subordinate organ of the Security Council, the executive body derives its effectiveness and authority from this close relationship, both in terms of political supervision and of providing support for its activities.[144]

236. At the same time the Panel stated its view that recourse to cost-free personnel (supplied by member States) should be limited and efforts should be made "to increase, wherever operationally possible, personnel employed directly by the United Nations", appointed on one-year terms as international civil servants subject to Article 100 of the Charter, i.e. staff obliged not "to seek or receive instructions from any government or from any other authority external to the Organization."[145]

237. The choice between a bilateral and an international basis for verification might be influenced not only by preferences as to whether inspectors' loyalty should be to an appointing national State or to an impartial organization. It might also be influenced by the circumstance that nationally appointed inspectors may be more easily given access to intelligence available to the appointing State. Some discussions within the IAEA in connection with a resolution concerning the possible establishment of a nuclear weapon free zone in the Middle East were instructive in this regard.[146] What emerged from this discussion and the resolution adopted was that the States concerned in the region seemed to envisage that adherence to the NPT - and NPT-type international inspection - should complement a nuclear weapon-free zone providing for more intrusive inspection, including the mutual right to challenge inspections[147] and employing inspectors directly responsible to the various participating countries. To quote one official concerned in the region:

> Under mutual verification the inspector goes to the field with the full backing of his or her country's institutional power. Put simply, if the

144. UN Doc. S/1999/356 , 30 March 1999.

145. Ibid.

146. Resolution adopted by the General Conference on 3 October 1997.

147. See infra, paras. 272 et seq.

country's intelligence service suspects anything, this information could be made available to help the inspector define what is wrong and where to go.[148]

### e. *One consolidated UN verification organization ?*

238. It should lastly be mentioned in this section that suggestions have sometimes been made that the various globally based verification organizations might be merged into one UN verification agency. Such a merger might appear superficially attractive and likely to offer some gains of synergy. It is also probable that if some State were trying to violate the commitment it has made with regard to one type of weapon, it might likely have done the same with other commitments (as Iraq did). One single organization might be more able to investigate the violations than several organizations acting independently of each other.

239. However, any merger would meet formidable difficulties, as the different organizations operate on the basis of treaties which are not harmonized and which will not easily be modified. Before the CTBTO was set up as a separate body there were suggestions that its functions could have been performed by the IAEA and that this would have saved many millions of dollars per year. However, for a variety of reasons the suggestion was strongly resisted by some and no one seems to have felt that economy and streamlining was worth insisting upon when it was difficult enough to get agreement on the treaty.

240. On the other hand, even though the various organizations - IAEA (for nuclear programmes), OPCW (for chemical weapons), CTBTO (for the comprehensive test ban) and soon, hopefully, a new organization to verify compliance with the Biological Weapons Convention - will be unable to exchange any confidential information, a

148. See IAEA, Personal Reflections, Vienna 1997, p.282.

measure of exchange of experience should be possible and useful and co-location of several organizations would appear desirable.

### *1. States' declarations as the starting basis for verification*

241. In many schemes of verification, like the IAEA safeguards system pursuant to the Non-Proliferation Treaty (1968), the system under the Chemical Weapons Convention (1993) and the system set up under the Ottawa Convention on Anti-Personnel Mines (1997) declarations by the State accepting verification about its possession of items to be declared - fissionable material, various chemicals, mines etc. - form the starting basis of the system. The preparation of such declarations may require considerable work by the government and industry of a State. There may also be some benefit in this to the governments: they may well, for their own purposes, want to have full knowledge of, say, various nuclear or chemical activities which take place within their borders. The international verification of such declarations may provide the State with a highly desirable quality control.

242. For the international organization receiving the declarations, the data provide vitally important starting points which can be checked for internal consistency and form the basis for requests for more information, if need be. Their correctness and completeness is checked inter alia through on-site inspection by international inspectors. However, both in view of the general wish of States to minimize the presence of inspectors and of the cost of such visits, reliance on remote monitoring and automatic data transmission and on other means of verification not requiring on-site inspection, are of increasing importance.

### 2. *Means of verification not requiring access to the State: "national technical means of verification".*

243. The expression "national technical means of verification" signals means which are under the full control of a State and which do not require any co-operation from the State on which the verification is focussed. These means can consequently be used without consent, even against the will of another State. Important examples are satellite observation, seismic monitoring and analysis of samples of water or air. "Intelligence", covering information obtained through clandestine means, interrogation of defectors, or the systematic scanning of open sources etc., may not literally fit under the expression "technical means", but in practical terms they do seem to be included.

#### *i. satellites*

244. Observations through the use of satellites have helped enormously to give States confidence that commitments made about arms control and disarmament measures are respected. They were of particular importance in East-West relations before on-site inspection was acceptable. While U 2 planes violated national airspace (and, as experience shows, could be shot down), international law told us that the satellites circled the world at levels above and beyond national sovereignty. When mutual confidence became a desirable commodity between the superpowers, the merits of satellite surveillance became evident. Several agreements referred to in this report even lay down bans on any interference with satellite surveillance and concealment from such surveillance.[149] Satellites go a long way to prevent surprises and they do it elegantly, with increasing precision and without intrusiveness on the ground or complex negotiations.

245. Satellites remain an important tool to assure a good deal of transparency in the arms control and disarmament area. A Soviet satellite discovered the South-African preparations for a nuclear test

149. See the CFE and INF treaties described supra, paras. 75 and 91.

in the Kalahari desert in 1977 and US satellite pictures were of great value in 1991 to show the Board of Governors of the IAEA relevant nuclear installations in the DPRK. At that time a few members of the Board were reluctant to accept this type of evidence. However, as satellite imagery becomes ever more precise and revealing and as it becomes available from several States and even on a commercial basis, the reluctance is likely to give way. Nevertheless one should not be lulled into confidence that everything of interest to arms control and disarmament is detected. Satellites photograph only that on which their masters train the cameras. The Argentine enrichment plant at Pilcanyio was not sighted before its existence was announced by the Argentine government and the large research reactor which China helped Algeria to build apparently was not spotted until several years into construction. The Indian nuclear test preparations in the spring of 1998 were evidently sufficiently well concealed for satellites not to spot them.[150]

*ii. analysis of samples*

246. The analysis of samples provides a powerful means of detecting the presence of various chemicals, biological substances or radio-nuclides. In order not to be so diluted that analysis becomes impossible, samples must in many cases be taken not too far away from where the source activity occurred. In practice this means that they need to come from the territory of a State, and this may involve the need of consent. However, in particular radio-nuclides are detectable even in very low concentrations, allowing detection even far away from the source.

247. For the detection of nuclear explosions in the atmosphere the radioactive fallout spreading with the winds is of decisive importance for detection. Samples of fallout taken far beyond the borders of the State initiating the explosion, will provide strong evidence of the

150. Perhaps it should be added that none of the activities mentioned were in violation of any international agreement

explosion. We find that the comprehensive CTBT relies on such samples (of air) as one method of verification.[151]

248. For the detection of other nuclear activities, e.g. enrichment of uranium or reprocessing of spent nuclear fuel, samples of water, air, soil or biota are becoming of great importance, but in most cases they must still be taken within the territory where the source activity occurred. Environmental sampling has been high on the verification agenda and has developed fast as a technique ever since the international community began to engage itself in mapping Iraq's programme to produce nuclear, chemical and biological weapons. What appears to have been the first evidence of Iraq's efforts to enrich uranium was obtained in 1990 when analysis was made of tiny particles stuck on the clothes of hostages who had been kept at the nuclear research centre Tuwaitha and who were released by Iraq. Since that time samples of water have been taken routinely in the waterways of Iraq by the IAEA under its Security Council mandate, to monitor that no unauthorized nuclear activity has been undertaken.

249. It should also be noted that the Model Protocol Additional to Safeguards Agreements, adopted by the IAEA in 1997 to strengthen the safeguards verification regime,[152] confirmed environmental sampling as an important tool. But here, as with Iraq, we are mostly concerned with samples taken within the territory of the State and with its consent. Even so these techniques may offer the great advantage that evidence (of compliance or non-compliance) can be obtained without a need for inspectors to have access to technologically sensitive parts of nuclear installations. The low level of intrusiveness of environmental sampling is a great asset. Yet, States which have had or still have nuclear weapon activities might turn out to be reluctant to give their consent to some such sampling, as it may give substantial information not only about the situation at the time of the sampling, but also about activities which took place long ago.

151. See supra, para. 159.

152. IAEA Doc. INFCIRC /540 Corr.

Indeed, it might be difficult to see from an analysis whether a nuclear activity which left traces was recent or from far back.

*iii. seismic monitoring*

250. The seismic effects of nuclear explosions underground will be detectable a long away from the site of the explosion and thus constitute evidence available without consent of the State. The CTBT relies on seismic monitoring as one of the main methods of verification and a widespread system of stations for such monitoring is established under the treaty.[153] While the development of the seismic techniques for the detection of nuclear underground explosions has helped to bring acceptance of the CTBT - and at the same time advanced seismic sciences - it is perhaps not likely that these techniques will be of use in any other arms control or disarmament context.

*iv. intelligence*

251. Intelligence is a broad term. Espionage, i.e. the compilation of information through illicit means, is only part of the concept. As noted above, intelligence may also comprise information through the interrogation of defectors, the monitoring of radio communications, the scanning of publicly available documents and prints, all of which is legal.

252. One of the conclusions of the IAEA after the discovery of the Iraqi illicit enrichment programme was that a systematic and continuous scanning of media could have given clues that Iraq was endeavouring to enrich uranium and could have prompted questions to Iraq. Such scanning was thereafter undertaken as a permanent feature of the safeguards system. This step met general support among member States and a scheme under which supplier States and importing States report to the Agency about their exports and imports of nuclear relevant equipment and material was also endorsed to strengthen the Agency's information base.

153. See supra, para. 159.

253. As might be expected, it is a more sensitive matter for international verification to make use of information which might have been obtained through clandestine means. The issue is not addressed directly in treaty texts. From reading these texts one might gain the impression that such information was not relevant.

254. The bilateral US-USSR INF Treaty of 1987 on the elimination of intermediate-range and shorter-range missiles provides that "each party shall use national technical means of verification at its disposal in a manner consistent with generally recognized principles of international law."[154] The rule is reinforced by providing that neither Party shall "interfere with national technical means of verification of the other Party operating in accordance with paragraph l of this Article."[155] Several other treaties contain the same type of clauses. In plainer language this should mean that information obtained through satellite observation and photography is recognized as relevant and permissible and must not be impeded. The same would evidently not go for information obtained through clandestine means, which are not "consistent with generally recognized principles of international law." Also, a party is free to interfere with such information gathering.

255. The more recent multilateral CTBT similarly allows a party to base a request for an on-site inspection "on any relevant technical information obtained by national technical means of verification in a manner consistent with generally recognized principles of international law."[156]

256. Under the CWC of 1993 a group of experts may be established to clarify a situation which may give rise to concern and such a group is authorized to examine "all available information and data

154. Art. XII (1).

155. Sub-para. 2 of the same Article.

156. Para. 37 of the treaty.

relevant to the situation causing the concern".[157] This provision seems more open-ended.

257. In the IAEA the issue never had any relevance before the Agency was mandated by the Security Council[158] to perform immediate on-site inspections "based on Iraq's declarations and the designation of any additional locations by the Special Commission" (i.e., UNSCOM). Although not articulated the idea was that intelligence organizations in member States should interface with UNSCOM and assist it with information which would help it to identify locations deserving inspection. It was UNSCOM's task to assess such information and decide whether it would designate a particular location for on-site inspection by the IAEA. The Agency was thus not contemplated as a direct recipient of intelligence. In practice direct briefings to the Agency often supplemented the designations made by UNSCOM.

258. There is no doubt that intelligence - in the broadest definition - has been of great importance to help both UNSCOM and the IAEA in their difficult task of mapping Iraq's clandestine programme for weapons of mass destruction. This experience raised the question to what extent, if any, a verifying organization would be justified in *other* cases to receive and make use of information coming from national intelligence. The question is not entirely academic. It is obvious that there will be significant restraints in the provision of intelligence by governments to verifying organizations, like the secretariats of the IAEA, the CWC and the CTBT. While satellite imagery might not be so difficult to share, information requiring the protection of sources might be hard to share with an organization which, as a matter of principle, recruits its international staff broadly. However, there are also some factors prompting offers of information. If hard and significant information were to exist in a national intelligence organization regarding a possible breach of a weapons commitment, and the responsible verification organization

157. Art. IX (4) (e).

158. Res. 687 of 1991.

were not somehow to be alerted, it would be difficult later to blame it for not being aware of what was going on.

259. No explicit guidance has been given to the IAEA Secretariat in these matters. That the Agency itself never engages in any clandestine information gathering goes without saying and there is scant guidance in government sponsored instruments. The 1995 NPT Review and Extension Conference expressed as one of its conclusions that:

> States parties that have concerns concerning non-compliance ... should direct such concerns, *along with supporting evidence and information*, to the IAEA to consider, investigate, draw conclusions and decide on necessary action in accordance with its mandate.

260. No restriction appears to have been set on what kind of information could be submitted to the Agency. Indeed, it would hardly be feasible to prevent a State - or, for that matter even a private individual, say a defector - from offering information to an international organization charged with the task of verification. If the organization routinely scans media, how could it reject information offered through other channels? Yet, it would appear that receiving intelligence - in the broadest sense - offered as a contribution to treaty-regulated verification by an international organization, rather than as a contribution to the specific Security Council-mandated regime of inspection and monitoring in Iraq,[159] would need to follow some strict ground rules, if it is to avoid objections from member States.

261. *First*, while the verifying organization might receive information from anyone, it should never use any but its own observations and data for conclusions. There is enough disinformation circulating to necessitate a critical analysis and assessment of all information volunteered and the avoidance of any conclusions based on data which the organization cannot independently verify. This is not to say that information proffered could not be of use. For instance,

159. Based on SC Res. 687 of 1991.

although not a basis for conclusions, it might help the verifying organization to look for relevant data or sites.

262. *Second*, the flow of information must be one way, i.e. the organization might receive, but cannot give anything back. An organization performing verification may acquire a great deal of confidential information and data from States accepting its verification. This confidentiality must continue to be scrupulously respected by the organizations, as is required by their rules. Indeed, in connection with the adoption in 1997 of the Model Protocol Additional to strengthen IAEA safeguards, the Board of the Agency requested a considerable strengthening of the rules on confidentiality of safeguards, as the new safeguards rules obliged governments to transmit much more information than was the case under the old rules.[160]

263. The apparent involvement of agents from national intelligence in UN and IAEA inspection operations under Security Council mandate in Iraq clearly damaged the international character of the operations. Although the two organizations were not under any obligation to observe confidentiality about their findings in Iraq and, indeed, were under a duty to report to the Security Council about them, it was for them and nobody else to make the findings and ensure that they related to the mandate given and nothing else. It would seem that the case shows, not that there should never be contacts between national intelligence and international inspectorates, but that such contacts must be handled prudently and with respect for rules and mandates given.

264. *Third*, intelligence passed to international verification organizations - such as information obtained through satellite observation - should preferably come from several countries, so that the input is balanced.

160. See IAEA Docs GOV/2897 and GOV/2959 of 1997 on the Agency's regime for the protection of confidential information.

### 3. *Means of verification requiring access*

#### i. *On-site routine inspection*

265. Although a number of very important bilateral US-USSR/Russia arms control agreements involve a considerable amount of routine on-site inspection, the focus here will be on the multilateral agreements relying on an international organization for inspection. As the States of the world become more closely woven together, verification of arms control agreements is likely increasingly to be a common international or regional task. As noted above, the CTBT was made for universal adherence, although for its effectiveness it would only have required acceptance by eight States which were not otherwise (through the NPT) debarred from testing. Similarly, a cut-off agreement prohibiting the production of highly enriched uranium and plutonium for weapons purposes could in theory be fully effective even if it were made only between the same eight States,[161] as all other States are already debarred from such production through their adherence to the NPT. However, it is generally assumed that such an agreement will be designed for adherence by all States, including those which are already, in effect, bound under the NPT to refrain from production of any nuclear material for weapons purposes.

266. The safeguards system of the IAEA was the first institutionalized on-site verification and inspection system that evolved. From its beginning as a tiny activity in the 1960s it has developed in little more than 35 years into a large professional operation engaging some 600 staff and costing some 100 million dollars per year. By the end of 1997, 931 nuclear facilities and other locations which contained nuclear material were subject to safeguards and during 1997 a total of 2499 inspections were carried out, requiring 10 240 person-days of inspection effort.

267. In the beginning the safeguards system, especially the on-site inspection, met with considerable resistance and scepticism. There

161. The five permanent SC members plus India, Israel and Pakistan.

was concern in some quarters that technical and commercial secrets in inspected non-nuclear-weapon States might be divulged by inspectors and that these States' nuclear industries would be at a disadvantage compared to their competitors in nuclear-weapon States which were not obliged to accept inspection. This is not the place to go into detailed technical descriptions of facility-specific safeguards verification,[162] nor of comprehensive safeguards verification created to respond to the requirements under the NPT and covering all present and future nuclear activities of a country[163] or the strengthened safeguards verification,[164] which it was deemed necessary to introduce after the failure of the old system to detect Iraq's programme for the enrichment of uranium. However, some features have more general interest and deserve description, comments and comparisons with similar features under the CWC and the CTBT.

268. A first comment is that nuclear industry's scepticism to inspection has largely subsided. No complaints have ever been heard about revelations of industrial or commercial secrets and the co-operation between industry and the inspectorate is mostly excellent. Yet, the experience of strengthening the traditional NPT-type safeguards verification[165] with a new additional protocol demonstrated that there was still reluctance among many governments to grant but the most evidently needed prerogatives and conveniences the inspecting organization. To take but one example: while the long negotiated CWC stipulates that visa shall be given to chemical inspectors for at least two years, the same provision to strengthen the independence of nuclear inspectors and to facilitate unannounced visit by them, was not accepted. One year was the best that could be had.

269. A second comment relates to the orientation of the verification system. As in the past, the system is based in the first place on ac-

162. IAEA INFCIRC/66/Rev.2.

163. Under IAEA INFCIRC/153 Corr.

164. Under IAEA INFCIRC/540 Corr.

165. Under IAEA INFCIRC/66 /Rev.2 and 153 Corr.

countancy (declarations) of nuclear material under the jurisdiction of the inspected party. The accounts are checked for consistency and - through on-site inspection - for reflecting the reality. Although a highly professional system, it has been criticized for being somewhat mechanistic, too much concerned with quantitative assessments and too little with qualitative judgments. At the root of this criticism lies a feeling among some that one should not have to devote so much effort to verify the numerous nuclear installations of advanced democratically organized States, where it would be unlikely that any clandestine programme would and could be hidden, but rather concentrate efforts on specific States with little or no democratic control and with possible motivation to acquire nuclear weapons.

270. This is obviously an important question of approach, which may have a more general bearing in the field of verification. It is true that the police in a big city may wisely put more efforts and resources into crime-ridden areas than in traditionally quiet neighbourhoods. However, an intergovernmental organization based on the principle of the sovereign equality of States cannot allow itself to assume that some members are lesser proliferation risks than others. It is more akin to airport controls which must treat all passengers in the same manner. It cannot act on trust vis-à-vis anyone.

271. A third comment relates to the scope of access for inspectors. Not entirely surprisingly governments will generally prefer that inspectors' access be limited to specific locations of undeniable relevance, while the inspecting organization will like to have maximum freedom of movement. Under the system of inspection elaborated for the verification of NPT obligations[166] governments as yet unaccustomed to inspection gave relatively limited on-site access to the inspectors. During routine inspections in declared nuclear installations they were limited to visiting so-called strategic points which were agreed. Whatever arguments could be adduced for this arrangement it certainly signalled that inspectors could be kept in place. True, in very special circumstances the system did not pre-

166. IAEA INFCIRC/153 Corr.

clude special inspections anywhere beyond declared facilities. However, in the absence of a system of information which could point to non-declared installations which would merit such inspection, no special inspections of such installations were ever asked before the revelations of Iraq's clandestine programme.

*ii. Special inspections (IAEA), challenge inspections (CWC) and on-site inspections (CTBT)*

272. At this point it might be of interest to examine some important differences between the IAEA's right to carry out special inspections,[167] the challenge inspections which can take place under the CWC[168] and the on-site inspections which can be requested under the CTBT.[169]

273. In the IAEA the Secretariat may request a special inspection when it considers that information made available by the inspected State party, including explanations, is not adequate. If the State rejects the request, such rejection can be overruled by a simple majority of the Agency's Board of Governors, deciding that it is essential and urgent to establish that nuclear material subject to safeguards is not diverted to nuclear weapons. Thus, a request for special inspection can only be made if the Secretariat has reason to believe that some nuclear material or facility which should have been declared, has not been so declared. In the case of the Democratic People's Republic of Korea such a request was made by the Director-General in 1992, upheld by the Board of Governors and rejected by the DPRK. As a result the matter was referred to the Security Council.

274. The IAEA model gives the Secretariat considerable power and responsibility to assess the situation and to decide in a politically sensitive matter. For the States involved this model might have the

167. Foreseen in paras. 73 and 77 of NPT-type safeguards agreement under INFCIRC/153 Corr.

168. Art. IX, para. 13et seq.

169. Art. IV, paras. 34-67.

advantage that a Secretariat will try to take a factual perspective and avoid politicization, if this is possible.

275. Under the CWC there is, as in the IAEA, a permanent inspectorate which pays periodic visits to the relevant installations. However, here any State party may request the "technical secretariat" to undertake a challenge inspection to clarify any questions concerning possible non-compliance with the Convention. Thus, the CWC Secretariat cannot itself take the initiative to conduct such an inspection. A request for a challenge inspection can only be rejected by a three quarters majority vote of all the members of the Executive Council.[170] This system takes the Secretariat out of the hot seat. On the other hand it could hold some risk for harassing challenge inspections.

276. As noted above, unlike the IAEA Secretariat which verifies States' compliance with safeguards agreements, the CTBT Secretariat is not to analyse the material obtained through the various monitoring methods employed with a view to discovering any anomalies to be followed up. Data are to be relayed to member States for analysis. If the States were to find data that need to be clarified, they can turn directly to the State on whose territory the relevant event appears to have taken place or to the Director-General or Executive Council of the CTBTO. If States members were not to be satisfied with the clarifications obtained, they - but not the Director-General - can ask for on-site inspection. Thirty affirmative votes would be needed - out of 51 members of the Council - to bring about such an inspection. A request can be based on "national technical means of verification in a manner consistent with generally recognized principles of international law", which would seem to make satellite observations acceptable, but not data obtained by clandestine means.

170. Art. IX (17).

### *4. Iraq as a watershed in the field of verification*

277. The revelations in 1991 about Iraq's success in concealing its clandestine programme for the enrichment of uranium and the development of a nuclear weapon became a watershed in the attitudes to safeguards verification. It was realized that to have a verification system which had serious deficiencies might be more dangerous than having none, because it might lull neighbours and the world at large into misplaced confidence. All understood that the system, to be meaningful, would have to be given more teeth. Modifications which until then would have been unacceptable now became possible, not least as regards access in connection with routine inspections. The limitation of access to strategic points which had existed in routine inspection under the NPT fell away and several other expansions occurred in the right to access and the possibility of unannounced inspections.

278. However, it has to be noted that even the rights of access under the strengthened IAEA safeguards look very modest when compared with the rights of access which the Security Council accorded UNSCOM and the IAEA to fulfil the mandate of inspection in Iraq. It might be of interest to see what a maximalist right of access can look like. In accordance with an exchange of letters of 14 May 1991 between the UN Secretary-General and the Iraqi Foreign Minister the inspectors working in Iraq have, for instance, unrestricted freedom of entry and exit without delay or hindrance; unrestricted freedom of movement without advance notice within Iraq; right to unimpeded access to any site or facility for the purpose of on-site inspection; right to request, receive, examine and copy any record, data, or information; right to install equipment or construct facilities or observation, inspection, testing or monitoring; right to take photographs whether from the ground or from the air; right to unrestricted communication by radio, satellite.

279. Under the plan for future ongoing monitoring and verification in Iraq, approved by the Security Council in October 1991, the rights listed above were confirmed and some additional prerogatives were

spelled out, e.g.: to stop and inspect vehicles, ships, aircraft or any other means of transportation within Iraq; to inspect imports or exports of material and other items upon arrival or departure; to conduct interviews with any personnel at any site.

280. An inspection regime with such extensive rights of access to sites and to information is unprecedented and will hardly be accepted by any State unless it is under severe pressure. That eight years of inspection in Iraq employing this regime have not been enough to give confidence that the mapping of Iraq's programme of weapons of mass destruction is "full, final and complete", points to a conclusion of great importance for all verification of arms control and disarmament, namely, that 100 percent certainty is hardly attainable.[171]

### 5. *The residue of uncertainty in verification*

281. The difficulty of verifying with full certainty that there is no fissile material, no chemical or biological substances which can be used in weapons, not a single antipersonnel mine on the territory of a State can perhaps be understood if the inspection and verification task is compared with the task of national police to ensure that no narcotic drugs are stored clandestinely in a country. The police can move anywhere and has extensive - though not unlimited - rights of access. It may perhaps tap telephones, subpoena witnesses and it may have many informers. Yet, it would be a successful police indeed if it could give absolute guarantees that there are no illegal drugs in the country.

282. In some respects the situation of the international weapons inspectors looking for undeclared material or installations is easier than that of the national police. Nuclear material is unique in leaving fingerprints and a national weapons programme for the enrichment of uranium or separation of plutonium will also call for rather large

171. See infra, para. 281.

industrial installations which may be visible from satellites or detectable from information about exports.

283. Nevertheless the freedom of movement and prerogatives of international inspectors will in most respects be much more limited than those of the national police. Furthermore, a few kilograms of plutonium are not larger than a fist; the same is true of an anti-personnel mine, while lethal chemicals or biological material can be stored in tiny containers. There is no way international inspection - or national police - could be sure to trace such small items hidden in a large country. Nor is there any way in which it could trace all documents, computer programmes, matrixes, prototype machines or, for that matter, engineers and scientists that may be part of a weapons programme. If this is what governments really "request", they cannot have it. Inspectors cannot monitor every inch of the territory of a State and it is not meaningful to go in blind and random search.

284. Although in public rhetoric governments may sometimes appear to be asking "complete" verification, they know that this is not possible. In normal verification under the NPT governments do not request an ambition to detect very small quantities of fissile material, but rather what is technically termed "significant quantities"; and they are aware that there must remain some measure of uncertainty. Indeed, governments are accustomed to basing their decisions and policies on some degree of uncertainty. Reducing that uncertainty as much as possible without incurring too high verification costs or too high intrusiveness, and accurately reporting on it, is the normal job of the verifier. Deciding on how far they will rely on such reports in their policies and actions is the business of governments. What level of uncertainty is acceptable may be different in different situations and under different regimes, e.g. under the NPT generally and under the inspection scheme for Iraq. Two examples may illustrate the point.

285. After dismantling its nuclear weapons and removing the fissile material from the weapons, South Africa asked the IAEA to verify

that there were no more weapons and that all the fissile material was accounted for. South Africa went out of its way to facilitate the task of the Agency's inspectors and invited them to visit "any place any time". The inspectors did a very thorough job. Yet, the conclusions of the Agency Secretariat which were accepted by the Board of Governors, reflect caution and a determination not give a greater assurance than strictly flowed from the inspections. As stated in a report of 3 September 1992, "The team found no evidence that the inventory of nuclear material included in the Initial Report was incomplete."[172]

286. And in a report of 8 September 1993 the following language is used:

> The team found no indication to suggest that there remain any sensitive components of the nuclear weapons programme which have not been either rendered useless or converted to commercial non-nuclear applications or nuclear usage.[173]

287. In the case of Iraq, where the Agency had unparalleled inspection rights and access to sites, documents and persons, had been working at full capacity for six years and had acquired a very extensive knowledge and understanding of the nuclear programme, but where there was hardly any genuine - and certainly no consistent - wish of the State authorities to fully co-operate, the reports to the Security Council, likewise show caution. A report of the IAEA of 6 October 1997 to the Security Council states[174] that there were "no indications" of significant discrepancies between the technically coherent picture that had evolved of Iraq's past nuclear programme and the information contained in Iraq's "Full, Final and Complete Declaration" (FFCD) of 7 September 1996 as supplemented since that date. However, the report goes on to say that:

172. IAEA doc. GOV/2609, para. 31.

173. IAEA doc. GOV/2684, para 31.

174. In para. 79.

> ...no absolute assurances can be given with regard to the completeness of Iraq's FFCD. Some uncertainty is inevitable in any country-wide technical verification process which aims to prove the absence of readily concealable objects or activities. The extent to which such uncertainty is acceptable is a policy judgment.[175]

288. In an informal briefing of the Council on 16 October 1997, the IAEA Director-General, commenting upon the quoted text, explained that:

> ... when the Agency reports that it has found no indication of activities, facilities or items, this does not amount to an assertion that there is none. The probability that "no indication" corresponds to "non-existence" depends upon how intrusive, extensive, systematic and skilful the investigation was that gave such result. Judging that probability is not a technical matter. Even less so deciding what level of probability is required.

289. In the case of Iraq the Security Council, too, will be aware that verification can never be 100 %, but its assumption is that Iraq will continue to conceal what it can and it will require a very high level of clarification. It should be kept in mind, however, that while the case of inspections in Iraq shows that it is possible to design verification systems that are extremely intrusive and fine-meshed, considerations regarding acceptability to States in general, regarding cost and the risk of setting off false alarms suggest some moderation in the devising of general systems. Inevitably then the level of assurance of full compliance by the inspected States is less high.

### 6. *"Managed access"*

290. An issue that ever more frequently crops up in the context of international verification of arms control and disarmament agreements is that of sensitive information or installations which the inspected party has a legitimate interest in keeping confidential and which

175. UN Doc. S/1997/779 of 8 October 1997.

should not be fully viewed by inspectors, e.g. to protect technical or commercial secrets or avoid any added risk of proliferation.

291. As was noted above, under traditional NPT-type verification the inspectors were limited in routine inspection to visiting strategic points in nuclear installations. The risk was then little that anything legitimately confidential would be revealed. Special arrangements had only to be made by the IAEA under the so-called hexapartite agreement regarding the inspection of enrichment plants, where access, notably to the cascade hall, by inspectors was subject to special arrangements to minimize the risk that proliferation-sensitive information should leak. However, when under strengthened safeguards the inspectors were to be given a much wider general freedom of movement in nuclear installations, a demand for special rules turned up and resulted inter alia in an article under which the Agency upon request by the inspected party would have to make:

> arrangements for managed access under this Protocol in order to prevent the dissemination of proliferation sensitive information, to meet safety or physical protection requirements, or to protect proprietary or commercially sensitive information.[176]

292. The Annex on Implementation and Verification to the CWC (which preceded the IAEA provision quoted above) provides that the inspected party is:

> under the obligation to allow the greatest degree of access taking account any constitutional obligations it may have with regard to proprietary rights or searches and seizures, the inspected State Party has the right under managed access to take such measures as are necessary to protect national security....[177]

293. Measures permitted under managed access include the removal of sensitive papers, the shrouding of sensitive equipment, the logging off of computer systems, restriction of sample analysis to the pre-

176. IAEA INFCIRC 540, Art. 7.

177. Part X pt. 41.

sence or absence of scheduled chemicals, random selective access to buildings and, only in exceptional cases, the granting of access only to individual inspectors to certain parts of the inspection site.

294. The provisions of the CWC and of the new protocol for strengthened IAEA safeguards show that fairly significant restrictions in access can be demanded by the inspected States. Of course, such a State may be restrained in any temptation to make use of available restrictions, lest an excessive demand appear unreasonable and draw suspicion.

295. It may be of interest to note that, curiously, even in the case of inspections in Iraq under Security Council mandate some restraints are observed despite the seemingly unlimited authority given to UNSCOM and the IAEA.[178] In early 1998 a full crisis erupted over the access by UNSCOM inspectors to "presidential sites" and it was widely speculated in the world press that the cause was that these sites were used to stock prohibited weapons of mass destruction. Eventually the crisis was defused by a visit of the UN Secretary-General, Kofi A. ANNAN. In the memorandum of understanding drawn up at his visit the following paragraph (3) occurs:

> The Government of Iraq undertakes to accord UNSCOM and IAEA immediate, unconditional and unrestricted access in conformity with relevant U.N. resolutions. In the performance of its mandate under the Security Council resolutions, UNSCOM undertakes to respect the legitimate concerns of Iraq relating to national security, sovereignty and dignity.[179]

296. Special procedures were designed involving the presence of foreign diplomats at inspections by inspectors of presidential sites apparently to satisfy the demands raised by "sovereignty and dignity". When considering that premises and documents of police, ministries, armed forces etc. were by no means excluded from inspection under the concept of "sovereignty", the protocol gesture

178. Recorded supra, para. 278.

179. UN Doc. S/1998 / 166 of 27 February 1998.

made to defuse the crisis seems to have been a modest price to pay. It is evident that the restraints as regards foreign presence that could be asked by Iraq in 1998 on the basis of respect for the notion of "sovereignty" were minimal compared to the restraints that Turkey read into the notion of sovereignty in the 19th century.

297. Regardless of any conceptual arguments that it might have invoked, Iraq's authorities would quite possibly have prevented inspector access to some point where inspection was demanded, long enough to enable the removal of small items or documents which would bring undesired revelations. For larger items, on the other hand, such conduct would be more difficult. Their removal would be likely to be spotted by satellite surveillance. At hospitals and religious premises the two inspecting organizations, while certainly not waiving their rights of inspection, observed appropriate decorum.

298. The above description of inspection problems which arose in Iraq should show that even when the inspecting organization is granted "unrestricted access", some restraint in the exercise of the right may be needed and a residue of uncertainty will inevitably remain as to whether everything has been disclosed.

### 7. *Compliance*

299. It is often remarked that a fundamental difference between international law and national law is that the latter but not the former is linked to means of enforcement ensuring compliance. While it is true that there is no international nuclear or other police, no courts that will automatically take jurisdiction in cases of violations of arms control or disarmament agreements, and certainly no automatic sanctions, the remark ignores many essential points.

300. *First*, rules of international law, like those of national law, are complied with in most cases because the subjects have accepted the rules as being in their own interest and because they have a habit of good-faith respect for treaty and other rules valid for them. The

peaceful settlement of disputes in accordance with agreed procedures avoids hardships and even bloodshed. The lowering of armament burdens under bilateral or multilateral agreements releases resources for development. The accepted ban on chemical and biological weapons prevents some of the most feared horrors and sufferings of war. And so on and so forth.

301. Sometimes it is the mutual or general adherence to the same norm that provides the advantage, sometimes the benefits gained by commitments may be different for different parties; there may be a direct quantitative *quid pro quo* as when two superpowers agree on specific but not identical steps of disarmament. Non-nuclear-weapon States have sometimes maintained that their renunciation of nuclear weapons under the NPT should be regarded as a "sacrifice" on their part and that the commitment of the nuclear-weapon States to pursue negotiations toward nuclear disarmament should be seen as a *quid pro quo*. However, upon analysis it is hard to maintain that there is much of a "sacrifice". Indeed, there may rather be a significant advantage for an individual State that many other States - especially neighbours and other States in the region - renounce nuclear weapons. The commitment of nuclear-weapon States, to be sure, may be perceived as another advantage gained, but it has hardly been the main motivation for any State to adhere to the NPT.

302. *Second*, where a State which has bound itself by a rule of international law feels that some new development has modified the situation, giving it some interest in disregarding the commitment, several considerations may restrain it from breaching its obligation. It may care for its own international reputation as a State respecting its commitments. It may be concerned about being singled out for condemnation. It may fear retaliation by neighbours, reactions by great powers or sanctions by the international community. In none of the cases would the reaction be as automatic and predictable as the reaction to violations of domestic law: States are mostly big and powerful subjects which, although not immune to reactions from the outside, cannot be thrown in jail, nor easily be fined. Even in the domestic sphere legal reaction to very powerful subjects, e.g. trade

unions waging illegal strikes or large religious or political groups pursuing some "civil disobedience", may be problematic.

303. With all this said, it must be squarely admitted that States breaking legal commitments often get away with it, especially if they are big and powerful. Moreover, precisely in the area of perceived national security interests, incentives may develop to disregard international obligations, especially if forceful reactions appear unlikely. This makes it all the more important to note the stronger leverages which are developing at the end of the 20th century and which are available to induce States to respect international obligations to which they are subject. The rapidly accelerating integration and organization of States into an international community makes States much more dependent on each other, e.g. in the area of trade, finance and development assistance.[180]

### 8. *What degree of uncertainty about compliance is tolerated ?*

304. Before some of the traditional and new means designed to induce compliance will be discussed, we must return to verification as fundamentally important to establish whether there is or is not compliance. We have seen how in some cases - the use of chemical weapons or dum-dum bullets - violations may be evident. Permanent verification procedures were not deemed necessary. However, for most rules in the field of arms control and disarmament technically advanced national or international means of verifying implementation are now needed. This report has described many of them in some detail. It has also shown that despite ever more developed means of verification there is normally and inevitably a residue of uncertainty about full compliance. The question must be asked: how do governments act in the face of this uncertainty?

305. It has been suggested above that the degree of uncertainty about full treaty implementation which governments may find acceptable

180. See supra, para. 22.

may vary, depending upon the importance of the rule to be respected and upon the country whose compliance is in question. Pragmatism rather than equal application of legal norms prevails. In the case of Iraq the tolerance of uncertainty about compliance with stiff obligations is very low in several governments, as they are convinced that Iraq will avoid to comply if it can and would be ready to use any undetected weapons of mass destruction. By contrast, as shown, an inevitable measure of uncertainty seems to be accepted with equanimity in the case of South Africa, as its government has much credibility and is not seen as having any motivation for a clandestine retention of nuclear weapons.

306. The inevitable residue of uncertainty in verification about compliance raises some other intriguing questions, which may be noted.

### *9. Compliance measures supplemented by possible counter-proliferation?*

307. Some experts have taken the view that as the organized international systems of verification fail to give complete reassurance about the absence of nuclear, chemical or biological weapons, States must retain a strong capacity to intervene by unspecified measures of "counter-proliferation" against suspect cases of non-compliance. They might develop not only means of rapidly identifying a use of biological weapons or chemical weapons and keep stocks of vaccines and antidote, but also technologically advanced means, like anti-missile systems to stop incoming missiles from possible low-capacity adversaries. Although such doctrines seem to supplement rather than compete with international means of inducement and enforcement, one is nevertheless tempted to ask if they can give 100 % protection against the development and use of prohibited weapons, and what is their cost.[181]

181. A working paper on "International Perspectives on Counterproliferation", was edited by M. Reiss and H. Muller in January 1995 under the auspices of the Division of International Studies at the Woodrow Wilson International Center for Scholars.

### *10. Verification of compliance with a cut-off agreement*

308. Another interesting question relating to the tolerable level of uncertainty of compliance in verification may surface in the negotiation of an agreement for the prohibition of production of highly enriched uranium and plutonium for weapons use: a cut-off agreement. Such an agreement would call for the inspection of at least all enrichment and reprocessing plants in the States parties to verify that none of the fissile material produced is for weapons use. An obligation of this kind exists already for non-nuclear-weapon States parties to the NPT and is verified under NPT-type safeguards (for instance in Brazil and Japan). However, the chief purpose of a cut-off agreement would be to oblige the five declared nuclear-weapon States parties to the NPT and States not parties to the NPT, notably India, Pakistan and Israel, if joining the agreement, to stop producing fissile material for weapons and subject their relevant plants to inspection and verification. As inspection in such plants is labour intensive and costly the argument has been made that it could be performed at lower intensity - and with less cost - in States which have nuclear weapons, as in these cases a higher residue of uncertainty about full implementation could be tolerated than in non-nuclear-weapon States. After all, these countries already have stocks of nuclear weapons and fissile weapons-usable material and it would not greatly affect security if inspection and verification failed to identify every single bit: it would only be a quantitative problem. By contrast, a verification failure to identify a quantity of plutonium in a non-nuclear State could be used by that State clandestinely to make a first nuclear weapon and thus achieve a qualitative change: to become a nuclear-weapon State. Against these arguments there is a fundamental argument about equality. How could it be justified that the same type of nuclear installation be verified for the same purpose at different levels of intensity in two different countries, say Japan and China? Equality - though not cost - speaks against the proposition.

*11. Compliance with a total ban on the possession of nuclear weapons*

309. If nuclear-weapon States can never be 100 % certain through verification that other nuclear-weapon States are complying with *their* obligation to eliminate all their nuclear weapons, how could they take the risk of standing "naked"? This is a problem of verification that will inevitably turn up in the coming discussions about the complete elimination of nuclear weapons. As this development is not imminent there will be time to ponder the issue. Perhaps nuclear weapons are not the only possible deterrence against nuclear weapons? Perhaps also a gradual increase in the transparency of States and development of an improved global security system will impact on the issue? The Report of the Canberra Commission on the Elimination of Nuclear Weapons (August 1996) provides valuable insights and ideas on the issue.

*12. Means of inducing compliance*

*i. Verification and detection as means of deterring non-compliance*

310. The standard safeguards agreements of the IAEA for the implementation of the NPT define the objective of safeguards as:

> the timely detection of diversion of significant quantities of nuclear material from peaceful nuclear activities to the manufacture of nuclear weapons or of other nuclear explosive devices or for purposes unknown, and deterrence of such diversion by the risk of early detection.[182]

311. The idea articulated in the agreement - to be accepted by the State - is clearly that the risk of early detection of any diversion of nuclear material will deter the State from attempting such diversion. Being found out as cheating would certainly be discrediting and damaging to a State's standing and would, moreover, very likely set

182. INFCIRC 153, Corr., para. 28.

in motion political, economic or even military pressures by other States.

312. In this context it might be noted that the nuclear test explosions carried out by India and Pakistan in the spring of 1998, without being violations of any legal commitment assumed by either country (as they had refused to join existing test bans), led to strong reactions by many States, including the cutting off of development aid, credit guarantees and support for loans in the World Bank. Here even conduct perceived by many States as defiance of an incipient rule of the global community provoked strong reactions.

*ii. Break-down of treaty relation likely result of non-compliance*

313. Article 60 of the 1969 Vienna Convention on the Law of Treaties provides that:

> A material breach of a bilateral treaty by one of the parties entitles the other to invoke the breach as a ground for terminating the treaty or suspending its operation in whole or in part.[183]

314. A party to a bilateral arms control or disarmament treaty will be aware that if it ceases to comply with its commitments, the other party is likely to declare itself free of any further obligation. This may act as a deterrent against breaches. The Convention defines the term "material breach" as a repudiation of the treaty or "the violation of a provision essential to the accomplishment of the object or purpose of the treaty". Evidently, a party to a treaty may choose to overlook minor departures from treaty obligations. However, as a party contemplating a breach is unlikely to know what will be tolerated by way of non-compliance, this uncertainty, too, might act as a deterrence against any non-compliance.

183. Sub-para. 1.

315. For multilateral treaties, the legal effects of non-compliance by one party are more complicated,[184] but they also allow suspension or termination by joint action of the other parties or even in several situations by another party specially affected by the breach. Thus under these provisions, too, a party tempted to breach an arms control or disarmament agreement would have to count on other parties freeing themselves of their obligations and taking whatever steps they consider appropriate and legal.

*iii. Non-compliance giving other treaty parties a right to withdraw*

316. As noted earlier, several arms control and disarmament treaties discussed in this report contain a clause along the following lines:

> Each Party shall in exercising its national sovereignty have the right to withdraw from the Treaty if it decides that extraordinary events, related to the subject matter of this Treaty, have jeopardized the supreme interests of its country...[185]

317. The right retained in this type of clause[186] is evidently broader than just covering a clear-cut breach of the treaties by other parties. It would enable a party to free itself from further obligations also in circumstances where the occurrence of a breach appears highly probable but may be difficult to prove, perhaps due to inconclusive verification. This type of provision may serve as a warning to a State contemplating non-compliance that even if it could make it difficult for anybody to prove non-compliance, it might trigger an undesired withdrawal by another party. On the other hand, the provision may also show another function of effective verification, namely, that this may help States which have complied to argue against unjustified attempts of withdrawal.

184. Sub-para. 2.

185. Art. IV of the 1963 PTBT.

186. Similar clauses are found, e.g., in Art. X (1) of the 1968 NPT, Art. XIX of the 1990 CFE, and Art. XV of the 1987 US-USSR Treaty on the elimination of their intermediate-range and shorter-range missiles.

318. It might be noted, lastly, that the DPRK at one point (on 12 March 1993) sent a notice of withdrawal from the NPT to the Security Council. However, on 11 June 1993, one day before the notice was to take effect, the DPRK "suspended" the "effectuation" of the notice.

*iv. Export control regimes*

319. Without doubt, bans or restrictions on the trade and export of weapons and of material and equipment relevant for the production of certain weapons can be a very important factor to prevent or at least impede the acquisition of arms or certain types of arms. Much effort was spent in the League of Nations period at least to subject all arms trade to licensing and to preventing illicit trade. More recently we have seen on several occasions how the UN Security Council imposed a complete ban on the transfer of weapons to a specific State, a decision that is legally binding on all member States if taken under Chapter VII of the Charter. In other cases there may be a legal duty to apply export restrictions as a result of provisions in arms control agreements[187] designed to strengthen the effectiveness of the conventions. In these cases trade and export restrictions may constitute implementation of broad treaty obligations.

320. In some other cases - missiles and conventional weapons - the "regimes" of export restrictions which have been jointly developed by limited groups of States are not even linked to a treaty. By and large the various "regimes" present themselves as informal mechanisms for harmonizing national rules and decisions on restrictions rather than hard-and-fast agreements.

321. Although still evoking some suspicion and controversy, regimes for weapons-related export restrictions may come to meet more general understanding and support, especially after the revelation of the extent to which Iraq's programme of weapons of mass destruction had been facilitated by imports of equipment and material. The value

187. E.g., Art. III (2) of the NPT and Arts. I, VII and XI of the CWC. On the general subject of the regimes, see the recent study by C. Ahlström, *The Status of Multilateral Export Regimes* (1999).

of multilateral weapon-related export control measures to a world increasingly devoted to arms control and disarmament can hardly be doubted. They will relate not only to weapons of mass destruction but also to conventional weapons, as can be seen in Articles 1 and 2 of the Ottawa Convention on Anti-Personnel Mines and in recent proposals to restrain the accumulation and proliferation of small arms. They may need to become more transparent and be subjected to broader international discussion and adjustment to gain general approval. In particular where they may affect possible rights of imports or affect dual use items there may be a need to assure that importers interests are heard.

### v. *Risk of retaliation as a means of inducing compliance*

322. The tit for tat, tooth for tooth and eye for an eye may be seen as a concept of revenge but just as well as a means of deterrence operating in a primitive community, where collective sanctions are unreliable or as yet underdeveloped. In the international community it has played and will continue to play a significant role until that community is better equipped authoritatively and impartially to establish cases of non-compliance with obligations and decide and perform reactions to such cases. Clearly the 1899 bans on use of dum-dum bullets and of asphyxiating and deleterious gases were sanctioned by the risk of retaliation, and it is believed[188] that the general compliance with the 1925 Geneva ban on the use of gas during the Second World War was due in large part to the fear of retaliation in kind. It is evident that although no prohibition of use has been agreed to concerning nuclear weapons, the risk of retaliation in kind has provided significant inducement for non-use.

### vi. *Risk of collective sanctions as a means of inducing compliance*

323. Arms control and disarmament treaties very often contain provisions about consultation between parties and measures of clarification in cases of suspected breaches. As we have seen, the right of

188. As noted supra para. 216.

termination or withdrawal may also exist implicitly or explicitly. The right of retaliation for breaches is never explicitly stated.

324. Some provisions on compliance in the CWC[189] enable the Conference of State Parties to restrict or suspend a State's rights and privileges until it returns from breach to compliance. It may also recommend State parties to take collective measures and in cases of particular gravity it is - as noted above - to bring the issue, relevant information and its own conclusions to the attention of the UN General Assembly and Security Council.

325. The Statute of the IAEA, which entered into force in 1957, likewise contains some sanction provisions. A member which has "persistently violated" the provisions of the statute or of any agreement entered into pursuant to the statute (notably a safeguards agreement) may be suspended from the exercise of the privileges and rights of membership.[190]

326. It is evident that although the IAEA has taken decisions depriving both Iraq and the DPRK of non-humanitarian technical assistance as a result of their non-compliance with safeguards agreements, neither the provisions of the IAEA nor those of the CWC form the basis for sanctions which bite. The two organizations are the watch-dogs but not the police of the organized international community. When the Board of Governors of the IAEA decided to terminate non-humanitarian assistance to the DPRK for its violation of the safeguards agreement, the DPRK withdrew from the Agency. The UN system's authority to take effective measures to bring about compliance with arms control and disarmament agreements is, of course, vested in the Security Council. Such measures - sanctions - can be taken only on the basis of Chapter VII of the UN Charter and require that the Council has determined the existence of a threat to the peace, breach of the peace or act of aggression.

189. Art. XII.

190. Art. XIX (B).

327. It is not, of course, certain that all cases of non-compliance with arms control and disarmament agreements constitute threats to the peace, nor is it by any means sure that all such cases will be brought before the Council. It is, nevertheless, a possibility in many cases and a statutorily required step in some cases.[191]

328. The Security Council, itself, has made it known how seriously it views any proliferation of weapons of mass destruction. In a Presidential Statement after a summit-level Security Council meeting in 1992 the following was said:

> The proliferation of all weapons of mass destruction constitutes a threat to international peace and security. The members of the Council commit themselves to working to prevent the spread of technology related to the research for or production of such weapons and to take appropriate action to that end.
> On nuclear proliferation, they note the importance of the decision of many countries to adhere to the NPT and emphasize the integral role in the implementation of that Treaty of fully effective IAEA safeguards, as well as the importance of effective export controls. The members of the Council will take appropriate measures in the case of any violations notified to them by the IAEA.

329. A remarkable feature of this statement is that it seems to lay down that any proliferation of weapons of mass destruction would be an event allowing the Council to take action under Chapter VII. However that may be, the statement can hardly have been meant to obviate the need to determine in each concrete case whether there is "a threat to the peace". How will the Council act in such cases?

330. The case of Iraq was brought to the Council as a case of clear-cut aggression and led to a massive armed intervention under the authority of the Council. In the Council-mandated inspections by the IAEA it was found that Iraq had violated its obligations under the NPT and the safeguards agreement with the IAEA. The Council has shown itself determined to ensure that all Iraqi weapons of mass

191. As for the IAEA under its relationship agreement with the UN.

destruction be eradicated, has given strong support to UNSCOM and the IAEA in their work to this end and has looked to its members to take enforcement measures on behalf of the Council when needed to ensure Iraqi compliance. It must be noted, however, that the bombings which took place in December 1998 and continued in "no fly zones" in 1999 did not aim at destroying any remaining weapons of mass destruction, as their locations were not known, but rather had the purpose of bringing pressure on Iraq to allow UNSCOM access which had been denied. The desired result was not achieved by May 1999; on the other hand, the departure of all inspectors was an unwanted result. The case illustrates limitations on what may be attained through the application of punishment by air strikes.

331. In the case of the DPRK, which was brought to the Council by the IAEA not as a breach of the NPT but as a case of non-compliance with its safeguards agreement with the DPRK, the action of the Council was very different. It encouraged its members to take steps to defuse the situation, and the United States reached what was termed an "agreed framework" under which the DPRK declared that it would "freeze" its existing nuclear programme and accept international verification on all existing plants; the United States would *inter alia* put together an international consortium to arrange financing for and the supply of two 1000 MW(e) light water reactors. When a significant portion of the light water reactor project was completed but "before delivery of key nuclear components", the DPRK would "come into full compliance" with its safeguards agreement.

332. The "agreed framework" reached between the US and the DPRK was endorsed by the Security Council, and the IAEA has been verifying the freeze as it was asked to do. Although no one has explicitly condoned the failure of the DPRK to comply fully with its safeguards agreement with the IAEA (and the General Conference of the IAEA has each year declared that the DPRK remains in non-compliance), it is evident that this degree of non-compliance is tolerated; presumably because any alternative course of action is deemed more problematic. One is driven to the conclusion that in its aim to avoid dangerous

confrontation, perhaps including armed force in a sensitive area of the world, the Security Council, including its permanent members, has not attempted to uphold a legal regime, judging it wiser to follow a pragmatic line.

## IV. Reflections on the future

333. This report has been a flashback, first, to view the aspirations and the results of the Hague Peace Conference 100 years ago and, then, to the aspirations and results which we have seen in the last 50 years: the period after the Second World War. Even though a report limited to some 100 pages inevitably gives a compressed and fragmented picture of the past, it prompts some reflections on the future.

334. Much of the tremendous change we have seen has been driven by technological evolution. With the expansion of production - including that of arms - population and communications everything seems to have become mega, except perhaps the micro chips. Yet, the aspirations of people for the world seem relatively constant: "the benefits of lasting peace", which translate into the absence of war and violence, resources for well-being rather than arms and every possible reduction of suffering when it occurs. Today we would sum these aspirations up as peace, sustainable development, human rights and democracy.

335. At all times governments and individuals need, and do, consider how to make reality of the rather constant aspirations. The flashback of this report may be supplemented by some thoughts as to what might be attempted in the short, medium and long term.

## IV.1 Short term

336. This report has given ample evidence how the détente after the Cold War facilitated effective joint action under the recognized authority of the Security Council. It has also pointed to the set-backs which détente has suffered for some time and how this is currently putting a break on the further successful process of *arms control and disarmament.* A first priority today should be to restore détente and thereby promote genuinely common efforts in the UN to preserve and restore peace and to *revive and accelerate the arms control and disarmament process.*

337. Considering that there are no conflicts about territory among the great powers, no crusading based on ideology and that none of them really fears that any other of them might launch a military attack, accommodation and restored détente ought to be within reach through prudent policies.

338. The larger and more serious armed conflicts which have taken place in recent years have not had any involvement of great powers and blocks and several of them have been more or less internal. The UN Charter, written over 50 years ago, did not contemplate for the Organization to intervene in such conflicts. Today, public opinion in many countries, alerted by modern communications to the brutal features of these conflicts, feels that the world organization cannot stand aside and must act to end them. In the UN, governments have mostly acted warily in reaction to these conflicts, well aware that although action is wanted, involvement that may be costly in human and financial resources, may not be. With an ever growing closeness between people it seems inevitable that the former barriers against international action will erode and that the evolution will go in the direction of more international action. Both for the legitimacy and success - though not assuredly promptness - of such action it would seem important that the action required be jointly decided or authorized at the UN. Disregarding such unity would risk stopping the development toward further cohesion between States in the organization - and in the world - increase tensions, raise fears among

the less powerful and raise obstacles to *arms control and disarmament*. Perhaps the time has come to reactivate the long-dormant Military Staff Committee of the Security Council.[192]

339. There needs to be international consideration of the special threat that is posed by various *sub-national and terrorist groups*, not least if there is a risk that any one of them might be equipped with *weapons of mass destruction*. In the view of some, the greatest threats in today's world come from such groups or from reckless *governments* that might be or might become so equipped. It is doubtful that many States will spend billions for measures against such hypothetical threats, and it would be serious if any measures designed for this purpose were to undermine or impede *disarmament* by the States that control huge stocks of arms. Indeed, it would be paradoxical if nuclear-weapon States felt they could lower the guard and maintain mutual vulnerability between themselves, thereby saving enormous resource at no greater risk, and at the same time feel constrained to erect costly barriers against existing or not existing low-capacity actors and, in the process, perhaps undermine disarmament. It would seem preferable that *joint* and urgent consideration be given among the nuclear-weapon States - and perhaps others - to policies and measures to guard against the possible low-capacity actors.

340. In the ongoing arms control and disarmament process there are many items for urgent attention. The CTBT needs to be signed and ratified by 44 States to enter into force this year. It must be ensured that all these States take the required action. The START II Treaty needs ratification, and START III needs to be brought to a conclusion, both matters that would be promoted by a revival of greater co-operation between the parties. The negotiation of the agreement on a prohibition of production of fissionable material for weapons purposes (cut-off) needs to get seriously started. Not least important would it seem to be that the countries on the Indian subcontinent join

192. Art. 47 of the Charter.

such an agreement to avoid a race between them to build up stockpiles of fissile material.

341. A review conference of the NPT will be held in 2000. After the attempt of the DPRK in 1993 to withdraw from the treaty and after the Indian and Pakistani nuclear weapons tests, fears were expressed that the treaty would fall apart. Fortunately these fears have not proved well-founded. For the maintenance of the broad and strong support which exists for the treaty, however, it would seem important that the nuclear disarmament between the nuclear-weapon States not come to a halt. These States can rightly hold that they have done a great deal in the last decade in fulfilment of their obligation under Article VI to negotiate toward nuclear disarmament, but they can ill defend a halt in that process.

342. As to the regions about which there is the greatest concern - the Middle East, the Indian sub-continent and the Korean Peninsula - it is inevitable that the prospects for non-proliferation and nuclear arms control are dependent upon the attainment of a measure of détente. Although any stable solutions need to be tailored to each area, one might nonetheless ask oneself whether *guarantees by the Security Council, both positive and negative*, might not be brought into the pictures. The incentive to develop nuclear weapons is almost always found in perceived security concerns and allaying such concerns is likely to be more effective than any appeals for international solidarity or, for that matter, punishments for not heeding the appeals. It is hard to overlook the fact that when so many States which would have had the technical capacity to develop nuclear weapons, have renounced it, this has mostly occurred against the background of positive security guarantees which have been available to them under various alliances.

343. Another rarely discussed and possibly intractable problem is that the NPT raises no bar to the construction of plants which can produce highly enriched uranium or plutonium for peaceful purposes. It simply requires such plants to be declared and placed under IAEA safeguards. With no need in the world for more plutonium for fuel

and an oversupply of enriched uranium for fuel, it is hard to see that any country could economically justify the construction of a new plant. Unquestionably attitudes to the development of "complete fuel cycles" were much more relaxed in 1968 than they are now. Today, brows would be raised - to say the least - if some State declared that it intended to construct a plant of this kind. It would seem that the only way to restrict the option which might now exist, would be to introduce some sort of international licensing of such plants and/or compensate a restriction by a scheme ensuring the supply of nuclear fuel and waste management services.

## IV.2 **Medium term**

344. The further development of the UN and its role to prevent or stop armed conflicts and to promote nuclear disarmament is an issue for the short and medium as well as long term. In the medium term maybe solutions could be found to the difficult and important issue of making the *Security Council more broadly representative* of the world and at the same time somewhat restrict the veto. In a world where economic and financial leverages will be increasingly important for the solution of differences it is natural that the economic power in the world should be represented in one way or the other. For the legitimacy of the Council's decisions, not least when it comes to authorize armed action, it would also be important that each of the developing continents - Asia, Africa and Latin America - be somehow permanently represented.

345. Another, possibly medium-term issue relates to the *regional* organizations. A role for them in the maintenance and restoration of peace is foreseen in Chapter VIII of the Charter and reliance has sometimes been placed on them in the past for these purposes. If, as seems likely, world public opinion and the States of the world will come to demand that the international community should play an increasingly active peacemaking and peace restoring role, and if, as also seems likely, many of the potential cases where action may be needed, would relate to national or regional rather than global con-

flicts, the greater reliance on regional organizations would seem a logical outcome. This will - already does - raise many questions. One concerns the future security architecture of Europe.

346. Yet another, possibly medium-term issue relates to the possibility of establishing a small professional rapid deployment force that could be deployed by decision of the Security Council, thus enabling the Council in some situations to avoid relying on national forces.

347. In the *disarmament field proper* one might regrettably expect that reaching arrangements for nuclear arms control on the Indian subcontinent and for regional non-proliferation in the Middle East and for the Korean peninsula will take time and keep governments busy also in the medium term!

348. Three other issues might, hopefully, also be ripe for action in the medium term. First, the unilateral commitments given by the United States and Russia in 1991 for the *withdrawal of sub-strategic (tactical) nuclear weapons* from theatres of deployment and ships should be transformed into legally binding form. Secondly, the efforts to reduce the trade and traffic in *small arms* should advance from the early stages in which they are now to more operative negotiations. And thirdly, there should be a further consolidation of the various export control regimes. Their transparency would need to be further improved, but, where they deal with-dual use items, there would also seem to be a need for ensuring some representation of the interests and possible rights of the importers.

## IV.3 Long term

349. The world today is sometimes said to be a "global village". In the sense that modern communications make everybody neighbour this may be true, but it would also be right to say that we live in a society which is still at a *primitive* level. We have no central authority claiming a monopoly on the possession and use of arms: the individual members of our society are still armed, keep order

within their territories, trade, quarrel, feud, make alliances and peace treaties. In an early society the concept of "the King's peace" stood for the idea that the King claimed a monopoly on the control of armed forces and their use and in return committed himself to protecting the subjects. The idea that the ruler should act under laws which have general approval of the citizens and that they should be equal before the law marks a further level of civilized development. Maybe one could see the Pax Romana as an attempt to establish the King's peace two thousand years ago? Maybe the Pax Britannica could be seen as another experiment about a hundred years ago? However, the idea of civilizing the international society by subjugating its members to one country is not what the world wants.

350. What is dreamt of is rather some gradual disarmament of the individual States, some gradual greater reliance on regional organizations for some purposes and some gradual vesting of specific world functions in an authority which is to act under laws adopted through some democratic procedure and which controls enough armed force to preserve peace in a world without national armies and without nuclear weapons.

351. Serious proposals for a complete eradication of nuclear weapons have been presented. They assume that there will remain other means and weapons which can be used against possible usurpers clandestinely developing nuclear weapons. They recognize formidable problems and assume a development in phases. They deserve serious study and consideration, also at the governmental level.

352. Proposals for general and complete disarmament were discussed for years between governments during the Cold War. It is hard to contradict the basic proposition that if weapons are eradicated, there can be no armed conflict. However, troubling questions present themselves. If all States disarm, would the United Nations be equipped with authority and military force to protect them? Should the Organization also have nuclear weapons? Would decisions be taken by a reformed Security Council? Would a veto remain for some? What guarantees would there be that commanders of UN

forces would not one day grab control? Questions like these can hardly be answered in the international community at its present level of development.

353. The issue of general and complete disarmament was quietly left aside and replaced by proposals for limited measures, some of which were agreed early, like the welcome PTBT and the NPT, the Antarctic Treaty and many others which have been discussed in this report. On this path the world has been moving at an accelerated pace in the last decade. That the pace may be kept up.

## V. Arms control and disarmament

*Elements for further discussion.*

354. Despite the efforts of many States and organizations and demands by the public and non-governmental organizations *the issue of disarmament* which was placed on the global governmental agenda at the First Hague Peace Conference in 1899 *moved at a very slow pace* for the larger part of the past hundred years. Worse still, in parallel with economic development ever larger resources were devoted to armaments of ever greater destructive capacity. Insecurity, especially between great powers and blocs, raised to ever higher levels of cost. Huge resources which could have been devoted to improving standards of living everywhere and helped developing countries to remove poverty were lost on arms races.

355. However, *in the last few decades* and especially after the end of the Cold War *doors have opened* to great new possibilities and a process has been initiated in which substantial reductions are being made in the military budgets of many States. Some new important factors have been driving this welcome evolution, above all a *reduction of tensions* between great powers and blocs. It is essential

that the current setbacks be overcome. Otherwise there is a big risk that the process will come to a halt.

356. Differences about *borders and the control of territories* only too often generated disputes and armed conflicts in the past. With a few significant exceptions they are now largely absent from the agendas of great powers and blocs.

357. Further, no State or group of States is seeking to *impose its ideology or social system* on other States. Rather, despite the fact that inequitable and inhumane social and economic conditions remain all too common, there is a growing global acceptance that the various conventions on *human rights* express *standards* which are not rooted in any specific region or religion but are truly universal in origin and relevant everywhere. There is an awareness that the tremendous inequality which exists in living standards between the richest and the poorest nations must be reduced. There is also an awareness that although conditions and traditions vary greatly on the globe and call for different institutions and practices, government everywhere must be *democratic*; be based on majority support while respecting the rights of minorities.

358. Another important factor which today influences the relations between States is the vastly increased interdependence in the fields of trade, economy, finance, technology and information, opening up means of inducement based on argument rather than armament. Moreover, in today's world an *array of institutions* in the political, judicial, trade, economic, financial and technical spheres are available to assist in the settlement of differences.

359. With all this said, it must be admitted that many factors may still provoke conflicts and, in the last resort, armed contests, and that few countries find it prudent at this stage to radically lower their military guards and follow the examples of some countries which have no military forces.

360. The tremendous *gap between the poorest and the richest* countries cannot remain without severe and potentially very dangerous strains resulting, unless the conditions of poverty are seen as a common challenge leading to common action. Evidently the huge *peace dividend* that would result from disarmament ought to yield significant resources to reduce the present gaps in the standards between the richest and the poorest and the dangers flowing from it.

361. *Competition about natural resources* - fresh water, arable land, fish, oil, minerals, etc. - is also likely to generate controversies in a world where the total population is still growing fast. *Environmental problems*, such as the need to reduce the global emissions of green-house gases or ozone-hole-creating gases, may also lead to severe differences between nations and groups of nations.

362. Lastly, in this open-ended list of sources of conflict, we must note that conflicts about *territorial control and borders* continue to exist in several parts of the world, not least in Africa, and are leading to armed conflicts which are severe even without the great power involvement which used to exacerbate conflicts in and between developing countries during the Cold War.

363. Humanity's entry into a world without armed conflicts between great powers and blocs, fewer regional and local armed conflicts and less armaments, is certainly no automatic journey, but one that will require much good will, sincere effort, prudence, pragmatism and patience. The great powers must themselves take great care that the largely constructive course which their relations have followed after the end of the Cold War is continued and is not jeopardized by any disregard for vital interests. While they may not always perceive the need for joint multilateral institutions and rules, being more able to fend for themselves than smaller States, no dictates by one or several great powers are likely to bring about harmonious international relations. The future world of ever closer interrelations between peoples, economies and cultures will require ever better functioning regional and universal institutions in which the difficult task of elaborating joint policies and actions is undertaken.

364. It is not difficult to draw up a long agenda for action and analysis in the field of arms control and disarmament. Many problems that need to be tackled in this field as the new century opens have not been discussed in the report submitted to the Hague Centennial; yet, many others have. Ten points are listed below in an agenda the length of which is limited only by our political experience and imagination:

1. Ratification and entry into force of the CTBT. Participation by India, Pakistan and DPRK. (action now)
- Ratification of the *Ottawa Convention on Anti-Personnel Mines.* (accelerated action)
- Initiation of active negotiations in the Conference on Disarmament of a *fissile material cut-off treaty (FMCT).* (action now)

2. Reduction in the possession of nuclear arsenals by declared nuclear-weapon States:
- Transformation into legally binding form of the 1991 US/ Russian commitments to withdraw tactical nuclear weapons from ships and foreign territories
- Ratification and entry into force of *START 2* and completion of *START 3* to further reduce the nuclear arsenals of the US and Russia. (action now)
- Action by the *three other declared nuclear-weapon States* formally to commit themselves to *further reductions in their nuclear arsenals.* (action now)

3. Non-proliferation of nuclear weapons:
- Negotiation of improved *positive and negative security guarantees* for States which legally commit themselves not to possess nuclear explosives. (action now)
- Study of *nuclear weapon free zones or zones free of weapons of mass destruction* for two areas of special tension, namely the Middle East and the Korean peninsula. (initiation)
- In this context, study of the use of specific *positive security guarantees* issued by the Security Council and of the possible

combination of verification performed by multilateral institutions and by the States participating in the zone.

4. Actions specifically relating to verification:
- Completion of a protocol regarding *verification* of the convention on *biological* weapons. (action now)
- Acceptance of *strengthened safeguards* by States parties to the NPT and other States which have concluded safeguards agreements with the IAEA. (action now)
- Development of methods of verification of the IAEA and agreements on *verification that nuclear material* - highly enriched uranium and plutonium - *which becomes redundant from the military sector*, notably through the dismantling of nuclear weapons is irreversibly removed from military use. (initiation)
- *Co-operation between multilateral professional institutions for verification* (nuclear, chemical, future biological and other) to exchange non-confidential data and experience to strengthen their detecting capacity. (initiation)

5. Study of the use of *restrictions on the trade and transfer of different types of arms* to minimize the risk of development of weapons of mass destruction (nuclear, chemical, biological) and certain missiles, without hampering legitimate peaceful technological development. Can the various existing regimes[193] be made more transparent and adjusted to become generally accepted or supported? (initiation)

6. Material and equipment relevant for the production of weapons of mass destruction or missiles must be *physically protected* by governments from being acquired by sub-national groups or terrorists and being the subject of trafficking. Governments need to establish multilateral mechanisms for technical assistance and co-operation to strengthen their capacity to prevent such acquisition and trafficking. (initiation)

193. Nuclear suppliers group, Australia group and Missiles technology control group.

7. Examination within the Conference on Disarmament of the question of commitments regarding the *no-first-use of nuclear weapons*. (initiation)

8. Examination within the Conference on Disarmament of measures leading toward the elimination of nuclear weapons. (initiation)

9. Discussion of the problem what measures are appropriate to meet the threat of reckless States, sub-national or terrorist groups which might control some missiles and small quantities of weapons of mass destruction. Are all to fend for themselves or should there be collective protection? Is it reasonable or risky to restrict the scope of the ABM? (initiation)

10. Discussion within the United Nations of *reforms strengthening its capacity* to cope, on behalf of the international community, with possible violations of agreements on disarmament and arms control, e.g. making the Security Council more effective by making it more representative while reducing the use of the veto, giving a greater role to regional organizations, and/or establishing rapid military deployment forces of the UN. (initiation).

# INTERNATIONAL HUMANITARIAN LAW (LAWS OF WAR)

Revised Report for the Centennial Commemoration of the First Hague Peace Conference 1899
by Christopher GREENWOOD[1]

## I. Introduction

1.1 The codification and revision of the laws of war, or, to use the term more widely employed today, "international humanitarian law",[2] proved to be one of the most important parts of the work of the 1899 Hague Peace Conference (referred to herein as "the Conference"). When the Conference convened, the laws of war were almost all unwritten, they covered only a comparatively small part of military activity and there was considerable controversy regarding their extent and manner of application even amongst States with otherwise similar views about international law. The Conference began the process, which has gone on throughout the 20th century, of developing a substantial body of written law for the conduct of hostilities. The results of that century of law-making are evident. In contrast to the position in 1899, most aspects of military activity are now regulated by treaty, or by rules of customary law which are authoritatively stated in treaty texts. The degree of detail is such that

1. Professor of International Law, London School of Economics and Political Science. The work on this Report was concluded in May 1999.

2. Not all parts of the laws of war can strictly be regarded as humanitarian but the doctrinal debate about which rules should be characterised as humanitarian and which should not falls outside the scope of this report. For the sake of simplicity, therefore, the terms "laws of war" and "international humanitarian law" will be treated as synonymous in this report. The term "law of armed conflict" is also treated as synonymous with "laws of war".



*F. Kalshoven (ed.),*
***The Centennial of the First International Peace Conference,*** 161–259.

any collection of the relevant agreements comprises hundreds of pages.

1.2 The Conference was held at a time when there was great optimism about the effect which scientific progress (including developments in the science of international law) could have upon the condition of humanity. Yet, as an eminent military historian has said, the undoubted progress which the 20th century has seen in tackling the problems of famine or sickness has not been matched by progress in reducing the threats posed by war.[3] While the subject of this Report is that part of the law which seeks to alleviate the effects of war, rather than to prevent war itself, the same note of caution applies. For all the undoubted progress which has been made during the last 100 years in developing the law in this area, the difficulty of preserving humanitarian values in time of war is, if anything, even more acute at the end of the century than it was at the beginning.

1.3 This sorry story therefore begs the question, why has compliance with this area of international law been so poor? Several answers suggest themselves. The ideological or tribal nature of much of 20th century warfare, the threat which defeat in warfare poses, the corresponding importance of victory and the sense that violations do not matter and can, in any event, be committed with impunity have all been factors.

1.4 It is this last consideration on which the present Report concentrates. The reason for that is that the other factors are to a large extent outside the control of those who seek to enhance respect for the laws of war without at the same time seeking, or feeling able, to change the nature of international society.

1.5 The centenary of the 1899 Peace Conference, coinciding as it does with the 50th anniversary of the adoption of the Geneva Conventions and the end of the UN Decade of International Law, thus provides an excellent opportunity to reflect on the development of

3. J. Keegan, *War and Our World* (BBC, 1998), p. 1.

the laws of war. The purpose of this Report will be to recall some of the achievements and failures of the last century and to attempt to identify those parts of the laws of war which stand in greatest need of attention at the end of the 20th century. The Report will focus on the analysis of four main subjects, or themes, which are of particular significance for the future of the laws of war. Most, though not all, of these themes were touched on at the Conference, even if developments during the succeeding hundred years have taken them in directions very different from those which might have been envisaged in 1899. The approach adopted, in respect of each of these themes, will be to conduct a stocktaking of the principal achievements and failures of the 20th century, to identify the principal problems which remain unresolved and, where appropriate, to suggest how such problems might be addressed.

1.6 At the end of a century which has seen so much of war and in which the laws of war have proved so comparatively ineffectual, it seems obvious that that law must be seen as deficient and the record of the last hundred years be adjudged one of failure rather than achievement. This Report will certainly identify deficiencies in several areas of the law. Yet the principal conclusion is not that the world needs new law, or different law, but that the law which we have needs to be made more effective. As Sir Franklin BERMAN has put it:

> It seems to many that the problem is not to discover what the law is, or how to apply it to the particular case, or even whether the existing rule is "satisfactory" or not, but rather how to secure or compel compliance with the law at all. It may be that we have now passed from a great phase of law-making to a period where the focus is not on new substantive law but on how to make existing law effective.[4]

1.7 As a preliminary to the main discussion, the Report begins (Part II) with a brief examination of the laws of war issues which came before the Conference, and its successor of 1907, and a survey

4. Sir Franklin Berman, Preface to H. Fox and M. Meyer (eds.), *Effecting Compliance* (1993), p. xii.

of the approach adopted at those conferences. Thereafter, the following themes will be examined in greater detail:

(1) *the scope and application of the laws of war* (Part III), a section which will examine the place of the laws of war in international law as a whole, their relationship with the prohibition on resort to force in the UN Charter and with other areas of law, such as the law of human rights, as well as considering the circumstances in which the laws of war become applicable;
(2) *the conduct of hostilities in international armed conflicts* (Part IV), which will discuss the substantive law applicable to armed conflicts possessing an international character, in particular the law relating to belligerent occupation, weapons, targets and combatancy and the law of naval warfare;
(3) *the conduct of hostilities in internal armed conflicts* (Part V), which will conduct a similar examination of the law applicable to armed conflicts occurring within a State;
(4) *methods for ensuring compliance with the law* (Part VI), which will look at the means of implementing the law considered in the earlier parts of the Report.

Finally, a concluding section (Part VII) will make some tentative suggestions regarding what should be considered the priorities for the future in this area of the law.

1.8 The present Report is a revised version of a preliminary Report issued in June 1998. It was always the intention that the Preliminary Report would be reconsidered and revised in the light of the discussions to be held as part of the commemoration process, with a final version of the Report being produced in 1999. There is, however, an additional reason why the Preliminary Report, and particularly Part VI required revision. At the time that it was drafted in 1998, the intergovernmental conference on the establishment of an International Criminal Court was opening in Rome. The work of this Conference has had a considerable impact on the laws of war and, in particular, on the methods for ensuring compliance with those laws. Until the outcome of the Rome Conference was known, it would obviously have been premature to engage in any detailed comment on the law in relation to war crimes.

1.9 Another most important development taking place in parallel with the 1899 Centennial has been the preparation by the ICRC of a study of customary international humanitarian law. At the time of writing, this study had not been completed, so it was not possible to incorporate any of its findings into the present Report. Nevertheless, a recurrent theme of the Report is that, notwithstanding the advances made in treaty law during the last one hundred years, the customary laws of war remain of great importance. The ICRC study is likely, therefore, to make a major contribution to clarifying the content of the customary law principles.

1.10 In preparing this Revised Report, the Rapporteur has been greatly assisted by the numerous comments which have been received on the Preliminary Report, from individuals, NGOs, the ICRC, and various regional and governmental bodies, of which are mentioned here the Government of the United Kingdom and the Advisory Committee on International Law Issues of the Netherlands. Where possible account has been taken of those comments.

1.11 I would also like to offer my gratitude to the Netherlands Ministry of Foreign Affairs, which commissioned this report and, in particular, to H.E. Ambassador Adriaan BOS, Mr. Teunis HALFF and Mr. Thijs BÜCHLI, who gave me much help and support and who patiently accepted the delays in delivery of the report. I would also like to thank the representatives of the Ministry of Foreign Affairs of the Russian Federation. The responsibility for any errors which remain is mine alone.

1.12 Reading the papers of the 1899 Conference after an interval of one hundred years is a sobering experience and in many respects a depressing one. It is impossible to avoid a feeling of disappointment when one compares the ideals of the 1899 and 1907 Conferences with most of what followed. It is certainly difficult to recapture the idea, widely held in 1899, that better law would invariably mean a better world.

1.13 Yet it is undeniable that the 1899 Conference and its successor in 1907 represented great advances in international humanitarian law. Those advances were built upon by the international community in a succession of subsequent international agreements, noticeably the Geneva Conventions of 1949 and the Additional Protocols of 1977. Despite all the disappointments, the 1899 Conference helped to launch a century of codification and development of the law which has given us a body of international humanitarian law which is far in advance of what existed in 1899. The problem is that this law is still ignored with impunity more often than not. It is the principal theme of this report that the challenge at the end of the 20th century is not to improve upon the law but to find ways of ensuring better compliance with that law.

# II. The Laws of War at the 1899 Peace Conference

## II.1 Background

2.1 When Count MOURAVIEFF first proposed the convening of an international peace conference,[5] the question of revision of the laws of war had been the subject of discussion in the international community for more than thirty years.[6] A number of treaties dealing with

5. Letter of 24 August 1898. The texts of many of the documents concerning the Conference can be found in *The International Peace Conference*, Netherlands Ministry of Foreign Affairs, 1907, and A. Pearce Higgins, *The Hague Peace Conferences* (1909) and J.B. Scott, *The Proceedings of the Hague Peace Conferences: The Conference of 1899* (Translation into English prepared by the Carnegie Endowment, 1920).

6. The laws of war themselves could, of course, be traced back to a much earlier date. It is important to realise that the requirement that certain humanitarian principles be observed in warfare was well established in all of the main cultures; see, e.g., E. Bello, *African Customary Humanitarian Law* (1980), M. Khadduri, *The Law of War*
(continued...)

specific topics had already been adopted. The Declaration of Paris, 1856, prohibited privateering and made a number of other provisions regarding the laws of naval warfare. The Geneva Convention, 1864, the first of the "Red Cross" conventions, established a legal regime for the protection of medical personnel in land warfare. In 1868 an attempt was made to adopt additional articles extending the 1864 Convention to naval warfare but these articles never entered into force. The St. Petersburg Declaration, 1868, outlawing projectiles of under 400 grammes in weight (i.e. rifle ammunition but not artillery shells) which were explosive or charged with fulminating or inflammable substances,[7] became the first agreement of modern times to prohibit the use of a specific category of weapons.

2.2 Moreover, there was considerable enthusiasm for the adoption of a comprehensive code of the laws of war, at least in relation to land warfare. The United States had issued such a code to its armed forces in 1863.[8] In 1874, at the Brussels Conference, representatives of fifteen States adopted the Project of an International Declaration concerning the Laws and Customs of War on Land, although this instrument never became binding.[9] The *Institut de droit international* published a Manual of the Laws of War on Land in 1880[10] which built upon the Brussels Declaration. All three texts were to prove influential at the Conference.

6. (...continued)
*and Peace in Islam* (1955), N. Singh, "Armed Conflicts and Humanitarian Laws of Ancient India" in C. Swiniarski (ed.), *Studies and Essays on International Humanitarian Law and Red Cross Principles* (1984), p. 531, and the essays in UNESCO, *International Dimensions of Humanitarian Law* (1988). See also the paper by V. Muntabhorn,"The 1899 Hague Peace Conference and the Development of the Laws of War: Asia's contribution to the Quest for Humanitarianism", delivered at the Asia-Pacific regional meeting in Melbourne in February 1999.

7. In the authentic French text, "tout projectile d'un poids inférieur à 400 grammes qui serait ou explosible ou chargé de matières fulminantes ou inflammables".

8. This was the famous "Lieber Code" drawn up by the jurist Francis Lieber for the Lincoln Government during the American Civil War and issued as General Order 100, D. Schindler and J. Toman (eds.), *The Laws of Armed Conflicts* (3rd ed., 1988), p. 3.

9. Schindler and Toman, p. 25.

10. 5 *Annuaire* (1881-2) p. 156; Schindler and Toman, p. 35.

## II.2 The Laws of War at the Conference

2.3 Although the proposal of the Russian Government for the Peace Conference originally focussed upon disarmament and the prevention of war, the detailed list of topics produced for the Conference was more heavily weighted towards the laws of war. The topics suggested for discussion were:
(1) the prohibition for a fixed term of any increase of the armed forces beyond those then maintained;
(2) the prohibition of, or limitation in the employment of new fire-arms or explosives;
(3) the restriction of the explosives already existing and the prohibition of the discharge of projectiles or explosives of any kind from balloons or by any similar means;
(4) the prohibition in naval warfare of submarine torpedo-boats or similar engines of destruction, and the ultimate abolition of vessels with rams;
(5) the application to naval warfare of the principles of the Geneva Convention of 1864 on the basis of the additional Articles of 1868;
(6) the neutralisation of ships and boats employed in saving those shipwrecked during or after an engagement;
(7) the revision of the unratified Brussels Declaration of 1874 concerning the laws and customs of war on land; and
(8) the acceptance in principle of the employment of good offices, of mediation and arbitration with the object of preventing armed conflicts between nations, and the establishment of a uniform practice in their employment.[11]

2.4 Items 1 to 4 on this list were allocated to the First Committee of the Conference, which concentrated on disarmament. That proved to be the least productive part of the Conference's work. The two Declarations agreed in the First Committee - on the prohibition, for a period of five years, of the discharge of explosive projectiles from

11. Pearce Higgins, op. cit. supra note 5, p. 40.

balloons[12] and the permanent prohibition of projectiles, "the sole purpose of which was the diffusion of asphyxiating or deleterious gases"[13] - are really laws of war instruments.[14] Items 5, 6 and 7, which clearly concerned the laws of war, were dealt with by the Second Committee, while the question of peaceful settlement of disputes was considered by the Third Committee.

2.5 In practice, it was in the area of the laws of war that the Conference made the greatest progress in developing the law. The foremost objective, of maintaining peace, gave rise to the Convention for the Pacific Settlement of Disputes but the undoubted importance of that Convention lay more in the creation of the institution of the Permanent Court of Arbitration than in the development of substantive law.[15] Very little was achieved in relation to disarmament. By contrast, the Conference took a number of important steps in what would now be described as the codification and progressive development of the laws of war.

2.6 The most striking achievement was the adoption of the Convention on the Laws and Customs of War on Land and the Regulations attached thereto. These Regulations built upon the Lieber Code, the 1874 Brussels Declaration and the 1880 Oxford Manual. The Convention was, however, much more than just an effort in codification. The task which the Conference set itself was the revision of the laws of war, with the aim both of making them more precise and laying down certain limits in order to modify the severity of war. On the whole, the Conference was successful in achieving these goals. The Regulations on the Laws and Customs of War on

12. Declaration No. I, 1899.

13. Declaration No. II, 1899. In the authentic French text, the passage quoted reads: "projectiles qui ont pour but unique de répandre des gaz asphyxiants ou délétères".

14. Captain Crozier, of the US delegation, made the point in his report that these subjects would more logically have been considered by the Second Committee for that reason; J.B. Scott (ed.), *Instructions to the American Delegates to the Hague Peace Conferences and their Official Reports* (1916), p. 29.

15. This subject is discussed in the Joint Report of Professors Orrego Vicuña and Pinto.

Land went beyond the earlier instruments in a number of ways. As one of the United States delegates put it:

> The code [i.e. the Regulations annexed to the Convention] in general presents that advance from the rules of General Order 100 [the Lieber Code] in the direction of effort to spare the sufferings of the population of invaded and occupied countries, to limit the acts of invaders to those required by military necessities, and to diminish what are ordinarily known as the evils of war, which might be expected from the progress of nearly forty years' thought upon the subject.[16]

2.7 The scope of the Regulations was ambitious, taking in most of the law of land warfare (with the exception of those issues covered by the 1864 Geneva Convention). Moreover, the fact that the Conference was not able to reach agreement on a number of important issues (noticeably, the question of combatant status for members of popular resistance movements) was mitigated by the incorporation in the Preamble of the Convention of the first version of the "Martens Clause", proposed by the Chairman of the Sub-Committee on Land Warfare of the Second Committee. This clause has attracted such a degree of attention over the course of the century that it is worthwhile reproducing it in full, together with certain other paragraphs of the Preamble:

> According to the view of the High Contracting Parties, these provisions, the wording of which has been inspired by the desire to diminish the evils of war, so far as military necessities permit, are intended to serve as general rules of conduct for belligerents in their relations with each other and with populations.
> It has not, however, been possible to agree forthwith on provisions embracing all the circumstances which occur in practice.
> On the other hand, it could not be intended by the High Contracting Parties that the cases not provided for should, for want of a written provision be left to the arbitrary judgment of military commanders.
> Until a more complete code of the laws of war can be issued, the High Contracting Parties think it expedient to declare that in cases not included in the Regulations adopted by them, populations and belligerents

16. Report of Captain Crozier, loc. cit. supra note 10, p. 46.

remain under the protection and the rule of the principles of the law of nations, as they result from the usages established between civilised nations, from the laws of humanity, and the requirements of the public conscience.[17]

2.8 While the 1899 Convention and Regulations were superseded in most respects by Hague Convention No. IV, 1907, and the Regulations annexed to that Convention, they remain an important landmark in the evolution of laws of war and many of the provisions which originated in the 1899 text and were carried over into the 1907 Regulations continue to be regarded as an authoritative statement of customary international law rules one hundred years later.

2.9 The Conference also adopted a Convention adapting the principles of the Geneva Convention to naval warfare, the project which States had failed to bring to completion in 1868. The Convention thus adopted was the forerunner of the Second Geneva Convention, 1949, which is still in force.

2.10 In addition, the Conference adopted three Declarations:

| | |
|---|---|
| Declaration No. I, | outlawing for a period of five years the discharge of explosive projectiles from balloons; |

17. The authentic French text stated:
Selon les vues des Hautes Parties contractantes, ces dispositions, dont la rédaction a été inspirée par le désir de diminuer les maux de la guerre, autant que les nécessités militaires le permettent, sont destinées à servir de règle générale de conduite aux belligérants, dans leurs rapports entre eux et avec les populations.
Il n'a pas été possible toutefois de concerter dès maintenant des stipulations s'étendant à toutes les circonstances qui se présentent dans la pratique.
D'autre part, il ne pouvait entrer dans les intentions des Hautes Parties contractantes que les cas non prévus fussent, faute de stipulation écrite, laissées à l'appréciation arbitraire de ceux qui dirigent les armées.
En attendant qu'un Code plus complet des lois de la guerre puisse être édicté, les Hautes Parties contractantes jugent opportun de constater que, dans les cas non compris dans les dispositions réglementaires adoptées par elles, les populations et les belligérants restent sous la sauvegarde et sous l'empire des principes du droit des gens, tels qu'ils résultent des usages établis entre nations civilisées, des lois de l'humanité et des exigences de la conscience publique.

| | |
|---|---|
| Declaration No. II, | prohibiting the use of projectiles, the sole purpose of which was the diffusion of asphyxiating or deleterious gases; and |
| Declaration No. III, | prohibiting the use of expanding bullets and other bullets which flatten easily or expand in the human body. |

While these Declarations straddle the boundary between the laws of war and disarmament, there is little doubt that the main motive behind their adoption was humanitarian. One of the United States delegates, for example, commented on Declaration No. I that:

> The action was taken for humanitarian reasons alone, and was founded upon the opinion that balloons, as they now exist, form such an uncertain means of delivery that they cannot be used with any accuracy.[18]

2.11 Finally, the Conference indicated, in a series of *voeux* adopted as part of the Final Act, that it considered it desirable that there should be discussion at a Second Peace Conference of a range of questions on the law of naval warfare and the law of neutrality which had not been before it in 1899, as well as suggesting a revision of the Geneva Convention, 1864.

## II.3 The 1907 Peace Conference and the Laws of War

2.12 The 1907 Peace Conference built upon the achievements of the 1899 Conference. Both of the Conventions on the laws of war adopted by the 1899 Conference were revised. In addition, the Second Conference adopted seven new Conventions on the laws of naval warfare, a Convention on the rights and duties of neutral powers in land warfare and a Convention relative to the commencement of hostilities.

18. Captain Crozier, loc. cit. supra note 10, p. 31.

# III. The Scope and Application of the Laws of War

3.1 In assessing the achievements of 1899 in the laws of war, two questions have to be addressed at the outset: when do those laws apply and what is their place in the structure of international law as a whole? These are not just theoretical questions - although they have considerable theoretical significance - for the answers have important practical implications. International law is not simply a collection of rules and principles, it is a legal system, within which no one body of law can exist in isolation from the whole and which is greater than the sum of its parts.

3.2 While the laws of war address the specific problems of the conduct of hostilities and are, to that extent, *lex specialis*, it is necessary to consider their relationship with the law governing the right to resort to force (the *ius ad bellum*) and also with other parts of international law which might have an impact upon the conduct of warfare, in particular the law of human rights and international environmental law. Moreover, the effectiveness of the substantive laws of war will be significantly reduced if there is constant controversy about the circumstances in which those laws are applicable. This Part of the Report will therefore examine the place of the laws of war in the structure of international law and the circumstances in which the laws of war become applicable.

## III.1 The Laws of War within the Structure of International Law

### (a) *Laws of War and Laws against War*

3.3 Even in 1899 there was something anomalous in a Peace Conference, summoned with the objective of preventing war, devoting so much attention to devising laws for the conduct of war. In the words of one contemporary commentator: "The Emperor of Russia might have said of it, 'I labour for peace, but when I speak to them thereof, they make them ready for battle.'"[19] Yet the delegates at the Conference evidently saw no inconsistency in seeking to prevent war while also drawing up codes of conduct for its regulation in the event that war should break out. Their attitude was succinctly stated in the Preamble to the Convention on the Laws and Customs of War on Land:

> Considering that, while seeking to preserve peace and prevent armed conflicts between nations, it is likewise necessary to have regard to cases where an appeal to arms may be caused by events which their solicitude could not avert;
> Animated also by the desire to serve, even in this extreme case, the interests of humanity and the ever progressive needs of civilisation;
> Thinking it important, with this object, to revise the laws and customs of war, either with the view of defining them more precisely, or of laying down certain limits for the purpose of modifying their severity as far as possible ...

3.4 That approach was plainly right, both as a matter of common sense and in principle, given that international law in 1899 did not prohibit recourse to war as an instrument of national policy and that the Conference did not attempt to alter that situation.[20] However, once international law - first through the Covenant of the League of Nations, 1919, and the Pact for the Renunciation of War, 1928, and latterly through Article 2(4) of the UN Charter - developed rules which severely limited the right of States to resort to force in their international relations, such an approach became more difficult to justify.

3.5 In particular, three issues arise. First, should international law continue to devote so much attention to the law on the conduct of war now that it has prohibited recourse to war as an instrument of national policy? Secondly, is it right – or even possible – to maintain the principle, which was taken for granted in 1899, that the laws of

19. Pearce Higgins, op. cit. supra note 5, p. 43.

20. The Convention for the Pacific Settlement of International Disputes merely required parties "before an appeal to arms ... to have recourse, as far as circumstances allow, to the good offices or mediation of one or more friendly Powers" (Art. 1).

war apply equally to all the warring parties, irrespective of which is the aggressor? Thirdly, quite apart from the principle of equal application, are the laws of war affected by the fact that they now co-exist with a law against war?

3.6 With regard to the first question, there have certainly been occasions during the 20th century when it has been argued that attention to the laws of war only serves to distract from the more important task of preventing war or even undermines the prohibition on resort to force. That was one of the reasons why the International Law Commission (ILC) did not place the reform of the laws of war on its agenda in 1949.[21] There can be no doubt, however, that the history of the 20th century has vindicated the approach of the delegates to the 1899 Conference in seeking to regulate the conduct of war at the same time as striving for its prevention. More than fifty years after the adoption of the UN Charter, it is all too apparent that prohibition of war has not meant prevention and that the need for legal regulation of warfare, "to serve, even in this extreme case, the interests of humanity" is greater than ever. There is no evidence whatsoever that the existence of laws designed to achieve that goal does anything to make war more likely or to undermine the prohibition on resort to force in the Charter and other instruments. On the contrary, recent UN practice - in particular, the determinations by the Security Council, in respect of the former Yugoslavia and Rwanda, that better enforcement of the laws of war could assist in addressing threats to international peace and security - strongly suggests that attention to the laws of war complements, rather than distracts from, the attempts to prevent war.[22]

21. 1 Ybk ILC (1949) pp. 51-53. A more practical reason was the fact that the Red Cross had already embarked upon a complete revision of the Geneva Conventions.

22. See SC Res. 827 (1993), establishing the International Tribunal for the Former Yugoslavia (ICTY), the preamble to which states the Council's view that the prosecution of persons responsible for serious violations of international humanitarian law would contribute to the restoration and maintenance of peace. See also Res. 955 (1994), establishing the International Criminal Tribunal for Rwanda (ICTR). The Council's view is reflected in the first decisions of the two Tribunals: *Prosecutor* v. *Tadic (Jurisdiction)* (Appeals Chamber, ICTY, 2 Oct. 1995) 105 ILR 419; *Prosecutor*
(continued...)

3.7 The second question poses more problems at both a theoretical and a practical level. The notion that the laws of war confer the same rights, and impose the same obligations, upon the aggressor and the victim of that aggression appears to run counter to the fundamental principle that no one should profit from their own unlawful act (*ex iniuria ius non oritur*). In particular, the laws of war confer upon belligerents extensive rights vis-à-vis not only other belligerents but also neutral States. Should a State be entitled to such rights when it has itself been responsible, in violation of its obligations under the UN Charter and customary law, for initiating a conflict?

3.8 The idea of distinguishing in the application of the laws of war between the aggressor and the victim (or, where, the UN undertakes or authorises the use of force, between the forces of a lawbreaker and those seeking to restore international peace and security) has been made on several occasions since international law developed a prohibition on recourse to force. In *United States* v. *List* (the Hostages case), the prosecution argued that, since Germany's invasion of the Balkan States had been an illegal use of force, the subsequent occupation was illegal in its entirety and those who commanded the German forces during that occupation could not rely, in their defence, upon the powers given by the laws of war to a belligerent occupant.[23] At the Diplomatic Conference on Humanitarian Law in 1974, it was argued by one State that soldiers who participated in an illegal war could derive no benefit from the laws of war, because of the illegality of their State's resort to force.

3.9 There are, however, compelling arguments, both of practice and principle, for rejecting such an approach. First, to hold that the laws of war applied in a different way to the different sides in a conflict would be likely to undermine the application of the law. As Sir Hersch LAUTERPACHT explained:

22. (...continued)
v. *Kanyabashi (Jurisdiction)* (Trial Chamber, ICTR, 18 June 1977) ICTR-96-15-T.

23. 15 *Ann Dig* p. 632 at pp. 636-7.

> ... unless the aggressor has been defeated from the very outset ..., it is impossible to visualize the conduct of hostilities in which one side would be bound by rules of warfare without benefiting from them and the other side would benefit from rules of warfare without being bound by them. Accordingly, any application to the actual conduct of war of the principle *ex iniuria ius non oritur* would transform the contest into a struggle which may be subject to no regulation at all. The result would be the abandonment of most rules of warfare, including those which are of a humanitarian character.[24]

3.10 Secondly, the overwhelming majority of the laws of war seek to benefit and protect not the belligerent States themselves but individuals caught up in the conflict. Even if the State to which they owe allegiance has acted unlawfully in resorting to force, the population of that State cannot be regarded as responsible for that illegality and should not, therefore, be deprived of the protection which the laws of war afford. The laws of war are directed to all individuals, in the sense that any individual at any level of authority may bear criminal responsibility for such violations of those rules as he or she may commit (e.g. the ill-treatment of prisoners or detainees), whereas the law against war is directed to the State itself and only the most senior decision-makers within a State have ever been convicted for the crime of waging aggressive war.[25]

24. H. Lauterpacht, "The Limits of the Operation of the Law of War", 30 BYIL (1953) p. 206 at p. 212.

25. Thus, the International Military Tribunal at Nuremberg acquitted Speer, Hitler's armaments minister, of crimes against the peace on the ground that he did not participate in taking the decisions to wage aggressive war, although he was convicted of war crimes, *Proceedings of the International Military Tribunal*, Part 22, pp. 521-3. Similar verdicts were reached in respect of a number of other defendants at Nuremberg. A US Military Tribunal in *United States* v. *Von Leeb* (the High Command case) (15 *Ann Dig* p. 620) held that the members of the German General Staff were guilty of war crimes but acquitted them of crimes against the peace. Similarly, in the IG Farben case, the US Military Tribunal stated that "we cannot say that a private citizen shall be placed in the position of being compelled to determine in the heat of war whether his government is right or wrong, or, if it starts right, when it goes wrong" (15 *Ann Dig* p. 668 at p. 670). ICTY has jurisdiction in respect of war crimes and crimes against humanity but not crimes against the peace.

3.11 Thirdly, except in those cases where the Security Council finds that a particular State is responsible for a threat to the peace, breach of the peace or act of aggression, the question which State is the aggressor in a particular conflict is frequently a matter of intense controversy. If the application of the laws of war varied as between the aggressor and the victim of aggression, the scope for abuse would be enormous. Each State would claim that it was not subject to the obligations of the laws of war and would deny the benefits of those laws to its opponent on the ground that that opponent was the aggressor. Indeed, a State keen to portray itself as the victim of aggression - whether or not with justification - might well feel that it had to deny the applicability of the laws of war, since to accept that they applied might be taken as weakening its stance on the question of aggression.

3.12 In this context, it is important to note that agreement regarding the criteria for determining what constitutes aggression and the application of those criteria in any particular case has hitherto proved elusive. The difficulty is illustrated by the fact that the Rome Conference of 1998, which adopted the Statute of the International Criminal Court, did not agree a definition for the crime of aggression, whereas it was able to adopt a detailed definition of war crimes.

3.13 It is, therefore, one of the achievements of the 20th century that the principle that the laws of war apply with equal force to all parties to a conflict has survived and been reaffirmed. The US Military Tribunal in *List* rejected the prosecution argument outlined above and held that, for the purposes of a war crimes trial, no distinction was to be made between an occupation resulting from a lawful use of force and one which was the product of aggression. The same view was taken in a number of other trials at the end of the Second World War. Proposals made at the 1974-77 Diplomatic Conference to depart from the principle of equal application received almost no support and the preamble to Additional Protocol I, 1977, reaffirms the principle of equal application when it states that:

> ... the provisions of the Geneva Conventions of 12 August 1949 and of this Protocol must be fully applied in all circumstances to all persons who are protected by those instruments, without any adverse distinction based on the nature or origin of the armed conflict or on the causes espoused by or attributed to the Parties to the conflict.

3.14 Most recently, the principle of equality of application of the laws of war was tacitly recognized in the Convention on the Safety of United Nations and Associated Personnel, 1994. That Convention provides that attacks upon United Nations and associated personnel in certain categories of UN operation are crimes which all States have a duty to make punishable under national law.[26] The Convention thus draws a legal distinction between the use of force by and against UN personnel. Article 2 (2) provides, however, that the Convention does not apply to a UN operation, authorized by the Council under Chapter VII of the Charter, "in which any of the personnel are engaged as combatants against organized armed forces and to which the law of international armed conflict applies." The inference is that once a UN force becomes subject to the laws of armed conflict, those laws apply equally to the UN force and its adversaries.[27]

3.15 The equal application of the laws of war does not, of course, mean that the illegality of the aggressor's resort to force produces no consequences. Since the aggressor's resort to force is unlawful, it incurs international responsibility for all the consequences of its use of force. It therefore has a duty to compensate not only those who have suffered loss as a result of the violations of the laws of war committed by its forces but also those injured by acts of the same

26. Art. 9. For discussion of the Convention, see E. Bloom, "Protecting Peace-keepers: The Convention on the Safety of United Nations and Associated Personnel" 89 AJIL (1995) p. 621, C. Bourloyannis-Vrailas, "The Convention on the Safety of United Nations and Associated Personnel", 44 ICLQ (1995) p. 560, C. Greenwood, "Protection of Peacekeepers: The Legal Regime", 7 *Duke Journal of Comparative and International Law* (1996), p. 185 and W.G. Sharp, "Protecting the Avatars of International Peace and Security", loc. cit. p. 93.

27. The problem of determining when the law of armed conflict becomes applicable to a UN operation is considered below.

forces which were not contrary to that law. In the latter case, the illegality which gives rise to the responsibility lies in the original wrongful resort to force. Moreover, since opposition to an illegal resort to force is an entirely foreseeable consequence of that unlawful act, the aggressor can also be held responsible for damage caused by lawful acts of war on the part of its opponents.

3.16 This was the approach adopted in the aftermath of the Gulf conflict, when the Security Council reaffirmed, in Resolution 687 (1991) that Iraq was "liable under international law for any direct loss, damage ... or injury to foreign Governments, nationals or corporations as a result of its unlawful invasion and occupation of Kuwait."[28] That has been interpreted by the UN Compensation Commission as including losses caused by military action or the threat of military action by the coalition forces.[29] In addition to the ordinary responsibility of the State for its unlawful act, the act of aggression may involve the criminal responsibility of those individuals responsible for taking the decision to initiate aggression and the responsibility of the State itself for an international crime.[30]

3.17 The third question posed in this section, namely whether the laws of war are affected by the fact that they now co-exist with a law against war, may also have considerable practical significance and has so far received comparatively little attention. It is clear that, under contemporary international law, the use of force by a State in its international relations will be lawful only if two requirements are satisfied:

28. Para. 16.

29. Governing Council Decision No. 7, para. 21(a), UN Doc. S/AC.26/1991/7/Rev. 1, 109 ILR 586, and the Report and Recommendations of the Panel of Commissioners in the *Well Blowout Control Claim* (18 December 1996), UN Doc. S/AC.26/1996/5, 109 ILR 479.

30. That responsibility will be delictual, although Article 19 of the ILC Draft Articles on State Responsibility raises the possibility of criminal responsibility of States. Whether the concept of criminal responsibility of the State, as opposed to the individuals, is a useful concept and what consequences follow from it are matters of controversy which cannot be considered here.

(a) the resort to force is compatible with the UN Charter and the relevant rules of customary international law; and
(b) the actual use of force is not contrary to the laws of war.

3.18 The first requirement will be satisfied if the resort to force is an exercise of the right of self-defence preserved in Article 51 of the Charter. For a State's use of force to constitute self-defence, however, it is not enough that the conditions for the exercise of that right existed at the time that the decision to use force was taken. The right of self-defence includes the limitations of necessity and proportionality[31] and the measures which the State actually takes must, therefore, meet the criteria of necessity and proportionality if the use of force is to be lawful. The implications were explained by Judge AGO in his Report to the ILC on the law of State Responsibility, when he said that:

> In fact, the requirements of the "necessity" and "proportionality" of the action taken in self-defence can simply be described as two sides of the same coin. Self-defence will be valid as a circumstance precluding the wrongfulness of the conduct of the State only if that State was unable to achieve the desired result by different conduct involving either no use of armed force at all or merely its use on a lesser scale.[32]

3.19 That does not mean that the degree of force employed in self-defence must be no greater than that used in the original armed attack. To quote Judge AGO once more:

> The requirement of the proportionality of the action taken in self-defence ... concerns the relationship between that action and its purpose, namely - and this can never be repeated too often - that of halting and repelling the attack or even, in so far as preventive self-defence is recognized, of preventing it from occurring. It would be mistaken, however, to think that there must be proportionality between the conduct

31. *Case concerning Military and Paramilitary Actions in and against Nicargua*, para. 176, ICJ Reports 1986, p.14 at p. 94; *Advisory Opinion on the Legality of the Threat or Use of Nuclear Weapons*, ICJ Reports 1996, p. 226 at pp. 244-5, paras. 40-41.

32. Eighth Report on State Responsibility, Ybk ILC, 1980, vol. II (i), p. 121.

> constituting the armed attack and the opposing conduct. The action needed to halt and repulse the attack may well have to assume dimensions disproportionate to those of the attack suffered.[33]

In other words, "the concept of proportionality referred to was that which was proportionate to repelling the attack, and not a requirement of symmetry between the mode of the initial attack and the mode of response."[34]

3.20 It then becomes necessary to determine whether the limitation of proportionality and necessity continues to apply when a State goes to war, or engages in an armed conflict, by way of self-defence. It has sometimes been suggested that "the limits inherent in the requirement of proportionality are clearly meaningless where the armed attack and the likewise armed resistance to it lead to a state of war between the two countries."[35] However, such an approach would mean that a State could free itself of some of the limitations of the right of self-defence by declaring war, or otherwise manifesting an intention to treat an attack as an act of war, something for which there is no warrant in the Charter and which would seem to be wholly contrary to principle. A further problem is that if "war" is here used as synonymous with "armed conflict" (as is now frequently the case), then the result would be that the proportionality and necessity limitation would apply only to isolated and low level instances of the use of force. If, on the other hand, "war" is in some

33. Loc. cit.

34. Dissenting Opinion of Judge Higgins, *Advisory Opinion on the Legality of the Threat or Use of Nuclear Weapons,* ICJ Reports 1996, p. 226 at p. 583. See also H. Waldock, "The regulation of the Use of Force by Individual States in International Law", 81 RdC (1952) p. 464 and A. Randelzhofer, Commentary on Article 51 in B. Simma (ed.), *The Charter of the United Nations: A Commentary* (1994), p. 677.

35. Ago, loc. cit. supra note 32, para. 121. See also Y. Dinstein, *War, Aggression and Self-Defence* (2nd ed., 1994) at pp. 232-3.

way to be distinguished from other kinds of "armed conflict" there is no agreement regarding the criteria by which that is to be done.[36]

3.21 Moreover, in its recent Advisory Opinion on the *Legality of the Threat or Use of Nuclear Weapons*, the ICJ considered that the requirements of necessity and proportionality as elements of the right of self-defence applied "whatever the means of force employed" and were thus applicable to the use of nuclear weapons.[37] It is difficult to imagine a use of nuclear weapons which would not amount to an act of war. It is suggested, therefore, that acts of force undertaken in self-defence must still comply with the requirements of necessity and proportionality, even if they occur in time of war or armed conflict.

3.22 Self-defence is not the only justification for resort to force in contemporary international law. Force may lawfully be used if it has been properly authorized by the Security Council in the exercise of its powers under Chapter VII of the Charter, as was done in the Gulf conflict in 1990-91 when those States which engaged in military operations against Iraq did so under an authorization conferred by Resolution 678. Once again, however, the use of force will be lawful only if it is confined to what is necessary and proportionate to the achievement of the goals set out by the Security Council.

3.23 In so far as other justifications which have been advanced for the use of force (e.g., humanitarian intervention or intervention to protect nationals) have become part of contemporary international law (a matter which falls outside the scope of this Report), they too are subject to the principle that, since they justify the use of force only in order to achieve a particular purpose, that justification is limited to what is necessary and proportionate to the achievement of that purpose.

36. See C. Greenwood, "The Concept of War in Modern International Law", 36 ICLQ (1987) p. 283.

37. Loc. cit. supra note 34, at para. 41. See also para. 105 (c).

3.24 It follows that the legality of the conduct of hostilities today cannot be judged solely by reference to the laws of war. The requirements of the law restricting resort to force must also be satisfied. The fact that a particular action might be considered a necessary and proportionate act of self-defence cannot justify it if it is contrary to the laws of war but the fact that a particular use of force does not contravene the laws of war no longer suffices to make it lawful if it fails to meet the criteria of being necessary and proportionate for the achievement of the goals of self-defence, the discharge of a Security Council mandate, the exercise of an authority granted by the Security Council or, perhaps, some other goal for which the use of force may be permitted by international law.

3.25 The acceptance of this principle, which is implicit in the Opinion of the ICJ in the *Nuclear Weapons* case, has important practical implications in several areas:

(a) It has an effect upon the duration of the period within which belligerent acts may be taken. While a cease-fire or armistice does not bring an end to a formal state of war, the continued assertion of belligerent rights after the conclusion of an armistice or cease fire will not normally be justifiable today, since it will not be a necessary measure of self-defence.[38] Even where there has been no formal armistice or cease-fire, such measures may be unjustified if hostilities have in fact ceased and there is no immediate danger of their recurrence.

(b) It may limit the geographical area within which hostilities may be conducted. Under the laws of war, there was a distinction between the "region of war", the area within which hostilities might lawfully take place, and the "theatre of war", within which they actually occurred. The region of war included the entire area of the high seas and the territory of the belligerents. While a State exercising a right

38. See SC Res. 95 (1951) which stated that the assertion by Egypt of belligerent rights against shipping two and a half years after the conclusion of an armistice and an end of active hostilities between Egypt and Israel could not be justified as a necessary measure of self-defence, notwithstanding Egypt's assertion that it was still in a state of war with Israel and the specific measures taken were not prohibited by the armistice agreement.

of self-defence is not obliged to confine its activities to the theatre of war selected by its assailant if broadening the area within which hostilities occur is necessary to repel the attack or to ensure the security of the defending State and its forces, it must be questioned whether it is any longer right to assume, especially in a conflict fought for limited objectives and of short duration, that it would be justifiable to initiate a military operation anywhere within the traditional region of war, no matter how remote from the scene of the actual fighting already taking place.

(c) It may have an effect upon what is to be considered a lawful target. The laws of war already contain detailed rules regarding targeting (which are the subject of discussion in Part IV, infra) and principles drawn from the law on resort to force cannot, of course, ever justify an attack upon something which the laws of war prohibit a belligerent from attacking. However, it is possible that an attack upon a particular target which is not protected by the laws of war may nevertheless go beyond what can be considered a necessary and proportionate act of self-defence and thus be unlawful.

(d) It may affect the weapons and methods of warfare which may lawfully be used. While a State resorting to force in self-defence or pursuant to a mandate from the Security Council is not required to limit itself to the level of weaponry employed by its assailant, a substantial escalation of violence will be justified only if it is necessary and proportionate. That was clearly recognized by the ICJ in the *Nuclear Weapons* opinion. Although the Court did not accept submissions that recourse to nuclear weapons was necessarily contrary to the principle of proportionality, it clearly considered that recourse to nuclear weapons was a step which had to be assessed by reference to the criterion of proportionality.[39]

(e) It will have an effect upon the relationship between belligerents and neutrals. The exact content of the law of neutrality today is, in any event, a matter for debate. Whatever that law may be, however, it is clear that it is affected in a number of ways by the principles of the Charter and the law on resort to force. Thus, where the Security Council imposes measures under Article 41 of the Charter, the

39. ICJ Reports 1996, p. 226 at p. 245, paras. 41-43.

obligation of States to comply with those measures[40] prevails over any inconsistent rights or obligations which may exist under the ordinary law applicable to relations between belligerents and neutrals.[41] Even where no such measures are taken, it is probable that a belligerent may exercise against neutral States the powers accorded to it by the law of neutrality only to the extent that such action is necessary for its own self-defence and proportionate to the threat which it faces.[42]

3.26 While these are, in the briefest outline, some of the implications which appear to follow from the fact that, in contrast to the position in 1899, the laws of war now exist within a framework of international law which significantly restricts the right of States to resort to force, the full implications of the relationship between the contemporary *ius ad bellum* and *ius in bello* have yet to be determined. Particularly in the area of relations between neutrals and belligerents, this is a subject which would repay further study.

## (b) *The Laws of War and other Areas of International Law*

3.27 The laws of war have not only been affected by the emergence of a law against war. Two other areas of international law - the law of human rights and international environmental law - have developed in a way which has potentially important implications for the laws of war.

3.28 While the matter is not entirely free of controversy, it appears that the principal human rights treaties were intended to apply in time

40. Arts. 2 (5) and 25 of the Charter.

41. Charter, Art.103. See also para. 4 of the resolution adopted by the Institut de droit international at its Wiesbaden session in 1975, 56 *Annuaire* p. 541.

42. See, e.g., the statement by the UK Government following the detention by the Iranian navy of the British vessel *Barber Perseus* during the Iran-Iraq War, 47 BYIL (1986), p. 583. However, not all States took this position, see A. de Guttry and N. Ronzitti, *The Iran-Iraq War and the Law of Naval Warfare* (1993).

of war or armed conflict, as well as times of peace.[43] The fact that some of these treaties contain provisions permitting States to derogate from some, though not all, of their obligations under the treaties in question in time of war or other national emergency implies that the existence of a war does not automatically terminate or suspend their application.[44] In its Advisory Opinion on *Nuclear Weapons*, the ICJ observed that "the protection of the International Covenant on Civil and Political Rights does not cease in times of war, except by operation of Article 4 of the Covenant whereby certain provisions may be derogated from in a time of national emergency."[45] The question, therefore, is what effect, if any, does the law of human rights have upon the application of the laws of war.

3.29 The effect of the law of human rights upon the conduct of hostilities is limited by two factors. First, a State party to a human rights treaty usually undertakes to ensure the rights guaranteed by the treaty only to persons in its own territory or subject to its jurisdiction. That concept is certainly broad enough to include territory occupied by a belligerent in time of armed conflict. The European Court of Human Rights has held that :

> the responsibility of a Contracting Party may also arise when, as a consequence of military action - whether lawful or unlawful - it exercises effective control of an area outside its national territory. The obligation to secure, in such an area, the rights and freedoms set out in the Convention, derives from the fact of such control whether it be

43. Space does not permit a more detailed examination of the relationship between humanitarian law and human rights law in this Report. The rapporteur has discussed the matter at greater length in his essay "Rights at the Frontier: Protecting Human Rights in Time of War" in B.A.K. Rider (ed), *Law at the Centre* (1999), p. 277.

44. See, e.g., European Convention on Human Rights, 1951, Art. 15 and the American Convention on Human Rights, 1969, Art. 27. The International Covenant on Civil and Political Rights, 1966, contains a clause providing for derogation in times of national emergency but does not mention war as such (Art. 4). However, in the course of the negotiation of Art. 6 of the Covenant, concerning the right to life, the deprivation of life by means of a *lawful* act of war was given as an example of a taking of life which would not be arbitrary within the meaning of that provision.

45. ICJ Reports 1996, p. 226 at p. 240, para. 25.

exercised directly, through its armed forces, or through a subordinate local administration.[46]

3.30 It is another matter, however, to treat persons in enemy territory as subject to the jurisdiction of a belligerent simply because those persons are present in territory which that belligerent subjects to attack. To say that in early 1991 the population of Baghdad was subject to the jurisdiction of those coalition States which were engaged in aerial bombardment of targets in Iraq would be to stretch the concept of jurisdiction well beyond the normal meaning of that term.

3.31 Secondly, many provisions in human rights treaties are of a very general nature and add little or nothing to the detailed provisions of the laws of war. This is particularly true of the provisions on the right to life. Thus, in the *Nuclear Weapons* Advisory Opinion, the ICJ, having stated that the right not arbitrarily to be deprived of one's life applies in hostilities continued:

> The test of what is an arbitrary deprivation of life, however, then falls to be determined by the applicable *lex specialis*, namely, the law applicable in armed conflict which is designed to regulate the conduct of hostilities. Thus whether a particular loss of life, through the use of a certain weapon in warfare, is to be considered an arbitrary deprivation of life contrary to Article 6 of the Covenant, can only be decided by reference to the law applicable in armed conflict and not deduced from the terms of the Covenant itself.[47]

What this passage suggests is that, instead of the treaty provisions on the right to life adding anything to the laws of war, it is the laws of war which may be of assistance in applying provisions on the right to

46. *Loizidou* v. *Turkey (Preliminary Objections)*, 103 ILR 622 (1995); 20 EHRR 99, para. 62 (European Court of Human Rights). See also the decision of the Court in the merits phase, 108 ILR p. 443 (1996); 23 EHRR p. 513, para. 56, and the decision of the European Commission on Human Rights in *Cyprus* v. *Turkey* (25781/94) 23 EHRR p. 244 at p.274.

47. I.C.J Reports 1996, p. 226 at p. 240, para. 25.

life.[48] There is, however, now a substantial body of case-law in the various human rights tribunals interpreting the provisions on the right to life and addressing such matters as what constitutes a proportionate use of force. Particularly in the context of internal armed conflicts, these decisions are likely to be of considerable importance and may help to shape the development of customary humanitarian law.

3.32 Nevertheless, there are a number of ways in which the law of human rights is likely to be of importance for the conduct of hostilities. First, the scope of human rights law is in some respects broader than that of the laws of war. Thus, the laws of war do not normally apply to a belligerent's treatment of its own nationals and some laws of war treaties do not apply to the treatment of nationals of neutral States.[49] The summary execution by a belligerent of deserters from its army or citizens accused of enemy sympathies, or the detention of nationals of a neutral State considered to favour an enemy would fall to be judged by reference to the relevant human rights law, rather than the laws of war.

3.33 Secondly, some human rights provisions might be used to assist in the interpretation of laws of war provisions. For example, the requirement in Article 84 of the Third Geneva Convention, 1949, which stipulates that "in no circumstances whatever shall a prisoner of war be tried by a court of any kind which does not offer the essential guarantees of independence and impartiality, as generally recognized" invites reference to the law of human rights as a guide to the guarantees which are generally recognized. While the Geneva Conventions and the First Additional Protocol themselves contain a

48. That was the approach taken by the Inter-American Commission of Human Rights in relation to alleged violations of the right to life occurring in what it held to be an internal armed conflict; *Abella* v. *Argentina*, Report No. 55/97, para. 161. See also hereafter, paras. 5.32 and 6.29.

49. For example, the definition of a protected person under Article 4 of the Fourth Geneva Convention, 1949, excludes nationals of a neutral State in the territory of a belligerent so long as the neutral State retains normal diplomatic relations with that belligerent.

number of due process safeguards, it is again likely that the jurisprudence of the human rights tribunals will assist in giving those provisions a contemporary interpretation.

3.34 Thirdly, human rights law is likely to be of particular importance in the case of belligerent occupation, where, as will be seen, the laws of war are somewhat outdated.

3.35 Finally, the enforcement machinery which forms part of some human rights treaties may offer an additional means for ensuring compliance with the laws of war, especially in non-international armed conflicts.[50]

3.36 It follows that while humanitarian law and human rights law should continue to be treated as distinct bodies of law, each may have more to contribute to the other than has generally been recognized.

3.37 The second area of relevance is international environmental law. There are, of course, specific provisions on the environment in the more recent treaties on the laws of war: the UN Convention on the Prohibition of Military or any other Hostile Use of Environmental Modification Techniques, 1977; Additional Protocol I to the Geneva Conventions, Articles 35 (3) and 55. In addition, a number of other treaty provisions regulate matters of direct environmental concern; e.g., the prohibition of wanton destruction of property in Article 23 (g) of the Hague Regulations on the Laws and Customs of War on Land and the rules on attacks on dams, dykes and nuclear electrical generating stations in Article 56 of Additional Protocol I.

3.38 The application of principles of general international environmental law to the conduct of hostilities, however, has recently been

50. This matter is considered further in Part VI of this report.

the subject of much comment.[51] Principle 24 of the Rio Declaration states that:

> Warfare is inherently destructive of sustainable development. States shall therefore respect international law providing protection for the environment in times of armed conflict and cooperate in its further development as necessary.

While the legal status of the Rio Declaration is far from certain, this provision has led to suggestions that a State engaged in an armed conflict must comply in full with the provisions not only of the laws of war but also the whole body of the environmental treaties to which that State is party.

3.39 This Rapporteur does not agree with such suggestions. In the *Nuclear Weapons* Advisory Opinion, the ICJ stated that the environmental treaties were not intended to deprive a State of its right to self-defence but went on to state that:

> Nonetheless States must take environmental considerations into account when assessing what is necessary and proportionate in the pursuit of legitimate military objectives. Respect for the environment is one of the elements that go to assessing whether an action is in conformity with the principles of necessity and proportionality.[52]

The notion that there is a general obligation to have regard to the protection of the environment in the conduct of military operations also finds support in the new edition of the United States Naval Commander's Handbook, which states that:

> It is not unlawful to cause collateral damage to the natural environment during an attack upon a legitimate military objective. However, the

51. See, e.g., UNGA Res. 47/37 and 49/50, UN Doc. A/49/323 ("Guidance for Military Manuals and Instructions on the Protection of the Environment in Times of Armed Conflict"), G. Plant, *Environmental Protection and the Law of War* (1992) and Grunawalt, King and McClain, *Protection of the Environment during Armed Conflict* (1997).

52. I.C.J Reports 1996, p. 226 at p. 242, para. 30.

> commander has an affirmative obligation to avoid unnecessary damage to the environment to the extent that it is practicable to do so consistent with mission accomplishment. To that end, and as far as military requirements permit, methods or means of warfare should be employed with due regard to the protection and preservation of the natural environment. Destruction of the natural environment not necessitated by mission accomplishment and carried out wantonly is prohibited. Therefore, a commander should consider the environmental damage which will result from an attack on a legitimate military objective as one of the factors during targeting analysis.[53]

3.40 The evolution of the law of human rights and international environmental law are obviously two of the most important developments in international law during the course of the 20th century. Their potential effect upon the laws of war has, however, only begun to be appreciated. It seems likely that this question is one which deserves further study if an approach is to be developed which respects the effect of those new bodies of law, while paying due regard to the special conditions of warfare.

## III.2 The Scope of the Laws of War

3.41 The two Conventions and three Declarations on the laws of war concluded at the 1899 Conference were intended to apply only in a formal state of war and only as between States party to the relevant agreement. That approach is summed up in a comment made by MARTENS at the Conference, when he said that "in order clearly to express what is, in the view of the Russian Government, the object of the Conference in this matter, I cannot find a better illustration than that of a 'Mutual Insurance Society against the abuse of force in time of war."[54] The parties to each Convention or Declaration undertook to observe the provisions thereof only vis-à-vis one another and only

53. US Navy, *Annotated Supplement to the Commander's Handbook on the Law of Naval Operations* (1997), para. 8.1.3.

54. Quoted in Pearce Higgins, op. cit. note 5, p. 259.

for so long as all of the belligerents in a particular conflict were parties to the relevant Convention or Declaration.[55]

3.42 During the course of the century, the international community has substantially modified its approach to the scope of application of treaties on the laws of war. First, the treaties adopted since 1945 are not confined to application in a formal state of war but apply to any armed conflict, irrespective of whether a formal state of war exists or not.[56] The practice of most States has also been to treat the older treaties which are still in force and which refer to "war" as applicable to any international armed conflict. This development has been of great importance and benefit. Even in 1899, it was not always easy to determine whether a conflict amounted to war in the formal sense or not.[57] During the 20th century, the task became increasingly difficult as hostilities were waged on a large scale by States which denied that they were at war.[58] The emphasis on the factual concept of armed conflict has removed an argument of great technicality and simplified the application of the law of war treaties.

3.43 Secondly, general participation or *si omnes* clauses of the kind employed in the 1899 and 1907 treaties have not been in general use since the 1929 revision of the Geneva Conventions. Although a State party to a treaty on the laws of war is bound to apply that treaty only with regard to other States party (or, in the case of the Geneva Conventions and Additional Protocol I, States which have undertaken to apply the provisions of the relevant agreement even though they have

55. See, e.g., Art. 2 of the Convention on the Laws and Customs of War on Land and Art. 11 of the Convention for the Adaptation of the Geneva Convention to Maritime Warfare.

56. See, e.g., common Art. 2 of the Geneva Conventions, 1949.

57. In 1883 a United Kingdom Government committee investigating the possibility of constructing a channel tunnel was informed that out of 117 conflicts occurring between 1700 and 1870, hostilities had been preceded by a declaration of war in only ten; Maurice, *Hostilities without Declaration of War* (1883). The tunnel was not built for another hundred years. See also F. Grob, *The Relativity of War and Peace* (1949).

58. For example, the hostilities in the 1930s between China and Japan. See Greenwood, loc. cit. supra note 36.

not formally become party), the entry into a conflict of a State not party to a particular convention no longer affects the relations between those belligerents which are parties. While the older treaties of 1907 (most of which remain in force) have not been amended, their importance today is as statements of customary international law and their general participation clauses have therefore become largely irrelevant.

3.44 In general, the changes which have occurred in the scope of application of the laws of war have given rise to few difficulties. Nevertheless, certain matters require comment.

(a) *The Concepts of War and Armed Conflict*

3.45 The existence of a formal state of war has now become almost entirely irrelevant for the application of the laws of war, although a declaration of war by a State which does not then engage in active hostilities (as was the case with some of the belligerents in the Second World War) will have the effect of bringing into force for that State the provisions of the Geneva Conventions and other rules of the laws of war, which may be of importance if that State interns enemy aliens or takes certain measures regarding enemy property.

3.46 The concept of an armed conflict is not defined in any of the treaties on the laws of war. There is, however, powerful support for the view that it should be given a very broad interpretation. The authoritative commentary on the 1949 Geneva Conventions, published by the ICRC, states that:

> Any difference between two States and leading to the intervention of members of the armed forces is an armed conflict within the meaning of Article 2 [common to the four Geneva Conventions], even if one of the parties denies the existence of a state of war. It makes no difference

> how long the conflict lasts, how much slaughter takes place, or how numerous are the participating forces ...[59]

A similar view has been expressed by the Appeals Chamber of ICTY in its decision in *Prosecutor* v. *Tadic (Jurisdiction)*, in which it stated that "an armed conflict exists whenever there is a resort to armed force between States".[60]

3.47 There is also some support for this approach in State practice. The United States, for example, considered that an armed conflict triggering the application of international humanitarian law had come into being between itself and Syria when Syrian anti-aircraft batteries in Lebanon shot down a United States naval aircraft in 1983 and captured the pilot.[61] The approach adopted by the ICJ in its decision in the *Nicaragua* case also points in this direction. It seems, however, that State practice is not always consistent on this point and that States have frequently disputed the existence of an armed conflict when they have been engaged in incidents of short duration involving the use of comparatively small numbers of troops.

(b) *United Nations Operations*

3.48 The question whether there is an armed conflict is particularly likely to cause difficulty when UN forces are involved.[62] The applicability of international humanitarian law to UN forces has been debated for many years. There are obvious difficulties in that the UN is not a party to any of the Conventions on the laws of war and that, not being a State, it lacks the capacity to carry out some of the obligations of the laws of war itself. For example, it has no courts or criminal law of its own and cannot itself punish a member of a UN

59. J.S. Pictet (ed)., *Commentary on Geneva Convention III* (ICRC, 1960), p. 23.

60. Decision of 2 October 1995, 105 ILR 419 at p. 453, para. 70.

61. *Digest of United States Practice in International Law* 1981-88, vol. III, p. 3456.

62. This issue is considered by the Rapporteur at greater length in C. Greenwood, "International Humanitarian Law and United Nations Military Operations", 1 YBIHL (1998) pp. 3-34.

force for a violation of the laws of war. Instead, it has to depend upon each State contributing troops to a UN operation to enforce the law amongst the members of its own contingent.

3.49 Nevertheless, it appears that there is no longer any doubt that the laws of war apply to a UN enforcement action which is designed to engage in hostilities in order to restore international peace and security. In the Korean conflict, after some initial hesitation, the UN Unified Command instructed its forces to comply with all four Geneva Conventions, notwithstanding that they were not then in force for some of the contributor States. While there remained an element of doubt as to whether the United Nations considered that its forces were bound by these treaties or were merely required to comply with the principles and spirit of the Conventions,[63] a leading study has pointed out that "there is, in fact, no known case in which the UN Command ever claimed exemption from any of the accepted rules of the laws of war, customary or conventional".[64] Since the time of the Korean conflict, the applicability of the laws of war to cases in which UN forces are a party to an international armed conflict has been generally accepted.[65] Similarly, when the United Nations authorizes military action (as in the Gulf conflict) by States which

63. S. Bailey, *How Wars End* (1982), vol. II, p. 444.

64. D. Bowett, *UN Forces* (1964), p. 56.

65. It is tacitly recognized by Art. 2(2) of the Convention on the Safety of United Nations and Associated Personnel, 1994, which provides that:

> This Convention shall not apply to a United Nations operation authorised by the Security Council as an enforcement action under Chapter VII of the Charter of the United Nations in which any of the personnel are engaged as combatants against organized armed forces and *to which the law of international armed conflict applies*. (emphasis added)

See also Bowett, op. cit., pp. 484-516, ICRC, *Symposium on Humanitarian Action and Peace-Keeping Operations* (Geneva, ICRC, 1994), D. Shraga in L. Condorelli and others, eds., *The United Nations and International Humanitarian Law* (1996), p. 321 and the two resolutions adopted by the Institut de droit international, on the Conditions of Application of Humanitarian Rules of Armed Conflict to Hostilities in which United Nations Forces may be Engaged (Zagreb, 1971, 54 (II) *Annuaire* (1971), p. 465) and on the Conditions of Application of Rules other than Humanitarian Rules, of Armed Conflict to Hostilities in which United Nations Forces may be Engaged (Wies-baden,1975, 56 *Annuaire* (1975), p. 540).

themselves become party to an armed conflict, there is no doubt that those States are subject to the laws of war.

3.50 The problem lies in determining when a UN force should be regarded as a party to an armed conflict. This task has become increasingly difficult as the United Nations has embarked upon operations which have elements of both enforcement action and more traditional peacekeeping. In some of these operations (noticeably those in the former Yugoslavia and Somalia), UN forces, and national or other forces associated with them, became involved in fighting on a scale which would undoubtedly have constituted an armed conflict under the criteria set out in the preceding section of this Report if States alone had been involved.

3.51 In principle, if the level of the fighting would be sufficient to amount to an armed conflict if the forces involved were purely national forces with no UN involvement, then the result should be the same when it is UN troops which become involved in that fighting. In other words, once a UN force, whatever its original mandate, becomes involved in fighting against organized armed forces, the situation should be classified as an armed conflict, to which the United Nations is a party, and the relevant principles of international humanitarian law applied. There is, nonetheless, great uncertainty regarding whether the UN forces and those associated with them are party to an armed conflict and, if they are, whether that armed conflict is international in character when the forces against which the UN contingents are engaged are not the forces of a State.

3.52 The reluctance to acknowledge that a UN force has become engaged in an armed conflict is likely to be increased by the entry into force of the 1994 Convention on the Safety of United Nations and Associated Personnel. In most circumstances, the effect of Article 2 (2) of that Convention is that if the law of international armed conflict (i.e. the main body of the laws of war, as opposed to the less extensive body of law applicable to non-international conflicts) applies to a UN operation, then the Safety Convention will not apply. Since that Convention is designed to protect UN and associated personnel from attacks, there will be an understandable reluctance to admit that a UN force has become involved in fighting to such an extent that the laws of war have become applicable and the protection afforded by the Convention has thus been removed.

3.53 The United Nations has accepted that UN forces should at all times comply with the "principles and spirit" of humanitarian law. This approach is now embodied in the model agreement drawn up for use between the United Nations and the States contributing contingents to the force. Article 28 of the model agreement provides that the operation:

> ... shall observe and respect the principles and spirit of the general international conventions applicable to the conduct of military personnel. The international conventions referred to above include the four Geneva Conventions of 12 August 1949 and their Additional Protocols of 8 June 1977 and the UNESCO Convention of 14 May 1954 on the Protection of cultural Property in the Event of Armed Conflict. [The contributor State] shall therefore ensure that the members of its national contingent serving with the [operation] be fully acquainted with the principles and spirit of these Conventions.[66]

The same agreement requires the contributing State to "exercise jurisdiction with respect to crimes or offences which may be committed by its military personnel" serving with the operation.[67] This requirement would include violations of the principles and spirit of the Conventions listed in Article 28.

3.54 More recently, the United Nations has included in the Status of Forces Agreements which it has concluded with host States in respect of certain operations a clause by which both the United Nations and the host State agree to act in accordance with the principles and spirit of these Conventions. The Agreement between

66. UN Doc. A/46/185 (23 May 1991). Similar provisions had been included in earlier agreements, see, e.g., the Exchange of Notes between the UN and Canada regarding the participation of Canadian units in UNFICYP, 1966, 555 UNTS p. 120.

67. Art. 25.

the United Nations and the Government of the Republic of Rwanda on the Status of the UN Assistance Mission for Rwanda (UNAMIR) of 5 November 1993, provided that:

> Without prejudice to the mandate of UNAMIR and its international status:
> (a) The UN shall ensure that UNAMIR shall conduct its operations in Rwanda with full respect for the principles and spirit of the general conventions applicable to the conduct of military personnel. These international conventions include the four Geneva Conventions of 12 August 1949 and their Additional Protocols of 8 June 1977 and the UNESCO Convention of 14 May 1954 on the Protection of Cultural Property in the event of Armed Conflict;
> (b) The Government undertakes to treat at all times the military personnel of UNAMIR with full respect for the principles and spirit of the general conventions applicable to the conduct of military personnel. These international conventions include the four Geneva Conventions of 12 August 1949 and their Additional Protocols of 8 June 1977;
> UNAMIR and the Government shall therefore ensure that members of their respective military personnel are fully acquainted with the principles and spirit of the above-mentioned international instruments.[68]

Similar provisions have subsequently been included in agreements with Haiti, Angola and Croatia.

3.55 There are, however, certain difficulties inherent in this approach. First, if events have reached the point at which a UN force is a party to an armed conflict, then it should apply the whole of the laws of war, not simply the principles and spirit of the Conventions cited. Secondly, it is not clear exactly what the duty to observe the principles and spirit of the Conventions means and how, if at all, it differs from the normal duty to comply with the Conventions in their entirety. Thirdly, the Conventions referred to in the model agreement and the status of forces agreements quoted above are not the whole

68. Quoted in Shraga, loc. cit. supra note 65, at p. 325, note 16. The Agreement was also communicated to the Rwanda Patriotic Front (at that time the forces fighting the Government of Rwanda, the RPF overthrew the then Government in 1994) "which confirmed its readiness to co-operate in the implementation of its provisions", Report of the Secretary-General of the UN, UN Doc. S/26927, 30 December 1993, para. 7.

of the laws of war. The model agreement and status of forces agreements are silent on the question whether there is a duty to comply with, for example, the customary law of war.

3.56 Several attempts have been made to give greater content to the undertaking to respect the "principles and spirit" of the international humanitarian law conventions. In 1995 the Special Committee on Peace-keeping Operations requested the Secretary-General to draw up a code of conduct for peace-keeping personnel consistent with applicable international humanitarian law, so as to ensure the highest standards of conduct.[69] That same year, a meeting of Experts convened by the ICRC produced a preliminary report on the subject.[70] In 1996 the ICRC submitted to the Secretary-General a 32 paragraph set of draft guidelines based on the proposals of the Meeting of Experts. Those guidelines in turn formed the basis for a draft directive on international humanitarian law prepared by the Secretariat of the UN in 1997. The draft directive has not yet been issued in final form.

3.57 The number of UN operations in the last ten years and the complexity of some of them mean that uncertainty about the legal regime applicable is potentially dangerous. The rapporteur is doubtful that a non-binding instrument such as the UN Guidelines, especially one which merely refers to the principles and spirit of international humanitarian law is sufficient. It is therefore suggested that the legal instruments applicable to UN military operations should be reconsidered. In particular, the priority should be:
(a) to clarify the circumstances in which a UN force is to be regarded as party to an armed conflict and to reaffirm that when it is to be so regarded, it is subject to the whole of the laws of war; and, as a minimum,
(b) where a UN force is not party to an armed conflict but is nevertheless engaged in hostilities, to give the greatest possible content to

69. UN Doc. A/50/230, 22 June 1995.

70. ICRC, *Report of a Meeting of Experts on the Applicability of International Humanitarian Law to United Nations Forces* (1995).

the obligation to observe the principles and spirit of humanitarian law and to do so in a form which is more than merely advisory.

## IV. The Conduct of Hostilities in International Armed Conflicts

4.1 The 1899 and 1907 Conferences considered almost the entire field of the law applicable to international armed conflicts. Much of that law was subsequently revised and refined in the 1949 Geneva Conventions and Additional Protocol I, 1977. For the most part the detailed legal regimes for the wounded, sick, shipwrecked and prisoners of war, which are now contained in the first three 1949 Conventions, have given rise to few problems and the development of this body of law can reasonably be regarded as one of the achievements of international law during the century which succeeded the 1899 Conference. A particularly important development in this regard was that the Conventions conferred rights upon the individuals whom they sought to protect and not just upon the States on whom those individuals depended.[71]

4.2 While it is not pretended that these Conventions are perfect, there is no need for any radical revision at this point in time. Such weaknesses as exist in this area of the law stem not from a deficiency in the basic legal regime itself but rather from the difficulty of ensuring compliance with that regime. The issue of compliance is considered in Part VI of this Report. It is not proposed, therefore, to consider the first three Geneva Conventions further in this Part of the Report.

4.3 Instead, attention will be focussed upon five areas of the law which were the subject of much discussion in 1899 and which continue to give rise to difficulties today:
(1) the entitlement to combatant status;

71. See, e.g., Convention No. III, Art. 7; Convention No. IV, Art. 8; Additional Protocol I, Art. 75.

(2) the law of weaponry;
(3) the law of targeting;
(4) belligerent occupation; and
(5) naval warfare.

## IV.1 Entitlement to Combatant Status

4.4 In considering the question who is entitled to take a direct part in hostilities and, consequently, to be treated as a prisoner of war upon capture, the 1899 Conference faced a dilemma which still exists today and which has become no easier to resolve. On the one hand, a clear distinction between combatants and civilians is essential if the latter are to receive the protection which the law requires. On the other hand, many States, especially those with comparatively small armed forces, rely upon popular resistance to an invader or an occupation army for their defence. Resistance movements of that kind are not organized in the same way or to the same degree as regular armed forces and frequently cannot be distinguished from the civilian population to the same extent. Should they, therefore, be treated as lawful combatants?

4.5 The 1899 Conference was unable to reach full agreement on this question. The test of combatancy which was laid down in Articles 1 and 2 of the Regulations on the Laws and Customs of War on Land made some concessions to the concept of popular resistance. Article 1 provided that:

> The laws, rights and duties of war apply not only to the army but also to militia and corps of volunteers, fulfilling the following conditions:
> 1. that of being commanded by a person responsible for his subordinates;
> 2. that of having a distinctive emblem fixed and recognizable at a distance;
> 3. that of carrying arms openly; and

4. that of conducting their operations in accordance with the laws and customs of war.[72]

4.6 In addition, Article 2 recognized the combatant status of members of a *levée en masse,* in territory not yet occupied, who "spontaneously take up arms to resist the invading troops without having had time to organize themselves in accordance with Article 1", provided that they respect the laws and customs of war. Nevertheless, more ambitious proposals to recognize the combatant status of irregulars in a wider range of circumstances were not adopted and it was the failure to agree upon these latter proposals which particularly prompted the inclusion in the Preamble of the Martens Clause.[73] Moreover, the extension of combatant status to volunteer groups and other irregulars in Article 1 is less significant than it might appear, since the conditions which that Article requires irregular combatants to meet are so exacting that few resistance movements have ever been able to comply with them.

4.7 The 1899 test of combatancy survived largely unchanged until 1977. The 1907 Regulations did not alter Article 1 but added the further requirement in Article 2 that members of a *levée en masse* had to carry arms openly. Article 4 A of the Third Geneva Convention, 1949, added that persons who met the criteria in Article 1 of the Regulations were entitled to be treated as prisoners of war on capture even if the movement to which they belonged was

72. The authentic French text reads:
Les lois, les droits et les devoirs de la guerre ne s'appliquent pas seulement à l'armée, mais encore aux milices et aux corps de volontaires réunissant les conditions suivantes:
1. d'avoir à leur tête une personne responsable pour ses subordonnés;
2. d'avoir une signe distinctif fixe et reconnaissable à distance;
3. de porter les armes ouvertement; et
4. de se conformer dans leurs opérations aux lois et coutumes de la guerre.

73. See supra, para. 2.7.

operating in occupied territory.[74] In practice, however, this change was of little importance, since the criteria in Article 1 have usually been interpreted in such a way that few, if any, guerrilla groups or resistance movements could comply with them. The British *Manual of Military Law*, for example, interpreted the requirement of a fixed, distinctive sign as meaning that "something less than a complete uniform will suffice", but went on to state that:

> ... it is reasonable to expect that the silhouette of an irregular combatant in the position of standing against the skyline should be at once distinguishable from the outline of a peaceful inhabitant, and this by the naked eye of an ordinary individual at a distance at which the form of an individual can be determined.[75]

It is difficult to imagine any guerrilla movement being able to comply with this requirement and survive.

4.8 Additional Protocol I, 1977, adopted an entirely new approach. It abolished the formal distinction between regular and irregular armed forces and provided that "the armed forces of a party to a conflict consist of all organized armed forces, groups and units which are under a command responsible for its subordinates".[76] Article 44 (3) then went on to provide:

> In order to promote the protection of the civilian population from the effects of hostilities, combatants are obliged to distinguish themselves from the civilian population while they are engaged in an attack or in a military operation preparatory to an attack. Recognizing, however, that there are situations in armed conflicts where, owing to the nature of the hostilities an armed combatant cannot so distinguish himself, he shall retain his status as a combatant, provided that, in such situations, he carries his arms openly:

74. The decision in *United States* v. *List,* 15 *Ann Dig* 632, had cast doubt upon the applicability of Art. 1 to groups in occupied territory, although it is only Art. 2 which expressly excluded such groups.

75. *Manual of Military Law,* Part III (1958), para. 92. This passage had first appeared just after the 1899 Conference.

76. Art. 43 (1).

(a) during each military engagement, and
(b) during such time as he is visible to the adversary while he is engaged in a military deployment preceding the launching of an attack in which he is to participate.
Acts which comply with the requirements of this paragraph shall not be considered as perfidious within the meaning of Article 37, paragraph 1 (c).

4.9 The second sentence of this Article was the product of a last-minute compromise negotiated between delegations which otherwise had little in common. It has been widely criticised both for its cumbersome structure and for reducing the requirement for a combatant to distinguish himself from the civilian population. Much of that criticism is justified. The two-tier test in the two sentences of Article 44 (3) is cumbersome. It leaves important questions about when the lower standard in the second sentence is applicable and what it actually requires. That has prompted some States to make declarations, upon ratification, that the second sentence is applicable only in occupied territory or wars of "national liberation"[77] and that sub-paragraph (b) applies to the time when the combatant is moving to a place from which an attack is to be launched.[78] Others have argued for a wider interpretation.

4.10 Nevertheless, the new Article 44 (3) is not unworkable. The lower standard in the second sentence is not of general application, for it operates only in conditions where compliance with the stricter requirements of the first sentence is impossible. Even where the standard in the second sentence is applicable, it requires that the irregulars carry arms openly during an attack and for some time prior to the attack. The interpretation, advanced by some groups, that all that is required is to produce weapons immediately before opening fire has no basis in law and is clearly contrary to the text. Moreover, if the provisions of Article 44 (3) go too far in relaxing the requirements of combatancy and may thus be said to endanger the civilian

77. As defined in Art. 1 (4) of Additional Protocol I.

78. Thus, most recently, the statements to this effect by the United Kingdom when it ratified the Protocol on 28 January 1998.

population, the 1907- 1949 test was also inadequate to protect that population, because it imposed conditions with which irregulars could not comply and thus offered no inducement to comply with other aspects of the law.

4.11 It must also be borne in mind that the new rules on combatancy do not involve any acceptance of terrorist methods of warfare - attacks upon the civilian population and indiscriminate attacks are outlawed by Article 51 of the Additional Protocol as well as by customary international law. It is important not to confuse the question of who may lawfully engage in hostilities with the quite different question of what methods of warfare they may employ when they do so engage.

4.12 The standards laid down in the Additional Protocol on this question have not really been tested in practice. While the second sentence of Article 44 (3) is far from ideal, the record of the negotiations of the Protocol suggests that it would be extremely difficult to secure agreement upon a better text today. Since the text is not unworkable, it is suggested that the best course is to leave it alone, seeking to interpret it in a rational way and to ensure that all combatants are encouraged to comply with the basic requirement to distinguish themselves from the civilian population during military operations. The controversy over Article 44 (3) shows that what was an intractable problem in 1899 remains difficult a century later.

## IV.2 The Law of Weaponry

4.13 The development of the law of weaponry and methods of warfare played an important part at the 1899 Conference.[79] In addition to the three specific Declarations (on asphyxiating gases, expanding

79. For an historical survey, see F. Kalshoven, "Arms, Armaments and International Law" 191 RdC (1985-III) p. 185.

bullets and projectiles discharged from balloons)[80] and the prohibition of poison and poisoned weapons (in Article 23 (a) of the Regulations on the Laws and Customs of War on Land), the Regulations on the Laws and Customs of War on Land stated three general principles:
(a) that belligerents do not have an unlimited right to choose the means of injuring the enemy;[81]
(b) that belligerents are forbidden to employ treacherous means of killing or injuring the enemy;[82] and
(c) that belligerents are forbidden to employ arms, projectiles or material of a nature to cause superfluous injury or unnecessary suffering.[83]

4.14 This statement of the general principles remains important and has been reaffirmed in Additional Protocol I, Articles 35 and 37. Although it did not include a provision to this effect in the Regulations, the Conference evidently considered that weapons which were inherently indiscriminate should also be prohibited and it was on this basis that it adopted the prohibition on projectiles discharged from balloons.[84]

4.15 Subsequent years saw the adoption of the Geneva Chemical and Bacteriological Weapons Protocol, 1925, prohibiting the use of asphyxiating, poisonous or other gases, all analogous liquids,

80. See supra, Part II.

81. Art. 22. The French text states: "les belligérants n'ont pas un droit illimité quant au choix des moyens de nuire à l'ennemi".

82. Art. 23 (b).

83. Art. 23(e), the French text of which reads:
Outre les prohibitions établies par des Conventions spéciales, il est notamment interdit:
(e) d'employer des armes, des projectiles ou des matières propres à causer des maux superflus.
The French term "maux superflus" has sometimes been translated as "superfluous injury" and at other times as "unnecessary suffering". The English text of Additional Protocol I, Art. 35 (2), which reaffirms the principle in Art. 23(e) of the Regulations on the Laws and Customs of War on Land, employs both terms.

84. See supra, para. 2.10.

materials or devices, and bacteriological methods of warfare. This prohibition on the use of chemical and biological weapons was re-inforced many years later by the Convention on the Prohibition of Development, Production and Stockpiling of Bacteriological and Toxin Weapons, 1972, which prohibited the possession of bacteriological and toxin weapons, and the Chemical Weapons Convention, 1993, which prohibited the possession and use as a means of warfare of chemical weapons. The UN Convention on the Prohibition of Military or any Other Hostile Use of Environmental Modification Techniques, 1977, prohibited the use of weapons intended to change the environment through the deliberate manipulation of natural processes.

4.16 Finally, a UN conference held in 1980 adopted the UN Convention on Prohibitions or Restrictions on the Use of Certain Conventional Weapons, 1981, the three original Protocols to which prohibited the use of weapons which injured with fragments which cannot be detected by X-rays (Protocol I) and imposed certain restrictions on the use of mines and booby traps (Protocol II) and incendiary weapons (Protocol III). A subsequent review conference in 1995-96 adopted an amended Protocol II on mines and a new Protocol IV on laser weapons. Finally, a convention outlawing anti-personnel land mines (which for some States will supersede the amended Protocol II to the Weaponry Convention in relation to anti-personnel mines, though not other types of mine and booby-trap) was adopted in 1997.

4.17 This record is not particularly impressive. In the century since the 1899 Conference, the advances in military technology have been enormous. The law, however, has changed little. Apart from the important developments of the law in relation to chemical and biological weapons (by the treaties of 1925, 1972 and 1993) and the recent developments in restricting or prohibiting the use of anti-personnel land mines, the treaty law has added little to the general principles. The general principles have remained significant and their continued validity was recently reaffirmed by the ICJ *Nuclear Weapons* Advisory Opinion. Yet a 1973 survey of the law on weaponry by the UN Secretariat cited bayonets or lances with barbs, irregular shaped bullets and projectiles filled with glass as examples of weapons considered to be outlawed by the unnecessary suffering principle.[85] Scarcely standard weapons at the beginning of the 20th century, these were museum pieces by its end. Similarly, leading text books still refer to the unnecessary suffering principle as meaning that "cannons must not be loaded with chain shot, crossbar shot, red-hot balls, and the like".[86] Such examples suggest that the law is firmly rooted in the 19th century.

4.18 Yet it would be wrong to underestimate what has been achieved. The use of chemical weapons was widespread during the First World War and the threat of biological weapons was a very real one. Although such weapons have not yet wholly disappeared from the battlefield, the record of compliance with the 1925 Protocol has been better than that of most treaties on the laws of war. Moreover, the 1972 and 1993 Conventions, with their provisions for disarmament and (particularly in the 1993 Convention) verification measures, offer a real prospect that these weapons of mass destruction can now be completely removed.[87]

4.19 The new regime for chemical and biological weapons is not only intrinsically important, it also suggests that the most effective way to proceed in seeking to rid the world of weapons which are particularly inhumane is by means of a disarmament approach, that is the prohibition of the *possession* of a category of weapon rather than a simple ban on *use* or restriction on the manner in which a weapon is used. Only in this way can States be given sufficient confidence that an agreement to relinquish a particular category of weapons will be honoured. While the complex and intrusive regime of the Chemical Weapons Convention is likely to prove acceptable only for weapons

85. *Respect for Human Rights in Armed Conflicts: Existing Rules of International Law concerning the Prohibition or Restriction of the Use of Specific Weapons*, UN Doc. A/9215, vol. I, p. 204 (1973).

86. H. Lauterpacht, *Oppenheim's International Law* (7th ed., 1952), vol. II, pp. 34-1.

87. This issue is dealt with at greater length in the report of Dr. Hans Blix.

of mass destruction and other weapons of particular military importance, the willingness of the international community to accept such a regime in respect of chemical and biological weapons and the insistence of the Security Council on Iraq's compliance with the disarmament requirements of Resolution 687 is an indication of what can be achieved.

4.20 It would also be wrong to dismiss the general principles as ineffective. It is true that there have been few cases in which a weapon with real military utility has been outlawed by the unnecessary suffering principle. Nevertheless, it must be remembered that this principle requires a balancing of the military advantage which may result from the use of a weapon with the degree of injury and suffering which it is likely to cause. As a Japanese court has stated "the use of a certain weapon, great as its inhuman result may be, need not be prohibited by international law if it has a great military effect."[88] The prohibition of weapons and methods of warfare the cruelty of which is not matched by the military advantages which they offer is an important step in preserving humanitarian values in war. Moreover, the principle of unnecessary suffering has also served as the inspiration for some of the specific prohibitions (such as those on blinding laser weapons and weapons which injure with fragments which cannot be detected by x-rays) which have been adopted. In addition, the unnecessary suffering and discrimination principles were also amongst the forces which inspired both the ban on chemical weapons and the recent ban on anti-personnel land mines, both of which are instances of bans on weapons regarded by many as being of real military utility.

4.21 With regard to the general principles, an important development was the articulation, in Article 36 of Additional Protocol I, of a duty for each State to examine proposals for new weapons and methods of warfare in order to determine whether their use would violate the principles of the laws of war. For this to be done effectively, it would

88. *Shimoda* v. *The State* 32 ILR p.34; see also the Opinion of Judge Higgins in the *Nuclear Weapons* case, loc. cit. supra note 34, at pp. 583-5.

be advantageous to have a clearer idea of the relevant considerations which have to be taken into account in assessing whether or not the employment of a particular weapon would be likely to cause unnecessary suffering. The unnecessary suffering test calls for a weighing of the military advantages offered by a particular weapon against the medical and other effects which that weapon produces. The debates on this subject amongst the Committee of Experts convened by the ICRC at Lucerne in 1974 and Lugano in 1975[89] demonstrated considerable disagreement about the factors to be taken into account on either side of this equation.

4.22 A report published in 1997 by the ICRC attempts to specify more precise criteria for determining whether a particular weapon causes unnecessary suffering.[90] The approach taken in this Report is to study the medical effects of existing weapons, the degree to which they cause death or particular types of injury and to suggest four criteria to be used in determining whether a new weapon is one which violates the unnecessary suffering principle:
(a) does the weapon foreseeably cause specific disease, specific abnormal physiological state, specific abnormal psychological state, specific and permanent disability or specific disfigurement;
(b) does the weapon foreseeably cause a field mortality of more than 25 % or a hospital mortality of more than 5 % (figures substantially in excess of those caused by weapons in use at present);
(c) are the weapons designed to cause particularly large wounds; or
(d) does the weapon foreseeably exert effects for which there is no well recognized and proven treatment?

4.23 The identification of these criteria and the medical study on which they are based is of considerable value in helping to show how the balancing act required by the unnecessary suffering principle can be made more precise and less anecdotal than at present. It is, how-

89. ICRC, *Report of the Conference of Government Experts on the Use of Certain Conventional Weapons, 1st and 2nd Sessions* (1975 and 1976).

90. R. Coupland (ed.), *The SIrUS Project: Towards a Determination of Which Weapons Cause Superfluous Injury or Unnecessary Suffering* (1997).

ever, important to realize that the fact that a particular weapon meets one of these criteria is not, in itself sufficient to brand it as unlawful without consideration of the military advantages which that weapon may offer. For example, the fact that soldiers cannot take cover from a particular type of weapon will, as the report points out, heighten the reaction of abhorrence produced by such a weapon[91] but it is also the very inability of soldiers to take cover that means that the weapon will, in the language of the 1868 Declaration, disable the greatest possible number of enemy combatants and which thus gives it its military effectiveness when compared with other weapons. Moreover, the Report considers only the "medical" or "humanitarian" side of the balance. Greater precision is also needed in determining what are the relevant factors to be taken into account on the military side of the equation.[92]

## IV.3 The Law of Targeting

4.24 The question of what is a legitimate target in warfare is obviously closely related to that of weaponry and methods of warfare. The 1899 Conference, however, had less to say on this subject. Articles 25-27 of the Regulations on the Laws and Customs of War on Land prohibited the attack or bombardment of undefended towns, villages or buildings (Article 25), imposed a limited obligation upon a commander to warn the authorities of a town before bombardment (Article 26) and required him to take all necessary steps to spare certain objects (e.g. hospitals, schools and charitable institutions) in the course of a bombardment (Article 27). These provisions are very limited in their scope and difficult to apply. The effectiveness of Article 25 is less than might appear, because a town can only be regarded as undefended if it is open to capture by the enemy without opposition. The provision is therefore inapplicable to towns situated behind enemy lines, because, even if they have no defences of their

91. Op. cit., p. 27.

92. See M. Bothe, J. Partsch and W. Solf, *New Rules for Victims of Armed Conflicts* (1982), pp. 196-7.

own, these cannot be occupied without sending forces through areas where resistance can be expected. Articles 26 and 27 have proved almost wholly ineffective.

4.25 The 1907 Conference left these provisions largely unchanged and the Fourth Geneva Convention, 1949, made only minor changes, designed to facilitate the creation of hospital and safety zones and neutralized zones.[93] Even this modest objective has not been realized, since almost no use has been made of such zones since 1949. The Hague Convention for the Protection of Cultural Property in the Event of Armed Conflict, 1954, and the Protocol thereto, built on the provisions of Article 27 of the Regulations on the Laws and Customs of War on Land but it was not until the adoption of Additional Protocol I that the customary law rules on targeting were reduced to writing and supplemented by the adoption of a number of new (and sometimes controversial) provisions.

4.26 It had long been accepted that the customary laws of war contained two cardinal principles regarding targeting:
(a) that attacks should be directed only at military objectives and not at civilians or civilian objects ("the principle of distinction"); and
(b) that in attacks upon military objectives there was a duty to avoid causing disproportionate civilian casualties and damage ("the principle of proportionality").[94]

4.27 The record of compliance with those principles during most of the 20th century has been dismal. They were almost universally disregarded during the Second World War and in most of the conflicts thereafter. Additional Protocol I attempted to give greater precision to these principles in a number of respects:
(1) Articles 48, 51 and 52 reaffirm the principles themselves - an important step in view of the scale of violations which had occurred.

93. Fourth Convention, Arts. 14 and 15.

94. See, e.g., the statement by the UK Prime Minister, Neville Chamberlain, at the time of the Spanish Civil War, 337 House of Commons Debates (21 June 1938), cols 937-8 and UNGA Res. 2444 (1968).

(2) Article 52 attempts to put flesh on the bare bones of the principle of distinction by defining what is meant by a military objective:

> Insofar as objects are concerned, military objectives are limited to those objects which by their nature, location, purpose or use make an effective contribution to military action and whose total or partial destruction, capture or neutralization, in the circumstances ruling at the time, offers a definite military advantage.

This definition avoids the pitfalls of the approach taken in, for example, the 1923 Draft Rules on Air Warfare [95] of seeking to list categories of military objectives.[96] Instead, it lays down a two-stage test: (1) does the object make an effective contribution (actual or potential) to the enemy's military action; and if so (2) is it, in the circumstances ruling at the time, one whose destruction, capture or neutralization would offer a definite military advantage. The reference to the circumstances ruling at the time is particularly important as it should avoid the approach of treating entire categories of items (such as bridges) as military objectives in all circumstances.[97]
(3) The Protocol also codifies the principle of proportionality, although it does not use that term. Article 51 (5) (b) defines as an indiscriminate attack (and therefore as one prohibited by Article 51 (4)):

> An attack which may be expected to cause incidental loss of civilian life, injury to civilians, damage to civilian objects, or a combination thereof, which would be excessive in relation to the concrete and direct military advantage anticipated.

95. A. Roberts and R. Guelff (eds), *Documents on the Laws of War*, 3rd ed. (2000) p. 139.

96. For criticism of the text in Article 52(2) as too vague and open-ended, see A. Randelzhofer, "Civilian Objects" in Bernhardt (ed.), 3 *Encyclopedia of Public International Law,* p. 93 (1982).

97. F. Kalshoven, 9 Neths YBIL (1978) p. 107, at p. 111.

This provision was welcomed at the time as a useful codification of the principle of proportionality.[98] While any attempt to determine the content of this principle is problematic, not least because it requires that a balance be struck between two such different considerations as military advantage and civilian losses,[99] the approach taken in the Protocol represents an advance in that it emphasizes that the military advantage must be "concrete and direct". Nebulous factors such as "breaking the morale of the enemy State" are not enough.[100]
(4) Article 57 translates these principles into a set of questions which must be asked by a commander in deciding whether, and how, to launch an attack.

4.28 Although Additional Protocol I was not, as such applicable in the 1990-91 Gulf Conflict (since Iraq was not a party to the Protocol), the Coalition States treated the provisions set out above as declaratory of rules of customary international law and announced that their targeting policy would comply with them. While this is not the place to evaluate that claim, the experience of the Gulf conflict suggests that the provisions on targeting in Additional Protocol I are workable. Rather, therefore, than seeking to refine those principles

98. See, eg, the statement by the UK Representative, VI Official Records p. 164.

99. The test is always a relative one in which the harm to the civilian population must be weighed against the military advantage. There is no justification for the attempt in the ICRC *Commentary* to introduce an absolute ceiling beyond which civilian casualties can never be justified. The passage in the *Commentary* which states that:

> The idea has also been put forward that even if they are very high, civilian losses and damages may be justified if the military advantage at stake is of great importance. This idea is contrary to the fundamental rules of the Protocol; in particular it conflicts with Article 48 '(*Basic rule*)' and with paragraphs 1 and 2 of the present Article 51. The Protocol does not provide any justification for attacks which cause extensive civilian losses and damages. Incidental losses and damages should never be extensive (para. 1980)

is misleading because it appears to confuse the term "extensive", which suggests an absolute test, with "excessive", a term which is clearly relative. However attractive the view in the *Commentary* may be from a humanitarian viewpoint, it does not accurately reflect the text of the Protocol or the underlying principle of customary law.

100. Breaking the morale of the enemy's armed forces, so that they will be less able to resist an attack is a different matter.

further at this stage, it is suggested that priority should be given to ensuring better compliance with them.

4.29 In this respect, an important step forward is the increased likelihood that those who violate the law relating to targeting, particularly those who deliberately target civilians, will face prosecution for those acts. ICTY already has jurisdiction over such acts[101] and it is likely that the International Criminal Court (ICC) will also do so if that body is established.

4.30 In passing, it should also be noted that the principles on targeting stated in the Protocol apply to any warfare which may affect the civilian population on land. Although usually discussed in the context of air bombardment and the use of regular forces, the duty to distinguish between the civilian population and the military and the requirement to observe the principle of proportionality apply just as much to those conducting guerrilla warfare as they do to the air force or artillery of the regular armed forces. Thus, the prohibition in Article 51 (2) of attacks "the primary purpose of which is to spread terror among the civilian population" applies to the planting of a car bomb as well as to the activities of a strategic air force.

## IV.4 The Law of Belligerent Occupation

4.31 The elaboration of a code for the government of occupied territory was one of the principal achievements of the 1899 Conference. Articles 42-56 of the Regulations on the Laws and Customs of War on Land, which were largely unchanged in 1907, laid down a framework of principles within which a belligerent occupant was required to act in governing occupied territory. Chief among these were:

(1) the occupant acquired only temporary control over the territory, not sovereignty, and was entitled, and required, to exercise the

101. See, e.g., the Rule 61 decision in *Prosecutor* v. *Martic* 108 ILR p. 39. At the time of writing, the Tribunal was hearing a case against *Blaskic* which involved allegations of unlawful bombardment.

powers of government while respecting, unless absolutely prevented, the laws already in force (Articles 42-3);
(2) the population of the occupied territory did not owe allegiance to the occupying power and could not be required to swear an oath (Articles 44-5), their lives, honour and property were to be respected (Articles 46-7); and
(3) the powers of the occupant to take or use public and private property in the occupied territory were restricted by Articles 48-56.

The underlying principle was that the *status quo* should be preserved as much as possible, so as not to prejudice either the population or the displaced sovereign in advance of the conclusion of a peace treaty, which would determine the future of the territory.

4.32 The emphasis in the Regulations on the Laws and Customs of War on Land was on the governance of the occupied territory and the powers of the occupant with respect to property, rather than the protection of the civilian population as such. The inadequacy of that approach was graphically demonstrated by the abuses committed by occupying powers during the Second World War (although the regime did not work particularly well during the First World War either). The Fourth Geneva Convention 1949 attempted to address this problem by adding a number of provisions (Articles 27-34 and 47-78) regarding the treatment of the population of occupied territory. These provisions prohibit reprisals against the population, collective punishments, deportations, hostage-taking and a number of other practices and are designed to give the civilian population and individual civilians a series of fundamental guarantees relating to freedom from arbitrary arrest and detention, conditions of detention, fair trial and the like.

4.33 The Fourth Convention does not, however, address the underlying questions about the governance of occupied territory or the powers of the occupant to requisition or make use of property in the occupied territory. On these questions, the 1899 and 1907 Regulations on the Laws and Customs of War on Land remain important as a statement of the customary international law.

4.34 The law of belligerent occupation has had a poor record of compliance for most of the 20th century. The principal problem has been the reluctance of States to admit that the law applies at all.[102] Particularly since the end of the Second World War, States which have occupied territory in the course of a military operation have denied that their subsequent governance of that territory was subject to the law of belligerent occupation on a number of grounds. In many cases, the State concerned maintained that it had a superior claim to title to the territory than did the State which it had displaced, so that far from becoming a belligerent occupant, it was merely regaining possession of its own territory. It was on this ground that Iraq denied the applicability of the law of belligerent occupation to its occupation of Kuwait in 1990-91, notwithstanding the universal opposition of the international community to its claims.[103] Similarly, Israel has denied the applicability, *de iure*, of the Fourth Geneva Convention to the West Bank and the Gaza Strip on the grounds that it did not accept that those territories had been part of the territory of another State prior to 1967. Israel has, however, agreed to apply the humanitarian provisions of the Convention on a voluntary basis.[104] The Security Council has, however, insisted that the Convention is applicable as a matter of law and has made a number of calls for Israel to comply with its provisions.[105]

102. A. Roberts, "What is a Military Occupation ?" 55 BYIL (1984) p. 249; E. Benvenisti, *The International Law of Occupation* (1993).

103. Iraq maintained that it had entered Kuwait at the invitation of the Provisional Government of Free Kuwait and that it had subsequently annexed the territory in accordance with the wishes of that "government" and to give effect to its own claims to title to Kuwait; see the Memorandum of the Government of Iraq, 12 September 1990, in E. Lauterpacht and Others (eds), *The Kuwait Crisis: Basic Documents*, vol. I (1991), p. 73. The annexation was condemned as invalid by the Security Council in Res. 662 (1990). The Council repeatedly insisted that Iraq should comply with the relevant provisions of the law of belligerent occupation, especially the Fourth Geneva Convention; see, e.g., Res. 666, 670 and 674.

104. E. Playfair, *International Law and the Administration of Occupied Territories* (1992).

105. See, e.g., Res. 605 (1987), 607 (1988), 636 (1989), 672 (1990), 681 (1990), 694 (1991). There are numerous other resolutions to this effect.

4.35 If the applicability of the law of belligerent occupation were to be dependent upon the resolution of the underlying question of title to the territory concerned, it would almost never be applicable. In fact, neither the Fourth Convention nor the Regulations on the Laws and Customs of War on Land makes it a precondition of the applicability of the law of belligerent occupation that the territory which is occupied must have been part of the territory of the displaced sovereign prior to the commencement of the occupation. Article 2 (2) of the Fourth Convention appears to point to such a conclusion:

> The Convention shall also apply to all cases of partial or total occupation of the territory of a High Contracting Party, even if the said occupation meets with no armed resistance.

4.36 That provision is, however, a residual one, since the applicability of the Fourth Convention is primarily determined by Article 2 (1), which provides that the Convention shall apply to "all cases of declared war or of any other armed conflict". In the event that, during an armed conflict, a State takes control, by military force, of territory which was not under its control prior to the conflict, then the Fourth Convention is applicable, whatever the underlying disputes about title. The same is true of the Regulations on the Laws and Customs of War on Land. Although the section on occupation is entitled "Military Authority over the Territory of the Hostile State", there is no requirement, express or implied, that the hostile State's title to the territory must be unchallenged or authoritatively established as a precondition to the application of this section of the Regulations.

4.37 The problem, therefore, is not one of a deficiency in the law but rather of the refusal of States actually to apply that law.[106] Any significant improvement, therefore, requires not new law but better enforcement of the law which already exists.

106. See E. Benvenisti, op. cit. supra note 102, for a discussion of this point with numerous historical examples.

4.38 That is not to say that the substantive law on belligerent occupation is entirely satisfactory. Two deficiencies are particularly apparent. First, the law of belligerent occupation, aiming as it does at a preservation of the *status quo* pending the conclusion of a peace settlement, is in some respects ill suited to the conditions of a prolonged occupation. It is difficult to see, however, how this problem can be addressed. Changes in the law to give the occupying power greater scope to change the law and practice in the occupied territory to take account of social, political and economic changes occurring during the occupation are unlikely to prove acceptable and would, in any event, come close to substituting the occupant for the displaced sovereign as the sovereign power. Substitution of a concept of trusteeship of the occupied territory for the existing regime of belligerent occupation seems likely to prove unworkable, given the inescapable fact that, unlike any normal concept of trusteeship, the relationship between the occupying power and the territory (as well as its population) rests on the successful use of force.

4.39 In so far as prolonged occupations are to be allowed to occur at all (a question which falls outside the terms of reference for this Report), the best that can be said is that the basic principles in the Regulations on the Laws and Customs of War on Land are sufficiently elastic to allow for a degree of evolution within the framework of an occupation regime which must be regarded as temporary. Accommodation of change in the case of a prolonged occupation must be within the framework of the core principles laid down in the Regulations on the Laws and Customs of War on Land and the Fourth Convention, in particular, the principle underlying much of the Regulations on the Laws and Customs of War on Land, namely that the occupying power may not exploit the occupied territories for the benefit of its own population.

4.40 Secondly, the provisions on the taking of property in occupied territory are now distinctly archaic. The rigid distinction between the powers of the occupant with regard to public property and private property is more difficult to apply in an era when the role of the State, both as owner and regulator, has become far greater than it was a century ago. The provision, in Article 55 of the Regulations on the Laws and Customs of War on Land, that the occupying power shall have the powers of a usufructuary of much public property[107] is exceptionally difficult to apply in the modern context.[108] Again, however, it is unlikely that agreement could be reached about a new body of law which would inevitably place considerable power in the hands of a belligerent occupant. Though less than satisfactory, the existing law is probably the best that can be obtained and the real challenge is to improve the record of compliance with it.

## IV.5 The Law of Naval Warfare

4.41 The nature of naval warfare in the 18th and 19th centuries was such that a substantial and sophisticated body of customary international law had already developed by 1899, in part due to the jurisprudence of prize courts. Under that law, belligerents could conduct hostilities everywhere except in the waters of neutral States. Most of the law concerned the circumstances in which it was legitimate for belligerent warships to capture enemy and neutral merchant vessels. So far as enemy merchant vessels were concerned, the better view (in spite of the strong opposition of the United States of America) was that enemy merchant vessels and their cargo were liable to capture and condemnation in prize. Neutral vessels, however, were liable to capture only in limited circumstances, such as when running a blockade. The emphasis was on capture rather than attack and the distinction between enemy and neutral shipping and waters was central to the operation of the law.

107. "L'Etat occupant ne se considérera que comme administrateur et usufruitier des édifices publics, immeubles, forêts et exploitations agricoles appartenant à l'Etat ennemi et se trouvant dans le pays occupé. Il devra sauvegarder le fonds de ces propriétés et les administrer conformément aux règles de l'usufruit."

108. It is, however, appropriate to bear in mind the provisions of Art. 53 of Geneva Convention No. IV, which do not distinguish between public and private property in prohibiting the wanton destruction of property.

4.42 The 1899 Conference took almost no action on this subject, beyond adopting the Convention for the Adaptation of the Principles of the Geneva Convention to Maritime War. It did, however, suggest that the question of naval warfare be considered at a subsequent Peace Conference. The 1907 Conference considered the law of naval warfare at length and, as well as revising the 1899 Convention on the wounded and sick, adopted seven new Conventions:

| | |
|---|---|
| Hague Convention No. VI | relating to the Status of Enemy Merchant Ships at the Outbreak of Hostilities |
| Hague Convention No. VII | relating to the Conversion of Merchant Ships into Warships |
| Hague Convention No. VIII | relating to the laying of Automatic Submarine Contact Mines |
| Hague Convention No. IX | concerning the Bombardment by naval Forces in Time of War |
| Hague Convention No. XI | relative to Certain Restrictions with Regard to the Exercise of the Right of Capture in Naval War |
| Hague Convention No. XII | relative to the Creation of an International Prize Court (which never entered into force) and |
| Hague Convention No. XIII | concerning the Rights and Duties of Neutral Powers in Naval War. |

4.43 While these treaties lay down a detailed code of rules, they have proved to be far from satisfactory. Parts were already anachronistic when they were drafted and they were largely disregarded in both World Wars, when the doctrine of reprisals was invoked to justify widespread departures from their provisions. Since only a minority of States are parties to the treaties themselves, it becomes important to know which provisions are to be regarded as declaratory of customary international law. That, however, is no easy task, given the comparative paucity of State practice which can be relied upon (much of the practice which does exist being referable to the reprisals claims and thus an uncertain guide). The only treaty for which substantial support can be found is the Mines Convention, which the ICJ has held is based upon "certain general and well-recognized principles, namely: elementary considerations of humanity, even more exacting in peace than in war."[109] In the *Nicaragua* case, the Court held that these principles prohibited the laying of mines without warning or notification in waters to which the vessels of another State had rights of access or passage.

4.44 There are several reasons why the law of naval warfare as stated in the 1907 treaties is difficult to apply in modern conditions. First, it presupposes a clear distinction between belligerents and neutrals. That distinction is far harder to draw today, since declarations of war or neutrality have been almost unknown since World War Two and States not directly involved in a conflict have frequently been strong supporters of one side or other in that conflict. In addition, the massive increase in the popularity of flags of convenience has meant that a very large part of the world's merchant shipping has come to fly the flags of States which are unlikely ever to be active belligerents, while the main naval powers are no longer the States with the larger merchant fleets. A further complicating factor, which has already been considered in Part III, is that the traditional concept of neutrality is difficult to reconcile with the law of the UN Charter in a number of respects.

4.45 Secondly, the Hague Conventions were based upon the assumption that the only part of the seas which was closed to belligerent naval operations was the waters of neutral States. While that proposition remains true today, the extent of those waters has greatly increased. Not only has the extent of territorial waters undergone a substantial increase since the Second World War, the concept of archipelagic waters means that large areas of what were formerly the High Seas are now considered to be part of the waters of the coastal State and thus, arguably, off limits to belligerents in a case where the coastal State is not directly involved in hostilities. Conversely, a

109. *Corfu Channel Case*, ICJ Reports 1949, p. 22; *Military and Paramilitary Activities in and Against Nicaragua*, ICJ Reports 1986, p. 112.

practice of belligerents in recent naval conflicts has been to proclaim exclusion zones, or war zones, in areas of the High Seas of strategic importance to them and to claim increased rights to control, and sometimes to attack, shipping within those zones.

4.46 Thirdly, the Hague Conventions treat interception, visit and search as the normal means of exercising belligerent rights in respect of merchant shipping. A merchant ship is treated as a legitimate target for attack only in exceptional circumstances (such as when resisting visit and search or travelling under convoy of enemy warships). Yet visit and search at sea is seldom a realistic option for States without substantial surface fleets and in an era of container shipping, visit and search at sea is unlikely to be particularly useful, since the contents of containers cannot be inspected without taking the ship into port. The Iran-Iraq War, in particular, saw both belligerents take a very broad view of the circumstances in which a merchant ship, even a neutral merchant ship, was a legitimate target. While some of these claims - for example, Iraq's claim that neutral merchant ships carrying exports of Iranian oil were a legitimate target for attack on sight - were almost certainly unjustified, there was a widespread feeling that uncertainty regarding the content of the law made it more difficult to resist such attacks.

4.47 These factors have led to a number of influential calls for a full-scale revision of the law of naval warfare.[110] That the 1907 treaties no longer provide sufficient guidance on their own is clear. That does not mean, however, that no satisfactory guide to conduct exists in the customary law. A recent initiative by the International Institute for Humanitarian Law has led to the publication of a text which, although it contains elements of progressive development, is in large part a restatement of the existing customary law in the San Remo

110. See, e.g., N. Ronzitti, "The Crisis of the Traditional Law Regulating International Armed Conflicts at Sea and the Need for its Revision" in Ronzitti (ed.), *The Law of Naval Warfare* (1988), pp. 1-58.

Manual on the law of naval warfare.[111] This Manual addresses the question of targeting by employing principles of targeting developed in the context of land warfare[112] and adapting them to the different context of naval warfare. It sets out the extent to which the law of neutrality at sea is still to be regarded as effective and it examines the question of where naval operations may lawfully be carried out in the light of the modern law of the sea.

4.48 While the case for a major revision of the law of naval warfare remains a strong one, any attempt to address this issue by means of an international conference would present considerable difficulties and would be doomed to fail unless it had the active support of the major naval States. In the circumstances, the personal view of the Rapporteur is that revision of the law of naval warfare, although desirable in the longer term, should not be considered an immediate priority. Instead, international efforts should be directed towards the further refinement of the customary law, using the San Remo statement as a starting point, and attempts to improve compliance with that law.

## V. Internal Conflicts

5.1 The 1899 Conference was concerned with the law applicable to conflicts between the States party to the Conventions which were there adopted and, ironically in view of the influence of the Lieber Code, which was drafted for use in the American Civil War,[113] did

111. L. Doswald-Beck (ed.), *San Remo Manual on International Law Applicable to Armed Conflicts at Sea* (1995); reprinted in *Documents* p. 573.

112. See Part IV, Section 3, of this report.

113. R. Abi-Saab, "Humanitarian Law and Internal Conflicts: The Evolution of Legal Concern" in A. Delissen and G. Tanja (eds), *Humanitarian Law of Armed Conflict: Challenges Ahead* (1991), p. 209, and *Droit Humanitaire et Conflits Internes* (1986).

not concern itself with conflicts occurring within a State.[114] One hundred years later, such conflicts have a far more prominent place on the international agenda, for it is here that the laws of war are arguably at their weakest and the case for revision consequently most pressing.

5.2 The existing treaty law on this subject is mainly contained in common Article 3 of the Geneva Conventions, 1949, and Additional Protocol II, 1977, although a number of other treaties are also applicable to internal conflicts.[115] Common Article 3 was adopted in 1949 after it became clear that a far more ambitious proposal that the four Conventions should extend in their entirety to civil wars would not be acceptable to the majority of States. The Article stipulates that in "armed conflict not of an international character occurring within the territory of one of the High Contracting Parties", the parties to the conflict (government and insurgent) were required to apply "as a minimum" certain basic humanitarian standards which are detailed in the Article. Article 3 also provided that "an impartial humanitarian body, such as the International Committee of the Red Cross, may offer its services to the parties to the conflict". That provision was undoubtedly a major step forward but the skeletal nature of common Article 3 is immediately apparent. The minimum humanitarian standards which it requires the parties to observe are concerned entirely with the protection of persons taking no active part in hostilities; there are no provisions on the actual conduct of hostilities and a single sentence - "the wounded and sick shall be collected and cared for" - does the work which in the case of international conflicts was done by two entire Conventions.

5.3 Common Article 3 was supplemented by Additional Protocol II in 1977. As in 1949, the original proposal from the International Committee of the Red Cross was more extensive than the text

114. See supra, Part II of this Report.

115. See, in particular, the Hague Convention for the Protection of Cultural Property, 1954, Art. 19, the amended Protocol II to the Conventional Weapons Convention, the Chemical Weapons Convention, 1993, and the Land Mines Convention, 1997.

eventually agreed at the Diplomatic Conference. Additional Protocol II is, however, far more detailed than common Article 3 and includes provisions for the conduct of hostilities, although almost all of these are designed to protect civilians rather than combatants.[116] It also lays down more detailed rules for the treatment of the wounded and sick and the protection of medical personnel,[117] as well as a series of provisions on basic humanitarian guarantees drawn from international humanitarian law and human rights law.[118]

5.4 It appears that there is also a body of customary international law applicable to non-international armed conflicts. Common Article 3 was itself treated as declaratory of custom by the ICJ in the *Nicaragua* case,[119] although the basis for this finding has been questioned.[120] In addition, at least some of the provisions in Additional Protocol II are also declaratory of customary international law. Far more striking, however, has been the decision of the ICTY Appeals Chamber in *Prosecutor* v. *Tadic (Jurisdiction),*[121] which found that there had developed an extensive body of customary international law applicable to non-international armed conflicts.

5.5 While these developments have meant that the law applicable to non-international armed conflicts has advanced considerably since 1899 (if, indeed, any such law existed at that date), a number of serious problems remain to be addressed.

116. Arts. 49 (1) and (2) and Arts. 13-18.

117. Arts. 7-12.

118. Arts. 4-6.

119. ICJ Reports 1986, p. 114, para. 218.

120. See, e.g., the dissenting opinion of Judge Sir Robert Jennings, loc. cit., p. 537.

121. 105 ILR p. 419.

## V.1 The Scope of Application of the Law on Internal Conflicts

5.6 The first such problem concerns the circumstances in which the law on internal armed conflicts becomes applicable. Common Article 3 merely refers to "armed conflict not of an international character", without any indication of what that term might mean. The term is, therefore, capable of a broad interpretation but it is clear that it does not apply to isolated acts of violence, such as sporadic acts of terrorism, or rioting. In that respect, Article 1 (2) of Additional Protocol II is probably stating the general law, when it provides that "situations of internal disturbances and tensions, such as riots, isolated and sporadic acts of violence and other acts of a similar nature" are not armed conflicts. The ICTY Appeals Chamber in *Tadic (Jurisdiction)* considered that there was an internal armed conflict whenever there was "protracted armed violence between governmental authorities and organized armed groups or between such groups within a State".[122] This definition was applied by the Inter-American Commission of Human Rights in the *Abella* case.[123]

5.7 Additional Protocol II, however, is subject to a higher threshold, Article 1 (1) providing that the Protocol applies to armed conflicts:

> which take place in the territory of a High Contracting Party between its armed forces and dissident armed forces or other organized armed groups which, under responsible command, exercise such control over a part of its territory as to enable them to carry out sustained and concerted military operations and to implement this Protocol.

The requirement of territorial control means that the majority of internal armed conflicts fall outside the scope of Additional Protocol II, the application of which is confined to full scale civil wars of the kind which occurred in Nigeria in the late 1960's. The Russian Constitutional Court in 1995 has held that Protocol II was applicable

122. Loc. cit., p. 488, para. 70.

123. Report No. 55/97, para. 160 et seq.

to the (first) conflict in Chechnya.[124] In addition, unlike common Article 3, Additional Protocol II does not apply to conflicts between warring factions within a State when none of these factions constitutes the government of that State.

5.8 The threshold for the application of the law of internal armed conflicts is unsatisfactory in a number of respects. First, it is difficult to find any justification today for the higher threshold for the application of Additional Protocol II. The provisions of Additional Protocol II are exclusively humanitarian in character. The provisions on the care of the wounded and sick should be uncontentious in any conflict, irrespective of its level of intensity. Those relating to fundamental guarantees are drawn in large part from human rights provisions, which are intended to apply in circumstances of normality, and the principles of common Article 3, which apply at the lower threshold in any event. The provisions on the conduct of hostilities are somewhat different, since these are derived from those of Additional Protocol I. Nevertheless, they are intended exclusively for the benefit of the civilian population and the limitations which they would impose upon government forces seeking to suppress a rebellion are minimal. There is no reason why a government should be obliged to observe these restraints towards its civilian population only in the circumstances specified in Article 1 of Additional Protocol II and not in all those to which common Article 3 applies and which are closer to a situation of normality within a State.

5.9 The higher threshold in Article 1 (1) of Additional Protocol II is, of course, explained in the text of that provision by reference to the need for an insurgent movement to control an area of territory in order to enable it to implement the Protocol. There is some force in that argument, since the provisions of the Protocol, like most of international humanitarian law, are more easily applied by those who have a territorial base than by forces which are constantly on the move. That is not to say, however, that the provisions of the Protocol cannot be implemented by an insurgent force which does not control

124. Judgment of 31 July 1995.

a clearly defined area of territory. Control of territory was not, for example, considered necessary for a national liberation movement to be able to apply the far more substantial provisions of the Geneva Conventions and Additional Protocol I.[125] Moreover, in any guerrilla conflict (and almost all internal conflicts are guerrilla conflicts for at least much of the time), the notion of territorial control is difficult to pin down. As a leading commentator has explained, it may vary between day and night.[126] In such circumstances, the existence of territorial control is thoroughly unsatisfactory to serve as a condition for the applicability of rules of international humanitarian law.

5.10 Secondly, contrary to what is provided in Additional Protocol II, it is important that the whole of the law of internal armed conflicts should be applicable to fighting between different non-governmental groups and not just to fighting between government and insurgent forces. In cases of civil war it is frequently difficult to determine which, if any, group can properly be regarded as the government of the State concerned.[127] Unlike Additional Protocol II, the test in common Article 3 avoids the need to address this question as a precondition for the applicability of international humanitarian law. Moreover, some of the most vicious internal conflicts of recent years have occurred between factions none of which could plausibly be regarded as the government of a State, the government either having ceased to exist or being unable to act.

5.11 Thirdly, with both common Article 3 and Additional Protocol II, there is a problem that, even where the conditions for their application have been met, governments are reluctant to admit that this is so. This reluctance is particularly evident in relation to Additional Protocol II, since for a government to admit the applicability of the Protocol is to concede that it has lost control of part of its

125. Additional Protocol I, Arts. 1(4) and 96(3).

126. G. Abi-Saab, "Wars of National Liberation", 165 RdC (1979-IV) p. 353. The remark was made in the context of an Art. 1(4) conflict under Additional Protocol I but is equally applicable to internal conflicts.

127. That was the case, for example, during part of the civil war in Liberia.

territory. It has, however, also been a feature of conflicts under common Article 3. As Judge KOOIJMANS has pointed out, this is a major weakness of the system of rules designed for internal armed conflicts.[128] In the absence of an acceptance on the part of the government, or of faction leaders, that an armed conflict exists, it is obviously less likely that the law will in fact be applied (although some governments have agreed to apply the standards in common Article 3 while denying that there is an armed conflict occurring on their territory). Yet the acceptance by a government that an armed conflict exists is not a legal prerequisite for the applicability of common Article 3 of Additional Protocol II. Both are stated to be applicable provided that certain objective criteria are met. It is therefore important that governments should not be allowed to escape their obligations by denying the existence of an armed conflict in circumstances where those criteria are met.

5.12 Finally, the comparatively high threshold for the applicability of the law of internal armed conflicts has opened up the threat of a gap between the coverage of human rights treaties and the rules of that law. Most human rights treaties permit derogation in cases of national emergency.[129] The question of exactly what constitutes such an emergency has frequently proved controversial but it is clear that the situation within a State can reach the stage at which that State may invoke the derogation clauses of the human rights treaties but still not amount to an armed conflict within the generally accepted sense of that term. It is possible, therefore, that a State might legitimately invoke the derogation provisions of the human rights treaties to which it is a party and thus remove some (though not all) of the protections afforded by those treaties, while still not being required to observe the limitations of the laws of war. There is no logical justification for this state of affairs, since there is no reason

128. P. Kooijmans, "In the Shadowland between Civil War and Civil Strife" in *Challenges Ahead*, op. cit. supra note 113, pp. 228-9.

129. See, e.g., Int. Covenant, Art. 4(1) ("public emergency which threatens the life of the nation"), Eur. Conv., Art. 15(1) ("war or other public emergency threatening the life of the nation"), Am. Conv., Art. 27(1) ("war, public danger, or other emergency that threatens the independence or security of a State Party").

why, in a state of emergency falling short of an internal armed conflict, a State should be permitted to engage in conduct which is forbidden to it in normal times and in the more serious conditions of civil war. The obvious desirability of closing that gap has led to the production of the Declaration of Minimum Humanitarian Standards ("the Turku Declaration") and other moves to elaborate a set of non-derogable standards drawn from both human rights law and the laws of war.[130]

5.13 Nevertheless, while the threshold for the application of Protocol II is set too high, a bigger problem is the refusal of governments to accept that that threshold has been crossed. The decision of the Russian Constitutional Court regarding the conflict in Chechnya is a rare example of a State formally recognizing the applicability of Protocol II.[131] In many other cases, however, the criteria for the application of that Protocol have been met but the State concerned has declined to acknowledge that fact. Similarly, States have been reluctant to accept that even the much lower threshold of common Article 3 has been crossed.

5.14 It is suggested, therefore, that the protection afforded to those not taking part in hostilities - and, in particular, to the civilian population caught up in an internal armed conflict - would be greatly enhanced if the international community were willing to take the following steps:
(1) make the threshold for the applicability of Additional Protocol II the same as that which currently exists for common Article 3;
(2) ensure that the threshold which will then be applicable to both sets of provisions is faithfully applied. The criteria for its application are, after all, objective ones and not a matter for the discretion of the State concerned and the international community has a legitimate

130. See, e.g., T. Meron and A. Rosas, "A Declaration of Minimum Humanitarian Standards", 85 AJIL (1991) p. 375.

131. See above, text at note 124. The Government of El Salvador applied the provisions of Protocol II during the civil war there, although without formally recognizing its applicability.

interest in ensuring that every State honours its international obligations in this respect; and
(3) harmonise the law of internal armed conflicts with the law of human rights by the identification of a set of standards common to existing human rights law and the law of internal conflicts which are to be applied at all points on the spectrum of internal unrest.

5.15 It is accepted that these proposals would involve a reversal of positions taken only just over twenty years ago when Additional Protocol II was adopted and would be seen by some States as a threat to sovereignty. In practice, however, no such threat would be involved. Violations of the law would not, of themselves, furnish a justification for intervention.[132] The restriction on the freedom of action of States would be small and the humanitarian gain potentially very considerable.

## V.2 The Substantive Law Applicable to Internal Armed Conflicts

5.16 A second problem concerns the comparative paucity of the substantive law applicable in internal armed conflicts. Even after the adoption of Additional Protocol II, this body of law is very limited, especially when one compares it with the substantive law applicable to international conflicts. There are indications that some States are prepared to apply the whole of the law of international armed conflict to internal armed conflicts as well.[133] The Appeals Chamber in *Tadic*, however, denied that the customary law of internal armed conflicts had yet reached the point where it was identical to that for inter-

132. Additional Protocol II, Art. 3.

133. See D. Fleck (ed), *The Handbook of Humanitarian Law in Armed Conflicts* (1995), p. 48, reproducing para. 211 of the German manual of the laws of war issued to the Bundeswehr.

national armed conflicts.[134] Moreover, some features of the law of international armed conflict - such as the law of belligerent occupation - are inappropriate for application in non-international conflicts and it is unlikely that the majority of States would be willing to accept the application of, for example, the underlying premise of the Prisoners of War Convention, that prisoners of war may not be subjected to punishment for the mere act of participating in hostilities, in conflicts between government and insurgent forces.

5.17 Nevertheless, there are other, less controversial principles of the law of international armed conflicts which could be applied to conflicts occurring within a State. The most obvious candidate is the provisions of the First and Second Geneva Conventions. Although Additional Protocol II, Articles 7-12, set out the main principles for the treatment of the wounded and sick and the protection of medical personnel, those provisions lack the detail of the First and Second Conventions, some of the provisions of which could usefully be extended to internal conflicts. While internal conflicts seldom have a naval dimension, it is not impossible that they might do so, in which case the extension of the principal provisions of the Second Convention to internal conflicts would be of great value.

5.18 The treaty law of internal armed conflicts also contains very few provisions on the conduct of hostilities themselves. Article 13 of Additional Protocol II states the basic principle that "the civilian population, as such, as well as individual civilians, shall not be the object of attack". This replicates the provision of Article 51 (2) of Additional Protocol I. However, unlike Additional Protocol I, Additional Protocol II contains no definition of the civilian population, a significant and damaging omission, since the distinction between civilians and combatants tends to be more difficult to draw in an internal conflict. There is no protection for civilian objects (other than that in Article 14 for objects indispensable for the survival of the civilian population). There is no definition of a legitimate military objective, comparable to that in Article 52 (2) of Additional

134. Loc. cit. supra note 121, para. 126.

Protocol I. Moreover, while outlawing attacks directed specifically against civilians, Additional Protocol II does not incorporate the principle of proportionality, i.e. that attacks may not be launched against a military objective if that attack may be "expected to cause incidental loss of civilian life, injury to civilians, damage to civilian objects, or a combination thereof, which would be excessive in relation to the concrete and direct military advantage anticipated".[135]

5.19 Another important distinction between Additional Protocol II and Additional Protocol I is that Additional Protocol I includes two provisions - Articles 57 and 58 on precautions in attack and defence respectively - which translate the main principles regarding the protection of civilians and civilian objects into rules of conduct for commanders. Article 57 is a particularly valuable provision, setting out, as it does, a "check list" for those who order an attack, to ensure that the provisions on the protection of the civilian population are properly observed. There are no comparable provisions in Additional Protocol II. Since, however, commanders in internal armed conflicts are required to observe the principles set out in Articles 13 to 16 of Additional Protocol II when they order an attack, a similar check list may be of great value in helping to develop a culture of compliance.

5.20 The evidence of the last fifty years is that the civilian population suffers at least as much in internal as in international conflicts. The extension to internal conflicts of more of the principles and rules for the protection of the civilian population from the effects of hostilities would offer a significant advance without unduly restricting the ability of a State to combat rebellion within its territory.

5.21 The laws of internal armed conflict also lack provisions for the protection of combatants. Apart from Article 4 (1) of Additional Protocol II, which prohibits orders not to give quarter, the only provisions regarding the treatment of combatants concern their treatment after capture.

135. Additional Protocol I, Art. 51 (5) (b).

5.22 The logic which lies behind the unnecessary suffering principle, however, is equally applicable to internal conflicts and it should be made clear that this principle is also applicable there. There is also good reason to apply to internal armed conflicts more of the provisions on weapons and methods of warfare which apply in international conflicts. As the ICTY Appeals Chamber has said, again in the *Tadic (Jurisdiction)* decision:

> ... elementary considerations of humanity and common sense make it preposterous that the use by States of weapons prohibited in armed conflicts between themselves be allowed when States try to put down rebellion by their own nationals on their own territory. What is inhumane, and consequently proscribed, in international wars, cannot but be inhumane and inadmissible in civil strife.[136]

Several of the more recent treaties on weaponry - the Chemical Weapons Convention, 1993, the amended Protocol II to the Conventional Weapons Convention and the Land Mines Convention, 1997 - are applicable in internal armed conflicts. The older treaties, however, are not, for the most part specifically applicable in internal conflicts (although the 1925 Chemical and Biological Warfare Protocol has been treated as laying down standards which are also applicable to conflicts within a State).

5.23 There is, therefore, a strong case for saying that these principles on the protection of the wounded and sick, the protection of the civilian population from the effects of hostilities and the law of weaponry should be applicable in internal armed conflicts.

5.24 Whether it is necessary to extend them by treaty is another matter. The decision in *Tadic* suggests that many of them may already be applicable as part of customary law. Since it is more than likely that the jurisprudence of ICTY and ICTR, as well as the ICC (if that body is established) will lead to the further elaboration of those customary rules, a treaty may well be unnecessary.

136. Loc. cit. supra note 121, para. 119.

5.25 If, however, it is accepted that the principles considered in this section of the Report should be applied in internal armed conflicts, there are certain advantages to achieving this goal by means of a new treaty, since that would make possible a systematic approach to the revision and codification of the law and would help in eliminating some of the uncertainty which undoubtedly exists at present regarding the content of the customary law:

> The emergence of the aforementioned general rules on internal armed conflicts does not imply that internal strife is regulated by general international law in all its aspects. Two particular limitations may be noted: (i) only a number of rules and principles governing international armed conflicts have gradually been extended to apply to internal conflicts; and (ii) this extension has not taken place in the form of a full an mechanical transplant of those rules to internal conflicts; rather the general essence of those rules, and not the detailed regulation they may contain, has become applicable to internal conflicts.[137]

5.26 It is noticeable, moreover, that only a year before the decision of the Appeals Chamber in *Tadic (Jurisdiction)*, the Commission of Experts appointed to investigate violations of international humanitarian law in the former Yugoslavia took a far more restricted view of the content of the customary law applicable to internal conflicts than that which was subsequently adopted by the Chamber.[138] It is also open to question whether, as Sir Hersch LAUTERPACHT commented many years ago, criminal trials are the best forum in which to resolve difficult questions about the content of the law regarding

137. Loc. cit. supra note 121, para. 126.

138. The Commission stated in its Final Report that:
The treaty-based law applicable to internal armed conflicts is relatively recent and is contained in common article 3 of the Geneva Conventions, Additional Protocol II, and article 19 of the 1954 Hague Convention on Cultural Property. It is unlikely that there is any body of customary international law applicable to internal armed conflict which does not find its root in these treaty provisions. (S/1994/674, para. 52.)

weapons, targets and the conduct of hostilities.[139] It is therefore of the utmost importance that the ICRC has embarked upon its study of the content of customary international humanitarian law, since this detailed project offers the best prospect of achieving a clear and comprehensive statement of the rules of customary law applicable to internal armed conflicts.

## V.3 Compliance with the Law of Internal Armed Conflict

5.27 The most serious problem with the law of internal armed conflict is, however, the very poor record of compliance. The reluctance of States to acknowledge that this law even applies to them has already been mentioned but even when its applicability is conceded, the record of compliance is poor. A marked improvement in compliance with the existing law would be a more significant step forward than would the revision of that law along the lines which have just been suggested. The topic of compliance with the laws of war in general is considered in Part VI. There are, however, a number of issues peculiar to compliance in internal conflicts which require brief comment here.

5.28 First, it has only recently been established that individuals who commit serious violations of the laws of internal armed conflict are guilty of war crimes under international law. As recently as five years ago, this proposition was doubted and when the Security Council established ICTR in 1994, giving it jurisdiction over violations of common Article 3, this act was described by the Secretary-General as an innovation, which "for the first time criminalizes common Article 3".[140] Since then, however, the fact that both the Yugoslavia and Rwanda tribunals have clearly been given jurisdiction over such offences by a Security Council which considered that it was acting within the existing law and respecting

139. H. Lauterpacht, "The Law of Nations and the Punishment of War Crimes", 21 BYIL (1944) p. 58 at p. 75.

140. UN Doc. S/1995/134, para. 12.

the principle *nullum crimen sine lege*, the decisions of ICTY,[141] and, most recently, the adoption of this principle in the Statute of the ICC[142] make it impossible convincingly to argue that the concept of war crimes does not extend to internal conflicts.

5.29 What does not so extend, however, is the special machinery for addressing grave breaches of the Geneva Conventions[143] and, in particular, the duty (as opposed to the right) of all States to make such conduct criminal under their own law, investigate alleged violations and, if there is sufficient evidence, to prosecute or extradite.[144] This part of the machinery for ensuring compliance with the laws of internal armed conflict would be greatly strengthened if (a) serious violations of the laws of internal armed conflict are included in the jurisdiction of the ICC, if that body is established, and (b) the machinery for the national prosecution of such offences were strengthened.

5.30 Secondly, it would be easier to develop and foster a culture of compliance with the law of internal armed conflict if there was a greater degree of external monitoring of compliance during a conflict (as opposed to prosecution of violations, which normally occurs after the conflict has ended and, in any event, long after the alleged violation has been committed). Two steps could be taken in that regard. First, the right of initiative which the ICRC currently possesses under common Article 3 could be strengthened. In particular, States could be required to accept the offer of services from the ICRC, if they have not accepted some other form of international supervision (as is already the case in international conflicts).[145] Secondly, the jurisdiction of the Fact-Finding Commission

141. In addition to *Tadic*, see *Prosecutor* v. *Martic*, 108 ILR p. 39.

142. Art. 8 (2) (c) to (f).

143. *Tadic*, loc. cit. supra note 121, paras. 79-85.

144. See, e.g., Geneva Convention III, Arts. 129-30.

145. See, e.g., Geneva Convention III, Art. 10.

established by Article 90 of Additional Protocol I could be formally extended to internal conflicts.[146]

5.31 Finally, as mentioned in Part III of this Report, it is possible that the monitoring mechanisms of human rights conventions could be used in an indirect way to assist in ensuring compliance with the law applicable in internal conflicts. While it is clear that a human rights monitoring body established by treaty possesses only the jurisdiction conferred by that treaty, the relationship between the law of human rights and the law applicable in internal armed conflicts is a close one. A human rights tribunal investigating alleged violations of the right to life in an internal armed conflict is likely, therefore, to be investigating conduct which will also involve alleged violations of the laws of armed conflict.

5.32 The potential for action of this kind is illustrated by the decision of the Inter-American Commission of Human Rights in the case of *Abella* v. *Argentina*, which concerned the fighting that followed a take-over of an army barracks. The Commission there stated that:

> ... the Commission's ability to resolve claimed violations of this non-derogable right [to life] arising out of an armed conflict may not be possible in many cases by reference to Article 4 of the American Convention alone. This is because the American Convention contains no rules that either define or distinguish civilians from combatants and other military targets, much less specify when a civilian can be lawfully attacked or when civilian casualties are a lawful consequence of military operations. Therefore, the Commission must necessarily look to and apply definitional standards and relevant rules of humanitarian law as sources of authoritative guidance in its resolution of this and

146. The Commission already takes the view that its jurisdiction extends to internal armed conflicts if the parties so agree. In one instance, the government of a State involved in such a conflict has formally invited the Commission to explore the willingness of the parties to accept a role of the Commission. This has not, however, led to any concrete results.

other kinds of claims alleging violations of the American Convention in combat situations.[147]

5.33 This approach, which builds upon the common ground between the law of human rights and the law of internal armed conflict should be encouraged as an aid to ensuring compliance, although, of course, it should be noted that human rights tribunals normally possess jurisdiction only in respect of alleged violations committed by the State.

# VI. Improving Compliance

6.1 The principal theme of this Report has been that, whatever the shortcomings of the laws of war, the most important objective is now to improve compliance with those laws, for it is here that the greatest weakness lies.[148] The recent fighting in the former Yugoslavia, Rwanda and Somalia, to take just three notorious examples, have shown the extent to which the most fundamental principles of the laws of war are disregarded in practice. While the substantive law is certainly capable of improvement, as this Report has endeavoured to show, it is curbing this tendency to flout the law which must be the priority. This Part of the report will therefore concentrate on some of the ways by which this might be done.

## VI.1 **Peacetime Measures**

6.2 Compliance with the law in relation to any activity is likely to be enhanced if those who engage in that activity are aware of their legal responsibilities and the steps which they must take to discharge them, in short, if a "culture of compliance" is developed, in which

147. Report No. 55/97, para. 161. See also para. 3.31 above and para. 6.29 below.

148. See the recent studies by H. Fox and M. Meyer (op. cit. supra note 4) and European Commission, *Law in Humanitarian Crises: How Can International Law be Made More Effective in Armed Conflicts* (1995).

respect for the law is seen as a normal and essential part of behaviour.[149] The development of such a culture can be a far more important factor in ensuring that the law is respected than the threat of prosecution or other measures taken after the conflict has started.

6.3 For example, Articles 48-57 of Additional Protocol I require that a commander who orders an attack should attempt to ensure that the target is a legitimate military objective, that civilians are not themselves targeted, that certain other objects subject to special regimes of protection (e.g. under Articles 54-56) are not attacked, that the attack will respect the requirement of proportionality and that, in choosing the methods and means by which the attack is to be carried out, he selects those which will be likely to avoid, or at least minimise, the civilian casualties. While prosecutions for failure to comply with these requirements are possible, it is likely to be far more difficult to bring a successful prosecution for, e.g., failure to comply with the proportionality principle or the selection of the wrong method or means of attack than for a crime such as the murder of prisoners. The best hope of ensuring that a commander will respect those principles laid down in Additional Protocol I (or the largely similar principles in customary law, where Additional Protocol I is not applicable) is if the commander is sufficiently well aware of his responsibilities that he or she instinctively takes such considerations into account in planning and taking decisions.

6.4 Central to the creation of such a culture of compliance amongst the military is the proper dissemination of the laws of war and training in their application in particular circumstances. The 1899 Conference recognized this need. Article 1 of the Convention on the Laws and Customs of War on Land, to which the Regulations are annexed, requires States to "issue to their armed forces instructions

149. L. Henkin, *International Law: Politics, Values and Functions*, 216 RdC (1989-IV), pp. 67-87.

which shall be in conformity with the Regulations".[150] The duty of States to disseminate the provisions of the relevant agreements to the members of their armed forces and their civilian populations is also stipulated in the Geneva Conventions and Additional Protocol I.[151]

6.5 Measures of this kind cannot be left until after the outbreak of a conflict, for then the belligerent States tend to have other priorities. It is important that all States provide appropriate education and training in the laws of war for the members of their armed forces in time of peace. That can, of course, be supplemented if the State concerned becomes involved in hostilities but a culture of compliance cannot be created overnight and, at least with regular armed forces, peacetime instruction is essential. In particular, that instruction has to be more than simply a presentation of the rules of the laws of war; it has to demonstrate how those laws form an integral part of military life and the business of fighting.

6.6 It is therefore important that assistance be given to those States which lack the resources to mount programmes of this kind or whose governments are unsure of what is required. The ICRC and the International Institute of Humanitarian Law at San Remo already perform valuable work in this respect. The expansion of these and similar programmes - something which would require greater resources - would be a simple and undramatic yet potentially very effective method of improving compliance with the laws of war.

6.7 Other measures which need to be taken in peacetime include, inter alia:
(a) the adoption of legislation and administrative practices in each State which are sufficient to ensure that that State can comply with its international obligations;

150. "Les Hautes Parties Contractantes donneront à leurs forces armées de terre des instructions qui seront conformes au Règlement ..."

151. See, e.g., Geneva Convention III, Art. 127; Protocol I, Art. 88; Protocol II, Art. 19; Hague Convention on Cultural Property, Art. 25.

(b) the scrutiny of new developments in weapons and methods of warfare to ensure that they will comply with the requirements of the laws of war (Additional Protocol I, Article 36);
(c) taking into account, in decisions about planning, the obligation in Additional Protocol I, Article 58 (b) to "avoid locating military objectives within or near densely populated areas"; and
(d) the establishment of systems for handling prisoners of war and other detainees in the event of armed conflict.

6.8 States need to be encouraged to take such measures and, where necessary, assisted to do so. In this context, one important development is the creation of the ICRC's Advisory Service to assist States in ensuring that their national legislation is adequate to enable them to meet their obligations under international humanitarian law.[152]

6.9 The possibility should also be considered of creating a system of periodic reporting to an impartial body (comparable to the system of periodic reporting to the UN Human Rights Committee by States party to the International Covenant on Civil and Political Rights, 1966). The system of periodic reporting has been a useful tool in encouraging States to ensure that they adopt the mechanisms necessary to meet their human rights obligations and the system could usefully be emulated in relation to international humanitarian law, although it must be recognized that the sensitivity of much military information is such that any reporting requirement would necessarily have to be limited in scope. A first step could usefully be made at the regional level.

152. See P. Berman, "The ICRC's Advisory Service on International Humanitarian Law and the Challenge of National Implementation", *International Review of the Red Cross* (1996) pp. 338-347 and the Annual Report for 1997 of the Advisory Service, *National Implementation of International Humanitarian Law* (ICRC, 1998).

## VI.2 The Protecting Powers and the Role of the International Committee of the Red Cross

6.10 The law is more likely to be respected if there is effective monitoring of compliance and if discreet pressure can be brought to bear upon States not to commit, or to tolerate the commission by those under their control, of violations. In particular, access to prisoner of war camps and detention centres, the exchange of reliable lists of prisoners of war and the fact that prisoners of war, detainees and the population of occupied territory have recourse to some outside body for their protection are all measures likely to encourage compliance with the laws of war. The Geneva Conventions and Additional Protocol I contain provision for the appointment by belligerents of Protecting Powers - neutral States which will oversee the treatment of prisoners of war and other nationals of one belligerent by its adversary. Protecting Powers played an important role, especially in relation to prisoners of war, during the Second World War.

6.11 The system of Protecting Powers has, however, scarcely been used at all since 1945. In part, the problem has been that a belligerent State is under no obligation to accept the nomination of a Protecting Power by its adversary. Article 5 of Additional Protocol I attempted to strengthen the system by providing for a series of steps to be taken in the event that agreement on the appointment of a Protecting Power proved difficult but it stopped short of imposing upon States a duty to accept a Protecting Power.

6.12 The international climate has undergone great changes since 1977 and some things which were unthinkable then are commonplace today. In particular, there appears to be a greater readiness to accept a degree of third-party settlement and outside intervention. It may be, therefore, that the imposition of a duty to accept the appointment of a Protecting Power is no longer unthinkable. If that is the case, it would be a valuable change in the law. If, however, it is necessary to work within the existing legal framework, much could still be done to encourage a far more widespread acceptance of the protecting power system. If life can be breathed back into this system, the machinery for ensuring compliance with the laws of war would be significantly strengthened.

6.13 In the absence of a Protecting Power, the Conventions and Protocol I require belligerents to accept the services of the ICRC, or another international humanitarian organization which offers all guarantees of impartiality and efficacy. It is, however, notorious that this is not always done. It is of the utmost importance that the international community makes clear that denial of access to the ICRC on the part of a State is both unlawful and wholly unacceptable. It has already been suggested, in Part V of this Report, that the duty to accept the services of the ICRC should be extended to internal armed conflicts.

6.14 It must also be recognized that impartiality and confidentiality are essential to the effectiveness of the ICRC. That means that the ICRC and those who work for it cannot be expected both to conduct the on-site inspections and visits which are currently their hallmark and which are so important to the prevention of violations of the law and to stand as public accusers of those who violate the law. This inescapable fact has important implications both for the relationship between this method of ensuring compliance and the public "naming and shaming" (considered in paragraphs 6.18 to 6.21, below) and for the ability of persons working for the ICRC to give evidence in criminal prosecutions, e.g. before the ICC (considered at paragraphs 6.31 et seq.).

## VI.3 The Fact-Finding Commission

6.15 Article 90 of Additional Protocol I established a Fact-Finding Commission with competence to:

> (i) enquire into any facts alleged to be a grave breach as defined in the Conventions and this Protocol or other serious violation of the Conventions or of this Protocol;

(ii) facilitate, through its good offices, the restoration of an attitude of respect for the Conventions and this Protocol.[153]

These two heads of jurisdiction are disjunctive, i.e. the Commission may use its good offices without holding an enquiry and vice-versa.

6.16 The competence of the Commission exists in respect of States which have made a declaration accepting its competence to enquire into allegations by any other Party accepting the same obligation.[154] There is also provision for the acceptance of the Commission's jurisdiction on an *ad hoc* basis.[155]

6.17 The establishment of the Commission was a modest but important measure, for the establishment of the facts, in the case of an alleged violation of the law, by the decision of an authoritative and impartial body may be of great assistance in putting an end to a continuing violation or in preventing a repetition of that violation. It is, therefore, a matter for great regret that, at the time of writing this Report, fewer than one in three of the States party to Protocol I had made declarations accepting its competence. In these circumstances, it seems unlikely that any proposal that acceptance of its competence should be made compulsory would be accepted. Nevertheless, States should be encouraged to accept the competence of the Commission at the earliest possible date and initiatives to that effect should be taken through the UN, the ICRC and regional organizations.

## VI.4 The Role of States and the United Nations

6.18 An important means of persuading belligerent States to demonstrate a greater respect for the laws of war is through the pressure of international public opinion. In part, this factor is a product of media coverage, the activities of non-governmental

153. Art. 90 (2) (c).

154. Art. 90 (2) (a).

155. Art. 90 (2) (d). See also supra, para. 5.30.

organizations and the interest of the public at large. Adverse publicity for violations of humanitarian law can sometimes have considerable influence. This is obviously a desirable development which should be encouraged wherever possible (e.g. through the enforcement of rules of law designed to protect journalists covering armed conflicts).

6.19 All States, however, have a measure of responsibility for ensuring compliance with the laws of war, even in conflicts in which they are not directly involved. Common Article 1 of the Geneva Conventions (and the corresponding provision in Protocol I) provides that "the High Contracting Parties undertake to respect *and to ensure respect*" for the Conventions in all circumstances.[156] It is going too far, however, to read this provision as imposing a legal obligation on neutral States to intervene in order to prevent or remedy violations of the Conventions.[157] What Article 1 does do is to make clear that a neutral State has the right, or standing, to make representations to a belligerent suspected of violations of the Conventions (or, as the case may be, of the Protocol). Certainly, representations of this kind cannot properly be regarded as constituting an interference in the internal affairs of another State, even when those representations relate to a non-international armed conflict.

6.20 In addition, Article 89 of Additional Protocol I provides that:

> In situations of serious violations of the Conventions or of this Protocol, the High Contracting Parties undertake to act, jointly or individually, in co-operation with the United Nations and in conformity with the UN Charter.

156. For a discussion of this provision, see L.Condorelli and L Boisson de Chazournes, "Quelques remarques à propos de l'obligation des Etats de 'respecter et faire respecter' le droit international humanitaire 'en toutes circonstances'", in C. Swiniarski (ed) *Studies and Essays in International Humanitarian Law and Red Cross Principles* (1984), pp. 17-36.

157. For a refutation of suggestions to that effect, see A. Roberts, "The Laws of War: Problems of Implementation in Contemporary Conflicts", in European Commission, *Law in Humanitarian Crises* (1995), pp. 13-82.

A more rigorous application of this provision could provide an effective means of improving compliance with the laws of war. There are indications, for example, that the inquiries conducted by the UN into conditions in prisoner of war camps during the Iran-Iraq war and into the use of chemical weapons by Iraq had an effect in improving conditions in the camps and (although this is obviously less susceptible of proof) in deterring further use of chemical weapons.

6.21 In part, the effectiveness of such measures lies in the generation of adverse publicity, acting as a catalyst for international political pressure on the law breaker. In recent years, however, the Security Council has gone further. In addition to condemning violations of the laws of war and calling upon the States concerned to respect the law, the Council has, on a number of occasions, determined that violations of the laws of war themselves constitute a threat to international peace and security and that measures to prevent or punish those violations have been ordered by the Council in the exercise of its powers under Chapter VII of the Charter.[158] Such action on the part of the Security Council, though obviously possible only in cases of particularly serious violations, is potentially a particularly powerful means of enforcement.

## VI.5 State Responsibility

6.22 Although not discussed in 1899, the question of State responsibility and the liability to pay compensation for violations of the laws of war was considered at length at the 1907 Conference, which added to the Convention on the Laws and Customs of War on Land a new Article 3, which provided that:

> A belligerent party which violates the provisions of the [Regulations on the Laws and Customs of War on Land] shall, if the case demands, be

158. See, in particular, the Council's resolutions on the former Yugoslavia, especially Res. 808 and 827.

liable to pay compensation. It shall be responsible for all acts committed by persons forming part of its armed forces.

6.23 Remarkably, it appears that this provision was not intended to be confined to claims between States but was to extend to a direct right to compensation for individuals.[159] This measure was seen at the time as an important inducement to States to comply with the Regulations and to ensure compliance by their forces.[160]

6.24 In practice, however, the payment of compensation for violations of the laws of war has been rare, most conflicts leaving the defeated party in such a weak economic state that it has not been considered feasible to press for compensation. The Gulf Conflict of 1990-91, however, is an exception. Iraq's duty to compensate those who suffered loss as a direct result of its invasion of Kuwait was expressly recognized by the Security Council which created a mechanism, the United Nations Compensation Commission (UNCC), by which effect could be given to that responsibility.[161]

6.25 The jurisdiction of the UNCC includes (though it is not limited to) the payment of compensation for violations of the laws of war. In particular, members of the civilian population in Kuwait are eligible for compensation in respect of loss or injury resulting from violations of the laws of war by Iraqi forces. Perhaps surprisingly, however, in the case of claims from members of the Coalition armed forces, the Governing Council of the UNCC has held that such claimants are eligible for compensation only if they were prisoners of war and their loss or injury "resulted from mistreatment in violation of international humanitarian law (including the Geneva Conventions of

159. F. Kalshoven, 'State Responsibility for Warlike Acts of the Armed Forces', 40 ICLQ (1991) p. 827.

160. See now, Additional Protocol I, Art. 91

161. SC Res. 687 (1991), para. 16. It is important to note that the Council recognized that Iraq was responsible under existing international law. Contrary to what is sometimes suggested, it did not impose a liability which would not otherwise have existed.

1949)."[162] It is difficult to see why other violations of the laws of war are excluded in the case of this category of claimants.

6.26 The duty of States to compensate the victims of their violations of the laws of war – quite apart from being something which should be enforced for its own sake – could prove to be an important means for encouraging compliance with the laws of war if States considered that there was a substantial likelihood of their being required to pay. While the mechanism established in the case of Iraq by Resolution 687 is likely to prove unique, consideration should be given to finding other means of ensuring that the normal duty of a State to compensate for its violations of international law is properly applied in the context of armed conflict.

6.27 It is important, however, to remember that the responsibility of the State is delictual in character and is in addition to, not in substitution for, the criminal responsibility of the individual State official who orders or commits violations of the laws of war.[163]

## VI.6 Human Rights Mechanisms

6.28 It is also possible that the various mechanisms for the enforcement of international human rights law may be able to offer a measure of assistance in improving compliance with the laws of war. Although such bodies have no jurisdiction to apply the laws of war as such, it is possible that in cases involving allegations of human rights violations during an armed conflict (international or internal), a human rights tribunal will look to the laws of war for guidance in relation to such issues as whether the deprivation of life in a particular case was arbitrary.

162. Governing Council Decision No. 11, UN Doc. S/AC.26/1992/11; 109 ILR 612. It is not clear why members of the armed forces who were the victims of violations of the laws of war while not prisoners of war are excluded.

163. ILC Draft Articles on the International Code of Crimes, 1996, Art. 4; UN Doc. A/51/10, p. 30; decision of the Supreme Court of Israel in *Attorney-General* v. *Eichmann*, 36 ILR p. 5.

6.29 That is what the Inter-American Commission of Human Rights did in its decision in *Abella* v. *Argentina*. The Commission was there faced with allegations that there had been violations of the right to life on the ground that the Argentine army had used excessive force in overpowering a group who had seized control of an army barracks. Finding that the situation had amounted to an internal armed conflict, the Commission argued that because "the American Convention contains no rules that either define or distinguish civilians from combatants and other military targets, much less specify when a civilian can be lawfully attacked or when civilian casualties are a lawful consequence of military operations," it needed to "look to and apply definitional standards and relevant rules of international humanitarian law as sources of authoritative guidance".[164]

6.30 It is not intended to comment here on the facts of that case or the Commission's findings in respect of them. Its approach to the relationship between human rights law and the laws of war is, it is submitted, in accordance with that of the ICJ in the *Nuclear Weapons* Advisory Opinion[165] and it is likely that a similar approach will be taken by other international human rights bodies. Provided that the relevant material on the laws of war and appropriate legal arguments are put before such a body, this approach may provide a further inducement to States to comply with the laws of war.

## VI.7 Prosecution of War Crimes

6.31 The most obvious, and currently the most studied, way in which the international community could improve compliance with the laws of war would be through strengthening the system for the prosecution of war crimes to the point where the likelihood of being brought to justice acted as a real deterrent to those contemplating the commission of war crimes.

164. Report No. 55/97, para. 161; see the full text quoted in para.5.32; see also supra, para. 3.31.

165. See paras. 3.28 to 3.36 of this Report.

6.32 The notion of individual criminal responsibility for violations of the laws of war is not a new one. Although the 1899 and 1907 Conventions contain no express provision for criminal responsibility, the concept was already well understood at the time and violations of the laws and customs of war, as enshrined in the Hague Regulations, were treated as a criminal offences at the end of both the first and second world wars, although it was only at the end of the second world war that any significant number of trials was held.

6.33 The present report is not the place to attempt a history of the law of war crimes. Suffice it to say that by 1945 two principles were well established. First, violations of the laws of war entailed the criminal responsibility of the individuals who committed or who ordered the commission of such violations even if there was no provision to that effect in the treaties concerned. Secondly, war crimes were crimes of universal jurisdiction, that is to say all States had the right, though not the duty, to prosecute war crimes, even if they were committed in another State by persons who did not have the nationality of the forum.

6.34 The Geneva Conventions of 1949 endeavoured to strengthen this regime by means of express provisions that certain violations of the Conventions were to be treated as "grave breaches" and that all States party to the Conventions had a duty to investigate allegations of grave breaches and either to prosecute or extradite anyone against whom a sufficiently credible allegation was made.[166] The system of grave breaches was further developed in Additional Protocol I.[167]

6.35 The adoption of these provisions (which, at least in the case of the Geneva Conventions, became binding on almost every State in the world) meant that most of the more serious violations of international humanitarian law committed in international armed con-

166. Geneva Convention I, Arts. 49-50; Geneva Convention II, Arts. 50-51; Geneva Convention III, Arts. 129-130; Geneva Convention IV, Arts. 146-7.

167. Arts. 85-88.

flicts[168] became subject to a regime in which all States not merely asserted a right to prosecute but accepted a duty to do so.

6.36 Yet for most purposes this regime existed only in theory. That is not to say that prosecutions for war crimes never took place. When they occurred, however, it was almost invariably the exercise of jurisdiction by a State over its own armed forces.[169] That is, of course, an important aspect of the enforcement of international humanitarian law. Yet the complete absence - until very recently - of any exercise of jurisdiction by other States is not only a negation of the enforcement system enshrined in the Geneva Conventions, it also removes a major incentive to States to exercise jurisdiction over their own service personnel. It is difficult, therefore, to escape the conclusion that in most States (though not all) the prospect of punishment for violations of the laws of war was not a serious deterrent.

6.37 The process of reviving criminal jurisdiction for war crimes began with the adoption by the Security Council of Resolution 827 (1993) creating ICTY and Resolution 955 (1994) creating ICTR. This Report is not the place to attempt a survey of the jurisprudence of those Tribunals.[170] There is no doubt, however, that they have played a major part both in the development of the law of war crimes and in reviving the concept of war crimes liability. In particular, the decision of the Appeals Chamber in the *Tadic* case,[171] while rejecting the applicability of the grave breaches regime to non-international

168. The system of grave breaches was held by the Appeals Chamber in *Tadic* not to apply to violations of the law committed in non-international armed conflicts, loc. cit. supra note 121.

169. As was the case in the My Lai prosecution. See, e.g., L. Friedman, *The Law of War, A Documentary History*, p. 1703 et seq.

170. The Rapporteur has attempted a brief survey of ICTY's jurisdiction to 31 December 1997 in "The Development of International Humanitarian Law by the International Criminal Tribunal for the Former Yugoslavia", 2 *Year Book of United Nations Law* (1998) pp. 97-140.

171. 105 ILR p. 419 (1995).

conflicts, made clear that violations of the laws of war in such conflicts were war crimes.

6.38 The process of enhancing the use of criminal jurisdiction as a means of enforcement of international humanitarian law was further advanced by the adoption in July 1998 of the Statute of the ICC. This act is without doubt the most important step forward in improving compliance with the provisions of international humanitarian law. This is not the place to attempt an analysis of all its provisions. Suffice it to say that the international community has provided for the creation of an international tribunal with jurisdiction to try those responsible for the most serious war crimes (as defined in Article 8 of the Statute) committed in internal or international conflicts, provided that the State of nationality of the defendant or the State in whose territory the alleged offence was committed has accepted the jurisdiction of the Court.

6.39 Provided that the States which voted for the adoption of the Statute of the ICC in 1998 follow their action through by becoming parties to that Statute and ensuring that the Court is able to operate efficiently, the stage is set for a very considerable enhancement of the means of enforcement of the laws of war. Those who violate that law will now, for the first time, face the serious prospect of being called to account before a standing international tribunal. Moreover, the creation of the ICC is likely to have an important effect in encouraging all States to take more seriously their obligations to prosecute such offences in their own courts, since a State which does so is less likely to find that those within its jurisdiction are prosecuted in the ICC.

6.40 While this Rapporteur therefore acknowledges the criticisms of the Court which have been made in certain quarters - many of which are dismissed too readily by the Court's supporters - he is firmly of the view that the Court is a step forward of the utmost importance and that every effort should be made to ensure that the largest possible number of States becomes party to the Statute.

6.41 The likelihood that there will now be a greater exercise of national jurisdiction should not be seen as detracting from the importance of the ICC but rather as an important parallel contribution to the enforcement of international humanitarian law. In this connection the work of the Advisory Service of the ICRC, of which mention has already been made, is likely to be particularly important in helping States to ensure that they have in place the legislation necessary to enable them to exercise that jurisdiction.

6.42 It is, however, important not to be starry eyed about what the ICC can achieve. In particular, two considerations need to be borne in mind. First, so long as the acceptance of its jurisdiction falls well short of universality, it would be quite wrong to use it as a means of developing the substantive law beyond the international consensus. No individual should be put at risk of prosecution before the ICC for breach of a norm not binding upon the State which he or she serves. An example - albeit a controversial one - is the recruitment of child soldiers.[172] At present, there is no rule binding on the generality of States prohibiting the recruitment into the armed forces of children aged over fifteen. If that age limit is to be raised, it should not be done through the amendment of the ICC Statute but through changes in the substantive law of armed conflict.

6.43 Secondly, the creation of the ICC should not be seen as a panacea. Prosecution of violations of the laws of war is an important means of encouraging compliance with the laws of war but it is not the only, or even necessarily the most effective, means. Indeed, prosecutions are, in one sense, an admission of failure, since they occur only after an offence has been committed. A strategy for improving compliance with the laws of war must pay at least as much heed to the prevention of crime as to its punishment. It would therefore be a great mistake to allow the creation of the Court to distract attention

172. The use of children in armed conflict is one of the most appalling features of modern warfare but this Rapporteur is of the firm view that what is called for at present is the enforcement of the existing laws prohibiting the recruitment of children below the age of fifteen, not a raising of the age limit.

or divert resources away from the other methods of ensuring compliance outlined in this Part of the Report.

# VII. Conclusions

7.1 This Report has not attempted to cover the whole of the laws of war. Some of the issues omitted from this Report, for reasons of space, are the subject of consideration elsewhere as part of the Commemoration process. The conclusions of the Report can be briefly stated.

7.2 The 1899 Conference began a great era of law making in relation to the conduct of warfare. The fact that the high hopes of a century of peace, which were entertained at that Conference, have been so cruelly and extensively disappointed by the realities of the 20th century should not be allowed to blind us to the achievements of that law-making process. As a result of the 1899 and subsequent conferences, the laws of war at the end of the 20th century are far more advanced than they were at its outset. Moreover, although this Report has emphasised the violations of those laws during the last hundred years, violations of the law have by no means been universal - the record of compliance is poor but it is not non-existent. Where the laws of war have been implemented, they have in large measure achieved the goal of the 1899 Conference "to serve, even in this extreme case, the interests of humanity and the ever progressive needs of civilisation".[173]

7.3 Nevertheless, the considerable achievement in law-making has not been matched by one of law enforcement. While the laws of war undoubtedly have their defects and difficulties, the most important weakness in the laws of war today lies not in their substance but in their implementation. It has therefore been the principal theme of this

173. Preamble to the Hague Convention with respect to the Laws and Customs of War on Land, 1899.

Report that the most urgent priority for the international community in relation to the laws of war is not the revision of that law but improving the record of compliance. To that end, the Report has made a number of suggestions in Part VI, although the subject is also considered throughout the Report.

7.4 One area of substantive law which, it is suggested, is in urgent need of revision is that relating to the conduct of internal armed conflicts, where Part V of the Report has made a number of proposals for consideration. Even here, however, revision of the substantive law is less important than achieving an improvement in compliance with the law which already exists. A substantial improvement in compliance even with the skeletal provisions of common Article 3 would do more to achieve humanitarian goals in internal armed conflicts than would the mere adoption of a new treaty, no matter how much that treaty improved the substance of the law.

7.5 The Report has also suggested that there is a need for further study (though not necessarily for a revision of the law) of the relationship between the law of the UN Charter and the laws of war. That need exists at two levels. First, the implications of the Charter for the conduct of warfare by States call for further thought. There remains a tendency to assume that the Charter has an impact only upon whether it is lawful for a State to resort to force, whereas the limitations inherent in the right of self-defence and the obligations flowing from the decisions of the Security Council also have serious implications for the way in which force is employed. Secondly, a more immediate concern is to determine and clarify the law applicable to the conduct of military operations by the United Nations itself. Both of these issues are considered in Part III of this Report. Further work upon these issues has the advantage that it will not require any change in the law or, therefore, the convening of a major international conference.

7.6 With regard to the law applicable to the conduct of hostilities in international armed conflicts, the Report suggests that the two areas in which the strongest case can be made for revision are the law of naval warfare and the law of belligerent occupation. These matters have been considered in Part IV. In each case, however, the Report suggests that, while it may be desirable to attempt a revision of the law at a later date, attempts to draw up a new body of law on either of these subjects is likely to prove of considerable difficulty. There is a consequent danger that a failed attempt at law reform may serve only to undermine the law which we already possess. The Report suggests that revision of the law in these two areas should not be regarded as a priority at the present time.

7.7 The law relating to nuclear weapons is the subject of discussion in other Reports. The present Rapporteur would, however, by way of a postscript, like to record his own view that this issue can be tackled only through the disarmament process.

# PEACEFUL SETTLEMENT OF DISPUTES
## PROSPECTS FOR THE 21ST CENTURY

Revised report prepared for the Centennial of the First International Peace Conference
by Francisco ORREGO VICUÑA
and Christopher PINTO[1]

## I. A changing international society

1. The Centennial Commemoration of the First Peace Conference of 1899[2] offers a unique opportunity to review the experiences arising from a century of efforts to achieve an adequate international dispute settlement system, as well as to discuss the trends and prospects that may be guiding the perfecting of such a system in the century ahead. Such an exercise is inextricably linked to the nature of international society as it evolves along time and to the characteristics of its governing legal order, perspectives that will be examined from the outset. In undertaking this examination and making proposals that may respond to the changing international outlook, the rapporteurs have considered that such innovations should not necessarily be restricted by the present legal framework, particularly the UN Charter, which is itself subject to the same pressures for change.

1. Professor Orrego Vicuña (Institute of International Studies, University of Chile) has undertaken responsibility for the writing of Sections I, III, and IV of the Report. Dr. Pinto (Secretary-General of the Iran-US claims Tribunal) has written Sections II, V and VI. The Rapporteurs took into consideration each other's views as expressed in the preparation of the report and in other publications; some parts are the outcome of joint undertakings. They are grateful for the many formal and informal comments received on the preliminary version of the report, many of which are reflected in this final version and duly cited as appropriate.

2. For the records of the 1899 and 1907 Hague Peace Conferences see James Brown Scott (ed): *The Reports of the Hague Conferences of 1899 and 1907* (1917).



*F. Kalshoven (ed.),*
*The Centennial of the First International Peace Conference,* 261–416.

## I.1 The transition from a Euro-centric society to the global society of the 21st century

2. The many changes that international society has experienced since 1899 mark the transition from the Euro-centric model that emerged with the establishment of the modern sovereign State and the Grotian legal order that gradually came into being, to the global society of the 21st century.[3] Because the 20th century has been the bridge between these two important historical periods, many features of the traditional order were still largely predominant while at the same time elements of change began to emerge, particularly in the past three decades. The sovereign State as a basic unity will not fade away in this context but its role in international society will be characterized by an interplay different from the past.

3. While the trends of change have prompted a variety of theories about the obsolescence of conflict, the absence of war and the decline of empires,[4] it regrettably does not appear realistic to exclude such elements from the discussion of future prospects of world society.[5] Nor do well-inspired utopian aspirations to a world government for the moment seem to find much support in the intricacies of human nature. Indeed, when the major developments and changes that are beginning to shape international society are examined in the context of the prospects for the 21st century, it may be realized that the main trend is not toward centralization as many have believed but, on the contrary, toward decentralization of the structure of society and the international legal order. At the same time strong links determine a greater integration among its component units, as is

3. The reader may again be referred to the records of the Peace Conferences (see note 2).

4. J. Mueller: *Retreat from doomsday: the obsolescence of major war* (1989); F. Fukuyama: "The end of history?", *The National Interest*, Summer 1989, pp. 3-18; P. Kennedy: *The rise and fall of great powers* (1987).

5. J. S. Nye: "The misleading metaphor of decline", *The Atlantic Monthly*, March 1999, 86-94; . P. Huntington: "No exit. The errors of endism", in "The future of History", *The National Interest*, Fall 1989, pp. 3-11.

evident from the operations of the global market, technology and communications.

4. A first notable change is that major contemporary developments are inspired by the need to ensure human freedom, dignity and welfare, matters which by their very nature tend to highlight the role of individuals and not that of superstructures. Second, while international society retains its universal nature, regionalism has become its main driving force, to such an extent that centralized action is no longer possible unless it relies on effective regional co-operation.[6] Third, the influence of non-State actors has become so prominent that sometimes it threatens the role of the State and certainly its traditional exclusivity.[7]

5. A fourth major change that follows from the above is that international society has become multi-centric and multi-cultural, thus also setting in motion a strong process of decentralization.[8] A particularly noteworthy phenomenon in this context is the assertion of a greater identity on the part of developing countries, which has contributed to new views about international society and international law. Fifth, enforcement of the law in international society continues to be highly decentralized and based more on solidarity than on a central enforcement mechanism, a trend that is most likely to continue and to rely increasingly on mutual convenience rather on commands, as it is already evident in environmental and trade matters. And sixth, the significant influence of contemporary international organizations, in itself a departure from the Euro-centric

6. W. W. Rostow: "The coming age of regionalism. A 'metaphor' for our time ?", *Encounter*, June 1999, pp. 3-7.

7. Société Française pour le Droit International: *L' État souverain à l' aube du XXIe siècle*, Colloque de Nancy, 1994.

8. E. Brown Weiss: "The new international legal system", in *Perspectives on International Law* (1995), p. 66.

model,[9] does not mean that it is substituting for a decentralized structure but rather that it is providing a common framework for the many forces and actors intervening in the shaping of international society. The effects of successive technological revolutions and of the dispersion of economic power are also strongly reinforcing a decentralized international society.[10]

6. In spite of the significance of all these changes international society is not likely to dramatically depart from its traditions and origins. It may be expected, therefore, that a situation of continuity and change will predominate throughout the 21st century and beyond, in which the diversified forces and actors referred to above will be seeking to balance and accommodate their respective interests. The need for such a balanced accommodation of interests will pose major challenges to the mechanisms for the settlement of disputes. Indeed, one such major challenge is how to keep a decentralized society that shares elements of integration united under the rule of law, while respecting its diversity and different traditions and cultures.

## I.2 The new structure of international law

7. The changes of international society have significantly influenced the nature of the governing legal order, which has evolved from relatively simple mechanisms for law-making to the highly complex contemporary arrangements. The will and consent of States[11] has come to be supplemented by a different view of the sources of international law,[12] including in particular the utilization of soft-law

9. L. B. Sohn: "The role of international law in the 21st century", Address at the Vrije Universiteit, Brussels, 23 March 1990, pp. 5-6.

10. Rostow, loc. cit. note 6, p. 3.

11. O. Schachter: *International Law in Theory and Practice* (1991), p. 10.

12. M. Bos: "Recognized manifestations of international law, A new theory of 'sources", *German Yearbook of International Law* (1977) p. 9; E. Jimenez de Aréchaga: "International Law in the Past Third of a Century", 159 RdC (1978-I),

instruments, a broader role for customary international law and a greater reliance on the general principles of international law and considerations of justice and equity.[13] While these developments have not altered the universal reach and nature of international law, nor its important differences with domestic law,[14] they have in fact searched for alternatives beyond the traditional consensus of States so as to ensure a timely and expeditious international legislation. This effort, however, has a limit in that it cannot substitute for the will of States and its expression in treaties and other legal acts. It follows that the progress of international law will in essence depend heavily on co-operation between States and their acceptance of the rules. In fact it is quite likely that this role of the State will be strengthened and not weakened.

8. The active participation of a limited number of States in the process of international law-making and the marginal intervention of others has to an extent eroded the assumptions of sovereign equality of the Grotian order,[15] while the emergence of non-State entities and individuals as actors in the making of the law has not only changed the characteristics of international negotiations but also the inputs into the formation of customary law.[16] However, here again the need for establishing a limit has become clear and the claim for sovereign equality is regaining strength, particularly in respect of dispute settlement. Because of the continuing need to address new subjects and issues under international law and solve new problems, the interaction between international and domestic law has significantly increased, just as the borderline between public and private inter-

12. (...continued)
pp. 11-34.

13. C. M. Chinkin: "The challenge of soft law: development and change in international law", 38 ICLQ (1989), pp. 850-866; G. Palmer: "New ways to make international environmental law", 86 AJIL (1992), pp. 259-283.

14. P. Weil: *Le droit international en quête de son identité*, 237 RdC (1992-VI), pp. 33, 87-88.

15. Brown Weiss, loc. cit. note 8, pp. 63-66; L. B. Sohn: "The shaping of international Law", 8 *Georgia Journal of International and Comparative Law* (1978), p. 3.

16. Brown Weiss, loc. cit. note 8, pp. 67-69.

national law is progressively fading. New approaches to compliance, the intertemporal dimensions of the law, inter-generational equity and accountability have also emerged in conjunction with this changing structure of international law.[17]

9. Precisely because international society is moving towards decentralization, a significant proliferation of law-making bodies is noticeable today both at the United Nations and the regional level. The vast activity emerging from these bodies has led to two additional difficulties in respect of the characteristics of present international law: the congestion of the international legal order by the existence of too many rules that do not always manifest a coherent approach, and the fragmentation of the law in a broad piece-meal structure that is not conducive to its orderly development.[18] A renewed emphasis on the role of the principles of international law has been a recent reaction related to this explosion of the international legal order, since such basic principles keep the structure together, allow for a relatively uniform interpretation of the law and, above all, ensure the universality of the legal system.

## I.3 Implications for dispute settlement mechanisms

10. The changes that are taking place in international society and international law have of course major implications in respect of the nature of dispute settlement mechanisms and their role in such a system.[19] This all the more so given the fact that judicial organs in domestic legal systems have many times preceded legislative organs,

17. Ibid., pp. 69-79.

18. Ibid., pp. 80-81.

19. H. Miall: *The Peacemakers. Peaceful Settlement of Disputes since 1945* (1992); C. Peck: *The United Nations as a Dispute Settlement System. Improving mechanisms for the prevention and resolution of conflict* (1996).

a situation still more evident in the case of international law.[20] It is therefore not to be expected that dispute settlement will be necessarily perfected as a result of the progress of international law, but rather to the contrary it is likely that on many occasions the perfecting of international law will follow the effectiveness of dispute settlement arrangements.

11. Because States held a major central role in the Euro-centric model and international institutions were limited, it was believed that an adequate dispute-settlement mechanism would require a strong degree of centralization. The comparison with domestic courts inevitably followed, particularly in terms of their prospective role, compulsory jurisdiction and forceful compliance, as well as in terms of the subordination of political power to courts in the model of liberal democracies.[21]

12. That approach, however, would not always harmonize with the features of a decentralized international system and would many times provide misleading terms of comparison. This is perhaps one of the most valuable lessons learnt from the experience of dispute settlement throughout the 20th century. The challenge lying ahead is to design a dispute settlement mechanism that will respond to the needs and realities of the evolving international society and its legal structure, including its trends towards a greater decentralization. At the same time, such mechanism has the duty to ensure that international law does not become an element of political power and manipulation and that its essential legal character remains within the strict bounds of a legal process.

13. In order to meet these new challenges and respect the necessary diversity, the new legal structure should ensure a broad freedom to opt for different dispute settlement methods and provide an ample

20. I. F. I. Shihata: *The power of the International Court to determine its own jurisdiction* (1962), p. 1.

21. D. S. Sullivan: "Effective International Dispute Settlement Mechanisms and the Necessary Condition of Liberal Democracy", 81 *Georgetown Law Journal* (1993) pp. 2370-2371.

choice of such methods.[22] In this context various aspects may be envisaged: the facilitation of dispute settlement through alternative options so as to avoid the complexities of judicial procedures;[23] the creation of mechanisms appropriate for the resolution of the more complex disputes involving non-State actors;[24] a new role for the ICJ, additional to its dispute settlement functions, to consist in handling the principles of international law as the guiding element of the legal order - in the order of a constitutional function;[25] arrangements for resolving institutional disputes involving political elements; and creating the necessary interlinkages between a variety of judicial and other mechanisms. All these aspects are dictated by the increasingly decentralized nature of international society and the broadening role of dispute settlement in it. These and other thoughts will be explored throughout this report.

## II. A century of efforts to ensure the peaceful settlement of international disputes

### II.1 Developing the available options

14. The first general multilateral agreement to provide its adherents with a range of dispute-settlement methods was the Convention for the Pacific Settlement of International Disputes, concluded at The Hague on 29 July 1899. It offers to "Signatory Powers" and, under prescribed conditions, to "non-Signatory Powers" facilities and services enabling them "[i]n case of serious disagreement or conflict"

22. UK Government comments on the Preliminary Report, Jan. 1999, para. 3.

23. P. H. Sand: "Transnational Environmental Disputes", in Daniel Bardonnet (ed.): *Le Règlement Pacifique des Différends Internationaux en Europe: Perspectives d'Avenir*, Colloque de l' Académie de Droit International (1991), p. 127.

24. T. Kamenov: "Bilateral Investment Agreements", in Bardonnet, op. cit. note 23, p. 121; Miall, op. cit. note 19, p. 185.

25. J. G. Merrills: *International Dispute Settlement*, 1991 (hereinafter: Merrills), p. 238.

to have recourse to the (1) *good offices* or (2) *mediation* of "one or more friendly Powers" in "differences of an international nature ... arising from a difference of opinion on points of fact"; (3) to institute an *International Commission of Inquiry*; and (4) in "questions of a legal nature, and especially in the interpretation or application of International Conventions", and indeed, any "international differences which it has not been possible to settle by diplomacy", to have recourse to *arbitration*. Although each of these four methods contemplates settlement through the involvement of third parties, the Convention implicitly, through references to preliminary efforts at settlement "by means of diplomacy", recognizes (5) *negotiation* as a fifth distinct method, and one *not* involving third-party intervention.

15. The Hague Convention of 1907, which revised the 1899 Convention, *inter alia* by expanding its provisions on International Commissions of Inquiry and Arbitration, and replacing the Convention of 1899 as between the parties to both Conventions, added no new method of settlement. The Covenant of the League of Nations introduced (6) *judicial settlement*, while (7) *conciliation* was first encouraged in a resolution of the Council of the League of Nations in 1922, and later provided for in the bilateral treaties (Locarno, 1925) concluded thereafter, and in the Geneva General Act of 1928, revised in 1949. The UN Charter added resort to (8) *regional agencies or arrangements* and (9) *other peaceful means of their own choice*, recounting the now familiar menu of methods when stating in Article 33 the general obligation undertaken by all Member States to settle their disputes amicably:

> 1. The parties to any dispute, the continuance of which is likely to endanger the maintenance of international peace and security, shall, first of all, seek a solution by negotiation, enquiry, mediation, conciliation, arbitration, judicial settlement, resort to regional agencies or arrangements, or other peaceful means of their own choice. .....

The Charter also provides elsewhere for (10) its own comprehensive dispute settlement system utilizing the Security Council, General Assembly, Secretariat and the ICJ.[26]

16. Resort to regional agencies or arrangements, to the political organs of the UN, or to the organs of other institutions can hardly be qualified as "methods" of settling disputes, but should rather be distinguished as "systems" or "arrangements" for that purpose. The consequence of resort to such systems or arrangements would be either (a) the application within the system or arrangement of one or more of the seven methods previously listed, or (b) submission of the dispute directly to an organ within the system that is itself competent to decide the dispute by reference to legal, political, technical or other considerations.

17. Methods of settlement are sometimes distinguished by reference to whether or not the disputants have accorded a role in the dispute to "third parties", or, in the words of the Hague Conventions, to "Powers strangers to the dispute". Negotiation would seem to stand alone in not requiring third-party assistance, although it could, and often does, benefit from such assistance, e.g. when a third State or a private individual brings together disputing States which have no mutual diplomatic relations, or when the disputants meet under the auspices of an international organization of which they are members. In general, however, a negotiation would take place directly between disputants, each of which would retain complete control over the process: the manner and level at which it takes place, its duration, regularity and outcome. By contrast, all the other methods listed above require the involvement of third parties. Settlement methods are also categorized by reference to the degree to which a third party is authorized to direct the settlement process and influence the outcome. Thus, good offices, inquiry, mediation and conciliation (sometimes characterized as "diplomatic" methods) call for varying degrees of third-party direction, ranging from merely bringing the

26. See generally, UN *Handbook on the Peaceful Settlement of Disputes between States* (1992) (hereinafter: UN Handbook); Merrills.

disputants together and organizing their interaction, to acting as an intermediary throughout the ensuing process; to determining or elucidating the facts in dispute, and reporting on them as an aid to arriving at a settlement; to taking the initiative to propose elements of a settlement to the disputants, and finally reporting to them on what elements would, in the opinion of the third party, be the basis of a fair and reasonable settlement. Whether the latter is called upon to engage in the full range of such activities or limit itself to some of them, would depend on the terms of reference agreed by the disputants. To label a method "good offices", "inquiry", or otherwise on the basis of objective criteria may present difficulty because of the flexible nature of the underlying concepts.

18. The disputants must agree on aspects of the appointment of the "third party", i.e. the constitution of the body to be charged with directing the process, and on the manner in which the process is to be conducted. The latter may be specified by the disputants in agreed terms of reference, or left to the discretion of the assisting third party. The settlement process may be relatively informal, provided always that the disputants are assured of equal treatment, including equal opportunities to present their views; or it may be governed by a set of rules (such as the model rules developed under the auspices of the United Nations, and by some dispute settlement institutions aimed at guaranteeing such treatment) which the disputants have agreed to apply.

19. When arbitration or judicial settlement (sometimes characterized as "legal" or "judicial" methods) is agreed to by the disputants, the third party - an arbitral tribunal, or a permanently constituted court - receives from them the broadest possible authority, *not merely to assist or direct the settlement process*, but also to *determine the outcome*. The proceedings are adversarial and characterized by a high degree of formality. Moreover, in the words of the Hague Conventions: "Recourse to arbitration implies an engagement to submit in good faith to the Award". An arbitral award is, by definition, binding on the disputants, and, subject to agreed procedures of judicial supervision or appeal, an arbitral award would be final.

However, the tribunal that rendered an award may be given the supplementary competence to correct or interpret it, or to make an additional award on some issue within its jurisdiction that has inadvertently been left unresolved. There may also be circumstances in which an award may be challenged as being null and void. Such rules apply with equal force to the judgements of international courts, which are similarly binding on the disputants, subject to the exercise of supplementary competences such as those granted to arbitral tribunals. The judgements of the ICJ are declared to be final and without appeal.

### II.2 **Methods of settlement**

#### (a) *Negotiation*[27]

20. Negotiation and its variants, sometimes distinguished as "consultation" or "exchange of views", are the methods most frequently used by States in attempting to settle disputes. Although often commenced voluntarily, at the initiative of a disputant, negotiation may also be obligatory, where it is commenced in implementation of a system of dispute settlement to which the disputants are committed,[28] or in implementation of the order of a court[29] or the decision or recommendation of some other body on which the disputants have by agreement conferred a measure of authority.[30] Negotiation presents no threatening aspect. It requires no involvement of a third party and

27. See generally, UN Handbook, pp. 9-24; Merrills, Chapter 1.

28. E.g., the 1959 Antarctic Treaty, Art. VIII (2); the 1975 Vienna Convention on the Representation of States in their Relations with International Organizations of a Universal character, Art. 84 (time bound); the 1978 Vienna Convention on Succession of States in respect of Treaties, Art. 41 (time bound); the 1979 Agreement governing the Activities of States on the Moon and Other Celestial bodies, Art. 15 (2); and the 1982 UN Convention on the Law of the Sea, Art. 283 (1).

29. Fisheries Jurisdiction Cases, ICJ Reports 1974, p. 32; Gabcikovo-Nagymaros Project case, ICJ Reports 1997.

30. E.g., the UN General Assembly, when acting pursuant to Arts. 10-14 of the Charter; and the Security Council when acting pursuant to Arts. 36-38, Art. 25 and Chapter VII of the Charter.

implies virtually no restriction on sovereignty. It offers the freedom to present and emphasize any element considered relevant by either disputant; allows confidentiality and cordial relations between the disputants to be maintained;[31] involves little extra expenditure, and is of proven efficiency,[32] since it is the means by which most inter-State disputes are resolved. That negotiation is in progress is not a bar to resort to some other method of settlement, and unless the contrary is specified by agreement, negotiation may continue in parallel with any other method.[33] When the negotiation is successful in settling the dispute, the former disputants may conclude an agreement embodying the terms of settlement. When the negotiation fails[34] and no settlement is reached, the disputants may resort to another method of settlement voluntarily, or in implementation of a prior treaty commitment,[35] the order of a court, or decision or recommendation of some other body on which the disputants have conferred a measure of authority. The confidentiality and privacy of the process create the conditions for preserving their mutual relations unimpaired. The salient trends of contemporary practice in respect of this and other methods will be examined in Section III below.

31. Free Zones of Upper Savoy and the District of Gex, P.C.I.J. Ser. A, No. 22 (1929), p. 13; North Sea Continental Shelf Case, ICJ Reports 1969, p. 48.

32. 1982 Manila Declaration on the Peaceful Settlement of International Disputes, Part I (10); Part II (3)(d).

33. United States Diplomatic and Consular Staff in Tehran, ICJ Reports 1980, p. 3, 24; Aegean Sea Continental Shelf Case, ICJ Reports 1978, p. 12; Military and Paramilitary Activities in and Against Nicaragua, ICJ Reports 1986.

34. Mavromattis Case, P.C.I.J., Ser. A, No. 2, p. 13; South West Africa Cases (Prelim. Obj.), ICJ Reports 1962, p. 346; Manila Declaration, Part I, par. 7.

35. For arrangements to resort to consultation see, e.g.: 1975 Convention on the Representation of States in Their Relations with International Organizations of a Universal Character, Arts. 84, 85; to resort to the ICJ failing agreement on another method of settlement: 1947 Convention on the Privileges and Immunities of the Specialized Agencies of the UN, Sec. 32; for exchanges of views, any method agreed by the disputants, conciliation, arbitration, judicial settlement (International Tribunal for the Law of the Sea, ICJ): UN Convention on the Law of the Sea (UNCLOS) Arts. 280, 283, 284, 286, 287.

(b) *Good offices, Mediation, Inquiry and Conciliation*

21. Unlike negotiation, these settlement methods require assistance or direction by a trusted third party. They may be commenced at the invitation or with the consent of the disputants, and cannot be imposed on them. However, the disputants may engage in them in implementation of a treaty obligation or of an order of a court, or the decision or recommendation of some other body on whom the disputants have, by agreement, conferred a measure of authority. Although differing from each other in form, the range of functions which these "diplomatic" methods require of a mutually agreed third party (one or more State representatives, international organization or official, one or more eminent private individuals), have much in common: investigating and clarifying the facts in dispute, ascertaining the limits of a disputant's position, making proposals to them that appear to the third party to represent a fair settlement of the dispute, and, if a settlement is achieved, helping to organize and oversee its implementation. The actual range of functions conferred on the third party would be determined by the disputants, possibly in consultation with the chosen third party. As with negotiation, the confidentiality and privacy inherent in these methods create the conditions for preserving the mutual relations of the disputants unimpaired.

22. While all third party-assisted and -directed methods require that the disputants be treated on the basis of equality and be allowed equal opportunities to state their case, good offices and mediation are generally conducted with a minimum of the formalities generally associated with maintenance of strict equality. Their aims and techniques are so similar that it is often difficult (and, from a practical standpoint, unnecessary) to distinguish between them. Both are directed at reducing tensions, opening or maintaining channels of communication between the disputants, giving them advice and helping them to understand each other's point of view, suggesting ways in which views could be reconciled and, in general, preventing aggravation of the dispute, while encouraging the disputants toward the goal of agreement on a negotiated compromise.

23. *Good offices and mediation.* Next to negotiation, good offices[36] and mediation[37] appear to be the most widely used third party-assisted methods of resolving disputes, or, if the processes are commenced early enough, *preventing* disputes from occurring. As with negotiation, these methods involve no restriction on sovereignty or freedom of action by either side and do not require the disputants to accept a decision or recommendation by the third party. All facts and contentions, whether legal or political, may be presented and will be faithfully conveyed between them. Although the expenses of a mediator or person using good offices must be met by the disputants,

36. Good offices is dealt with together with mediation in Arts. 2-8 of the Hague Conventions of 1899 and 1907. Although no separate mention is made of good offices in Art. 33 of the UN Charter, it is referred to in the 1982 Manila Declaration (Part I, par. 5) and in the 1988 Declaration on the Prevention and Removal of Disputes and Situations which may Threaten International Security and on the Role of the United Nations in this Field (par. 12). The 1948 American Treaty on Pacific Settlement (Pact of Bogota) provides for, and distinguishes the two methods (Chapter II). The UN Secretary-General has been called upon to "lend his good offices" in resolving numerous international disputes, including those in Indonesia, Palestine, Tunisia, Cyprus, Kampuchea, Central America and Afghanistan. His good offices have also been used in connection with questions relating to East Timor, the Falkland Islands (Malvinas), Western Sahara, the Comorian Island of Mayotte, Namibia, and the continental shelf between Libya and Malta. See generally, UN Handbook, pp. 33-40; Merrills, Chapter 2.

37. Mediation is dealt with together with good offices in Arts. 2-8 of the Hague Conventions of 1899 and 1907, and is mentioned in Art. 33 of the UN Charter, in the Pact of the League of Arab States, the OAS Charter, the 1948 American Treaty on Pacific Settlement, the 1964 OAU Protocol of the Commission of Mediation, Conciliation and Arbitration, and the 1959 Antarctic Treaty; as well as in the 1970 Declaration on Principles of International Law concerning Friendly Relations and Co-operation among States in accordance with the Charter of the United Nations, the Final Act of the 1975 Conference on Security and Co-operation in Europe, and the 1982 Manila Declaration. Mediation has been undertaken by the UN Secretary-General on several occasions on the instructions of the Security Council, e.g. during the Falklands (Malvinas) war; by State representatives, e.g. the Soviet Foreign Minister in the dispute between India and Pakistan over Kashmir (1965), by Algerian representatives during the Iran-Iraq war (1975), and again in 1980 during the critical situation between the US and Iran over the taking of hostages; by intergovernmental organizations, e.g. the World Bank in 1960, in the Indus Basin dispute between India and Pakistan; by NGOs, or humanitarian mediation on numerous occasions by the ICRC; and by individuals, e.g. Alexander Haig between Argentina and the UK during the Falklands (Malvinas) war. See generally, UN Handbook, pp. 40-45; Merrills, Chapter 2.

this would seem to involve them in only minimal extra expenditure. When the functions are performed by an international organization of which the disputants are members, or by its representatives, all or a substantial portion of these costs would be absorbed by the organization and thus borne by the membership as a whole. With a view to minimizing the significance of cost in considering whether to resort to a method of settlement available under the auspices of the Permanent Court of Arbitration (PCA), its Administrative Council decided in October 1994 to establish a Financial Assistance Fund with approved Terms of Reference and Guidelines for its operation. The Fund, to which contributions are made on a voluntary basis, provides financial assistance to qualifying States to enable them to meet, in whole or in part, the costs involved in international arbitration or other means of dispute settlement offered by the Hague Conventions.[38]

24. As with direct negotiations, which may proceed while other settlement methods are being tried, it would seem that good offices and mediation may also continue while the disputants engage in some other third party-assisted or -directed procedure.

25. *Inquiry and conciliation.* Inquiry and conciliation, two other methods of dispute settlement requiring the assistance and direction by trusted third parties, may be commenced only at the invitation or with the consent of the disputants, and cannot be imposed on them. However, as with good offices and mediation, the disputants may be obligated to engage in them in implementation of a treaty commitment, a court order, or the decision or recommendation of some other body on which the disputants have, by agreement, conferred a measure of authority. These are also "diplomatic" methods. In form, they are "inquisitorial" rather than "adversarial" and they conclude with written reports containing conclusions as to the facts, and recommendations concerning a fair resolution of the dispute, and not decisions that are binding and enforceable. However, they are

38. For information on the operation of the Fund, see 94th *Annual Report of the Permanent Court of Arbitration* (1996), paras. 2-4, 53 and Annex 10.

generally conducted by a "Commission", in accordance with agreed rules, so that they are clearly more formal than the processes of good offices and mediation.

26. *Inquiry.* While Title III of the Hague Convention of 1899 provided for "International Commissions on Inquiry", Part III of the Hague Convention of 1907 contains greatly expanded provisions on the subject, rivalling in detail those dealing with arbitration. Thus, the 1907 Convention provides for the constitution of a Commission of Inquiry and the filling of vacancies, in terms virtually identical with its provisions on arbitral tribunals. It makes provision also for venue, languages of proceedings, representation and assistance of parties, on-site investigation, compelling of witnesses and their examination, recording of evidence, privacy of deliberations and decisions, authentication of the Report of the Commission, and its presentation "*at a public sitting* ". Article 35 of the Convention provides that:

> The Report of the commission is limited to a statement of facts, and has in no way the character of an Award. It leaves to the parties entire freedom as to the effect to be given to the statement.

27. On the other hand, the "Optional Rules for Fact-finding Commissions of Inquiry" drawn up by the International Bureau of the PCA in 1996 cover similar ground, but state categorically that "[t]he report of the Commission is not binding on the parties, unless the parties have agreed",[39] adding that "[u]nless the parties decide to make it public, *the report shall remain confidential.*"[40]

39. Art. 14 (2). The disputants may agree to recognize the Report as binding. See the Ruling Pertaining to the Differences between France and New Zealand Arising from the Rainbow Warrior Affair, 71 ILR (1986), p. 256.

40. Art. 15. Similarly, Art. 10 provides: "Unless the parties agree otherwise, or unless disclosure is required by the law applicable to a party, the members of the Commission and the parties shall keep confidential all matters relating to the fact-finding proceedings, including the investigations, hearings, deliberations and findings of the Commission. Unless the parties agree otherwise, the Commission shall meet in camera." See generally, UN Handbook, pp. 24-33; Merrills, Chapter 3.

28. Inquiry, as a procedure for investigating the facts of a dispute, has been provided for in bilateral treaties, as well as multilateral treaties such as the Covenant of the League of Nations,[41] the UN Charter, and the constituent instruments of some international organizations.[42] Of the virtues of the process, the League of Nations Committee of Experts for the Codification of International Law wrote:

> In most cases the enquiry may be expected to end the dispute without creating any abiding bitterness between the two States concerned. Neither party has reason to regard itself as victor or vanquished; neither has had to bow to the peremptory dictates of a judicial sentence. The Commission merely submits its report and the parties concerned are free to draw their conclusions therefrom and to order their actions accordingly.[43]

29. This feature has been repeatedly endorsed by the General Assembly, at least since 1963, and most recently in 1991.[44] The Convention on the Law of the Non-navigational Uses of International Watercourses, adopted by the General Assembly on the basis of a draft elaborated by the International Law Commission (ILC) and opened for signature on 21 May 1997, provides in Article 33 that if a dispute remains unsettled six months after a request has been made for negotiations, it may, at the request of any disputant, be submitted

41. Arts. 12 (1) and 15 ("enquiry" by the Council or the Assembly of the League).

42. Constitution of the ILO, Art. 26; 1982 UNCLOS, Annex VIII, Art. 3. See also 1977 Additional Protocol I to the 1949 Geneva Convention relating to the Victims of International Armed Conflict.

43. Report of the Sub-Committee (Guerrero, Rapporteur, Wang Chung Hui) on "State Responsibility for damage done in their territories to the person or property of foreigners", reprinted in 20 AJIL (1926); Supplement (Special Number) p. 199.

44. Res. 1967 (XVIII) of 16 December 1963; Res. 2329 (XXII) of 18 December 1967 (Register of experts: most recent update 18 December 1970, doc. A/8108); Declaration on the Prevention and Removal of Disputes and Situations which may Threaten International Peace and Security and on the Role of the United Nations in this Field, Res. 43/51 of 5 December 1988, annex; Declaration on Fact-finding by the United Nations in the Field of the Maintenance of International Peace and Security, Res. 46/59 of 9 December 1991, annex; and see the studies by the UN Secretary-General in 1964 (doc. A/5694) and 1966 (doc. A/6228).

to "impartial fact-finding" by a Commission constituted as specified in that Article. Reference of the dispute to the ICJ or to arbitration is mentioned as possible methods of settlement.

30. Four cases in which commissions of inquiry were established pursuant to the Hague Conventions, have been documented and are frequently cited as models of this method of settlement.[45] The UN Secretary-General has sent out missions to investigate situations at the request of disputing parties[46] and more often on the instructions of the Security Council.[47] Its character as a "diplomatic" method of settlement not requiring the disputants to accept the outcome (Report) has made it the subject of frequent favourable consideration by States, although its application in practice (except in the context of the United Nations) remains relatively rare. As presently conceived, the organization and operation of this method of settlement would appear to be more "invasive" than those earlier considered, besides being potentially more costly if initiated by the disputants alone and without international institutional support.

31. *Conciliation.* Neither Hague Convention made provision for a procedure called "conciliation". However, some distinguished internationalists after World War I conceived "inquiry" as a "method of conciliation".[48] The distinction may have derived from the emphasis imparted by each term: "inquiry" emphasized the investigative aspect of the process ("elucidating the facts by means of an impartial and

45. Incident of the North Sea Dogger Bank (Great Britain and Russia, 1904-5); the Tavignano case (France and Italy, 1912); the Tubantia case (Germany and the Netherlands, 1921-2); the Red Crusader case (Denmark and Great Britain, 1961-2). See International Bureau of the PCA, 96th *Annual Report to the Administrative Council* (1996), Annex 3.

46. e.g. Iran and Iraq, 21 July 1988.

47. e.g. Security Council res. 384 (1975) on the situation in Timor.

48. "We should not forget the immense service which was rendered to the cause of peace by this method of conciliation in the Dogger Bank affair between Russia and Great Britain..." (emphasis added). Report of the Sub-Committee cit. note 43.

conscientious investigation"),[49] while "conciliation" emphasized facilitating the reconciliation of the disputants' positions that could follow that process. It was perhaps the apprehension that statements of facts, however "impartial and conscientious", might not be value-free, that led to a shift in emphasis to reconciling opposing views, and the establishment of "conciliation" as a distinct procedure that has maintained a certain acceptability over the decades.

32. It was not until 1937 that the Administrative Council of the PCA authorized the International Bureau to place its offices and organization at the disposal of "Conciliation Commissions". Conciliation was, however, provided for in the Locarno treaties (1925) and the Geneva General Act 1928/49. It was also the subject of a recommendation addressed to States by the *Institut de Droit International*, with annexed to it a set of Regulations on the Procedure of International Conciliation.[50] Since World War I, conciliation has been provided for in a large number of global and regional treaties, as *one of a number of methods* from which disputants might choose; as the *only method* for resolving disputes; as a *preliminary means of achieving settlement*, coupled with the obligation to proceed to arbitration or judicial settlement if the conciliation effort were to fail, and as *the residual method* of settlement when other methods have not been agreed, or have failed. On the basis of this endorsement we may conclude that the majority of States would be willing to accept an obligation to submit prospective disputes to conciliation, in preference to any method from which a binding award or judgement would result, possibly even in preference to its "next of kin" so to speak, "inquiry".[51] Conciliation is listed in Article 33 of the UN

49. Hague Convention of 1907, Art. 9. See generally, UN Handbook, pp. 45-55; Merrills, Chapter 4.

50. 49 *Annuaire* (1961-II) pp. 385-91.

51. Global (since 1949): 1969 Vienna Convention on the Law of Treaties; 1969 International Convention relating to Intervention on the High Seas in Cases of Oil Pollution Casualties; 1975 Vienna Convention on the Representation of States in their Relations with International Organizations of a Universal Character; 1978 Vienna Convention on Succession of States in respect of Treaties; 1982 UNCLOS; 1983 Vienna Convention
(continued...)

Charter; it has been endorsed early by the UN General Assembly,[52] which has recommended later the use of the conciliation rules of the UN Commission on International Trade Law, and, at its Fiftieth Anniversary Session in 1995, adopted Resolution 50/50 with, annexed to it, the United Nations Model Rules for the Conciliation of Disputes between States. The International Bureau of the PCA has prepared its own Optional Conciliation Rules (1996), as have other dispute settlement institutions.

33. Conciliation appears to combine in a felicitous manner most of the attributes sought by most States when choosing a method of settlement they could engage in with confidence. The outcome places no limits on a State's freedom of action; it is free to present any and all elements it considers relevant; orderly presentation of evidence and witnesses is assured by the Commission by application of agreed rules. Any agreement reached is the surest guarantee of the effectiveness of the process, and confidentiality and privacy contribute to the maintaining of friendly relations. Cost might be a negative factor, unless the process takes place within an international organization. An eminent scholar and internationalist outlines some of those attributes as follows:

51. (...continued)
on Succession of States in respect of State Property, Archives and Debts; 1985 Vienna Convention for the Protection of the Ozone Layer; 1986 Vienna Convention on the Law of Treaties between States and International Organizations or between International Organizations. Regional: 1948 American Treaty of Pacific Settlement; 1957 European Convention for the Peaceful Settlement of Disputes; 1964 Protocol to the OAU Charter on the Commission of Mediation, Conciliation and Arbitration (amended 1970); 1976 Treaty of Amity and Co-operation in Southeast Asia; 1981 Treaty establishing the Organization of Eastern Caribbean States; 1994 OSCE Convention on Conciliation and Arbitration. Conciliation is the method provided for more often than any other in the overwhelming majority of treaties listed in successive surveys of dispute settlement arrangements carried out by the League of Nations (1927) and the United Nations (1949, 1966).

52. In 1949 the General Assembly established a panel of experts from which disputants might select, in implementation of their commitment under Art. 33 of the Charter, members of commissions of inquiry and conciliation. The facility has not been used. In 1949 it established a Conciliation Commission for Palestine, and in 1960-61 a Conciliation Commission for Congo.

> What [international] society most needs now, it is said, is peace and stability; it is more important to obtain a friendly settlement than a just settlement which might leave hard feelings. Conciliation, it is said, on the one hand, gives a safeguard for national sovereignty, and on the other hand builds up the desire for pacific settlement; when this desire is sufficiently established, it will be time enough to impose justice upon unwilling states. ..... It is to be recalled, too, that arbitration results in a decree and that the decree is binding judicially, while conciliation merely recommends, leaving the state free to accept or reject the recommendation as it pleases, or as it feels the pressure of public opinion. Conciliation therefore harmonizes better, it is said, with a society based upon voluntary co-operation. It permits a state to concede its whole position, for the sake of peace, but without surrendering its principle. Since the conciliation commission is not limited to law, it has a wider range within which to find a solution. ..... On the whole, the argument of those who prefer conciliation asserts that an amiable solution is to be preferred to litigation, and that peace weighs more than justice.[53]

34. The UN General Assembly, in the preamble to its 1995 Resolution containing Model Rules for the Conciliation of Disputes between States, notes that numerous bilateral and multilateral treaties for the settlement of disputes provide for conciliation, and observes that the method has "proved its usefulness in practice". It further observes that the Model Rules incorporate the results of experience in international conciliation as well as "a number of innovations which can with advantage be made in the traditional practice". Conciliation was originally conceived as an entirely voluntary method of settlement, so that its commencement and continued operation were dependent on the consent of the disputants. The reference in the Resolution to "innovations" may include those procedural rules which are intended to foster the use of conciliation as the sole or residual method of settlement, e.g. the rules that would make the process sustainable in the absence of co-operation by one of the disputants, and thus make it more attractive as a method of last resort. Such provisions include those designed to resolve constitutional problems, such as designation of an "appointing authority" who would nominate a member of the Conciliation Com-

53. C. Eagleton: *International Government* (1957) p. 226.

mission if a disputant failed to do so within a specified period. Provisions of this kind were included in Article 66 of the 1969 Vienna Convention on the Law of Treaties and in paragraphs 1 and 2 of the Annex to that Convention which deals with settlement of disputes by compulsory conciliation upon the unilateral application of a disputant. Procedures for compulsory conciliation were further refined in section 2 of Annex V to the 1982 UNCLOS, which provides, in addition, for continuance of conciliation proceedings despite "failure of a party or parties to the dispute to reply to notification of institution of proceedings or to submit to such proceedings".

35. However, despite such innovations, the outcome of conciliation proceedings as conceived under the Model Rules remains essentially "traditional" and does not limit the freedom of action (sovereignty) of the disputants: the Commission's report does no more than record any agreements reached and, failing agreement, the Commission's conclusions on all questions of fact or law relevant to the matter in dispute, as well as any recommendations it may deem appropriate for an amicable solution. An earlier convention, while reaffirming the non-binding nature of a commission's recommendations, expressly contemplates that the disputants could accept them as binding.[54] In another innovative provision, the 1985 Vienna Convention for the Protection of the Ozone Layer requires the Conciliation Commission to "render a *final and recommendatory award* ",[55] a phrase which, if interpreted in a traditional manner, would appear to be self-contradictory. While both "recommendation" and "award" may be "final", an "award" by definition is binding on the parties, while a "recommendation" is not. The provision goes on to require the parties to do no more than consider the "recommendatory award" in good faith.

36. As with Commissions of Inquiry, the proceedings of Conciliation Commissions as well as their concluding reports and recommen-

54. 1975 Vienna Convention on the Representation of States in their Relations with International Organizations of a Universal Character, Art. 85 (7).

55. Art. 11 of the Convention.

dations are, in principle, confidential and may not be made available to the public except with the consent of the disputants.[56] Article 28 of the UN Model Rules provides the following:

> 1. Except as the parties may otherwise agree, neither party shall be entitled in any other proceedings, whether in a court of law or before arbitrators or before any other body, entity or person, to invoke any views expressed or statements, admissions or proposals made by the other party in the conciliation proceedings, but not accepted, or the report of the commission, the recommendations submitted by the commission or any proposal made by the commission, unless agreed to by both parties.
> 2. Acceptance by a party of recommendations submitted by the commission in no way implies any admission by it of the considerations of law or of fact which may have inspired the recommendations.

Article 16 of the PCA Optional Conciliation Rules provides, in addition, that:

> The parties undertake not to initiate, during the conciliation proceedings, any arbitral or judicial proceedings in respect of a dispute that is the subject of the conciliation proceedings, except that a party may initiate arbitral or judicial proceedings where, in its opinion, such proceedings are necessary for preserving its rights.

37. Although conciliation has been provided for in a wide variety of treaties for more than 70 years, and was the method broadly acceptable to opposing sides even during the Cold War, its use to resolve individual disputes has not been frequent (some 20 times) and has

56. Art. 14 of the PCA Optional Rules requires the Conciliator and the parties to "keep confidential all matters relating to the conciliation proceedings" unless the parties agree otherwise, "or the disclosure is required in connection with judicial proceedings" which are necessary for preserving a party's rights (as contemplated under Art. 16), and extends confidentiality to the settlement agreement "except where its disclosure is necessary for purposes of implementation and enforcement". By Art. 19 of the Rules, the Conciliator and the parties undertake that, unless the parties agree otherwise, the Conciliator will not act as an arbitrator or as a representative or counsel of a party in any arbitral or judicial proceedings in respect of the dispute that is the subject of the conciliation proceedings, nor will the parties present the Conciliator as a witness in any such proceedings.

not always been successful. Yet, as one authority observes, "conciliation offers a procedure adaptable to a variety of needs and demonstrates the advantage to be derived from the structured involvement of outsiders in the settlement of international disputes.".[57]

38. The dispute-settlement system of the World Trade Organization (WTO), as the most recently established, calls for special mention as it provides for models that are both new and different from those described above. It provides for submission of a dispute to negotiation, consultation, good offices and mediation at the option of the disputants and, if no settlement is reached, for referral of the dispute to a Panel appointed for the purpose by the Dispute Settlement Body (DSB). The Panel's "rulings and recommendations" may be adopted by the DSB, enabling pressure for implementation to build among the membership. The DSB is empowered to supervise implementation, and when appropriate, may authorize categories of action in retaliation for non-compliance. Arbitration is maintained as a possible alternative within the dispute-settlement system. Many features of the WTO system are instructive, including the manner in which the membership's opinion may be mobilized to secure compliance with Panel "rulings and recommendations", expeditious treatment of disputes by the application of time limits, and the special consideration accorded to developing countries in meeting the demands of the system. Some other trends arising from the WTO procedures will be discussed further below. These developments have been properly characterized as a new kind of quasi-judicial settlement, where diplomatic means interact with panel proceedings that have a close relationship with arbitration.

### (c) *Arbitration and judicial settlement*

39. Arbitration and judicial settlement are frequently classified together as "judicial" methods of settlement, as contrasted with the

57. Merrills, pp. 76-79.

"diplomatic" methods dealt with above since, by definition, they require termination of the dispute by a decision (judgement, award) that is binding upon the parties and enforceable in accordance with its terms. Arbitration as a method of dispute settlement between States is concisely described in Article 37 of the Hague Convention of 1907:

> International arbitration has for its object the settlement of disputes between States by judges of their own choice and on the basis of respect for law.
> Recourse to arbitration implies an engagement to submit in good faith to the Award.

40. However, the requirement that there must be privity of contract between the disputants in order to give an arbitral tribunal jurisdiction over a dispute may now be in the process of modification. Thus, while the Washington Convention on the Settlement of Investment Disputes (establishing ICSID) in Article 25 gives its tribunals jurisdiction over a legal dispute "which the parties to the dispute [i. e. an investor and a host State] consent in writing to submit to the Centre", tribunals in two cases[58] found that a promise by a host government to refer disputes to ICSID arbitration contained in a bilateral agreement between it and the investor's government was sufficient to give the tribunal jurisdiction over a dispute between the corporate investor and the host government. These interpretations of the "consent" requirement in the Washington Convention may have encouraged a trend toward securing greater protection for the foreign investor under dispute settlement systems which provide for what has been called "arbitration without privity",[59] reflected in some

58. *Asian Agricultural Products Ltd.* v. *Republic of Sri Lanka*, ICSID Case No. ARB/87/3 (1990); *Southern Pacific Properties (Middle East) Ltd.* v. *Arab Republic of Egypt*, ICSID Case No. ARB/84/3 (1992).

59. J. Paulsson: "Arbitration without privity", 10 *ICSID Review Foreign Investment Law Journal* (1995), pp. 232 et seq.; B. Stern: "Some reflections on ICSID", paper presented at the Kuwait International Commercial Arbitration Conference, 1997; T. Wälde: "Investment Arbitration under the Energy Charter Treaty-from Dispute Settlement to Treaty Implementation", 12 *Arbitration International* (1996), pp. 429 *et seq.*

multilateral agreements: the *North American Free Trade Agreement* (NAFTA) 1992, and the *Energy Charter Treaty* (1994).

41. As one commentator[60] observes:

> Through this new type of investment convention, whether bilateral, regional or multilateral, we enter the era of arbitration without contractual relationship between the parties to the dispute - or arbitration without privity. It is nothing short of a revolution of the classic arbitration theory, which postulates that arbitration is the product of a contract: either an arbitration clause for future disputes or an arbitration agreement for existing disputes. The classic theory also postulates the equal situation of both contracting parties: each of them can initiate arbitration proceedings, and each of them, if a defendant, can counterclaim. Under the new generation of investment conventions, it is not so: only the aggrieved investor can bring a claim, and whether the defending State can bring a counterclaim is unclear.

42. One of the most attractive features of international arbitration has been the obligation undertaken by the disputants to submit to and implement the award duly rendered by the arbitral tribunal that was composed in accordance with their agreement, and which they recognize as bringing the dispute to an end. This is of particular importance in international commercial arbitration, where the finality of the award may be seen as an investor's ultimate assurance that a dispute will remain insulated from the uncertainties connected with submission to a host State's legal and judicial system. Thus, recent, international effort has sought to secure enactment of national legislation facilitating enforcement of awards through domestic courts, narrowly defining the grounds on which international awards might be challenged, while the 1958 New York Convention on the Recognition and Enforcement of Foreign Arbitral Awards provides treaty support in the same direction. The now widely accepted and emulated 1976 UNCITRAL Arbitration Rules makes express

60. J. Werner: "The Trade Explosion and Some Likely Effects on International Arbitration", 14 *Journal of International Arbitration* (1997), p. 6.

provision only for "interpretation"[61] of an award, the correction of clerical and arithmetical errors, and for the rendering of an "additional award" intended to deal with claims presented to the tribunal but not covered in its award. While the Rules provide in some detail for the challenge of arbitrators, they make no express provision for the challenge of an award or for its annulment.

43. Omission of express provision for challenge of an award reflects a relatively recent trend. Thus, the 1899 and 1907 Hague Conventions make provision for a disputant's "right to demand the revision of the Award"; the ILC 1958 Model Rules on Arbitral Procedure provide for challenges to the validity of an award, and its annulment; and the 1965 ICSID Convention offers procedures for "revision" and "annulment" of an award. The International Bureau of the PCA, when developing in the period 1992-1996 a series of Optional Rules for the arbitration of different types of dispute, chose to follow UNCITRAL's lead in omitting express provisions on revision and annulment, despite support for such provisions among some of those participating in the preparatory work.[62]

44. However, the trend away from express provision for challenge to an arbitral award may itself be coming under scrutiny, as considerations of stability of international decisions continue to be weighed against notions of fairness. It seems reasonable that a challenge to the validity of an award by an international tribunal should not be directed to domestic courts, particularly where public law questions must be determined and such a course may present the prospect of divergent decisions, but rather toward an independent and impartial international body. Recent proposals by eminent authority may foreshadow future institutionalized international review of arbitral

61. R. D. A. Knutson: "The Interpretation of Arbitral Awards: When is a Final Award not Final?", 11 *Journal of International Arbitration* (1994), pp. 99-109.

62. Final Report and Recommendations to the Administrative Council by the 1999 Steering Committee, PCA *97th Annual Report*, 1997, at 89.

awards: proposals for an International Arbitral Court of Appeal,[63] and for an International Court of Arbitral Awards.[64] Judge HOLTZMANN's proposal, endorsed by Judge SCHWEBEL, President of the ICJ, is

> "to create a new international court that would take the place of municipal courts in resolving disputes concerning the enforceability of international commercial arbitration awards".[65] Under the treaty establishing the Court, applications to set aside or enforce awards would be within the sole jurisdiction of the new international court.[66]

45. Arbitration may, in principle, be engaged in only on the basis of an agreement between the disputants. Such agreement may take the form of a prior general undertaking to submit disputes to arbitration, or concluded *ad hoc* in order to resolve a dispute that has arisen. The agreement would cover all aspects of the arbitration including the choice, appointment and challenge of arbitrators or judges, the procedure to be followed, and the applicable law. The tribunal would generally be invested with the power to determine its own competence, and to fill lacunae in the agreed procedures. Up to the moment the agreement is concluded, these matters would be within the joint control of the disputants.

46. As with all other dispute-settlement methods open to States that are "sovereign" and "equal", judicial settlement may be engaged in only on the basis of prior agreement between the disputants. In contrast to arbitration, "judicial settlement" implies reference to a pre-constituted court, the composition and operation of which would

63. See generally M. Rubino-Sammartano: *International Arbitration Law* (1990).

64. H. Holzmann: "A Task for the 21st Century: Creating a New International Court for Resolving Disputes on the Enforceability of Arbitral Awards", in M. Hunter et al.: *The Internationalization of International Arbitration* (The LCIA Centenary Conference) (1995) pp. 109-114; S. M. Schwebel: "The Creation and Operation of an International Court of Arbitral Awards", ibid., pp. 115-123.

65. Holtzmann, loc. cit. note 64, p. 112.

66. For a critique of this proposal see G. M. B. Hartwell: Statement made at the *Seventh Geneva Global Arbitration Forum*, 2 December 1998.

generally be beyond the control of the disputants. Since the end of World War I and the entry into force of the Protocol to the Covenant of the League of Nations which established the Permanent Court of International Justice, that Court, and its successor, the ICJ, have represented the archetype of courts to which States may refer their disputes for judicial settlement. Thus, in contrast to the method of arbitration, disputants have no choice in the matter of the judges[67] who would hear and determine their case, nor as to the procedures which would apply.[68]

47. While the classic statement of the object of arbitration is "settlement of disputes ... on the basis of respect for law", the function of the Court is "to decide [disputes] in accordance with international law".[69] This has been seen by several commentators as an additional basis for distinguishing the two procedures. Thus, it has been remarked that "the arbitrator desires to settle the dispute to satisfy the parties through a decision which will ensure peace. He decides the matter not according to law, but disposes of it *ex aequo et bono* ".[70] OPPENHEIM, then Whewell Professor of International Law at Cambridge, himself confirms that:

> ..... an arbitral tribunal is not a court in the real sense of the word, for its decisions are not necessarily based on rules of law, and it does not necessarily deal with legal matters. An arbiter, *unless the terms of*

67. Two provisions of the Statute of the ICJ do introduce some element of choice: Art. 31 on the appointment of judges ad-hoc, and Art. 26 on the formation of a chamber of the Court "for dealing with a particular case". While the number of judges to constitute such a chamber will be "determined by the Court", it will do so "with the approval of the parties". See also Rules of the ICJ (14 April 1978), Arts. 7-8 (judges ad-hoc) and 17 (formation of a Chamber to deal with a particular case). Commentators have noted a possible similarity between provision for the formation of a chamber to hear a particular case, and the selection of the members of an arbitral tribunal from a list of potential arbitrators as provided under the Hague Convention of 1907.

68. Procedures applicable in cases before the Court are specified in the Statute and in the Rules of the Court.

69. Art. 37 of the 1907 Hague Convention, Art. 38 (1) of the ICJ Statute.

70. H. Wehberg: *The Problem of an International Court of Justice* (1918) p. 14, quoting Pohl.

*reference otherwise provide* [emphasis added], decides *ex aequo et bono*, whilst a judge founds his decision on rules of law and is only applied to on legal issues ... The experience which we have so far had of arbitral tribunals shows that they make praiseworthy efforts to arrive at a finding which shall as far as possible satisfy both parties, and that they have in view a compromise rather than a genuine declaration of law.[71]

48. Interestingly, another authority, himself soon to be Whewell Professor, disagreed. LAUTERPACHT, who believed that international arbitration fulfils "the same function as normal judicial settlement within the state" and that "the true nature of international arbitration" was indistinguishable from that of judicial settlement, was critical of:

the tendency to provide for recourse to arbitral tribunals on the vague but persistent assumption that arbitral tribunals, although bound to apply law, need not somehow apply strict law; that their function lies midway between the application of law and adjudication *ex aequo et bono*; and that, therefore, the reference to these of disputes other than those concerning respective rights introduces the possibility of the law being changed in accordance with justice and political requirements.[72]

49. *Arbitration.* Although this difference of view continues,[73] initiatives within international dispute-settlement institutions have sought to recreate arbitration in the image of judicial settlement, substituting what some characterized as a flexible process (implying that there could be an appeal to the autonomy of the will of the parties at

71. L. Oppenheim: *The Future of International Law* (1921) p. 46.

72. H. Lauterpacht: *The Function of Law in the International Community* (1933) p. 379. See also M. Masahiro: "Recent trends in the jurisprudence of the Interrnational Court of Justice and international arbitral tribunals, with special reference to territorial and boundary cases, 6 *Asian Yearbook of International Law* (1996) pp. 3-27.

73. Representative of the Netherlands, quoted in 5 Yb ILC (II), 1953, p. 235. Julius Stone expressed a similar opinion: "The features of arbitration law which offer so many avenues of escape and which serve in the Commission's eyes as excuses for 'shirking' international undertakings may be the very features which attract States to enter into social undertakings", *Legal Controls of International Conflict* (1954) p. 736. See also C. Pinto: "Structure, process, outcome: thoughts on the 'essence' of international arbitration", in *Leiden Journal of International Law*, Special Issue, 1993, pp. 241-264; and H. Holtzmann, op. cit. note 64, pp. 265-277. See generally UN Handbook, pp. 55-65; Merrills, Chapter 5.

all stages of the process prior to issue of the award, thus leaving it vulnerable to interruption) with what one Government representative described as "setting up some water-tight rules rendering impossible any future attempt at evasion by a state which once accepted binding arbitration". Commenting on the ILC Model Arbitration Rules, the same representative said:

> However praiseworthy this ambition is, yet some doubt may arise whether in this way arbitration will not be divested of one of its specific characteristics and whether this may not entail the impossibility for arbitration to maintain itself beside international judicature. In other words: may not arbitration lose its attractiveness for the states?[74]

50. Those initiatives have resulted in several sets of arbitration rules,[75] all directed at safeguarding the "integrity" of the process, a term which contemplates continuity of the arbitration in good order in accordance with the original undertakings of the disputants objectively interpreted. Such rules relate to the filling of initial or casual vacancies in a tribunal by an appointing authority pursuant to agreed procedures,[76] and remedies for other consequences of the failure of one of the disputants to co-operate, as in the case of the "truncated tribunal",[77] or default of appearance by a party.[78]

74. H. Fox: "Arbitration", in *International disputes: the legal aspects*, Report of a Study Group of the David Davies Memorial Institute of International Studies, p. 102.

75. See, e.g., the Model Arbitration Rules drafted by the ILC (1957); the Arbitration Rules of UNCITRAL (1979), and the modified version thereof adopted and applied effectively by the Iran-United States Claims Tribunal (1983); the Optional Arbitration Rules of the PCA (1992, 1993) and the 1998 Arbitration Rules of the International Chamber of Commerce.

76. This is the case, for example, under the UNCITRAL Arbitration Rules, Arts. 6-13.

77. See UNCITRAL Arbitration Rules, Art. 32, par. 4; UNCLOS Annex VII, Art. 8: "The absence or abstention of less than half of the members shall not constitute a bar to the tribunal reaching a decision". See S. M. Schwebel: *International Arbitration: Three Salient Problems* (1987).

78. See UNCITRAL Arbitration Rules, Art. 28, par. 2; UNCLOS Annex VII, Art. 9.

51. Several treaties, bilateral and multilateral, provide for recourse to arbitration in the event of a dispute as *one of a number of methods* from which disputants might choose, as an *alternative* to recourse to the ICJ, as the *sole method* of settlement, or as the *residual method* if other settlement efforts fail. However, it seems that the number of inter-State agreements providing for recourse to arbitration concluded, say, each decade since the beginning of the 19th century, having reached a kind of apogee in the decade 1891-1900 in which some 74 arbitration agreements were recorded, has since declined steadily to less than 10 in the decade 1981-90, without prejudice to the fact that a number of inter-state agreements provide for the arbitration of future disputes. It appears that the overwhelming majority of arbitration agreements were concluded between the countries of Western Europe and America.[79]

52. The PCA records nine arbitrations that have taken place under its auspices since 1945, five of them since 1994; there is also an increase in the number of arbitrations between State and non-states parties, six of which have been administered by the International Bureau of the PCA in the last decade. This wider scope of the PCA's involvement in arbitration and its role as designator of appointing authorities under the 1976 UNCITRAL Arbitration Rules, indicate a promising development in the PCA's activities.[80] The recent conclusion of the Eritrea/Yemen arbitration is a further evidence of this trend.[81] Other arbitrations after World War II include those by the Arbitral Tribunal for the Agreement on German External Debts and by the Arbitral Commission on Property Rights and Interests in Germany; the *Palena* case (Argentina/Chile Frontier case, 1966); the *Lac Lannoux* case (France/Spain, 1957); the *Rann of Kutch* case (India/Pakistan, 1968); the *Delimitation of the Continental Shelf* case

79. See the comprehensive work by A. M. Stuyt: *Survey of International Arbitration* (1990); C. Gray and B. Kingsbury: "Developments in dispute settlement: inter-State arbitration since 1945", BYIL (1992) pp. 97-134. See also Pinto, loc. cit. note 73.

80. 96th Annual Report of the PCA (1996) p. 33. See also the Initial Comments of ITS International Bureau on the Preliminary version of this Report, June 1998, p. 1.

81. See the Eritrea/Yemen (Territorial Sovereignty and Scope of the Dispute) Award of 9 October 1998.

(UK/France, 1977); the *Beagle Channel* (Argentina/Chile, 1977); the *Sharjah/Dubai boundary* case (1981); the *Maritime Delimitation* case (Guinea/Guinea-Bissau, 1985); the *La Bretagne* case (Canada/France, 1986); the *Taba* case (Egypt/Israel, 1988); the *St. Pierre and Miquelon* case (Canada/France, 1992); and the cases decided and to be decided by the Iran-United States Claims Tribunal (established 1981, and continuing).

53. In general, arbitration leading to a final and binding award has been the method of choice for resolving disputes in which legal or technical elements predominate, when the disputants' legal cultures and technical resources are comparable, and when the disputants themselves are of roughly equivalent political and economic influence. In such cases, the outcome is likely to be implemented, even if disagreed with by the "losing" party, and if resentment were to threaten a harmonious relationship, this would not be the case for long. The method may not have the same efficacy when a substantial asymmetry exists between the disputants. In that case, all the concerns outlined below that give rise to different approaches to "binding" methods of settlement may be expected to result either in failure of the disputants to agree upon arbitration as the method of settlement, or in substantial difficulties being encountered in the successful conduct of the arbitration. The situation obviously will be different when arbitration is available as an option or as a residual method in the context of highly institutionalized dispute settlement arrangements, as is the case, for example, of UNCLOS.

54. If asymmetric disputants were to agree to engage in arbitration, their agreement to apply one or another of the recently developed model arbitration rules would go far toward ensuring the orderly and proper conduct of the process. This would still leave possible problems associated with execution of the Tribunal's award, currently moderated through international agreement[82] and implementing national legislation. The ideal would be for the disputants to

82. See, e.g., the 1958 New York Convention on the Recognition and Enforcement of Foreign Arbitral Awards.

conduct the arbitration within an organizational framework in which the award would be self-executing, or themselves to agree at the outset upon a method that would achieve that result. One such method agreed and successfully operated relatively recently, is the so-called Security Account established by and with the consent of the Iranian Government, out of which awards rendered against Iran by the Iran-United States Claims Tribunal are paid merely upon furnishing proof of their authenticity to the Account Holder, the Central Bank of Algeria. It is not clear why the Algiers Accords provided for establishment of a Security Account for payment of awards against Iran, but made no corresponding provision that would ensure payment of awards rendered against the United States. However, the reason for this additional guarantee of payment of awards by Iran may have been that most of the claims before the Tribunal had been brought against that country by private parties (natural or legal persons) whose guarantees of payment through attachments of Iranian property in claims before US Courts had been nullified by President Carter as part of the arrangement for resolving the crisis in relations between Iran and the United States, which included the transference of those claims to the Tribunal for arbitration. The amount of the Security Account (initially US$ 1 bn., to be regularly replenished at the level of 500 mn.) may indicate its association essentially with the private claims, since intergovernmental claims could be for substantially larger sums.

55. While the device of automatic payment out of the Security Account has accomplished its purpose, it is doubtful whether the circumstance of its negotiation could ever be replicated, or whether it would be possible to establish such a Security Account along the same lines to guarantee payment of government claims which could be larger by several orders of magnitude.

56. The costs of arbitration could also be a factor deterring recourse to this method of settlement. In addition to the fees of counsel, advocates and technical advisers, the hire of premises and staff, including, where necessary, translators and interpreters, could be considerable, depending on the venue and duration of proceedings. In

this connection the Fund established by the PCA, from which a substantial part of such expenditures might be reimbursed to qualifying States, could greatly facilitate recourse to arbitration under the auspices of that body.[83] The PCA has also been concerned about the cost and length of arbitrations, emphasizing strict limits for the exchange of memorials and other steps and suggesting that instead of hourly fees the parties could agree in fixing beforehand the total amount of fees to be paid.[84]

57. *Judicial settlement.* The ICJ is one of the "principal organs" of the United Nations. The Statute of the Court, to which all UN Members are *ipso facto* parties, declares that the Court is the "principal judicial organ" of the United Nations. As stated in Article 34, paragraph 1, of the Statute: "Only States may be parties in cases before the Court." And all States, whether Members of the UN or not, may have access to the Court. Its jurisdiction, which is stated to comprise not only "all matters specially provided for in the Charter ... or in treaties or conventions in force" but also "all cases which the parties refer to it", is, in principle, unlimited *ratione materiae* . While disputes as to its jurisdiction may arise for one reason or another, the Court is itself empowered to settle the matter by decision.

58. The ICJ is available as a court of first and last instance; its judgement is binding on the parties to the dispute and is "final and without appeal". In the performance of its functions, it is governed by its Statute, by the Rules of the Court (1978), and by the Resolution concerning its internal judicial practice it adopted in 1976 pursuant to Article 19 of its Rules. All of these provisions are published and apply without a need for further acceptance by potential litigants submitting to the Court's jurisdiction. A range of incidental competences enable the Court to indicate provisional measures, to decide prelimi-

83. See note 38. See also: Report of a meeting (London, 31 Jan.-1 Feb. 1997) on "Funding of and Access to International Courts and Dispute Settlement Bodies", organized jointly by the Program on International Law and Sustainable Development of the Foundation for International Environmental Law and Development (FIELD) and the Center on International Co-operation, New York University.

84. Initial comments cit. note 80, p. 4.

nary objections, to decide counter-claims, to permit third parties to intervene in proceedings, to act as a court of reference in specified circumstances, and to interpret or revise its judgements. Equipped with this comprehensive range of competences, composed of 15 independent, highly qualified jurists of the highest moral character, and so organized as to "remain permanently in session", the ICJ is conceived as empowered to deal with any and all inter-State disputes brought before it, either by way of a judgement or, when requested to do so, by issue of an advisory opinion.

59. An analysis of the jurisprudence of the Court and of its predecessor, the Permanent Court of International Justice, indicates that many of the cases referred to them involved questions of interpretation or application of treaties, or related to specific legal problems, including (a) sovereignty over certain territories, and frontier disputes; (b) maritime delimitation and other law of the sea disputes; (c) the diplomatic protection of nationals abroad; (d) circumstances arising from the use of force, and (e) enforcement of contracts and violation of certain principles of customary law.[85]

60. The ICJ is the pinnacle of the dispute-settlement mechanisms discussed, as was the Permanent Court of International Justice before it. As a permanent body of experts chosen in accordance with rigorous standards and maintained by the United Nations as a whole, the Court offers several advantages over *ad hoc* arbitration: it can act with a minimum of delay in dealing with urgent matters, including requests for interim measures of protection; its administrative costs are charged to the budget of the United Nations, thus reducing the financial burden on litigants; and it may rely on a Registry and administrative facilities that could rarely be matched by those of *ad hoc* arbitration. From the overall standpoint of development of international law, the Court's permanence and the prestige of its members are the surest guarantee of validity and consistency in the interpretation and application of international law, both customary and

85. See UN Handbook, pp.68-69, for a comprehensive list of cases in these categories.

conventional, thus fostering integrative tendencies throughout a diverse "population" of States.

61. The cost involved in engaging experienced counsel, producing witnesses and experts, preparing written pleadings and other steps required in an action before the Court could, however, be a factor of considerable weight to many States. Taking into account the United Nations special role in the maintenance of international peace and security, as well as Charter provisions (e.g. Article 36, paragraph 3) and General Assembly resolutions encouraging States to refer legal disputes to the Court, the Secretary-General on 1 November 1989 announced the establishment of a Trust Fund financed through voluntary contributions, to assist States in the settlement of disputes through recourse to the Court. The purpose of the Fund is to provide financial assistance to enable qualifying States to meet certain expenses incurred in connection with (i) disputes submitted to the Court by way of special agreement, or (ii) the execution of a judgement of the Court resulting from such special agreement.[86] Consideration should be given to broadening the financial base of the Fund, through contributions from States as well as other entities. The establishment of funds similar to those of the ICJ and the PCA should be considered in relation to other permanent courts and tribunals, such as the International Tribunal for the Law of the Sea.

62. The Security Council, in the exercise of its primary responsibility for the maintenance of international peace and security, has established three organs which carry out judicial functions, one dealing with claims against an invading State and the compensation due in respect of them; and two dealing with international crimes and punishment of those who are individually responsible for these crimes.

86. For the text of the Trust Fund Rules and Terms of Reference see 28 ILM (1989) p. 1589. The Trust Fund has been used in the cases of Burkina Faso/Mali, Chad/Libya, and Senegal/Guinea-Bissau, and it has been suggested to increase the size of the Fund and the amount of the assistance awarded; see Comments by Roy S. Lee on the Preliminary Report, 30 November 1998, pp. 2-3.

63. The first of these organs relates to Resolution 687 of 3 April 1991 which reaffirmed Iraq's liability under international law for loss, damage, injury and other consequences resulting from the unlawful invasion and occupation of Kuwait. By Resolution 692 of 20 May 1991 the Security Council established a UN Compensation Fund to provide compensation for qualifying losses and to meet the expenses of the UN Compensation Commission; the latter functions at the level of a Governing Council and of expert Commissioners assisted by a Secretariat. As described by the Secretary-General, "...the Commission is not a court or an arbitral tribunal before which parties appear; it is a political organ that performs an essentially fact-finding function of examining claims, verifying their validity, evaluating losses, assessing payments and resolving disputed claims. It is only in this last respect that a quasi-judicial function may be involved".[87] In practice, however, while the Governing Council, composed of States representatives, performs a political role in guiding the process, the Panels, composed of independent Commissioners from the legal community, perform an eminently legal work close to a judicial function. It would appear that claimants before the Commission are not precluded from asserting their claims in other fora.

64. The work of the Compensation Commission is making a major contribution to the development of innovative methodologies for dealing in an efficient and fair manner with a multitude of cases ranging from claims for relatively small amounts (US $ 2,500-100,000) which are submitted by governments after consolidation, to claims for very large sums (e.g. for environmental damage) which are dealt with individually.

65. The Security Council by Resolution 827 of 25 May 1993 established an International Tribunal for the sole purpose of prosecuting persons responsible for serious violations of international humanitarian law committed in the territory of the former Yugoslavia

87. Report of the SG pursuant to para. 19 of SC Res. 687 (1991), UN Doc. S/22559, 2 May 1991.

(ICTY), and adopted the Statute of the Tribunal attached to the Resolution. ICTY held its inaugural session on 17 November 1993, adopted Rules of Procedure and Evidence which entered into force on 14 March 1994, and has since indicted and tried several persons within its jurisdiction. By Resolution 955 of 8 November 1994 the Security Council established a similar International Tribunal for the prosecution of persons responsible for genocide and other serious violations of international humanitarian law committed in the territory of Rwanda (ICTR), and Rwandan citizens responsible for such offences in neighbouring States between 1 January and 31 December 1994. Although the Security Council thus chose to establish a separate tribunal for Rwandan cases, it decided that ICTR's co-existence with the Yugoslav Tribunal "dictated a similar legal approach", as well as "certain organizational and institutional links", so as to ensure "a unity of legal approach, as well as economy and efficiency of resources".[88] Thus, members of the Appeals Chamber of ICTY also serve as members of the Appeals Chamber for ICTR, and a single Prosecutor serves both Tribunals, assisted by separate staffs. It should be noted that ICTR's jurisdiction is somewhat wider than that of ICTY and includes violation of Article 3 common to the 1949 Geneva Conventions and the 1977 Additional Protocol II (protection of victims of non-international armed conflict).[89] Although not engaged in resolving disputes between States, both Tribunals are judicial organs of the United Nations which, through administering justice by punishing those guilty of the criminal offences within its jurisdiction, contribute to the avoidance of conflict and the maintenance of international peace and security.

66. The work of both Tribunals has shown that the investigation and prosecution of individuals accused of serious violations of international humanitarian law is feasible. Although some accused occupying very high political positions remain at large, a significant number of suspects have been taken into custody and await trial. Both Tribunals have contributed to an extent that would have been

88. Report of the UN Secretary-General, UN Doc. S/1995/134, para. 7.

89. Art. 4 of the Statute of ICTR.

difficult to contemplate a decade ago, to the creation of an impressive body of international humanitarian law, for example, clarifying and expounding the nature of "crimes against humanity", and establishing that individuals may be tried, convicted and held into account, whether such conduct is connected with international armed conflict, with internal conflict, or not connected with any conflict at all.[90] No less has been their contribution to the development of the procedures to be followed and the rules of evidence applicable in international criminal cases, drawing on both common law and civil law traditions.

67. The General Assembly, at its 47th Session in 1992, requested the International Law Commission to undertake the elaboration of a draft Statute for an international criminal court as a matter of priority (Resolution A/47/10). Thus began a process whereby the draft Statute presented by the ILC in 1994 became the subject of consideration and revision by the Assembly's Ad Hoc Committee on the Establishment of an International Criminal Court in 1995 and 1996; and in 1997, by a Preparatory Committee[91] open to participation by all States Members of the UN and its Specialized Agencies and IAEA. The revised Statute was, after further negotiation and revision, adopted by a UN Diplomatic Conference in Rome on 17 July 1998,[92] and has now been signed by more than 70 States.

90. *Tadic case*, Appeal on Jurisdiction, 35 ILM (1996) p. 32.

91. Resolution A/50/639, 5 December 1995.

92. UN Doc. A/CONF.183/9. For the text of the Statute see 37 ILM (1998) p. 999. The Conference *inter alia* called for the establishment of a *Preparatory Commission* for the Court consisting of representatives of States signatories of the Final Act and other States invited to the Rome Conference; and, as observers, representatives of the international organizations which receive standing invitations from the UN General Assembly, of interested regional intergovernmental organizations, of ICTY and ICTR, and, within specified limits, of non-governmental organizations. The mandate of the Preparatory Commission is to prepare proposals for practical arrangements for the establishment and coming into operation of the Court, including, before 30 June 2000, the finalization of the draft texts of the rules of procedure and evidence and of the elements of crimes.

68. The new International Criminal Court, which will be brought into being upon entry into force of the Rome treaty,[93] builds upon the pioneering experience of ICTY and ICTR. Its many innovative features have already been described elsewhere,[94] and discussion and analysis of those features will deservedly continue to attract scholarly attention in the future. Only a few of them will be referred to briefly here.

69. The ICC is to consist of 18 judges elected by States Parties from among their nationals, for a term of nine years, the first election being followed by a drawing of lots to select one-third of their number to serve for periods of 3, 6 and 9 years. In addition to the stipulated criteria relating to professional competence, the electors are required to take into account representation of the principal legal systems of the world and equitable geographical distribution. Unlike the statutes of other international tribunals, the ICC Statute specifies and additional criterion: "fair representation of female and male judges". Re-election of individual judges is not permitted except for those who are elected to serve for 3 years or less in accordance with the provisions of the Statute (Part 4).

70. The jurisdiction of the ICC is limited (Article 5) to "the most serious crimes of concern to the international community as a whole", i.e. (a) the crime of genocide, elaborated in Article 6; (b) crimes against humanity, elaborated in Article 7; (c) war crimes, elaborated in Article 8; and (d) aggression, when that crime is eventually defined in accordance with Articles 121 and 123 of the Statute. Its jurisdiction is not "universal", in the sense that *universal jurisdiction* confers on each State the competence to prosecute

93. The Statute will enter into force on the first day of the month after the 60th day following the date of deposit of the 60th instrument of ratification (Art. 126).

94. See e.g. G. Sluiter: "An International Criminal Court is Hereby Established", 16 *Netherlands Quarterly of Human Rights* (1998) pp. 413-420; B. S. Brown: "Primacy and Complementarity: Reconciling the Jurisdiction of National Courts and International Criminal Tribunals", 23 *Yale Journal of International Law* (1998) pp. 384-436; Papers presented at *Symposium on the International Criminal Court: A Critical Review of the Results of the Rome Conference*, convened in honor of Judge Antonio Cassese, Erasmus University, Rotterdam, 5 November 1998.

persons suspected of crimes under international law, such as piracy. Rather, its jurisdiction with respect to the crimes specified is qualified in a variety of ways, generally reflecting the emphasis placed by all governments on the priority accorded to national jurisdiction and existing treaty obligations.

71. Thus, a precondition is that its jurisdiction has been accepted (Article 12) by (a) the State Party in whose territory the conduct in question occurred; or (b) the State Party of which the accused is a national; or (c) in the case of exercise of jurisdiction in relation to a State which is not a party to the Statute, that this State has lodged a declaration with the Registrar accepting jurisdiction with respect to the crime in question.

72. An important feature is that its jurisdiction is to be "complementary" to national criminal jurisdiction (Preamble and Article 1). Unlike ICTY and ICTR, whose jurisdictions are concurrent with those of national courts and are given a certain priority, in that they may request the latter to defer to their competence (Article 9, ICTY), national investigation and prosecution of crimes over which the ICC has jurisdiction is to be the rule. However, the ICC may exercise jurisdiction over such crimes if it determines that a national judicial system is "unwilling or unable" to carry out investigation or prosecution, or has collapsed (Article 17, "Issues of admissibility"). The principle of "complementarity" gains emphasis from the Statute's complex provisions on preliminary rulings regarding admissibility (Article 18) and challenges to the jurisdiction of the Court or the admissibility of a case (Article 19).

73. The ICC may exercise jurisdiction if it is invoked by a State Party's referral of a situation to the Prosecutor pursuant to Article 13 (a); or by the Prosecutor initiating action with respect to a crime under Article 13 (c); or by referral of a situation to the Prosecutor by the Security Council under Article 13 (b). In the case of referrals by the Security Council, it is open to speculation whether the ICC would be able to exercise a range of powers similar to those exercised by the *ad hoc* Tribunals for the former Yugoslavia and Rwanda, and

whether the provisions of Article 103 of the UN Charter would then operate to extend its powers beyond the limits otherwise laid down in its Statute. Article 15 is particularly noteworthy:

> "The Prosecutor may initiate investigations *proprio motu* on the basis of information on crimes within the jurisdiction of the Court".

74. Observing that the Statute's many jurisdictional complexities would not operate in the cases of referrals by the Security Council, one commentator foresees that the business of the ICC might be largely determined by the Security Council's readiness to use the Court when exercising its powers under Chapter VII of the Charter.[95] In that context he notes with concern the negative votes of two permanent members of the Council (China, USA) when the Statute was adopted at Rome.

75. A noteworthy transitional provision permits a State, on becoming a party to the Statute, to exclude by declaration the Court's jurisdiction over war crimes committed by its nationals or on its territory, for seven years from the date the Statute enters into force in respect of that State (Article 124).

76. The International Tribunal for the Law of the Sea, established pursuant to part XV and Annex VI of UNCLOS, is one of four "compulsory procedures entailing binding decisions" among which a party to the Convention is free to choose for the settlement of disputes concerning its interpretation or application. Within the limits specified, the Tribunal has a broad general jurisdiction *ratione materiae* and *ratione personae*, the latter including international organizations and natural and legal persons. However, Part XV, Section 5, of UNCLOS specifies certain "limitations and exceptions" with respect to the application of those procedures. The law to be applied by the Tribunal (or by the ICJ or an arbitral tribunal, if chosen by the parties) in resolving a dispute within its jurisdiction, comprises the "Convention

95. Papers presented by T. Van Boven on "Some remarks on the operation of the International Criminal Court, and procedural aspects" and by A. Bos on "Report" at the Symposium referred to in note 94.

and other rules of international law not incompatible with this Convention". The Tribunal (or any other chosen body) may decide *ex aequo et bono* if the disputants so agree.

77. The Tribunal's 21 judges having been elected at a meeting of States Parties on 1 August 1996, it had by the end of 1997 adopted its Rules of Procedure and constituted, in addition to the Seabed Disputes Chamber required by Section 5 of Part XI, and Section 4 of annex VI to the Convention, and a Chamber of Summary Procedure required by Article 15, paragraph 3 of annex VI to the Convention, two other "standing chambers" pursuant to paragraph 1 of the same Article to deal respectively with fisheries disputes and marine environment disputes.

78. The rule of the exhaustion of local remedies applies to disputes between States Parties "where this is required by international law" (Article 295). Any decision by a court or tribunal having jurisdiction under Section 2 of Part XV of the Convention is stated to be final and binding upon the disputants, and must be complied with by them (Article 296).

79. In the first case to come before the Tribunal, the *M/V/SAIGA*, an oil tanker flying the flag of St. Vincent and the Grenadines, had been arrested by Guinean customs authorities and taken to Conakry, Guinea, where the ship and its crew were detained and a cargo of 5000 tons of gasoil of an estimated value of US$ 1 million off-loaded. St. Vincent and the Grenadines alleged that Guinea, as detaining State, had failed to comply with its obligations under the UN Convention on the Law of the Sea concerning the prompt release of the vessel and its crew. The Tribunal was unanimous in finding that it had jurisdiction. Having determined the admissibility of St. Vincent's application and a number of other issues concerning interpretation of the Convention's provisions on the prompt release of vessels, by a majority of 12 to 9, the Tribunal, having taken into account the value of the gasoil off-loaded, held that upon the posting of a bond for US $ 400,000 Guinea must promptly release the vessel and those members of the crew in detention. The Tribunal dealt with

the case with exemplary speed: proceedings commenced on 13 November 1997 and judgement was delivered on 4 December 1997.

80. Provision for resort to judicial settlement has also been made on a regional basis. Thus, the Court of Justice of the European Union is a court with broad compulsory, and for some cases exclusive, jurisdiction, statutorily required to "ensure that in the interpretation and application of [the EEC/EU Treaty] the law is observed" (Article 164). Other regional courts have been established with specialized jurisdiction: the European Court of Human Rights established by the European Convention on Human Rights (1950) and the Inter-American Court of Human Rights established by the American Convention on Human Rights (1969) have jurisdiction in regard to violation of the provisions of their respective conventions.[96]

## II 3 **Systems of settlement**

### (a) *Resort to regional agencies or arrangements*

81. "Resort to regional agencies or agreements", mentioned in Article 33 of the Charter, is dealt with more extensively in Chapter VIII (Articles 52-54), whereby UN Members entering into such arrangements or constituting such agencies are required to make every effort to achieve pacific settlement of local disputes through such arrangements or agencies before referring them to the Security Council. Although the Charter requires the Security Council to encourage regional dispute settlement by these means, that function is not to impair its right under Article 34 of the Charter to investigate any dispute or situation in order to determine whether its continuance is likely to endanger the maintenance of international peace and security; nor the right of a State under Article 35 of the Charter to

96. For other examples of regional courts and tribunals dealing with disputes in such fields as trade and nuclear energy, see UN Handbook pp. 69-70.

bring any such dispute or situation to the attention of the Security Council or the General Assembly.

82. The term "regional arrangements" in Article 52 is interpreted to mean agreements on dispute settlement which do not create a permanent institution with international legal personality (e.g. the 1957 European Convention for the Peaceful Settlement of Disputes), while the term "regional agencies" refers to permanent regional institutions with international legal personality established by treaty to perform broader functions, including the settlement of disputes, e.g. the League of Arab States,[97] the Organization of American States (OAS),[98] the Organization of African Unity (OAU)[99] and the Associa

97. The League of Arab States is a regional agency, the purpose of which is to strengthen relations and promote co-operation among its member States *inter alia* in economic, social and cultural affairs. It has an important dispute-settlement function as well: under the Pact of the League of Arab States (1945), the League's Council (composed of one representative from each Member State) "shall mediate in all differences which threaten to lead to war between two member States, or a member State and a third State with a view to bringing about their reconciliation". The dispute must be referred to the Council by the disputants, and the Council will then decide the dispute in the absence of the representatives of the disputants, by majority vote. The Council's decision is declared to be "enforceable and obligatory", which suggests that the Council's function is conceived as arbitration rather than conciliation or mediation according to the meanings assigned to those terms above. Excluded from the Council's action, are disputes that "concern a state's independence, sovereignty, or integrity". For examples of dispute settlement by the Arab League see UN Handbook, pp. 92-93.

98. Arts. 23-26 and 82-90 of the Charter of the OAS (1948) deal with settlement of disputes. Art. 23 (as amended in 1985), provides that "All international disputes that may arise between American States shall be submitted to the peaceful procedures set forth in this Charter before being referred to the Security Council of the United Nations". Art. 24 contains a list of settlement methods similar to that of Art. 33 of the UN Charter, while Art. 26, which contemplates a "special treaty" on dispute settlement, was eventually implemented through conclusion of the American Treaty on Pacific Settlement (Pact of Bogotá, 30 April 1948). Arts. 82-90 of the Charter had provided until 1985 a central role for the Inter-American Committee on Peaceful Settlement, consisting of five member States elected by the Council, which upon activation by the Permanent Council could exercise its power to offer good offices, carry out investigation of the facts in dispute, and make recommendations to the disputants. Non-co-operation by a disputant could be reported by the Committee to the Council which could make suggestions for remedying the situation. It should report persistent non-co-operation to the Assembly. This Committee, however, was abolished
(continued...)

tion of South East Asian Nations (ASEAN). [100] Other types of

98. (...continued)
by the 1985 Protocol of Amendments to the OAS Charter, which now confers on the Secretary-General of the OAS powers similar to those of the UN Secretary-General, enabling him to undertake initiatives in the matter of dispute settlement. The Permanent Council and the Secretary-General of the OAS have, through their initiatives, several times brought about amicable settlement of disputes in Latin America. For examples of dispute settlement under the American Treaty on Pacific Settlement, see UN Handbook, pp. 93-94.

99. Article XIX of the Charter of the OAU (1963), records the pledge of the membership to settle all disputes among themselves by peaceful means, and foresees the establishment of a Commission of Mediation, Conciliation and Arbitration by means of a separate Protocol to form an integral part of the Charter. The Protocol, signed at Cairo in 1964, establishes a Commission of 21 members of different nationalities elected by the OAU Assembly of Heads of State and Government, and prescribes general principles and procedures to apply in mediation, conciliation and arbitration. A dispute may be referred to the Commission by the parties jointly who are free to agree on one or more of the three procedures, by unilateral application by a party, by the Council of Ministers or by the Assembly of Heads of State and Government. In order to provide a quicker response to settlement requests, the OAU in 1977 suspended elections to the Commission and established a committee of 9 representatives of States and three others to be appointed by the Chairman. In practice, the OAU has adopted a variety of procedures when undertaking dispute settlement initiatives, acting through its Council of Ministers, the Assembly of Heads of State and Government, special or ad hoc committees, and eminent statesmen. For examples of OAU settlement initiatives, see UN Handbook p. 95.

100. The Treaty of Amity and Co-operation in Southeast Asia (1976) (as amended in 1987) provides for pacific settlement of disputes in Arts. 14-17. To settle disputes through regional processes, the parties to the Treaty constitute, as a continuing body, a High Council comprising a representative at ministerial level from each of them "to take cognizance of the existence of disputes or situations likely to disturb regional peace and harmony." If such a dispute were to arise, and "direct negotiation" does not resolve it, the High Council may, if all the disputants so agree, apply Art. 15 of the Treaty, which empowers the High Council (a) to take cognizance of the dispute or situation and recommend appropriate means of settlement; (b) to offer its good offices; or (c) upon agreement of the disputants, to constitute itself into a committee of mediation, inquiry or conciliation; and (d) to recommend interim measures of protection. The Treaty encourages all the parties to it to "offer all possible assistance" to settle the dispute. These provisions are to apply to States outside South-East Asia which may be parties to the Treaty of Amity, only if they are "directly involved in the dispute to be settled through the regional processes." The Asia-Pacific Economic Co-operation Forum (APEC) has also considered the establishment of a voluntary mediation service to supplement the WTO dispute settlement mechanism; see B. P.
(continued...)

organizations, such as the OSCE,[101] can also qualify as regional arrangements for the purposes of dispute settlement and other functions. The term "regional agencies" may also refer to some institutions (court, tribunal, commission) created by treaty on a regional basis to deal with disputes arising with respect to the subject dealt with in the treaty, e.g. protection of human rights (European and American Courts of Human Rights); or management of shared natural resources (International Commission to Protect the Moselle from Pollution).[102] Most regional agencies and arrangements provide for systems of dispute settlement offering a choice of one or more of the settlement methods listed in Article 33 of the UN Charter.

100. (...continued)
McGivern, 35 ILM (1996) p. 1102.

101. At the Helsinki Summit in July 1992, the OSCE declared itself to be a "regional arrangement" within the meaning of that term in Chapter VIII of the UN Charter. It thus shares with the UN, in the non-enforcement field, responsibility for maintaining peace and security in the region, and is actively involved in dispute prevention, dispute and dispute resolution, besides strengthening the membership's commitment to these processes, and confidence building. At weekly meetings of the OSCE Permanent Council in Vienna, the organization offers a forum for frank dialogue on any political issue. The Chairman (changing annually) takes initiatives for conflict prevention and crisis management. The 1992 Helsinki Summit, recognizing that many disputes in the region had roots in ethnic issues, acknowledged that questions of human rights "are matters of direct and legitimate concern to all participating states, and do not belong exclusively to the internal affairs of the state concerned". A High Commissioner on National Minorities is charged with acting early through quiet diplomacy to relieve ethnic tensions. The OSCE Convention on Conciliation and Arbitration, entered into force on 5 December 1994, establishes a framework for obligatory conciliation leading to non-binding settlement proposals, and a "directed conciliation" procedure when disputants are instructed to engage in conciliation by the OSCE Ministerial Council. Arbitration is based on agreement of the parties, and leads to binding decisions. See W. Höynck: "From CSCE to OSCE", in *Helsinki Monitor* (1995 No. 3) p. 11 et seq; and L. Caflisch: "The OSCE Court of Conciliation and Arbitration: some Facts and Issues", in M. Bothe, N. Ronzitti, and A. Rosas (eds.): *The OSCE in the Maintenance of Peace and Security*, pp. 381-397. For a discussion of the trends arising from these procedures of conciliation and arbitration, see below, Section III.

102. The Commission was established by the 1956 Convention on the Canalization of the Moselle and the 1961 Protocol on Prevention of the Pollution of the. For more examples of regional "arrangements" and regional "agencies" see UN Handbook p. 81 et seq.

83. As a result of a long-standing tradition[103] and on the occasion of the 1999 Centennial Conference, the OAS, at the initiative of the Inter-American Juridical Committee, has begun to consider ideas to perfect its regional mechanisms for the settlement of disputes and their connection with global trends. Among other ideas, the following have been proposed: to enable regional organizations to request advisory opinions from the ICJ; to create a regional Inter-American Court of Justice in the tradition of the old Central American Court of Justice; to attain an hemispheric understanding for the referral of certain kind of disputes to the ICJ; to revise the Pact of Bogotá on the Peaceful Settlement of Disputes; and to strengthen fact-finding dispute settlement arrangements.[104]

84. Other regional discussions held on the occasion of the Centennial Conference have emphasized traditions relating to dispute settlement which are deeply rooted in the multi-cultural background of those regions. At the meeting of the Afro-Asian Legal Consultative Committee held in New Delhi on 11-12 February 1999, for the discussion of the 1999 Preliminary Reports, the principle of non-use of force in international law and relations was specifically linked to the concept of peaceful settlement of disputes, wherein the role of regional organizations should be strengthened, among other means by the establishment of regional courts to supplement the working of the ICJ.[105] The role of negotiations and other methods of dispute avoidance was also emphasized.[106] Also the Asia-Pacific Regional Conference on the 1899 Hague Peace Conference, organized by the University of Melbourne Faculty of Law and held in Melbourne

103. F. Galo Leoro: "Peaceful Settlement of Disputes. An Overview", Inter-American Juridical Committee,OAS Doc. CJI/SO/II/doc. 34/94, rev.1, 13 August 1994.

104. Inter-American Juridical Committee, OAS: "Report to the Co-sponsors of the 1999 Centennial Commemoration", Report on the Peaceful Settlement of Disputes, Doc. OEA/Ser. Q, CJI/doc. 79/98, 27 August 1998, pp. 11-12.

105. AALCC Meeting to consider the Preliminary Reports on the Themes of the First International Peace Conference, New Delhi, 11-12 February 1999, Report of the Rapporteur, S. M. Confiado, on the proceedings of the session on settlement of disputes, para. 5.

106. Ibid., paras. 6-8.

18-20 February 1999, contributed a number of important aspects on the approaches of this broad region to dispute settlement, including the role of peace-making and other preventive methods, the need to pay special attention to internal conflict with international implications as the source of major contemporary disputes, and the importance of considering appropriate dispute settlement procedures for conflicts involving indigenous peoples and natural resources issues.[107] Negotiation and other non-adversarial methods of dispute settlement were identified as more appropriate choices in the light of the traditions of the Asia-Pacific Region.[108]

85. *Relationship of regional arrangements and agencies to the organs of the United Nations.* Where States have entered into regional arrangements or constituted regional agencies, they are required to "make every effort" to have their "local" disputes settled through such arrangements or by such agencies before referring them to the Security Council (Charter, Article 52, paragraph 2), and the Council is required to encourage such practice (paragraph 3). On the other hand, it is the right of every Member of the UN to bring to the attention of the Security Council (or of the General Assembly) any dispute or any situation which might lead to international friction or otherwise give rise to a dispute, and the right of the Security Council to investigate such dispute or situation.

86. To guard against the possibility of unwarranted or premature approaches to the Security Council regarding what may prove to be a dispute or situation better settled at the regional or "local" level, the Security Council will, having inscribed the matter on its agenda, consult with the disputants with a view to ascertaining whether or not the dispute has become sufficiently acute as to endanger international peace and security. If the Council then determines that this is not the

107. Asia-Pacific Regional Conference for the Commemoration of the Centenary of the 1899 Hague Peace Conference and the 50th Anniversary of the 1949 Geneva Conventions, University of Melbourne Faculty of Law, Melbourne, 18-20 February 1999, Summary of the proceedings presented by Professor Gillian Triggs.

108. See, for example, Kening Zhang: "China and Peaceful Settlement of International Disputes", Paper prepared for the Asia-Pacific Regional Conference (see note 107).

case, it may decide to refer the dispute to the regional forum and to await the latter's report, but nevertheless keep the matter on its agenda. Should the dispute later ripen into one that, in its opinion, endangers international peace, or regional efforts to resolve the dispute fail, the Security Council could resume dealing with the dispute at short notice, and without prior discussion of the advisability of including it on the agenda.[109]

87. In practice it is likely that a State will only seek to bring a situation or dispute before the Security Council or the General Assembly *in extremis*, since the grave consequences that could attend the decision to engage in third-party assisted or directed dispute settlement (in particular, a method which would conclude with a binding decision) would *a fortiori* exert powerful negative pressures in this context as well. This would be particularly true where the prospective complainant is relatively small, with a developing economy and militarily weak; and the prospective responding State a large and/or powerful State in the same region and therefore a "neighbour", and one whose continued goodwill would be of incalculable value. If the dispute or situation were to be of any real consequence, it seems highly unlikely that any regional "arrangement" or "agency" could be found to command the confidence of such a complainant, given the respondent's economic and political influence. On the other hand, inviting the attention of a "foreign" player like the Security Council (or the General Assembly) to the dispute, which would inevitably engage inadequately informed media comment and speculation and possibly result in polarization of opinion within the organization, could so incense the respondent as to exacerbate the dispute and lengthen indefinitely the time needed for eventual resumption of mutually gainful economic relations, more likely to be important to the complainant than the respondent.

109. UN Handbook, pp. 96-97.

(b) *Other "peaceful means" of the disputants' choice*

88. Universal multilateral treaties provide for a variety of dispute settlement systems devised by participating States. Such systems (other than those provided for in the UN Charter dealt with in Section V below) seem to fall into two broad categories: (i) treaties which establish permanent inter-governmental institutions (e.g. the World Bank group of organizations and the World Health Organization), and (ii) treaties which do not establish such institutions (e.g. the four 1958 Geneva Conventions on various aspects of the law of the sea and the 1969 Vienna Convention on the Law of Treaties). All of them deal with highly specialized activities, and in most cases establish regimes often of a more or less technical character.

89. *(i) Treaties establishing permanent institutions.* These treaties include the constituent instruments of the specialized agencies of the United Nations. Those dealing with financial matters provide for self-contained dispute settlement procedures. Thus, a dispute arising between members of the organization or between a member and the organization are to be submitted to an organ of restricted membership (e.g. the Executive Directors of the World Bank) for decision. In any case where that organ has given a decision, any member may require that the question be referred to the plenary organ (e.g. the Board of Governors of the Bank) whose decision shall be final. Disputes between the organization and a former member, are to be submitted to arbitration.[110] A member that does not fulfil its obligations under the constituent instrument may be suspended from membership by the plenary organ.[111] In the case of the IMF, a member in breach of its

110. See e.g. the Articles of Agreement of the International Bank for Reconstruction and Development, Art. IX; Art. XVIII of the Articles of Agreement of the International Monetary Fund.

111. Art. VI of the Articles of Agreement of the Bank. Two highly innovative dispute resolution mechanisms have been established by the Bank: ICSID (1966) and the Bank's Inspection Panel (1993). The *Inspection Panel*, an independent forum established by resolution of the Executive Directors on 22 September 1993 (IBRD Resolution No. 93-10; IDA Resolution No. 93-6) consists of three persons nominated by the President of the Bank and appointed by the Bank's Executive Directors, who (continued...)

obligations may be declared ineligible to use the resources of the Fund or may be required to withdraw from the Fund.[112]

90. The constitutions of other international organizations provide for a variety of dispute settlement procedures.[113] In general, if a question or dispute concerning the interpretation or application of the constituent instrument is not settled by negotiation or other "diplomatic" method, or by reference to the plenary organ, it must be submitted to the ICJ unless the disputants agree to another mode of settlement.[114] Such treaties would also generally provide that the organization may, when so authorized by the UN General Assembly, request the Court for an advisory opinion on any legal question arising within the competence of the organization.[115]

111. (...continued)
hold office for a specified term and may not be re-appointed. The procedure which may lead to a Panel investigation commences with receipt of a request from (a) an affected party (which must be a community of persons, not a single individual) in the territory of a borrower, (b) in special cases an Executive Director of the Bank, and (c) at any time, the Bank's Executive Directors acting as a Board. The request must allege that the Bank has failed to comply with its "operational policies and procedures", and before hearing a request the Panel must satisfy itself that the alleged failure to comply has, or threatens to have, a material adverse effect on the rights or interests of an affected party; that the alleged violation is serious, and that the subject-matter of the request has been brought to the attention of the Bank's Management. The Panel is empowered to issue (a) decisions on procedural matters, (b) recommendations to the Bank's Executive Directors, and (c) reports to the Executive Directors setting forth its findings. A Panel's decision, recommendation or report are to be reached by consensus. If consensus cannot be reached the majority and minority views are to be stated. See also Section III below.

112. Art. XV of the Fund Agreement; for other examples, see UN Handbook, pp. 136-140.

113. For numerous examples, see UN Handbook, pp. 143-146.

114. See Art. 75 of the Constitution of the WHO.

115. See Art. 76 of the WHO Constitution; *Advisory Opinion on the Legality of the Use by a State of Nuclear Weapons in Armed Conflict*, ICJ Reports 1996.

91. The constitutions of the ILO and the ICAO provide procedures both for securing compliance with international standards[116] and for resolving disputes[117] among the membership, which allow legal measures and membership-influence roles in achieving those purposes.

92. New agreements concluded to establish and administer complex environmental regimes incorporate collective performance management systems designed to *avoid* the actual occurrence of disputes. Many of the environmental protection agreements share basic characteristics, aimed in particular at attaining universal participation in achieving the object and purpose of such "umbrella" treaties. Their provisions must therefore be able to accommodate the interests of States with widely different levels of capability in the scientific, technological and financial domains, while ensuring at the same time that the commitments undertaken will not lead to denunciation or withdrawal. All participants must be fully convinced that problems of non-compliance will result in severe forms of environmental damage. Normally these agreements provide for an assembly as a deliberative organ and an executive council empowered to adopt rules, standards

116. See ILO Constitution, Arts. 19-25; ICAO Constitution, Arts. 37-42.

117. Under the ILO procedure, if a member "is not satisfied that any other Member is securing the effective observance of any Convention which both have ratified", it may file a complaint with the International Labor Office. The Governing Body may also do so *proprio motu* or on receiving a complaint from a delegate to the Conference. The complaint may be referred to a Commission of Inquiry, which makes a report to the Governing Body, containing recommendations on how to deal with the complaint. If the disputants accept the report, the dispute is resolved on that basis; if the report is not accepted, either government may refer the complaint to the ICJ, whose decision will be final. If any member fails within specified time limits to carry out the recommendations of a Commission of Inquiry or the decision of the Court, the "Governing Body may recommend to the Conference such action as it may deem wise and expedient to secure compliance therewith." (ILO Constitution, Arts. 26-34). The ICAO Council is empowered to decide any dispute between member States relating to the interpretation or application of the ICAO Convention. Either party to a dispute may appeal from the Council's decision to the ICJ or to an ad hoc arbitral tribunal. The decision of the Court or the tribunal is final and binding (ICAO Constitution Arts. 84-88). In 1971, India's appeal to the ICJ from a Council decision in favour of Pakistan, was rejected (Appeal relating to the Jurisdiction of the ICAO Council, ICJ Reports 1972, p. 46 et seq).

and practices leading to the implementation of the objectives pursued. Also organs composed of scientific and technical experts participate in the decision-making arrangements, and a secretariat provides for the necessary legal and administrative services.

93. A complaints procedure established under the 1987 Montreal Protocol on Substances that Deplete the Ozone Layer has provided a pioneering system aimed at the prevention of injury or damage resulting from non-compliance, and avoiding the "disagreement on a matter of fact or law" which is the essence of a dispute. Under such a system, and related models, a complaint about actual or potential default might be initiated by a Member State[118] and will be the subject of deliberation by the political organs of limited or universal membership.[119] The *case-in-context approach* followed by these organs ensures that all circumstances[120] and not only those legally admissible are taken into account, with particular reference to the problems faced in compliance by developing countries or countries in transition and the fulfilment by industrialized countries of their financial and technology transfer commitments. The procedure is essentially

118. It has been noted that under the Basel Convention an alleged treaty violation was brought to the attention of the Secretariat by a non-governmental organization and led to an amicable solution to the problem; I. Rummel-Bulska: "Implementation Control: Non-compliance Procedure and Dispute Settlement: From Montreal to Basel", in *Österreichische aussenpolitische Dokumentation*, Special Issue, in W. Lang (ed.): *The Ozone Treaties and their Influence on the Building of International Environmental Regimes* (1996) p. 51.

119. On reporting and deliberation on non-compliance by a designated organ: Montreal Protocol on Substances that Deplete the Ozone Layer, 1987, Arts. 7, 8, 9 (3), 12 and Annex IV; Basel Convention on the Control of Transboundary Movements of Hazardous Wastes and their Disposal, 1989, Arts. 12, 13, 19; Protocol to the Antarctic Treaty on Environmental Protection, 1991, Art. 13; Framework Convention on Climate Change, 1992, Arts. 7 (2) (i), 10-13; UN Convention on Biological Diversity, 1992, Arts. 23 (4) (a) and (g), 26; Protocol to the Convention on Long-range Transboundary Air Pollution on Further Reduction of Sulphur Emissions, 1994, Arts. 5, 8; Convention to Combat Desertification, 1994, Arts. 26, 27; International Tropical Timber Agreement, 1994, Arts. 30-34.

120. Protocol on Further Reduction of Sulphur Emissions, Art. 7 (2); Montreal Protocol, Art. 5; Framework Convention on Climate Change, Arts. 4 (7)-(10), 7 (2) (b), 13.

consultative, informative (fact-finding and conciliatory) and inquisitorial rather than adversarial, seeking to establish the intention to perform and aimed at determining the capability to do so.[121] To this end, the preservation of harmony is pursued through co-operation among the membership; requires a consensus as to the "appropriate action to be taken", particularly in terms of assisting the party in default in order to enable it to carry out its treaty obligations,[122] and is inspired by the principle of "common but differentiated responsibility". The aggregate of these provisions *mobilizes peer pressure* directed at securing performance of and compliance with the specific treaty commitments.

94. *(ii) Treaties which do not establish permanent institutions.* Universal multilateral treaties not establishing permanent institutions contain a wide variety of dispute settlement provisions. These may be entirely optional, leaving it to a participating State whether or not to accept a procedure contained for example in an optional protocol; or they may provide a system that combines free choice among the seven traditional methods with a residual procedure to be followed in the event that the parties cannot agree on a method, or the method agreed upon by them did not result in settlement. Such residual

121. On the less adversarial nature of non-compliance procedures and their greater use under the Montreal Protocol as compared to dispute resolution procedures, see D. G. Victor: "The Montreal Protocol's Non-compliance Procedure", in Lang, op. cit. note 100, p. 69. See also Abram and A. H. Chayes: *The New Sovereignty: compliance with International Regulatory Agreements* (1995) pp. 25, 110. On the operation of the Implementation Committee of the Montreal Protocol it has been observed that "...the Committee sees its role as helping to avoid disputes, to seek solutions, and to promote focussed discussion about non-compliance rather than as a judicial enforcement system"; Victor, op. cit. p. 67.

122. It has been noted that "With a more constructive approach based on a recognition that non-compliance is frequently the consequence, not of malice or greed, but rather of technical, administrative or economic problems, a regime that worked with, rather than against, Parties in difficulty was sought"; P. Széll: "Implementation Control: Non-compliance Procedure and Dispute Settlement in the Ozone Regime", in Lang, op. cit. note 100, p. 46. See generally M. Koskenniemi: "Breach of treaty or non-compliance? Reflections on the enforcement of the Montreal Protocol", in 3 *Yearbook of International Environmental Law* (1992) pp. 123-162.

procedures may range from negotiation, through compulsory conciliation to arbitration and recourse to the ICJ.[123]

(c) *United Nations system*

95. The UN Charter, offering the most comprehensive integrated system available for the settlement of international disputes, is dealt with in Section V below.

# III. Innovation and privatization in dispute settlement arrangements: expanding the available options and the role of an Alternative Dispute Resolution mechanism

96. The experience gathered along the 20th century shows that States and other entities have a preference for solving their disputes by recourse to negotiations and other non-adversarial methods, while the judicial option is kept many times as an alternative of last resort. This explains the evolution that these other methods have undergone and the many innovations that are still being introduced, a situation likely to gather momentum as the 21st century moves on. This variety of options is also necessary to allow States to exercise their freedom of choice. In addition, as international society is no longer exclusively an inter-State domain and other actors have forcefully come to the fore, international disputes are no longer solely a matter involving States. The various methods available need also to accommodate their use by such new actors. The traditional methods of judicial settlement have in many respects reached their limits in both the domestic and international ambits, requiring supplementary arrangements. Well established alternative dispute-settlement methods have been reshaped to respond to the new challenges in this field, while a

123. For examples of these treaties see UN Handbook, pp. 146-153.

variety of new approaches have also been introduced for this purpose. The salient features of these developments will be examined in this section.

## III.1 Evolving approaches to international dispute settlement

97. *(i) A preventive approach.* A first important characteristic of contemporary approaches to dispute settlement is to aim at prevention rather than resolution of ongoing disputes.[124] The preventive emphasis is found in both political and legal disputes and it reaches both State and non-State actors. The many recent experiences relating to peace-keeping, peace-building and peace-making, together with the intensification of monitoring techniques and other elements associated to these efforts, are important indications of this new emphasis on prevention. The fact that disputes have also evolved from purely inter-State claims to internal strife with international implications, is also pointing to the need to ensure a broader approach to dispute settlement. This approach will become paramount as the 21st century advances, but of course formal dispute settlement will need to be available in case the preventive efforts fail.

98. *(ii) Increasing number of submissions.* As a result of a preventive legal environment, that in addition is likely to reduce the legal risks involved,[125] and of the availability of formal procedures, a significant increase in the number of disputes submitted to prevention and resolution is to be expected. Furthermore, just as the exclusion of disputes affecting "vital interests" was subsumed in the traditional

124. I. F. I. Shihata: "Implementation, enforcement and compliance with international environmental agreements: Practical suggestions in light of the World Bank's experience", 9 *Georgetown International Environmental Law Review* (1996) pp. 37-51.

125. G. W. Coombe: "The Future: Implementing New Approaches to the Settlement of Transnational Commercial Disputes", 17 *Canada-United States Law Journal* (1991) p. 535.

distinction between legal and non-legal disputes,[126] so the theoretical line separating legal from political disputes will continue to fade, if it ever was clear, thereby also increasing the types of disputes to be submitted to such arrangements. This will also result in new pressures on the availability of dispute settlement options.

99. *(iii) Institutionalization and the rule of law.* Two other positive consequences are also to be expected: a greater institutionalization of dispute settlement will continue to gather momentum in order to handle the new functions and volumes involved; and dispute settlement will be increasingly governed by rules of law rather than by considerations of political power as in the past.[127]

100. *(iv) New requirements of market economies.* The 21st century will also witness the consolidation of a process well under way in terms of the transition from command economies to market economies,[128] that having originated in domestic experiences has inspired major changes in the international economy as well. This process is having and will increasingly have a strong influence in the characteristics of dispute settlement. First, individuals, who are the major actors in a market economy, will require direct and expeditious access to the settlement of disputes with other participating entities, whether State or non-State. Second, private property and individual rights are today an essential element of the liberal democratic State,[129] and are also shaping international society, thereby requiring protection in terms of both equality under the law and control of arbitrariness. And third, the rule of law becomes the key factor in ensuring the climate

126. C. Gray and B. Kingsbury: "Developments in Dispute Settlement: Inter-State Arbitration since 1945", BYIL (1992) p. 103.

127. Ibid., p. 103.

128. I. F. I. Shihata: *Complementary Reform* (1997) p. 33.

129. D. S.Sullivan: "Effective International Dispute Settlement Mechanisms and the Necessary Condition of Liberal Democracy", 81 *Georgetown Law Journal* (1993) p. 2373.

of stability and predictability required by the adequate functioning of a market economy.[130]

101. *(v) Privatizing international justice.* The dispute settlement demands of an international society based on market economy and the role of individuals is leading to various innovative arrangements and also to forms of privatization of international justice.[131] This in itself is not an entirely new phenomenon in international society since, as a result of the less structured nature of international law, methods such as inquiry, conciliation, mediation and arbitration have been used in it for long, and particularly since 1899-1907. It is rather the scope of these methods that is changing, together with the introduction of a number of other alternatives. In order to meet these new demands, a creative role is to be expected from dispute-settlement bodies that need to clarify the meaning of rules of international law that are not always precise or specifically binding,[132] a task that will require more stringent standards as to the independence and dedication of dispute settlers and a greater transparency in the procedures followed.

## III.2 Reshaping traditional methods in a new international context

102. *(i) Strengthening consultations.* While at this stage of the development of international law it would appear that negotiations and consultations are an ordinary occurrence in view of their simplicity and, as noted in Section II, because of being the least invasive method of dispute settlement and prevention, this is regrettably not yet the case. In fact, negotiations and consultations are on occasion difficult to engage because of the unwillingness of one party to start a

130. Shihata, op. cit. note 128, p. 34.

131. Ibid., p. 44, with reference to J. B. Weinstein: "Some Benefits and Risks of Privatization of Justice Through ADR", 11 *Ohio State Journal on Dispute Resolution* (1996) p. 241; see also M. R. Wilkey: "International Trade and Foreign Direct Investment", 26 *Law and Policy in International Business* (1995) p. 615.

132. Shihata, op. cit. note 128, p. 36.

procedure that could lead to a compromise solution or other type of commitment along the way.

103. It follows that there is a need to strengthen this option in the context of new arrangements for the settlement of disputes. A first step to this end is to develop the requirement of *notification* of such actions that are likely to affect the rights of another party,[133] and eventually to *associate other interested States* with the domestic decision-making process that is likely to have such an effect.[134] A second step is the *broader undertaking of consultations* so as to prevent the emergence of a dispute or ensure its early solution.[135] To refrain from actions likely to aggravate the situation and eventually to adopt interim measures are also significant aspects of this approach.[136]

104. In view of the preventive function of these methods other related steps might also be usefully considered. The *monitoring* of situations that might result in disputes has been emphasized lately in the context of political affairs,[137] but it is equally possible in respect of other types of both public and private relations, including questions of

133. See, e.g., the Canada-United States Free Trade Agreement, 22-23 December 1987 and 2 January 1988, 27 ILM (1988) p. 281, Art. 1803, and comments by L. B. Sohn: "Bipartite Consultative Commissions for Preventing and Resolving Disputes Relating to International Trade Treaties", in *International Law in an Evolving World, Liber Amicorum Eduardo Jiménez de Aréchaga* (1994) p. 1183.

134. *Institut de Droit International*, Resolution on "Responsibility and Liability under International Law for Environmental Damage", Art. 29, Session de Strasbourg, 4 September 1997, 37 ILM (1998) p. 1473.

135. OSCE, Convention on Conciliation and Arbitration in the Framework of the OSCE, 15 December 1992, 32 ILM (1993) p. 557, Preamble; see in particular the Principles adopted by CSCE at La Valette, 8 February 1991, and the principle on prevention of disputes; and comments by Sohn, loc. cit. note 133, pp. 1184-1185.

136. OSCE, Convention cit. note 135, Art. 16; see also North American Free Trade Agreement (NAFTA), 17 December 1992, 32 ILM (1993) p. 694, Art. 2006; and comments by Sohn, loc. cit. note 133, pp. 1183-1185.

137. UN Secretary-General: *An Agenda for Peace: Preventive Diplomacy, Peace-making and Peace-keeping*, UN Doc. S/24111, 1992, para. 27.

compliance.[138] Availability of *information* becomes a particularly important requirement in this respect.[139]

105. Given the greater complexity of these arrangements, *institutionalization* of procedures will necessarily follow.[140] The prominent role that bilateral commissions have had[141] is being supplemented by the action of both regional and global international organizations. A UN agreement on consultations has been specifically proposed to facilitate the operation of this particular method.[142] The obligations relating to this method and related aspects might be strengthened first as a general principle of international law, but in addition this can be done more effectively in the context of specific and more detailed international regimes on settlement of disputes.

106. *(ii) Enhancing the role of inquiry.* The role of inquiry has also been enhanced lately as a result of the needs of information associated with the prevention and settlement of disputes. As discussed in Section II, this classic method has proven to be particularly helpful in dealing with highly technical disputes where the facts need to be clearly established and understood. But again in this respect the new demands of international society have evidenced the need for innovation. As with other methods, *institutionalization* of inquiry has significantly developed and this will no doubt be the essential feature

138. *Institut de Droit International,* Resolution on Procedure for the adoption and implementation of rules in the field of the environment, Session de Strasbourg, 4 September 1997, 67-II *Annuaire de* (1998) p. 514.

139. NAFTA cit. note 136, Art. 2006, and comments by Sohn, loc. cit. note 133, p. 1184.

140. Sohn, loc. cit. note 133, pp. 1196-1197.

141. Ibid., p. 1189.

142. L. B. Sohn: *The use of Consultations for Monitoring Compliance with Agreements concluded under the auspices of International Organizations* (1993) pp. 80-82. See also the extensive discussion on settlement of disputes in the context of the Manila Declaration on the Peaceful Settlement of International Disputes adopted by the UN General Assembly in November 1992, 19 *United Nations Chronicle* (Dec. 1982) pp. 80-81; and comments by L.B. Sohn: "Draft General Treaty on the Peaceful Settlement of International Disputes: A Proposal and Report", American Bar Association, Committee on World Order Under Law, 20 *The International Lawyer* (1986) p. 261.

of its further evolution. Important steps have been taken in this respect by the Security Council as far as peace and security are concerned,[143] and by a number of technical organizations, notably GATT and WTO.[144] The PCA too has prepared Optional Rules for fact-finding commissions of inquiry.[145] The traditional model of bilateral commissions of inquiry continues to have a useful role.[146]

107. *(iii) New orientations in conciliation.* Conciliation has been well developed under international law since the period 1899-1907 and new innovations are periodically introduced as the demand for this alternative continue unabated. An interesting example of current trends is found in the 1992 Convention on Conciliation and Arbitration of the OSCE.[147] The process of institutionalization is again noticeable in this experience, not by the intervention of standing bodies but, like in the PCA, by the availability of a *roster of conciliators* and arbitrators,[148] which is a more effective alternative. While in this case appointments are made by member States it might be appropriate in other cases to *enlarge the appointing authority.*

108. Another important feature of this model is that conciliation is linked up with other choices, notably arbitration. Such a linking, which is also within the historical tradition, will certainly be developed in the years ahead in order to provide a variety of choices within a broad institutional framework. The role of *good offices*

143. L. B. Sohn: "Broadening the Role of the United Nations in Preventing, Mitigating or Ending International or Internal Conflicts that Threaten International Peace and Security", *International Rule of Law Center Occasional Papers*, Second Series, No. 1, 1997, p. 35.

144. See for example GATT, Art. XXIII (2).

145. PCA Optional Rules of Procedure for Fact-finding Commissions of Inquiry, 1997.

146. See, for example, the 1914 Chile-US Treaty for the Settlement of Disputes.

147. OSCE, Convention cit. note 135, and comments by L. Cuny: *L'OSCE et le règlement pacifique des différends: La Cour de conciliation et d'arbitrage*, IHEI, 1997; L. Caflisch: "Vers des mécanismes pan-européens de règlement pacifique des différends", 97 *Revue Générale de Droit International Public* (1993) pp. 1-36.

148. OSCE, Convention cit. note 135, Art. 3.

should also be considered in this context. It should also be noted that the OSCE Convention develops the principle of subsidiarity so as not to impair the jurisdiction of the ICJ, the PCA and the major European Courts.[149] This is an important principle for the introduction of priority in dispute settlement methods or jurisdictions in the context of a highly structured system for dispute settlement.

109. *Compulsory recourse* to conciliation has also been an important feature of dispute settlement found in both bilateral[150] and multilateral treaties.[151] Some other interesting innovations concerning conciliation are found in the experience of the Chile-United States Commission for the Settlement of Disputes, the only treaty of the Bryan network that has ever been invoked.[152] Although this is in essence a commission of inquiry and conciliation that after difficult arrangements can lead to arbitration, an ad-hoc agreement between the parties mandated it to arrive at a *binding decision* on compensation, thereby in fact transforming it for that case into an adjudicatory body.[153] Such developments evidence quite vividly that even old treaties and mechanisms might be put to an entirely new use in the context of changing international relations and needs.

110. As noted above, a good number of recent and present disputes originate in situations of internal conflict that become directly or indirectly internationalized. New approaches to deal with such internal conflicts have recently been developed and on occasion interrelate with or have implications for dispute settlement under international

149. Ibid., Art. 19, and comments by L. Caflisch and L. Cuny: "La Cour de Conciliation et d'arbitrage de l'OSCE: Problèmes d'Actualité", *OSZE Jahrbuch* (1997) p. 4.

150. Chile-Argentina, Treaty of Peace and Friendship, November 29, 1984, Annex 1, Art. 2, 24 ILM (1985) p. 11.

151. UNCLOS, Art. 284; OSCE, Convention cit. note 135, Art. 18.

152. Chile-US Treaty cit. note 146; Commission decision in the matter of compensation for the deaths of Letelier and Moffitt, 31 ILM (1992) p. 1; and comments by Gray and Kingsbury, loc. cit. note 126, p. 100, note 17.

153. Chile-US Agreement to settle dispute concerning compensation for the deaths of Letelier and Moffitt, 30 ILM (1991) p. 422.

law or other arrangements. The model of a Truth and Reconciliation Commission followed by both Chile and South Africa in connection with their respective transitions to democracy, or the discussion of this approach in the Cambodian situation as an alternative to an International Criminal Tribunal, are recent examples to be taken into account. The establishment of International Truth and Reconciliation Commissions might prove an adequate alternative in some situations, particularly where the important issue is to set a truthful historical record of events and responsibilities that may lead to conciliation and not to punish individuals.

111. *(iv) Developing flexible mediation.* As discussed in Section II above, mediation has followed an evolution similar to conciliation but it is not used as much in view that it usually entails a proposal made by the mediator to the parties; in the case of conciliation recommendations may also be made but most often this is not done so as to keep the procedure entirely flexible.[154] Although the parties are of course free to accept or not such a proposal, on occasion they would prefer to avoid any element in the process that might constitute a precedent or affect the desired flexibility; the barring of information that might be used later in an adjudicatory settlement has been identified as an important element to this end.[155] This is why recent examples of mediation, in particular the Papal mediation between Chile and Argentina,[156] have proceeded with great flexibility, with the mediator making suggestions to the parties when he felt this useful, or otherwise helping the parties to negotiate directly under his guidance. In fact, this is a practical combination of mediation and conciliation, which is the feature likely to predominate in the future.

112. The essential feature of mediation or other third party intervention will be to have an individual, commission or institution that

154. H. M. Holtzmann: "Dispute resolution in Europe under the UNCITRAL conciliation rules", in Bardonnet, op. cit. note 23, pp. 297-298.

155. Ibid., pp. 302-303.

156. S. Benadava: "La mediación de la Santa Sede en el diferendo chileno-argentino sobre la zona austral", in *International Law at a time of perplexity: essays in honour of Shabtai Rosenne* (1989) pp. 33-50.

the parties are prepared to *trust*.[157] In certain types of difficult disputes, however, the mediator must also have a particularly *strong moral or political authority* in respect of the parties so as to provide weight to his opinions, thus turning the alternative of not arriving at a settlement into an unlikely event. This again was the salient element of the Papal mediation where the authority of His Holiness JOHN PAUL II, the Holy See and the Catholic Church in Chile and Argentina were crucial for a successful outcome. Future trends also indicate an increasing search for highly authoritative mediators and conciliators in respect of disputes involving sensitive political questions, as is apparent in the role of the President of the United States in the Middle East peace process or of Russian diplomacy in the efforts to end sanctions against Iraq. This trend also explains the increasing *institutionalization* of these procedures in regional or global international organizations.[158] The authority required from a mediator in such types of conflict is of course a different matter than the recent experiences with mediation backed by the threat of the use of force if the effort fails to produce an agreement. A suggestion has been made to the effect that dispute settlement mechanisms should also have an intermediary to bring the parties together and encourage them to choose a mode for settling their dispute without waiting for the parties to take the initiative, an approach which would allow for a special pro-active role of mediation.[159]

113. *(v) Adapting existing facilities.* The relevance of the methods discussed above in contemporary dispute settlement is further evidenced by the continuing *adaptation of the available rules and facilities* to this effect. The 1950 Revised General Act for the Pacific Settlement of International Disputes,[160] the 1980 UNCITRAL Conciliation rules, the 1988 Rules of Conciliation of the International Chamber of Commerce, the 1995 UN Model Rules for the Conciliation of Disputes between States and the 1996 PCA Optional Concili-

157. Merrills, p. 231.

158. Holtzmann, loc. cit. note 154, p. 303.

159. Comments on the Preliminary Report by R. S. Lee, 30 November 1998, pp. 1-2.

160. Holtzmann, loc.cit. note 154, pp. 297-298.

ation Rules[161] are examples of this important updating which is also evident in specialized areas.

114. Particularly noteworthy is the effort undertaken by the *PCA* in this respect. In spite of the fact that conciliation was not included in either the 1899 or 1907 Conventions, the PCA developed a practice allowing for such procedure[162] and has succeeded in establishing the rules noted above. The fact that facilities have been made available to both international organizations and private parties is also a significant indication of the current evolution in dispute settlement[163] and updates the Conventions in a practical manner not requiring the difficult process of formal amendment.[164] This approach also provides an important precedent how to update other treaty arrangements that have fallen behind time, as it is rather dramatically the case with the Inter-American System.[165]

115. *(vi) Reference procedures to technical bodies*. The use of inquiry, conciliation and mediation in the context of technical bodies has also found a most successful experience in the "reference" procedure established under the 1909 Boundary Waters Treaty between Great Britain and the United States.[166] With the consent of both parties a dispute may be formally referred to an International Joint Commission, and if this body is unable to decide the matter it is then

161. PCA, 1999 Steering Committee: Final Report and Recommendations to the Administrative Council, June 1997, pp. 4, 13.

162. Ibid., pp. 12-14.

163. Ibid., pp. 10-12.

164. Ibid., pp. 6-7.

165. On the settlement of disputes in the Inter-American System, with particular reference to the 1948 Pact of Bogotá, see generally F.V. Garcia Amador: *The Inter-American System* (1983).

166. US-UK, Treaty Relating to Boundary Waters and Questions Arising Between the United States and Canada, January 11, 1909, 36 Stat. 2448, *T.S.* No. 548; and see Great Lakes Water Quality Agreements of 1972, 23 U.S.T. 301, T.I.A.S. No. 7312, and of 1978, 30 U.T.S. 1383, T.I.A.S. No. 9257.

submitted to an umpire.[167] However, under a more practical approach either party can also bring a question or difference to the Commission, which may issue a report and recommendations, relying to this effect on factual inquiries by experts and other arrangements.[168] Formal dispute settlement eventually leading to arbitration is combined in this experience with more flexible arrangements, which allow for inquiry and forms of conciliation and mediation. This approach is most appropriate for dispute settlement in the context of specialized areas of co-operation, and this or similar combinations of method should be particularly encouraged in future bilateral or multilateral arrangements of this kind.

## III.3 Emerging opportunities for international arbitration

116. *(i) Consensual arbitration.* As international arbitration is the oldest and perhaps the most well established method for the settlement of disputes under international law, it will remain a viable alternative to judicial settlement in the future.[169] However, as with judicial settlement, it is not to be expected that a truly compulsory jurisdiction of arbitral tribunals will be any more acceptable than in the past as far as disputes involving general rules or issues of international law are involved.[170] Arbitral jurisdiction will in essence continue to be built on the consensual acceptance of the parties, whether this is given on

167. E. Brown Weiss: *Managing International Water Conflicts: The Great Lakes (US-Canada)*, February 1997, at 1-2.

168. Ibid., pp. 1-2; see also E. Brown Weiss: "New directions for the Great Lakes Water Quality Agreement: A commentary", 65 *Chicago-Kent Law Review* (1989) pp. 375-386.

169. Gray and Kingsbury, loc. cit. note 126, p. 109.

170. Ibid., p. 109. See in general M. C. W. Pinto: "Structure, Process, Outcome: Thoughts on the 'essence' of International Arbitration", 6 *Leyden Journal of International Law* (1993) pp. 241-264.

*ad hoc* basis or in anticipation of a dispute by means of an optional clause.[171]

117. *(ii) Opportunities for improvement.* In spite of this overall limitation, progress is to be expected in respect of a number of other aspects and trends. First, *compulsory jurisdiction* is finding increasing application in specialized and technical matters.[172] Second, the possibility of preparing *lists of subjects* in respect of which arbitration might be obligatory continues to attract authors, just as it was proposed in the 1899-1907 negotiations,[173] an approach which could well be linked, not to general questions of international law, but to the specialized fields in which it could better prosper. Third, *general clauses for the exclusion of arbitration* in respect of certain categories of disputes are, as noted above,[174] either obsolete or fading away. And fourth, like with other methods, increasing *institutionalization* will continue to develop so as to make this alternative more effective.

118. *(iii) Solving legal obstacles.* A number of legal problems that have haunted arbitration in the past might also find prospective solutions in this new context. The discussion about *arbitrability* and the existence or non-existence of a dispute that has often been raised in connection with the recourse to arbitration,[175] could in itself be submitted to decision by an independent body or authority in the context of institutionalized proceedings. A particular role for the President of the ICJ could be envisaged to this effect.

119. Increasing recourse to *international law as the law applicable in arbitration* will significantly facilitate the task of tribunals in identi-

171. Institut de Droit International: *"Projet de règlement pour la procédure arbitrale internationale"*, 1875, discussed by S. Torres Bernárdez: "L'Arbitrage Interétatique", in Bardonnet, op. cit. note 23, pp. 213-214. With respect to the OSCE Convention, see also Cuny, op. cit. note 147, pp. 68-69.

172. Torres Bernárdez, loc. cit. note 171, p. 263.

173. Scott, op. cit. note 2, pp. 60-61, 392-393; Sohn, loc. cit. note 142, pp. 282-284; Torres Bernárdez, loc. cit. note 171, pp. 263-264.

174. See note 126 and associated text.

175. Torres Bernárdez, loc. cit. note 171, pp. 222-223.

fying the general or specialized governing rules, including the role of equity as a principle of international law and where appropriate to decide *ex aequo et bono*. It is of interest to note that in the 1957 European Convention an arbitral decision *ex aequo et bono* may be adopted in the silence or absence of a *compromis*, but with the added safeguard of taking into account the general principles of international law and of respecting conventional commitments and international decisions binding the parties.[176] It is in fact a kind of international law governed by the *ex aequo et bono* principle that can provide the necessary *flexibility within legal limits*. Problems relating to *compliance* with arbitral awards may also be addressed in the framework of institutionalized proceedings. This is no longer a matter to be left solely to the good faith and honour of the parties,[177] since these have on occasion been breached: measures related to domestic enforcement and other features will need to be established. The law and practice of commercial arbitration under the UNCITRAL rules, the International Chamber of Commerce[178] and other experienced bodies, is most relevant in this respect and in itself provides an insight of what future trends are likely to be in terms of international arbitration generally. The experience of the ICSID Convention in respect of the enforcement of arbitral awards must also particularly be noted in this context.

120. *(iv) Institutionalized arbitration in the PCA.* The process of institutionalization again offers interesting opportunities for the PCA. apart from its functions in inter-State arbitration under the Hague Conventions, the important practice and adaptation of various procedures it has undertaken could well place it in the position of effectively handling the new tide of general international arbitration

176. European Convention for the Peaceful Settlement of Disputes of 29 April 1957, Art. 26; and comments by Torres Bernárdez, loc. cit. note 171, pp. 247-248.

177. Torres Bernárdez, loc. cit. note 171, pp. 251-252.

178. International Chamber of Commerce, Rules of Arbitration, 36 ILM (1997) p. 1604. See also the Mediation, Arbitration ans Expedited Arbitration Rules of the World Intellectual Property Organization, 36 ILM (1995) p. 559; Commercial Arbitration and Mediation Center for the Americas, Mediation and Arbitration Rules, 35 ILM (1996) p. 1541.

that could be expected in the future, but not quite that appertaining to specialized areas which is being directed to other bodies. The 1992 Optional Rules for arbitration between two States and the 1993 Optional Rules established for arbitration between two parties of which only one is a State, like those adopted in 1996 for arbitration involving international organizations and States and for arbitration between international organizations and private parties,[179] illustrate well the link between the PCA and the new trends in the field, as well as the ability to adapt the Hague system to new times. It is suggested in this respect that a further revision of the PCA rules could be undertaken with the participation of legal experts from major international organizations, such as the World Bank, so as to adapt these procedures to the operational needs of such organizations; the end result of this effort would be to make available the PCA rules to thousands of contracts entered by such organizations with their clients and other entities.

121. In addition, the PCA could perform useful *functions in respect of many arbitral systems* that have occasionally lacked adequate institutional support in their own regional contexts, such as the 1948 Pact of Bogota in the ambit of the OAS or the 1964 OAU Protocol on mediation, conciliation and arbitration.[180] In such situations the PCA would not replace regional organizations but supplement their functions if needed, for example by providing a choice to the parties; this in itself would greatly encourage a more efficient action of the regional organizations concerned. Similar roles could be performed in the context of various UN Resolutions on arbitration or other treaties. These opportunities for the PCA would require, however, a *broad choice of arbitrators* beyond the listed members, as provided for under the Optional Rules and prior practice, since appointment to the list by member States has not always proven to be adequate; on the other hand, it has been rightly suggested that a broad evaluation of the effectiveness of international arbitration and of the mechanisms of the

179. Report cit. note 161, pp. 10-12.

180. For a reference to regional and other relevant arbitration treaties, see Torres Bernárdez, loc. cit. note 171, pp. 209-210.

PCA could be undertaken as a result of the 1999 Conference with a view to its enhancement.[181]

## III 4 Innovating in specialized fields of international law

122. Some of the shortcomings of dispute settlement in cases involving questions of general international law are no longer found in certain key specialized fields, such as trade, investment and the law of international organizations, where the same States have been willing to accept innovations of significance. These experiences offer interesting insights into the trends that are beginning to predominate.

123. *(i) A structured system of dispute settlement.* Dispute settlement under GATT and WTO is still confined to inter-State disputes, but even in this limited context it has significantly improved over past approaches to the settlement of such disputes. The GATT system was largely the result of an accepted successful practice rather than of detailed negotiated arrangements.[182] Interestingly enough, it was this very practice that marked the evolution from "power-oriented" to "rule-oriented" policies,[183] enabling, first, the greater role of international law in dispute settlement in this area and, next, the development of a *quasi-judicial mechanism under the WTO.* This process has led to a greater *"legalization" and "de-politization"* of dispute settle-

181. See E. Vio Grossi: Observations on the Document "Peaceful Settlement of Disputes: Prospects for the XXI Century", Inter-American Juridical Committee, OAS Doc. OEA/Ser. Q. CJI/doc. 53/98, 24 August 1998; for the choice of arbitrators under the optional rules, see Report cit. note 161, p. 8.

182. E.-U. Petersmann: "The dispute-settlement system of the World Trade Organization and the evolution of the GATT dispute-settlement system since 1948", 31 *Common Market Law Review* (1994) p. 1224.

183. Ibid., p. 1187.

ment,[184] except in some specific areas such as dispute settlement under the Antidumping and Subsidies Code.[185]

124. Problems relating to "forum shopping" and "norm shopping" among eight different dispute-settlement procedures, delays in the establishment of panels and the adoption of panel reports, problems of non-compliance with the rulings reached and criticism about the lack of transparency in procedures,[186] led to an *integrated dispute settlement system* under WTO. The salient feature of the new system is the *multiple combination of political and legal methods* available to the parties. As noted in Section II above, the former include consultations, good offices, conciliation, mediation, recommendations by panels, the Appellate Body or the Dispute Settlement Body, surveillance in the implementation, and compensation and suspension of concessions. The legal choices include Panel procedures, the Appellate Review Procedure, Rulings of the Dispute Settlement Body on the reports of the prior two, arbitration and domestic court proceedings.[187] In some respects, in particular with arbitration, the parties are allowed a greater autonomy to establish the procedure to be followed, but always within the guidelines and requirements of the governing system.[188] It should be noted, however, that although a quasi-judicial system offers the advantage of a structured arrangement, it also involves the risk of somewhat detracting from the flexibility that made the GATT experience successful in the first place.

125. A number of other innovations have been introduced to overcome problems of the prior experience under the GATT. The most

184. R. Hudec: *Enforcing International Trade Law. The Evolution of the Modern GATT Legal System* (1993) p. 138, and discussion by Petersmann, loc. cit. note 182, p. 1188.

185. Petersmann, loc. cit. note 182, p. 1225; see also T. M. Rief: "Coming of Age in Geneva: Guiding the GATT Dispute-settlement system on Review of Antidumping and Countervailing Duty Proceedings", 24 *Law and Policy in International Business* (1993) pp. 1185-1200.

186. Petersmann, loc. cit. note 182, pp. 1203-1205.

187. Ibid., p. 1210.

188. Ibid., p. 1221.

important of these is the introduction of the "*inverted consensus*", a principle under which the panel reports must be adopted by the Dispute Settlement Board unless there is a consensus to reject them. This dramatically overturns the GATT procedure that required consensus for the adoption of such reports.[189]

126. In spite of these improvements, important shortcomings still remain in this system of dispute settlement.[190] One of its most significant limitations is that *individuals and corporations continue to be barred* from access to it in spite of their being the principal actors of the international trading system.[191] While in this respect pressure may be expected to continue to mount, in the meantime some other alternatives could be pursued. First, like with the ICJ, individuals can participate in proceedings with the agreement and co-operation of the States which are the formal parties to the dispute, or, like in the PCA, Optional Rules could be developed by WTO itself. The modest step envisaged by the Dispute Settlement Understanding of WTO for requesting information from individuals[192] should be supplemented by strengthened rights of participation in the near future.

127. *(ii) International control of domestic legislation.* A second model of important innovations in dispute settlement arrangements is found in both the Canada-US States Free Trade Agreement (FTA)[193]

189. P. Pescatore: The GATT Dispute Settlement Mechanism", 27 *Journal of World Trade* (1993), p. 18.

190. E.-U. Petersmann: *The GATT/WTO Dispute-settlement system: International Law, International Organizations and Dispute Settlement*, 1997. See also Societá Italiana di Diritto Internazionale: *Diritto e Organizzazione del Commercio Internazionale dopo la creazione della Organizzazione Mondiale del Commercio*, Il Convegno, Milano, 5-7 Giugno 1997, in particular the presentation by Treves (pp. 323-351) and Lafer (p. 1).

191. Pescatore, loc. cit. note 189, p. 19; Petersmann, loc. cit. note 182, p. 1243.

192. B.-R. Killmann: "The Access of Individuals to International Trade Dispute Settlement", 13 *Journal of International Arbitration* (1996) p. 166.

193. Canada-US Free Trade Agreement, 2 January 1985, 27 ILM (1985) p. 281.

and the North American Free Trade Agreement (NAFTA). [194] Three types of mechanisms are provided under the latter. First, disputes concerning investments can be submitted to the ICSID facility, its Additional Facility or UNCITRAL arbitration rules, thereby opening direct access to the private investor concerned.[195] Second, disputes between the parties can be submitted to a panel mechanism which reaches a non-binding decision that cannot be appealed or challenged, but which may ultimately lead to forms of retaliation.[196] Although there are differences with the FTA and the GATT arrangements, the NAFTA mechanism may be used as a substitute for the latter. [197]

128. The most interesting mechanism is that relating to *antidumping and countervailing duties disputes* under Chapter 19 of NAFTA and its precedent in the FTA. Under this mechanism each country may keep its legislation on the matter, but amendments may be challenged before a panel in respect of compatibility with the GATT/WTO and its effects upon prior decisions of a panel.[198] More importantly, the question of whether national legislation has been correctly applied is subject to challenge before binational panels that come to replace national judicial review of final determinations on the matter.[199] Equally significant is that this procedure is open to private parties and that panel decisions are binding. A procedure for Extraordinary Challenge of panel decisions is available to State parties within

194. NAFTA cit. note 136.

195. NAFTA Chapter 11, and comments by G. N. Horlick and F. A. DeDusk: "Dispute Resolution under NAFTA. Building on the U.S.-Canada FTA, GATT and ICSID", 27 *Journal of World Trade* (1993) pp. 22-27.

196. Ibid., pp. 34-41.

197. Ibid., p. 34.

198. K. Moody-O'Grady: "Dispute Settlement Provisions in the NAFTA and the CAFTA: Progress or Protectionism?", 18 *The Fletcher Forum of World Affairs* (1994) p. 127.

199. Ibid., p. 128.

limited grounds. Consultations can also be undertaken in case of domestic interference with the panel process.[200]

129. Although questions of constitutionality[201] and other points of criticism[202] have been raised in connection with this mechanism, it is nonetheless a precedent-setting arrangement to avoid trade protectionism and arbitrariness. A final international review of the appropriate application of domestic legislation is a most attractive alternative for the future of dispute settlement in general, as the availability of this procedure to private parties is also likely to influence developments in the matter,[203] perhaps even beyond trade mechanisms. Suggestions for dispute settlement in other trade arrangements have included an APEC dispute mediation service and a voluntary pre-GATT panel system.[204] More traditional methods have been adopted in MERCOSUR.[205]

130. *(iii) Direct access by affected parties.* A third model of innovation in dispute settlement is found in the Convention on the Settlement of Investment Disputes between States and Nationals of other States, setting up the International Centre for Settlement of

200. Ibid., pp. 131-132.

201. Ibid.

202. Wilkey, loc. cit. note 131, pp. 629-631.

203. A. F. Lowenfeld: "Binational Dispute Settlement Under Chapter 19 of the Canada-United States Free Trade Agreement: An Interim Appraisal", 24 *New York University Journal of International Law and Politics* (1991) p. 355.

204. C. J. Green: "APEC and Trans-Pacific Dispute Management", 26 *Law and Policy in International Business* (1995) pp. 726-727. The development of dispute-settlement mechanisms for trade and investment in the Pacific Rim was also discussed at the Commemoration of the Centenary of the 1899 Hague Peace Conference, convened by the University of Melbourne Faculty of Law, 18-20 February 1999, as a part of the regional developments that are to be expected in dispute settlement.

205. MERCOSUR: Protocol of Brasilia for the Settlement of Disputes, 36 ILM (1997) p. 691. See also Costa Rica, El Salvador, Guatemala, Honduras, Nicaragua, Panama: "Statute of the Central American Court of Justice", 34 ILM (1995) p. 921.

Investment Disputes (ICSID).[206] Submission of disputes to ICSID requires the consent of the parties, which is usually given in advance in the context of bilateral and multilateral investment treaties that have come to provide an impressive network of jurisdictional clauses and matters covered by it. Arbitration and Conciliation Rules govern the proceedings to be conducted under the Centre. An Additional Facility has been enacted to allow for the submission of disputes when one party is not a Contracting State or a national of a Contracting State, thus broadening the access beyond the actual contracting parties; to allow similarly access when the dispute does not arise directly out of an investment; or to institute fact-finding proceedings.[207] Besides the broad scope of this system, two of its features are important to retain: the direct participation by foreign investors, and the obligation of Contracting States not to undertake diplomatic protection or bring claims in respect of their nationals when the dispute has been submitted to arbitration under the Convention. An effective dispute settlement arrangement has thus preempted one of the major sources of political and legal conflict in the history of international law, an approach that could well be followed in other areas. Since the consent to ICSID arbitration is exclusive of any other remedy, the system is in fact insulated from the control or interference of national courts.[208]

131. Special arrangements for the submission of claims by individuals to international procedures have also been successfully implemented in the framework of the Iran-United States Claims Tribunal and of the UN Compensation Commission. The Governing Council of the latter body has developed a comprehensive approach to the question of remedies, allowing for governments to submit consolidated claims and receive payments on behalf of individuals affected, including

206. Convention on the Settlement of Investment Disputes between States and nationals of Other States, March 18, 1965, *ICSID Basic Documents*, 1985; see also note 111.

207. ICSID, Rules Governing the Additional Facility for the Administration of Proceedings by the Secretariat of the International Centre for Settlement of Investment Disputes, September 27, 1978, Document ICSID/11, June 1979.

208. Shihata, op. cit. note 128, pp. 47-52.

claims on behalf of third parties.[209] The Commission itself may intervene as a trustee on behalf of certain categories of claimants.[210] In the case of a corporation that is barred from making a claim because of its nationality, its partners are allowed to do so in proportion to their interest if not affected individually by the nationality requirement,[211] an approach which innovates in relation to some of the problems discussed by the ICJ in the *Barcelona Traction* case.

132. *(iv) Private entities in international organizations.* A fourth model that needs to be kept in mind concerns dispute settlement mechanisms and associated procedures devised in the context of international organizations or highly institutionalized arrangements. These include notification and reporting, monitoring, conditionality of financial assistance, financial and other sanctions, independent supervisory bodies, administrative tribunals and other alternatives concerning supervision and enforcement.[212] A noteworthy development is the creation of the World Bank Inspection Panel that allows for the review of operations, not as a commission of inquiry or implying a mediation or adjudication function, but as a mechanism that enhances quality control in the design and implementation of projects, ensuring a greater institutional transparency and accountability.[213] A most significant feature of this mechanism is the direct legal access to bring complaints before an international forum by private parties affected by a given project, such as an organization, association or other grouping of individuals,[214] a procedure that has been rightly described as "a progressive step in the development of both the law of

209. UN Compensation Commission: *Criteria for expedited processing of urgent claims*, UN Doc. S/AC.26/1991/1, 2 August 1991.

210. Ibid., UN Doc. S/AC.26/1991/5, 23 October 1991.

211. Ibid., UN Doc. S/AC.26/1991/4, 23 October 1991.

212. Petersmann, loc. cit. note 182, p. 1170.

213. I. F. I. Shihata: *The World Bank Inspection Panel. A Background Paper on its Historical, Legal and Operational Aspects*, November 1997, pp. 4, 8; see also note 111.

214. R. E. Bissell: "Recent Practice of the Inspection Panel of the World Bank", 91 AJIL (1997) pp. 741-744.

international organizations and the international law of human rights".[215]

133. The jurisdiction and work of the Administrative Tribunals established within major international organizations such as the United Nations and the World Bank again set an important precedent in respect of the direct access of given categories of individuals to international tribunals, an approach which could well be followed in other types of arrangements involving individual rights and interests.

## III.5 Towards a global Alternative Dispute Resolution system

134. *(i) Court directed ADR procedures*. Early third-party intervention has been identified as the key factor in dispute prevention and resolution both in domestic and international procedures.[216] This reality has led to significant developments in the use of Alternative Dispute Resolution (ADR) in national and international practice. Well established organizations, such as the Center for Public Resources,[217] provide ADR services to broad business sectors in the United Sates at the national and regional levels, as well as in other countries, including mediation, arbitration and other methods. Even more significantly, courts themselves have enacted ADR procedures that are conducted under the guidance and with the encouragement of the judiciary, thereby directing the parties to a whole range of alternatives that in most cases will remove the need for the litigation before the court, a process that will result in diminished costs, greater expediency and more time available for the court to conduct its regular business. The "Michigan Mediation" procedure has made mandatory the use of mediation before court proceedings can com-

215. Shihata, loc. cit. note 213, p. 25.

216. Miall, op. cit. note 19, p. 189.

217. Center for Public Resources, Institute for Dispute Resolution, 1979.

mence,[218] while the United States District Court for the Northern District of California offers a variety of choices to the parties and counsel.[219]

135. *(ii) Domestic ADR options.* Among the methods recommended in the latter court are: *Early Neutral Evaluation*, in which a prestigious private lawyer will assist the parties in evaluating the strength, weakness and value of the case, preparing the ground for settlement negotiations; *Court-Annexed Arbitration*, which is a mandatory but non-binding arbitration for cases involving relatively small amounts of claim, while voluntary and non-binding arbitration is encouraged in other cases; *Summary Jury or Bench Trials*, which involves a non-binding advisory verdict or judgment, as well as the opportunity to question the judge and the jurors, thus providing guidance to the settlement negotiations that follow this procedure; *Consent to Jury or Court Trial before a Magistrate*, which follows the ordinary procedure before a magistrate chosen by the parties and not the assigned judge; *Settlement Conferences* conducted by the Judge or Magistrate, in which the judge or magistrate presiding over a case will help the parties as a mediator or facilitator; and *Special Master*, usually involving a high degree of expertise, in which a prestigious lawyer will help the parties in managing the case, fact-finding and settlement.[220]

136. *(iii) A structured ADR international system.* A number of these methods and experiences can be of interest in international dispute prevention and resolution, a field where they occasionally have been used under different names and in a rather isolated manner. It is really important to insert these alternatives in a relatively structured system of dispute resolution. To this end it might be appropriate for the ICJ, other Tribunals and eventually the Security Council, to provide encouragement and guidance for such a structured system of alternatives available to the parties.

218. Shihata, op. cit. note 128, p. 41.

219. Coombe, loc. cit. note 125, p. 538.

220. Ibid., p.538-540.

137. For instance, the ICJ before actually admitting a case, or at some stage in the proceedings, might conceivably require the parties to undertake some form of alternative dispute resolution, including those that are highly developed under international law, such as consultations, conciliation, mediation or arbitration, or even those that might be adapted from national practice, to the extent of course that this might be deemed helpful to the settlement of the dispute in question. The Court in fact has occasionally encouraged the parties to negotiate and settle in the course of the proceedings,[221] and the suggestion made here would simply provide a more systematic approach and a greater variety of choices conducive to the same end. A Committee of Jurists (that will be discussed in conjunction with the Court further below) could also be of help in this context. Furthermore, this may prove to be an essential device if the number of judicial cases continue to increase.

138. This ADR system should not lead to a strict hierarchy of international tribunals or methods, since this could detract from the necessary freedom and flexibility that the parties and the system must have. It is rather a question of bringing to the parties' attention in an organized way the various choices at their disposal and how they could take advantage of these alternatives. In the domestic experiences mentioned above material is prepared to this effect by the court itself.

139. *(iv) A global ADR system.* To the extent that such approach is organized, guided and encouraged, the ADR system that has been gradually emerging will become a truly global undertaking in the 21st century. Each method in itself has been evolving toward the satisfaction of new needs and realities and additional methods are at hand.

221. Presentation by Judge Mohamed Bedjaoui, in C. Peck and R. S. Lee (eds.): *Increasing the effectiveness of the International Court of Justice* (1997) p. 23. See also W. M. Reisman: "The supervisory jurisdiction of the International Court of Justice: International Arbitration and International Adjudication", RdC, 1996, p. 9. For the guidance of the Court in respect of legal issues in the Gabcikovo-Nagymaros case and the commitment of the parties to further negotiate on these bases, see the Report of the ICJ presented by President Stephen M. Schwebel to the UN General Assembly, 52nd Session, 36th Plenary Meeting, 27 October 1997, Doc. A/52/PV.36, pp. 2-3.

Private institutions are already providing global facilities in certain respects and it is to be expected that international courts and other bodies will provide or arrange for similar functions. In this manner, the administration of international justice broadly conceived will become fully integrated with and supplemented by a privatized system of alternative methods,[222] which is in fact the only viable alternative to do justice to the growing demands of the international community.

## IV. A central role for the ICJ in the new structure of international law

140. If non-judicial options do not succeed or are not available, or the parties to a dispute prefer a judicial settlement in view of the nature of the controversy or the high prestige of a given court, or are bound to accept a court's jurisdiction because of legal commitments, the availability and strengthening of the judicial settlement of disputes shall always be a major need of the international community. In addition to the dispute settlement function that a court such as the ICJ has, it is possible to foresee a new function which relates more to a constitutional role. Precisely because international society is becoming more decentralized, the need to identify the basic principles of international law governing the international community becomes more evident since it is this element that ensures its integration and coherence. While it may not yet be a question of adopting a Constitution for the world community - although the time will come for that step - it certainly is a question of developing such principles that an author has rightly described as essential for the integration of the law, transformation, delegation of power, intrinsic limitation of power, the supremacy of law, the supremacy of the social interest and social

222. Wilkey, loc. cit. note 131, p. 615.

responsibility.[223] A Constitutional Court for the world community will have to be established in the not too distant future. The UN Charter and a few selected treaties have thus far performed the task of providing for some of such basic principles, but this has been a rather limited exercise.[224] As with many of the first steps of international legal development, authors and learned institutions have also contributed to this exercise.[225] There is a need, however, for a broader undertaking in the matter which for the time being would seem to be more a judicial than a legislative function.

141. The question that follows is whether the ICJ might perform this type of constitutional function in the meanwhile or might itself evolve towards a Constitutional Court in addition to its regular dispute settlement role. To a meaningful extent this objective can be accomplished without recourse to lengthy and difficult procedures of reform and amendment, particularly in view of the reluctance that States have shown thus far to undertake a reform of the Charter or the Court,[226] but if amendments should prove indispensable States may wish to consider them at some point in time.

223. P. Allott: Eunomia. *New Order for a New World* (1990) pp. 167-168.

224. On the constitutional role of the UN Charter, see P.-M. Dupuy: "The Constitutional Dimension of the Charter of the United Nations Revisited", 1 *Max Planck Yearbook of United Nations Law* (1997) p. 1. For a critical view of the Charter as compared to a federal constitution, see G. Arangio-Ruiz: "The 'Federal Analogy' and UN Charter Interpretation: A Crucial Issue", 8 *European Journal of International Law* (1997) p. 1.

225. I. Brownlie: *Principles of Public International Law*, 1990; *Oppenheim's International Law*, 1992.

226. See, for example, the comments by Professor Shabtai Rosenne on the Preliminary Report of 24 November and 7 December 1998, with reference to GA Res 52/161 of 15 December 1997, para. 4; references are made hereafter to this last comment unless noted. See also the comments by Judge Gilbert Guillaume on the Preliminary Report of 22 September 1998.

## IV.1 The evolving role of the ICJ

142. The role of the Court has traditionally been conceived as one directed at solving specific conflicts among States in the context of the complex jurisdictional ambit of international law.[227] This is indeed one important aspect of its role, but by no means the only one. If the needs of the international community are put in the perspective of the 21st century, the kind of constitutional function described above gains in importance. The Permanent Court of International Justice was inserted in the still more limited scenario of its time since its role was largely related to the post-war settlements and arrangements and did not always find support in the principal powers.[228] As a result, most of the cases submitted to the Permanent Court did not lend themselves to judicial pronouncements that would have a "forward reach beyond merely deciding the dispute before that Court".[229] In spite of these limiting circumstances or conceptions, both the past and the present Court gradually developed and continue to develop the law in the context of both judgements and advisory opinions,[230] as is evident, e.g., in the fields of navigation, fisheries, and maritime delimitation. These trends of change have been reinforced as the transition from the old period of autocratic international relations gradually leads to a pattern of democratic international relations,[231] and again the need for such developments will become more apparent as the 21st century progresses. This evolving role of the Court is still more evident when its role is examined in the light of its Advisory Opinions, that have

227. M. Virally: "Le champ opératoire du règlement judiciaire international", *Revue Générale de Droit International Public* (1983) No. 2, p. 285.

228. Rosenne, Comments cit. note 226, with ref. to L. Lloyd: *Peace through Law: Britain and the International Court in the 1920s* (1997); M. Pomerance: *The United States and the World Court as a Supreme Court of the Nations: Dreams, Illusions and Disillusion* (1996).

229. S. Rosenne: "Lessons of the past and needs of the future", in Peck and Lee, op. cit. note 221, p. 468.

230. Comments by the Government of China on the Preliminary Report, p. 3; Comments by the United Kingdom Government on the Preliminary Report, para. 8.

231. Rosenne, loc. cit. note 221, p. 468.

greatly contributed to the development of the principles of international law in selected areas.[232]

143. The present full docket of the ICJ has been generally interpreted as a sign of strength and as an indication that its appeal to solve disputes is unrelated to the reluctance of States to accept its compulsory jurisdiction.[233] Indeed, the fact that the number of submissions to the Court is increasing must be welcome as an indication of greater reliance on its dispute-settlement functions. However, it should not pass unnoticed that the very same States forming its constituency have also been increasingly seeking to solve their disputes by different means, establishing new and more effective arrangements to this effect. These alternatives will inevitably contrast with the possibilities offered by the Court,[234] thus creating a delicate medium and long-term situation which not necessarily will favour its role. The so-called proliferation of international tribunals is an eloquent expression of this phenomenon,[235] as is the greater specialization of a number of the new emerging arrangements. This is not so much a question of overlapping jurisdictions, which treaties and courts generally tend to avoid, but rather one of separate alternatives which may lead disputant States away from the Court.

144. On the other hand, it has been rightly remarked that the type of disputes that States are willing to submit to the Court is in itself rather limited since, in spite of the variety of matters brought before it, they often do not include questions that have important domestic political

232. Hans Corell: "The feasibility of Implementing The Hague/St. Petersburg Centennial Recommendations Under the UN System", Consultation on the Peaceful Resolution of Major International Disputes, London, 11-15 December, 1998, pp. 9-10.

233. Mohammed Bedjaoui, presentation in Peck and Lee, op. cit. note 221, p. 20.

234. L. Condorelli: "La Cour Internationale de Justice: 50 ans et (pour l'heure) pas une ride", 6 *European Journal of International Law* (1995) pp. 393-394. See also T. Treves: "Recent trends in the settlement of international disputes",1 *Cursos Euro-mediterráneos de Derecho Internacional* (1997) pp. 395-436.

235. L. Boisson de Chazournes et al. (eds.): "Implications of the proliferation of international adjudicatory bodies for dispute resolution", *ASIL Bulletin*, No.9, November 1995.

implications or affect significant aspects of international relations.[236] Here again, however, the situation has been undergoing some changes since, as it has been appropriately commented, cases dealing with nuclear weapons and major cases concerning territorial sovereignty and maritime delimitation do relate to important issues of international relations or may have significant domestic implications.[237] This evolution does not, however, derogate from the fact that many cases which States decide to bring before the Court are cases of "*importance moyenne*",[238] neither major questions nor small issues, particularly if examined from the perspective of the need to develop some major areas of the governing principles of international law. More importantly, the vast areas of international law dealing with trade, finance, investment and other matters are never brought before the Court. If questions of major interest and priority for States and other entities are systematically kept away from the Court, this could result in a critical situation that could affect the institution,[239] particularly if a perception of "*vieillissement*" takes hold.[240] To the extent that the Court supplements its traditional dispute settlement role with one associated to the principles of constitutional law and the law of international organizations[241] its central function in the international community might be better asserted and relied on.

145. Various crises of the Court have been attributed to the decline of the optional clause, to the mistrust of the Third World or to Western indifference,[242] but the problem seems to be more complex than that. Its limited functions in settling disputes between States, which is its main role in the 20th-century perspective of States, means in practice

236. Virally, loc. cit. note 227, p. 309.

237. Rosenne, Comments cit. note 226, p. 5.

238. Virally, loc. cit. note 227, p. 309.

239. Ibid., p. 309-310.

240. Condorelli, loc. cit. note 234, p. 399.

241. Virally, loc. cit. note 227, pp. 294, 303.

242. G. Abi-Saab: "De l'evolution de la Cour Internationale. Reflexions sur quelques tendances recentes", *Revue Générale de Droit International Public* (1992) No. 2, pp. 276-281.

that "the court is seized of a matter and that the Court does not seize a matter".[243] While in so doing the Court has significantly contributed to the law of international litigation,[244] its contribution to the broader functions outlined above has been restricted by the nature of the matters submitted to it and has therefore been more indirect or occasional.

146. Because the Court has not been enabled to systematically develop its guiding role in respect of the basic principles of international law, the legal order governing international society is every passing day less structured and even a minimal hierarchy of its rules is beginning to fade, a situation that will only become worse as new tribunals enter the international scene.[245] However, to the extent that cases or requests for advisory opinions have enabled the Court to exercise this guiding role, it has in the past decade significantly asserted a noticeably greater emphasis on this aspect, particularly in respect of the interpretation of the United Nations law, the necessary orientation of the international legal system and of the judicial functions related thereto. It does not today have a choice and has to deal with cases as they come. In the adjudication of specific disputes the Court will often be able to develop its views about principles, even as an obiter dictum and the identification of rules of *jus cogens,*[246] but this will not always be possible, or not to the extent required by the evolution of the international community. A broader function for the Court as the central judicial body of the international community should be built in the future.

243. Afro-Asian Legal Consultative Committee: "Report of the First Session of the meeting held to consider the Preliminary Reports on the themes of the First International Peace Conference", New Delhi, February 11, 1999, para. 12.

244. Rosenne, loc. cit. note 229, pp. 472-473; and see generally S. Rosenne: *The Law and Practice of the International Court, 1920-1996* (1997); M. N. Shaw: "The International Court of Justice: A Practical Perspective", 46 ICLQ (1997) pp. 831-865.

245. R. Y. Jennings: "The Judiciary, International and National, and the Development of International Law", 45 ICLQ (1996) p. 5.

246. Guillaume, Comments cit. note 226, p. 2. See also the Comment on the Preliminary Report by Prof. Barbara Kwiatkowska, 16 November 1998, pp. 1-2.

## IV.2 A new constitutional role for the ICJ: managing the evolving principles of international law

147. Many of the efforts directed at revitalizing the Court have been inspired in the traditional approach and, therefore, have put greatest emphasis on improvements that might facilitate the handling of occasional disputes.[247] In not few occasions such efforts have aimed to curtail actual or potential competition with the Court in the handling of disputes, as it is quite evident in respect of the law of the sea[248] and the environment.[249] There is of course merit in many of the proposals made in respect of this approach, since the dispute settlement function of the Court will always need to be available in the most effective terms possible.

148. As noted above, however, a different approach has gradually emerged to strengthen the Court's functions in respect of its role as the central judicial body of the international community, a role that reaches beyond dispute settlement and puts it in a position to contribute to the development of the principles of international law governing the international society generally or some of its major organizations in particular. The Court itself has been quite aware of this capability and indeed has already advanced in its implementation. One distinguished writer of international law has identified the turning point with the advisory opinion on *Reservations to the Convention on the Prevention and Punishment of the Crime of Genocide*, the interim protection in the *Anglo-Iranian Oil Company* case and the

247. See generally Peck and Lee, op. cit. note 221; see also D. W. Bowett, J. Crawford, I. Sinclair and A. D. Watts: "The International Court of Justice. Efficiency of Procedures and Working Methods", Supplement to 45 ICLQ (1996) pp. 1-35.

248. S. Oda: "Dispute Settlement Prospects in the Law of the Sea", 44 ICLQ (1995) pp. 863-872. See also A. E. Boyle: "Dispute Settlement and the Law of the Sea Convention: Problems of Fragmentation and Jurisdiction", 46 ICLQ (1997) pp. 37-54.

249. Comments by P. H. Sands, in Peck and Lee, op. cit. note 221, p. 439.

*Anglo-Norwegian Fisheries* case,[250] another with the case on *Military and Paramilitary Activities in and against Nicaragua*.[251]

149. While the conclusions of the Court in some of these cases and opinions may be controversial, what matters is the different nature of such pronouncements as compared with the traditional approach discussed above. This other function of the Court has been compared to that of the US Supreme Court deciding on a point of constitutional interpretation as opposed to that of a domestic judge with a routine case, particularly in view of the greater complexity of international law.[252] This constitutional role has also been discussed lately in the specific context of the UN Charter,[253] to which no doubt the Court has contributed in providing stability and integrity to the Charter regime.[254]

150. In light of the above it may be suggested that the outlook of the Court for the 21st century might be further strengthened if it develops a new judicial policy directed to assert its central role in international society. This is not a question of exclusivity of the Court since it already faces severe competition from various dispute settlement arrangements which must be welcome. It is rather a question of envisaging the Court "not in isolation, but as one major partner in a general complex of different kinds of decision-making under the rule of law".[255] Either in terms of its advisory opinions, where competition is not significant, or in the handling of cases involving questions of

250. Rosenne, loc. cit. note 221, pp. 468-470.

251. Abi-Saab, loc. cit. note 242, p. 295.

252. Merrills, p. 238.

253. Presentation by M. C. W. Pinto on "The Court and other international tribunals", in Peck and Lee, op. cit. note 221, p. 285.

254. Rosenne, loc. cit. note 229, p. 481. For evidence of this contribution see the Court's reasoning in upholding its jurisdiction in the Lockerbie Case (Preliminary Objections), Decision of 27 February 1998.

255. Presentation by Sir Robert Jennings on "Contributions of the Court to the Resolution of International Tensions", in Peck and Lee, op. cit. note 221, p. 79. See also the Report presented by ICJ President Stephen M. Schwebel, op. cit. note 221, p. 3.

identification and interpretation of the governing principles of international law, it can develop this new judicial policy which can lead to the incorporation within its jurisdiction of vast domains of international law that are still *terra nullius*.[256]

151. This new role has been aptly described as one directed to "confirm and articulate the aggregate of principles of international law in respect of present conditions of international society, contributing more to the establishment and consolidation of the international legal system and even peaceful relations between States than a variety of cases dealing with secondary aspects which rather serve to inflate the statistics".[257] Or, in the writings of a most experienced author, the transition of the Court "marks the end of an international court as an instrument for applying Euro-centered inherited international law and the start of its conversion into the organ of truly universal international law applied in an international community for which the Charter is the controlling instrument".[258]

### IV.3 The issue of compulsory jurisdiction in the light of a new role of the ICJ

152. The question of compulsory jurisdiction has haunted both the Permanent Court and the present Court, all sorts of equations being proposed to strengthen the judicial capacity of the respective Courts.[259] This is not the occasion to examine such proposals but a fundamental issue needs to be raised. Is international society likely to evolve towards the establishment of a truly compulsory jurisdiction of the Court? The answer, even in the medium and long term, seems to be negative. The possibility of having an international court based on

256. For the concept of *terra nullius* see Condorelli, loc. cit. note 234, pp. 399-400.

257. Abi-Saab, loc. cit. note 242, p. 295 (translation by the Rapporteur).

258. Rosenne, loc. cit. note 221, p. 470.

259. See generally L. Gross: "Review of the role of the International Court of Justice", 66 AJIL (1972) pp. 479-490; L. Damrosch (ed.): *The International Court of Justice at the Crossroads* (1987).

a system of compulsory jurisdiction similar to that known in domestic courts does not appear to be in the reach of the 21st century. But not even the limited form of voluntarily accepted compulsory jurisdiction embodied in the optional clause or some other similar mechanism appears to be much in the favour of the international community, although there have been specific acceptances in certain areas and regional groupings. The fact that only one third of the UN Member States, and only one of the permanent members of the Security Council, have accepted the compulsory jurisdiction of the Court under the optional clause seems to confirm this perspective. The situation might be different if the acceptance of jurisdiction is discussed in terms of the listing of a limited number of particular issues or matters, an approach that was extensively discussed in the period 1899-1907 and at other times.[260] It is suggested that this limited option should be further explored.

153. This outlook might appear to be contradictory to the trend of States to accept many forms of compulsory jurisdiction under other arrangements for dispute settlement, security affairs and other questions. Yet, no such contradiction exists in fact since the reluctance of States to accept compulsory jurisdiction is related to the nature of the respective tribunals or arrangements. Unlike the case of specialized courts and tribunals, or unlike the particular situation of regional courts,[261] it is highly improbable that States would be willing to submit their disputes in a generally compulsory manner to a Court of general nature under international law, such as the ICJ. The uncertainties surrounding international law in many respects conspire against a general court deciding on those very issues in a compulsory manner, while this uncertainty is significantly reduced in the case of

260. For list of matters subject to compulsory arbitration in the Russian proposal and amendments in 1899 and the British and Portuguese proposals in 1907, see Scott, op. cit. note 2, pp. 60, 392. See also L. B. Sohn: "Draft General Treaty on the Peaceful Settlement of International Disputes", 20 *The International Lawyer* (1986) pp. 281-284.

261. On the compulsory jurisdiction of the ICJ as accepted in the European Convention for the Peaceful Settlement of Disputes of 29 April 1957, see I. Seidl-Hohenveldern, "Le règlement des différends en Europe au-delà du Marché Commun", in Bardonnet, op. cit. note 23, pp. 177-179.

specialized and regional legal orders. Moreover, the consensual nature of the jurisdiction of the Court is further reinforced by the need of States to protect themselves from frivolous lawsuits and the abuse of rights inspired in political purposes.[262] Acceptance of the Court's compulsory jurisdiction continues to be perceived as a political decision, unlike the situation with respect to specialized tribunals where this decision often is of a more technical character.

154. This conclusion is not to be considered as a discouraging sign for the prospects of dispute settlement. On the contrary, to the extent that consensual jurisdiction reflects the reality of international society,[263] it can contribute to achieve a system in which States will have greater confidence for the submission of their disputes. In fact, the interminable discussions about objections to jurisdiction in order to escape judicial action contribute little to the effectiveness of dispute settlement.[264] Consensual jurisdiction and the particular mechanism of the present optional clause are not bad in themselves in the context of international society, although they would be hardly conceivable in the structured organization of a domestic legal system.[265]

155. The above considerations do not mean at all that things should remain as they are. First, the mechanisms for consensual jurisdiction can be greatly improved and a number of interesting proposals have been made to this effect, particularly in order to avoid self-judging reservations related to domestic jurisdiction and to introduce reciprocity and other qualifications into the termination of the optional clause.[266] Second, special agreements can be greatly encouraged as the expression of consensual jurisdiction, particularly in the context

262. Rosenne, Comments cit. note 226, p. 8.

263. Bedjaoui, loc. cit. note 233, p. 19.

264. Shihata, op. cit. note 20, p. 3.

265. Comments by P. Weil, in Peck and Lee, op. cit. note 221, p. 94.

266. J. E. Noyes (ed.): *The United Nations at 50. Proposals for improving its effectiveness*, American Bar Association, Section of International Law and Practice, 1997, pp. 11-15.

of disputes between neighbours, the greatest source of disputes.[267] And third, compulsory jurisdiction will significantly advance in any event in the context of specialized disputes, regional arrangements and other situations already quite evident in contemporary practice. Furthermore, the limited option of compulsory jurisdiction mentioned above could provide an encouraging development. Since treaties will still be the principal source for the acceptance of the jurisdiction of international courts,[268] a number of developments could also be meaningful in this respect. It has been suggested, for example, that States should be encouraged to ratify the 1907 Hague Convention establishing the PCA, that some reservations to dispute settlement clauses in major multilateral treaties could be withdrawn, and that new treaties should include appropriate dispute settlement clauses.[269]

156. On the other hand, account should be taken of the fact that discussion of compulsory jurisdiction was a very different matter in 1899-1920, with a very limited number of participating States and hence of potential disputes to be submitted to the Court, than it is today with close to 200 States active in the international community. If the Court has difficulty handling the number of cases in its current docket, all of them submitted under some form of consensual jurisdiction, it would not appear a wise suggestion to dramatically increase the potential number of submissions under a general system of compulsory jurisdiction. In addition, judicial settlement continues to be a rather exceptional type of dispute settlement since most conflicts are resolved by means of other procedures,[270] a situation that is not likely to change in the foreseeable future. In this connection, it would seem more appropriate to emphasize the strengthening of the general rule rather than the exception. Because of this exceptional nature of judicial dispute settlement, the absence of compulsory jurisdiction in a Court of general nature does not seem to affect the thrust of the evolution of the international legal order and society itself.

267. Merrills p. 233.

268. Comments by the Government of China to the Preliminary Report, p. 3.

269. Comments by the Government of the UK to the Preliminary Report, pp. 2-3.

270. Shihata, op. cit. note 20, p. 1.

157. All of the above relates to the contentious jurisdiction of the Court, which as noted is not likely to be the only feature of its evolution. If the matter is looked upon from the perspective of its suggested new constitutional role in respect of the principles of international law, then compulsory jurisdiction might acquire a different meaning. The attitude of the international community towards the perfecting of the basic principles governing the international legal order should be more open than in respect of procedures that directly involve a disputed matter. This step of course assumes a further isolation of the decision at the domestic level from political perceptions about the Court's intervention in dispute settlement. Although some questions of a constitutional kind might reach the Court by way of the submission of a dispute, this would probably be limited by the same restrictions affecting contentious jurisdiction generally. It follows that such a new role of the Court can be better achieved in part by the strengthening of its advisory functions and in part by the participation of the Court in a more structured and institutionalized process of dispute resolution.

## IV.4 Expanding the advisory functions of the ICJ

158. In the light of past experience and the record of the Court, the exercise of its advisory function has proven to be an effective manner to deal with questions involving the basic principles of international law. A number of interesting proposals have been made to expand this function of the Court, some of which entail simultaneously access of entities other than States to the Court. Some of these proposals could further contribute to the strengthening of its place in an international society increasingly shaped by both States and other actors. This enhanced role, always to be exercised with judicial prudence, would strengthen significantly the final authoritative interpretation of the law by the Court.

159. The proposal to authorize the UN Secretary-General to request advisory opinions from the Court on legal questions connected with

the discharge of his or her responsibilities[271] has been received with mixed feelings and some criticism.[272] Some of this criticism is well-founded, particularly where it concerns giving the control of such a powerful tool to the Secretary-General, of risking requests on secondary issues and, above all, of eventually upsetting the delicate balance between the primarily administrative functions of the Secretary-General and the political functions of the Security Council and the General Assembly. While the Secretary-General has important political power under Article 99 of the Charter, he has exercised it sparingly because of these difficult balances. Because of these problems, it is feared that he might be put in an impossible political situation, in addition to the fact that the very political organs of the United Nations have not favoured this initiative. The possibility has also been raised of the Secretary-General requesting advisory opinions in matters that fall clearly within his authority[273] and that consequently would be deprived of political connotations. Important questions of law fall in fact under his responsibility, for example in terms of the immunities of UN officials, in respect of which the power to request advisory opinions should be recognized.[274] It is suggested accordingly that the power to request advisory opinions be given to the Secretary-General within the scope of his administrative functions. To this end, the independent advice of a Special Committee of Legal Experts (that will be explained below) could be helpful.

271. UN Secretary-General, op. cit. note 137, para. 38.

272. For comments on this proposal see S. M. Schwebel: "Fifty Years of the World Court: A Critical Appraisal", *Proceedings of the American Society of International Law*, 1996, p. 347. For critical views see A. Pellet: Report on "Strengthening the role of the Court as the Principal Judicial Organ of the UN", in Peck and Lee, op. cit. note 219, p. 245, and the literature cited in note 269 thereto. See also Comments Rosenne cit. note 226, p. 9; Corell, note 232, p. 12; China, note 268, p. 4, and UK, note 269, p. 5.

273. Corell, Comments cit. note 232, p. 12.

274. Such a request might have an important role in strengthening the immunities of experts on mission in respect of legal process, as evidenced e.g. by the 1989 *Mazilu* advisory opinion and by the ECOSOC request for an advisory opinion in the case of lawsuits filed in Malaysian Courts against a Special Rapporteur of the UN Commission on Human Rights; see ICJ, Communiqué No. 98/26, 10 August 1998, and No. 98/27, 12 August 1998.

160. Additional UN organs and specialized agencies might also be so authorized, as well as other inter-governmental organizations.[275] The development of the concept of UN organs has led to the establishment of various autonomous institutions, but none of these have thus far been authorized to request advisory opinions, a situation that could be remedied without particular difficulty.[276] It has also been suggested that treaty organs composed of representatives of States could be similarly authorized, unlike the case of treaty organs composed of individuals.[277] Under this last suggestion, organs such as the Assembly of States Parties to the Statute of the ICC or the Meeting of States Parties under UNCLOS could be authorized to request advisory opinions from the Court on legal questions relating to their activities.[278] In a number of these situations there will be no need for an amendment of the Charter, while in other cases the necessary legal authority may be found by way of interpretation rather than of formal amendments. Similar developments as to the power to request advisory opinions might be expected in the context of other Tribunals, notably the International Tribunal for the Law of the Sea. Major regional organizations, such as the OAS or the OAU might also be empowered to request advisory opinions from the Court. A most promising suggestion has also been made to the effect that States and intergovernmental organizations might be authorized to request advisory opinions from the PCA under a new optional rule for this purpose, a development that would not contradict the 1907 Convention.[279] In all such developments, however, it should be first ascertained that the organization or organ in question has a role of significance so as to require the eventual clarification of major points of international law.

275. Pinto, loc. cit. note 253, pp. 292-293.

276. Rosenne, Comments cit. note 226 (24 November), p. 2.

277. Ibid., p. 2-3.

278. Ibid., p. 3.

279. Ibid., at p. 4.

161. Proposals have also been made to authorize NGOs and individuals to request advisory opinions.[280] In this respect, however, there is a serious concern about the risk of introducing heavily politicized issues within the ambit of the Court or else of distorting the nature of the judicial system envisaged. This option might be justified in the future to the extent that such entities find a clearly established role in the international community and satisfy accepted standards of professionalism, accountability and transparency. The distinction made in the Antarctic Treaty System, as to granting the status of observer, between non-governmental organizations of a scientific or professional character and those engaged in activities of a political nature, might be useful to keep in mind in this context of access to the advisory functions of the Court. Once again, the advice and reporting of a Special Committee appears to be a necessary condition for the request of advisory opinions.

162. States themselves could also be authorized to request advisory opinions from the Court following the model of the American Convention on Human Rights.[281] In the case of an individual State this option might be combined with the possibility of a referral mechanism by its highest court (as will be discussed further below).[282] The joint request of an advisory opinion by two or more States as an alternative to the submission of a contentious case is also a useful approach.[283] However, as with any request for an advisory opinion, it should be first ascertained that the position of other interested parties is not circumvented. These alternatives may be combined appropriately with the practice of binding advisory opinions which is already available in the context of disputes involving international

280. See, for example, Pinto, loc. cit. note 253, p. 292.

281. L. B. Sohn: "Important Improvements in the Functioning of the Principal Organs of the United Nations that can be made without Charter Revision", 91 AJIL (1997) p. 660, for a reference to Art. 64 of the 1964 American Convention on Human Rights allowing OAS members to consult the Court on the interpretation of the Convention and related treaties.

282. Comments by the Advisory Committee on International Law Issues of the Dutch Ministry of Foreign Affairs on the Preliminary Report, para. 4. 3. 3.

283. Sohn, loc. cit. note 281, p. 660.

organizations,[284] including the difficult question relating to disputes on rules of *jus cogens*.[285] Nothing prevents either that two States might apply to the Security Council for this organ to request an advisory opinion in the context of the settlement of a dispute between such States.[286] Also, as noted above, a new procedure might be made available under the PCA.

163. The interesting precedent set by the advisory opinions associated with the work of the UN Administrative Tribunal, which in fact allowed for individuals to bring their case before the Court, would also make possible the extension of similar procedures to other disputes involving individuals, an alternative which in due course might be useful in the light of the trends of international society.[287] While in these cases individuals did not personally appear before the Court, nothing should prevent a special procedure to this effect if needed.

164. The expansion of the advisory functions of the Court might also be associated with important institutional arrangements. UNCLOS provides for advisory opinions of the Sea-Bed Dispute Chamber of the International Tribunal for the Law of the Sea, at the request of one-fourth of the members of the Authority, when an issue arises about the conformity with the Convention of a proposal before the Assembly. This precedent might be adapted to a similar situation and vote requirement in the UN General Assembly and the role of the Court in a parallel context.[288] Proposals to lower the two-thirds majority currently required to request an advisory opinion by the

284. See, e.g., 1946 Convention on the Privileges and Immunities of the United Nations, Section 30; 1947 UN Headquarters Agreement, Section 21; for discussion: H. Corell, in Peck and Lee, op. cit. note 221, p. 10.

285. 1986 Vienna Convention on the Law of Treaties between States and International Organizations or between International Organizations, Art. 66 (2); discussion by Corell, loc. cit. note 284, pp. 10-11.

286. Rosenne, Comments cit. note 226, p. 11.

287. Sohn, loc. cit. note 281, p. 659; Pinto, loc. cit. note 253, p. 293.

288. Sohn, loc. cit. note 281, pp. 659-660.

General Assembly have also been advanced.[289] It has been rightly noted, however, that at present advisory opinions may be requested by the General Assembly or other bodies with a majority that falls short of an absolute majority of States Parties, a situation that would require correction as in the Rome Statute of the ICC by introducing special voting requirements and quorums.[290]

165. As mentioned before, the establishment of a Special Committee of Legal Experts could be a useful tool to facilitate the expansion of the advisory functions of the ICJ and help the development of its constitutional role as suggested. A proposal to have a body of this kind linked to the General Assembly has been advanced, particularly with a view to decide which requests should be forwarded to the Court.[291] This is an aspect that should be further elaborated upon. It might be suggested, for example, that such a body should be attached to but independent from the Court and its members appointed by the Court among distinguished jurists. Alternatively it could be attached to the United Nations itself. Its main task would be that of providing independent legal advice about the issues embodied in a given request for an advisory opinion, not to substitute for the independent judgement of the organ requesting such opinion or of the Court itself,[292] but simply to contribute a technical legal assessment about the nature of the request. Three main functions can be suggested in this respect: (i) advising on the appropriateness of a request for an advisory opinion by the Secretary-General so as to ensure that it falls clearly

289. Comment by L. Sohn, in Peck and Lee, op. cit. note 221, p. 67, suggesting a one-third vote requirement.

290. Rosenne, Comments cit. note 226 (24 November), pp. 1-2.

291. Sohn, loc. cit. note 281, p. 660; see also L. B. Sohn: "Broadening the Advisory Jurisdiction of the International Court of Justice", 77 AJIL (1983) p. 124; Pinto, loc. cit. note 253, pp. 293-294; Rosenne, Comments cit. note 226,pp. 11-12, pointing out that such a mechanism effect exists in the Rules of Procedure of the General Assembly (A/520/Rev.15), Annex II, Part I, paragraph 1 (a), but has never been utilized.

292. Concerns in this respect have been expressed by Guillaume, Comments cit. note 226, p. 3. See also the Report prepared by the Inter-American Juridical Committee of the OAS on the Preliminary Report, as the outcome of a Study Group for which the Rapporteur was K. Highet; Doc. OEA/Ser.Q,CJI/doc.79/98, 27 August 1998, pp. 4-12.

within his authority under the Charter, or in connection with requests made by certain categories of authorized entities;
(ii) reporting on the legal issues embodied in a request made by the authorized entities so as to clearly separate such issues from political questions, a report that might be annexed to the request for consideration by the Court; and
(iii) providing it with a kind of *amicus curiae* brief in matters that the requests for advisory opinions raise in connection with issues of substance in the development of principles of international law, interpretation of basic treaties or other significant rights and questions. The Committee might indeed constitute a roster of qualified jurists the Court could call upon as *amicus curiae*. The specific role and modalities of such a body should be defined in the context of the new functions envisaged for the dispute-settlement system and the role of the Court therein.

166. The identification and precision of the guiding principles of international law, even in terms of the discussion of customary international law, is often done today by means of the legal opinions of the UN Legal Counsel, who is called upon to perform this task by organs or governments. The Special Committee of Legal Experts could also have a role in this respect, in connection with matters the Legal Counsel might wish to submit to it for consultation and advice. When such opinion of the Legal Counsel is required with urgency, it could be issued as a preliminary opinion subject to further consultation with the Committee if the circumstances so justify.[293]

## IV.5 Toward a greater role of the ICJ in institutionalized dispute settlement arrangements

167. The central role envisaged for the Court can also be strengthened by means of its greater participation in institutionalized arrangements

293. Conversation with Mr. Thijs Büchli, Executive Secretary of the 1999 Centennial of the First International Peace Conference, 16 February 1999.

for dispute settlement. This aspect may of course refer both to advisory functions and contentious jurisdiction as the case may be.

168. The institutionalization of dispute settlement under the United Nations is perhaps the most obvious arrangement of this kind. To the extent that a greater linkage might be developed between Chapters VI and VII of the Charter, for example, the possibility for the Security Council to recommend a referral of a legal dispute to the Court under Article 36 (3) of the Charter will become a more common procedure, and may even be considered as a new basis for its jurisdiction.[294]

169. Questions concerning the maintenance of international peace and security, while posing difficult issues in terms of the eventual concurrent intervention of political and judicial bodies,[295] also provide for an opportunity of reciprocal referrals by means of which one body will refer to the other a dispute more related to the latter's principal functions, either judicial or political. However, just as political bodies are not supposed to interfere with judicial decisions, not even in the case of action by the Security Council in a situation of non-compliance,[296] judicial bodies are not supposed to interfere with decisions of the political organs.[297] Desirable is that both be brought together in an institutionalized procedure for the performance of their respective roles.[298] An effort of this kind has been undertaken in the context of the interaction between the Security Council and the ICC. Possi-

294. Commentary by P. H. Kooijmans, in Peck and Lee, op. cit. note 221, pp. 63-64. On recourse to dispute settlement as a requirement for the lawfulness of countermeasures, see the proposals at the ILC and discussion in O. Schachter: "Dispute Settlement and Countermeasures in the International Law Commission", 88 AJIL (1994) pp. 471-477. See also Sohn, Draft General Treaty, cit. note 260, p. 281, art. 27.

295. Pellet, loc. cit. note 272, p. 243.

296. P. Magid, "The Post-Adjudicative Phase", in Peck and Lee, op. cit. note 221, p. 329.

297. Pellet, loc. cit. note 272, p. 247.

298. F. Orrego Vicuña: "The settlement of disputes and conflict resolution in the context of a revitalized role for the United Nations Security Council", in R. J. Dupuy (ed.): *The Development of the Role of the Security Council*, Colloque de l'Académie de Droit International (1993) pp. 41-49.

bilities of contradictory situations will always exist, in the context of which recourse to an advisory opinion of the ICJ might also be useful.

170. The institutionalized structure devised for these issues should generally ensure harmonious participation by both political and judicial bodies, thereby providing a useful precedent for the participation of the Court in other similar arrangements. The development of preventive forms of dispute resolution in the UN and other bodies will certainly provide new opportunities for the Court in this institutionalized context. In fact, on several occasions cases have been withdrawn from the Court or proceedings suspended so as to allow for negotiations or other forms of settlement, thereby combining various options conducive to the best arrangement of conflict prevention.[299]

171. An intriguing proposal along this line of ideas is to develop an *actio popularis* when fundamental interests of the international community and questions of international law are involved in a situation,[300] with particular reference to *erga omnes* obligations.[301] Not only would access to the Court be significantly broadened but also the effect of its decision would extend to the international community as a whole.[302] The practical result of this initiative would be to establish an international class action before the Court.[303] The General Assembly, States and international organizations have been suggested as entities that should be provided with the competence to bring such actions before the Court,[304] or to allow for a special right of intervention to this effect.[305] A number of pro

299. Bedjaoui, loc. cit. note 233, p. 23.

300. C. Chinkin, "Increasing the use and appeal of the Court", Peck and Lee, op. cit. note 229, pp. 50-55.

301. Rosenne, loc. cit. note 221, pp. 488-489.

302. Ibid., p. 489.

303. Rosenne, Comment cit. note 226 (24 November), p. 1.

304. Chinkin, loc. cit. note 300, p. 52.

305. Suggestion by Judge Stephen M. Schwebel in his dissenting opinion on the *Declaration of Intervention in the case of Military and Paramilitary Activities in and*
(continued...)

cedural safeguards would have to be provided in this context, particularly in order to protect minority rights and so as not to prejudice the consensual nature of the Court's jurisdiction in contentious cases.[306] Here again, the alternative of advisory opinions seems to be the best suited.[307] While such proposals have been received with caution,[308] it has been considered that while today an *actio popularis* may be brought by any State in respect of the violation of obligations *erga omnes* in the context of a case under the jurisdiction of the Court,[309] the broader concept of an *actio popularis* might be justified in the light of the needs of the international community provided adequate safeguards are built into its operation.

172. The appointment of an Advocate-General at the Court has also been discussed.[310] The intervention of this official could be justified in the context of the procedure for an *actio popularis* and similar innovations. The purpose of a function of this kind is to bring the fundamental issues and interests of international law and society to the attention of the Court, a development that might become necessary in the context of its new role. This is to an extent the role of the Advocate-General in the European Court of Justice, which of course responds to a more integrated system of administration of justice. In the case of the ICJ a similar function has been exercised in respect of advisory opinions by the UN Legal Counsel.[311] This aspect could be developed further in conjunction with the suggested Special Committee of Legal Experts, which as mentioned above could have a

305. (...continued)
*Against Nicaragua,* ICJ Reports 1984, p. 215, at p. 223; and see Chinkin, loc. cit. note 300, at p. 52, note 33.

306. Rosenne, Comment cit. note 226 (24 November), p. 1.

307. Ibid.

308. Corell, Comment cit. note 232, p. 13.

309. Guillaume, Comments cit. note 226, pp. 2-3.

310. Chinkin, loc. cit. note 300, pp. 52-56.

311. Rosenne, Comment cit. note 226, p. 13.

role in presenting before the Court relevant *amicus curriae* briefs in cases that would so justify.[312]

## IV.6 Broadening access to the ICJ

173. The advisory functions of the Court and the many modalities and prospects discussed above, clearly indicate that international organizations and other entities may have direct access to it in that context. This still leaves contentious jurisdiction closed to entities other than States in the strict terms of Article 34 of the Statute. Yet, to the extent that States are no longer the exclusive actors of the international community there is no fundamental reason why this restriction should not be relaxed to that very extent. Indeed, there is an opinion supporting some degree of broader access to the Court by international organizations.[313] Any such development would of course have to be restricted to the ambit of competence of the qualifying international organizations. Access to the Court for other entities, such as NGOs, corporations and individuals, has also been suggested,[314] but this could only become a likely development once these entities would satisfy the conditions discussed above and their role would have become recognized in the international community.

174. It should be noted that the development of a system of international criminal justice is directly concerned with the submission of individuals to those jurisdictions, an element that will probably have a strong influence in the role of individuals before other types of international jurisdictions. Such a system, as embodied in the ICC,

312. See the role of the independent body of experts in the context of the 1988 Convention against Illicit Traffic in Narcotic Drugs and Psychotropic Substances and the 1971 Convention on Psychotropic Substances, and discussion by Michael Bothe: "Conflict settlement in the field of international drug control", in Bardonnet, op. cit. note 23, p. 155.

313. Bedjaoui, loc. cit. note 233, p. 27; Schwebel, loc. cit. note 272, p. 347. The initiative does not seem to find political favour at the UN: see GA Res 52/161 of 15 December 1997.

314. Pinto, loc. cit. note 253, pp. 292-294.

obviously relies for the most on the acceptance and co-operation of the States concerned.

175. Interesting interpretations have been advanced how to broaden access to contentious proceedings before the ICJ without necessarily amending the Statute. First, it has rightly been argued that Article 34 does not have to be understood as referring only to independent States but can also include any defined political entity with power to conduct its own foreign affairs, even in limited spheres.[315] Second, it has also been pointed out that even if individuals cannot appear as parties before the Court, they may participate in contentious proceedings and present their own case with the assistance of the parties.[316] Questions of diplomatic protection, denial of justice[317] and generally the protection of human rights[318] lend themselves well to this approach. Access by States generally, and eventually by other entities, might also be facilitated by recourse to ad-hoc chambers, particularly in view of the fact that a summary procedure limited to a single pleading by each party is to be utilized, or the parties may agree to, or the Chamber decide on, further limited pleadings, thus expediting the time required for a decision,[319] and in view of the role of the litigants in selecting the members of the Chamber, a matter in which the Statute has been liberally interpreted.[320] The organization of the Court in chambers of a binding nature might also be considered, but this would probably require an amendment of the Statute.

315. Rosenne, loc. cit. note 221, p. 487.

316. Ibid., at 487-488. For the participation of individuals in proceedings before the European Court of Human Rights, see J. A. Carrillo Salcedo: "Le système de Strasbourg. Reformes à apporter au système", in Bardonnet, op. cit. note 23, p. 409.

317. Rosenne, loc. cit. note 221, p. 488.

318. P. Leuprecht: "Protection internationale des droits de l'homme et répression des crimes individuels internationaux", in Bardonnet, op. cit. note 23, p. 67; and C. Salcedo, loc. cit. note 316, pp. 401-402.

319. Art. 92 of the Rules of the Court. A summary procedure limited to two pleadings by each party was agreed in the *Frontier Dispute (Burkina Faso/Mali),* ICJ Reports 1986.

320. S. M. Schwebel: "Ad Hoc Chambers of the International Court of Justice", 81 AJIL (1987) pp. 831-854.

176. The precedents established in terms of direct access of individuals by the Court of Justice of the European Union, the International Tribunal for the Law of the Sea, the PCA, ICSID, the Iran-United States Claims Tribunal[321] and other arrangements, will no doubt have an influence when the time comes for considering access of individuals to courts dealing with the broader views of international law. Indeed, nothing prevents that the Court might wish to use its powers under the present Statute to ascertain directly the position of an individual in a case at hand.[322]

## IV.7 A Court of reference for international law

177. Two further attractive lines of thought have been advanced to strengthen the role of the ICJ. One is the referral by other international tribunals of issues of general international law that are not within the sphere of their specialized jurisdiction.[323] The other is a similar referral by high domestic courts.[324] In both cases Article 177 of the Treaty of Rome (1950) offers an important precedent, particularly in terms of ensuring the uniform interpretation of the community law where a variety of courts are likely to intervene in its application.[325] However, the point has been made that this procedure bears no analogy with the ICJ.[326]

321. Pinto, loc. cit., note 252, at 292.

322. Rosenne, Comments cit. note 226, p. 14.

323. G. Guillaume, "The future of international judicial institutions", 44 ICLQ (1995) p. 848, and discussion by R. Y. Jennings: "The proliferation of adjudicatory bodies: Dangers and Possible answers", in Boisson de Chazournes, op. cit. note 235, p. 2.

324. Pinto, loc. cit. note 253, p. 294, referring to early works by H. Lauterpacht. See also S. M. Schwebel, "Preliminary Rulings by the International Court of Justice at the Instance of National Courts", 28 *Virginia Journal of International Law* (1988) p. 495; S. Rosenne, "Preliminary Rulings by the International Court of Justice at the Instance of National Courts: A Reply", 29 *Virginia Journal of International Law* (1989) p. 401.

325. Merrills, p. 251.

326. Rosenne, Comments cit. note 226, p. 15.

178. Referral by international tribunals by way of a request for an advisory opinion of the Court[327] appears to be a feasible alternative that ought to be encouraged. Even if these tribunals may lack authority to do so under their own statutes,[328] such authority may be provided by the UN General Assembly or other policy-making bodies, within the broader authorization to request such opinions discussed above, particularly if the Tribunal in question is related to the United Nations. The alternative of an appeal before the Court[329] or some form of review or cassation[330] appear lesss feasible because it assumes a formal judicial hierarchy that is not available nor likely to be available in the future in a decentralized international society.

179. Referrals by national tribunals should follow a similar distinction. The request of an advisory opinion appears to be a viable procedure, unlike a formal appeal or other recourse that will be closely linked to the question of compulsory jurisdiction and the reluctance of States to accept such alternative from the Court.[331] Emulating an important precedent, the Court could be requested to give an advisory opinion on the compatibility of domestic laws with given treaties or rules of international law.[332] Normally such referrals would be concerned with questions relating to the interpretation of treaties, customary law and the general principles of international law, and national courts would not be obliged to make this referral and

327. Sohn, loc. cit. note 281, p. 660.

328. Pinto, loc. cit. note 253, p.t 295.

329. Schwebel, loc. cit. note 272, p. 347. For an appeal to the Permanent Court of International Justice by mixed arbitral tribunals, see.Manley O. Hudson: *Permanent Court of International Justice 1920-1942* (1943).

330. Jennings, loc. cit. note 323, p. 6.

331. L. Caflisch: "Reference procedures and the International Court of Justice", in L. Gross (ed.): *The future of the International Court of Justice*, Two vols., 1976, Vol. II, p. 591; and discussion by Pinto, loc. cit. note 253, p. 295.

332. Under Art. 64 of the American Convention of Human Rights any OAS member may request the Inter-American Court on Human Rights to provide an opinion "regarding the compatibility of its domestic laws, with the aforesaid international instruments"; see also Sohn, loc. cit. note 281, p. 660.

would only do so if they consider it useful for the resolution of cases before them.[333]

180. A number of procedural guarantees might be considered in order to facilitate the acceptance of this referral function of the Court. First, the Committee of Legal Experts suggested above might be requested to provide an advice on the relevance of the referral from the point of view of international law. Second, the requesting national court or international tribunal might be entitled to appoint a judge ad-hoc for the proceedings at the Court, particularly in order to ensure that the context of the case or some particular legal tradition be duly taken into consideration.[334] Third, in the context of regional courts various additional mechanisms may be considered in order to ensure the harmonization of the law with the decisions taken by a court of reference.[335] One particular problem that has been rightly pointed out and needs to be clarified is how to make sure that an advisory opinion in a referral procedure does not have an *erga omnes* effect.[336]

181. The suggestions discussed above, like many other views that aim at enhancing the role of the Court,[337] inevitably give rise to questions about its composition and structure, an aspect that will be considered in Section VI below.

333. Advisory Committee, Comments cit. note 282, para. 4. 3. 6.

334. During the negotiations for an European Economic Area an integration of the European Court of Justice and the EFTA States was considered in the context of dispute settlement; Christophe Reymond: "Institutions, decision-making procedure and settlement of disputes in the European Economic Area", 30 *Common Market Law Review* (1993) pp. 455-456. A Greek ad-hoc judge at the Court of Justice of the European Community was also discussed for the settlement of disputes in the agreement of association; Seidl-Hohenveldern, loc. cit. note 262, p. 187.

335. For the mechanisms of the European Economic Area in this respect , see Reymond, loc. cit. note 334, pp. 472-476.

336. Corell, Comments cit.. note 232, p. 15.

337. See, for example, C. G. Weeramantry: "Expanding the potential of the World Court", in N. Jasentuliyana (ed.): *Perspectives on International Law* (1995) p. 309, and the literature cited by Pinto, loc. cit. note 253, pp. 290-291.

## IV.8 Proposals aiming at reducing the uncertainties of international law

182. Many of the problems discussed above in connection with dispute settlement under the ICJ, arbitration or other similar means, are closely related to the uncertainties still surrounding international law. Indeed, States have sometimes given as a reason for their reluctance to engage in dispute settlement processes where the outcome is to be based exclusively on legal rules, that there are certain inadequacies in the nature of international law. This is of particular concern when the outcome of the process is to be a final and binding decision by a third party as in the case of arbitration and judicial settlement. Thus, it has been suggested that many core principles and rules of international law are vague or equivocal and capable of multiple interpretations. Some criticize the rules on the ground that they fail to supply adequate answers to current problems, while others find that the rules and processes offered by international law are ineffective and open to manipulation by the more powerful litigant. The following proposals on questions of codification and making of international law, teaching and research and availability of sources could help to overcome some of these constraints.

183. *(i) A new role for the ILC in the codification of international law and the research on its implementation and effectiveness.* The ILC is the body charged by the UN General Assembly with primary responsibility for promoting the progressive development of international law and its codification, and the latter function would seem to include, by definition, any necessary clarification of the rules to be codified. However, rapid technological, political and social developments in the second half of the 20th century have led to the creation of additional bodies commissioned to formulate international regulatory concepts and rules. Thus, new concepts and rules were elaborated at the Third UN Conference on the Law of the Sea, under pressure essentially from new technologies available for military and resource exploitation purposes. Similarly, international agreements in the field of human rights, and more recently, agreements regulating

activities having an impact on the environment, have been successfully formulated and negotiated outside the Commission.

184. Such a proliferation of bodies for the formulation of new legal norms and rules, while the ILC continues with its assigned tasks, in some ways mirrors developments in the field of dispute settlement, where specialized international courts and tribunals are established to function in parallel with the Court as the principal judicial organ of the United Nations. In both fields, the proliferation of bodies should be seen as a natural and logical development in response to the growing feasibility of the legal regulation of human activity for the benefit of all. In both cases "proliferation" is an essentially supplementary and complementary phenomenon, not to be seen in any way as adversely affecting the primacy of either body in its field. However, the very supplementary nature of "proliferation" must lead to consideration of new responsibilities for both the Court and the Commission.

185. Over some fifty years of its existence, the Commission has seen its role as essentially that of codifying the law on topics that were "sufficiently ripe" for its consideration, and doing so by elaborating draft articles on each selected topic for eventual adoption at a diplomatic conference. The result has been the production of meticulously researched and elegantly crafted texts which, in many instances, have become "the law" on the topic dealt with. In addition, when requested to do so by the General Assembly, the Commission has not hesitated to produce draft articles that became the foundation for urgently needed innovative legal rules and institutions, such as the Draft Code of Crimes against Peace and Security of Mankind and the Draft Statute for an International Criminal Court.

186. In addition to its function of clarifying, codifying and developing the rules of international law, a broad interpretation of the Commission's Statute might allow it to play a more comprehensive and penetrating role. Thus, the late Julius Stone, convinced that worthwhile codification activity, to be effective, required a vast extension of "our understanding of international law in the full context of its

contemporary operation", urged that the Commission be authorized "to plan, to supervise, and, in part, to carry out a wide and flexible program aimed at extending our knowledge and understanding of the operation of international law as a means of social control."[338]

187. Accordingly, he suggested that the Commission might assume the role of an "International Law Research Centre", to which could be channelled material from privately financed national research centres the world over. Such a role could materially assist and facilitate international dispute resolution in all it forms. The Commission could, for example, through a permanent working group on the subject *keep under review the implementation and effectiveness of multilateral treaties*. A report, published annually, could cover adherence to such treaties (signature, ratification, accession) and disseminate information concerning compliance, including the application of remedies for breach, ranging from collective management measures to dispute settlement.

188. Another task for a second working group might broadly be described as *co-ordination*. This group could gather current, if not advance, information on all multilateral treaty-making activity with at least four main objectives: (i) bringing to light possible duplication of effort; (ii) calling attention to inter-related studies or initiatives of relevance to ongoing treaty negotiations; (iii) noting any inconsistencies in emerging treaty provisions; and (iv) recording *lacunae* which might need to be studied with a view to coverage on a priority basis.

189. The focus of a third working group might be described as *fundamental studies*. The group would gather material and carry out studies in depth concerning the *implementation and effectiveness of international law*, evaluating its impact (or lack thereof) on the quality of life of the individual human being. The latter studies would be conceived as interdisciplinary, requiring the Commission to seek the

338. J. Stone: "On the vocation of the International Law Commission", 57 *Columbia Law Review* (1957) p. 16.

assistance of outside experts on such matters as municipal law and legislative practice, sociology, psychology and legal anthropology. Information from these studies, given wide distribution, could facilitate resolution of the delicate issues involved in the settlement of international disputes.

190. *(ii) A World School of International Law.* Just as there is a need to perfect the making of international law so as to contribute to the clarity of its rules, there is also a need for perfecting the research, teaching and training in this discipline. It is accordingly proposed that a World School of International Law be established in The Hague, drawing on the scholarly and professional resources of the various international courts and tribunals in that city as well as of the Academy of International Law and other academic institutions.

191. The World School would envisage undertaking two main tasks. First, to provide for a high-level research centre that would be at the forefront of the evolution of international law. Second, to provide for high-level teaching and training for advanced students, practising lawyers, law professors, judges, diplomats and other professions. related to the implementation and advancement of international law. Different programmes might be devised for each of these tasks, including doctoral and masters programmes for those pursuing academic interests.

192. The World School by necessity would rely on a broad network of qualified scholarly and professional institutions on a world-wide basis, which would be linked for the purpose of undertaking particular programmes. Parts of these programmes could be undertaken at such associated institutions. Advanced communications and electronic technology would be made available to this network. The World School would also work in close association with those institutions mandated to codify or develop international law so as to provide a high-quality input and contribute to satisfy their research needs.

193. Particular priority should be assigned to the active participation in the World School of scholars and qualified professionals and insti-

tutions from the developing world, so as to prevent a one-sided and exclusionary view of international law and its cultural background.

194. *(iii) A Code of International Law in the Internet.* What has been called the "congestion in the international legal order", where hundreds of different instruments deal with similar or interrelated subjects, needs to be rationalized, in part to avoid the unnecessary proliferation of rules and interpretations and in part to reduce the costs involved in negotiations, enforcement and establishment of different bodies.[339] A computerized database of the international legal order has been suggested to this effect.[340] It is accordingly proposed to organize the preparation and development, also under the guidance of the ILC, of a Code of International Law following the model of Restatements of the Law and taking advantage of the Internet legal information services and similar facilities.[341] In this context the basic principles of international law, as evidenced in State practice and international legislation, could be systematically examined in order to refine their meaning and extent and, above all, to produce the necessary commentaries on them,[342] an initiative that has been repeatedly suggested for the Commission,[343] with the advantage that a view representing more broadly the world community could be assured.

339. E. Brown Weiss: "The new international legal system", in *Perspectives on International Law* (1995) p. 66.

340. Ibid., at 81.

341. F. Orrego Vicuña: "Complexities in international law making: challenges for the International Law Commission", in United Nations: *Making better International Law, The International Law Commission at 50*, Proceedings of the UN Colloquium on Progressive Development and Codification of International Law (1998) pp. 223-225. For a model of a Restatement of the Law, see American Law Institute: *Restatement of the Law. The foreign relations law of the United States* (1987).

342. For a proposal to undertake a systematic collection of international law with commentary, see L. B. Sohn: "Making international law more user-friendly", Address to the UN Congress on Public International Law, New York, March 17, 1995, as cited by Brown Weiss, loc. cit. note 339, p. 81, note 50.

343. F. Cede: "New Approaches to Law Making in the UN-System", 1 *Austrian Review of International and European Law* (1996) p. 59.

# V. Dispute Settlement under the Charter of the United Nations

195. Three political organs of the United Nations, the Security Council, the General Assembly and the Secretary-General, share the responsibility for implementing its main purpose, viz., the maintenance of international peace and security. They each are thus equipped with important functions in connection with the peaceful settlement of disputes between States. Together with the ICJ, they offer Member States an integrated system for the settlement, and very importantly, for the prevention, of disputes.

196. Article 24 confers on the Security Council "primary responsibility" for the maintenance of international peace and security. When the Council acts in discharge of that responsibility, it does so pursuant to specific powers granted to it by all the Members of the Organization. When carrying out these duties on behalf of the membership, the Council is enjoined to act in accordance with the purposes and principles of the United Nations. To facilitate the discharge of its responsibility, the General Assembly may call its attention to situations likely to endanger international peace and security (Article 11 (3)); any Member State may bring to its attention any situation which might lead to international friction or give rise to a dispute (Article 35 (1)); and the Secretary-General may bring to its attention any matter which, in his opinion, may threaten the maintenance of international peace and security (Article 99).

197. Since modern communication systems enable information to be received in all capitals simultaneously, the usefulness of these provisions is not so much that they encourage report to the Council of the mere existence of situations, but rather that they enable it to be informed that, in the judgment of the reporting entity, those situations are threatening and, if left unheeded, could endanger peace and security. It is thus open to the Council, if it makes a like evaluation of the facts, to act at an early stage of a threatening situation, possibly

early enough to *prevent the occurrence* of open disagreement (a dispute), but more likely, given the speed with which such situations develop, to *prevent aggravation* of a dispute, and assist in resolving it.

198. The Council is empowered to act by various provisions of the Charter, and does not always indicate under which of them it is doing so. Its role in the peaceful settlement of disputes derives mainly from Chapter VI of the Charter which empowers it *inter alia* to investigate any dispute or situation which might lead to international friction or give rise to a dispute, to call on disputants to settle their dispute by peaceful means, and to recommend to the parties involved, at any stage, appropriate procedures or methods of settlement, including resort to regional arrangements and agencies.[344]

199. The power of the Security Council to act under Articles 36 and 37 when a particular dispute or situation has arisen is not dependent on a request by one or other of the States involved, or on their consent at that stage. Every Member State by the mere fact of its adherence to the Charter is deemed to have given its consent to the Council's acting *proprio motu* in such cases. The States involved in a particular dispute or situation are thus expected to accord due weight to, and eventually comply with, "any procedures or methods of settlement" recommended by the Council, including reference of "legal disputes" to the ICJ (Article 36 (3)), with the prospect of further action by the Council under Article 94 if a party to a case fails to perform the obligations incumbent upon it under a judgement rendered by the Court; and reference of "local disputes" to regional arrangements or agencies under Article 52.

200. Chapter VII of the Charter confers on the Council, should it determine the existence of any threat to the peace, breach of the peace or act of aggression, the power (1) to call upon the parties concerned to comply with any provisional measures it deems necessary or desirable (Article 40); and (2) to make recommendations or decide

344. Charter Arts. 33 (2), 36, 37, 38 and 52.

upon (Article 39) the further measures not involving the use of armed force (Article 41), or involving the use of such force (Article 42) that must be taken to restore peace. Nor are the latter powers of the Council limited by the general "domestic jurisdiction" exception contained in Article 2 (7) of the Charter, since it is clear that even a dispute or situation within the territory of a State may lead to "*inter-national* friction", and thence to a dispute or situation that may "endanger international peace and security". States Members of the UN are required to carry out the decisions of the Council for the maintenance of international peace and security (Articles 25, 48), as are other States in certain circumstances (Articles 2 (6) and 35 (2)).

201. In the discharge of its responsibilities the Security Council investigates disputes and situations in order to determine whether they are likely to endanger international peace and security, and makes recommendations to States in specific or general terms regarding settlement of their disputes. It does so by applying the methods of good offices, inquiry and mediation which are carried out on its behalf by the Secretary-General, or by a commission composed of State representatives or eminent individuals found to be acceptable to the disputants, and acting in accordance with terms of reference worked out within the Council. Given its capacity to act under certain circumstances without invitation from the disputants, it may, in theory, act very early in order to prevent the occurrence of a disagreement among States. In practice, however, this is hardly likely to happen, and the Council's more usual role is to act to prevent aggravation of a dispute and recommend the terms, or procedures (e.g. reference to the Court or regional arrangements or agencies) for achieving a settlement, or to take more forceful measures under Chapters VI or VII of the Charter to end physical manifestations of the dispute, including the disposition of armed forces to prevent clashes between disputants, bring about disengagement of opposing forces and monitor a cease-fire, and, where domestic administration has broken down, to set up a temporary international administration while assisting local

authorities to restore order and resume control and commence reconstruction.[345]

202. Several ways in which the role of the Security Council might be developed and enhanced have been suggested by the membership and by the Secretary-General. These include making greater use of fact-finding and good offices missions or establishing various forms of UN presence; making wider use of subsidiary organs established by the Council; acting at an early stage of a dispute, if necessary, on a confidential basis, and avoiding or minimizing delay especially where disputes may develop into armed conflict; holding high (ministerial) level meetings from time to time to review the international situation; appointing the Secretary-General as rapporteur for a specified question; and recommending reference of disputes to the ICJ, or to regional arrangements or agencies.[346]

203. The Charter confers on the General Assembly the broadest powers to discuss "any questions or matters" (excluding only those coming within the "domestic jurisdiction" exception in Article 2, paragraph 7) and to make recommendations to Members or to the Security Council (Article 10). Among such questions or matters are disputes and situations which may lead to international friction, whether or not they are questions relating to the maintenance of international peace and security, of which special mention is made in Article 11. The broad scope of the Assembly's dispute-settlement powers is further confirmed by Article 14, which empowers it to "recommend measures for the peaceful adjustment of any situation, regardless of origin, which it deems likely to impair the general welfare or friendly relations among nations ...". However, Article 12 of the Charter prohibits the General Assembly from making any re-

345. For numerous examples of SC action see UN Handbook pp. 111-118; Merrills pp. 196-201.

346. See: 1982 Manila Declaration, 1988 Declaration or the Prevention and Removal of Disputes, and 1991 Declaration on Fact-finding by the United Nations in the Field of the Maintenance of International Peace and Security; also the 1989 and 1990 Reports of the Secretary-General on the Work of the Organization, docs. A/44/1, Suppl. No. 1, and A/45/1, Suppl. No. 1.

commendation with regard to a dispute or situation in respect of which the Security Council is exercising the functions assigned to it by the Charter, unless the Council were so to request.

204. In the exercise of its functions in the field of peaceful settlement of disputes, the General Assembly has on numerous occasions discussed questions and made recommendations to States which were engaged, or might engage in a dispute.[347] Soon after the inception of the United Nations, the General Assembly in 1947 established an Interim Committee to deal with disputes and situations referred to it during periods when it was not in session, and if the Security Council was unable to act because of the veto. Although the Assembly did take action occasionally on the basis of a report from the Interim Committee, the procedure has rarely been used. One of the Committee's recommendations, to use the Secretary-General as "rapporteur" for a specified question, was revived recently in the 1988 Declaration on the Prevention and Removal of Disputes. The Assembly's "Uniting for Peace" resolution[348] also aimed at being prepared to act for the event that the Security Council, then frequently paralyzed by the negative vote of a permanent member, failed to exercise its primary responsibility for the maintenance of international peace and security. The resolution established a "Peace Observation Commission" which could observe and report on the situation in any area where international tension had developed and was likely to endanger the maintenance of international peace and security; and a "Collective Measures Committee" to study and report to the Council and the Assembly on methods which might be used to maintain and strengthen international peace and security. Neither subsidiary organ appears to have been used in recent times.

205. The role of the Secretary-General in dispute settlement derives from Article 98 of the Charter, which enables him to draw attention to areas of tension and conflict, e.g. in his annual report to the General Assembly on the work of the organization, and requires him to

347. For examples see Merrills, pp. 183-184.

348. Resolution 377 (V) of 3 November 1950.

perform other functions entrusted to him by its organs; as well as from Article 99 which authorizes him, on his own initiative, to bring to the attention of the Security Council any matter which, in his opinion, may threaten the maintenance of international peace and security. The Secretary-General has used these powers with significant effect on numerous occasions to reduce tensions or prevent aggravation of a conflict, e.g. during the Cuban missile crisis in 1962, in the crisis in relations between Iran and the United States in 1979, in the Middle East, in Central America, in Cyprus, Kampuchea, Namibia, Afghanistan and Iraq.[349] Acting personally or through his representatives, on his own initiative or on the instructions of the Security Council, he carries out functions ranging from good offices and mediation and, at least in one instance, conciliation with a quasi-arbitral role[350] (peace making), to implementing the Security Council's peacekeeping and peace building initiatives.

206. Successive Secretaries-General have maintained the independence and discretion essential for the exercise of the delicate functions assigned to, or inherent in, their office. Accordingly, the 1982 Manila Declaration, the 1988 Declaration on the Prevention and Removal of Disputes and the 1991 Declaration on Fact-finding by the United Nations, all foresee an enhanced role for the Secretary-General, in general urging utilization of his authority to the fullest extent and in a timely manner, emphasizing the tension-reducing and dispute prevention aspects of his functions.

207. Although the Security Council, the General Assembly and the Secretary-General function essentially on the political plane, they are expected to do so in accordance with such legal limits as are prescribed by the treaty which brought them into existence. Indeed, the Charter emphasizes such limits when, in Article 24, it reminds the Security Council that in the discharge of its undoubtedly heavy "primary responsibility" for the maintenance of international peace and

349. See the examples in Merrills, pp. 185-191; UN Handbook pp. 128-33.

350. Ruling pertaining to the Differences between France and New Zealand arising from the Rainbow Warrior Affair, 1986, 74 ILR (1986) p. 241; 81 AJIL (1987) p. 325.

security, a responsibility clothed with broad discretion in the evaluation of emotionally charged situations, it must nevertheless "act in accordance with the Purposes and Principles of the United Nations".

208. Inevitably, therefore, tension may develop between a political organ in the exercise of its functions, and the ICJ as the "principal judicial organ of the United Nations" to which the entire membership may have direct access and which they recognize as competent in the matter of the "interpretation of treaties", the Charter being one such treaty. Although no court is likely to find it appropriate to substitute its own discretionary decision for a decision taken by an organ given the authority to exercise that discretion and engaged in doing so while dealing directly under pressure of time with the facts as they unfold, there seems no reason why a court may not evaluate the exercise of a discretion, and decide whether or not the constitutional limits placed on that discretion were observed, taking into account of course the terms of Chapter VII of the Charter.[351]

209. The Court has had occasion to consider whether it is precluded from dealing with a question or situation when the Security Council is exercising its functions in respect of it, as well as whether the efforts of another political organ to settle a dispute could proceed parallel with reference of that dispute to the Court. On the first question, the Court has declared:

> Whereas Article 12 of the Charter expressly forbids the General Assembly to make any recommendation with regard to a situation while the Court is exercising its functions in respect of that dispute situation, no such restriction is placed on the functioning of the Court by any provision of either the Charter or the Statute of the Court. The reasons are clear. It is for the Court, the principal judicial organ of the United Nations, to resolve any legal questions that may be in issue between parties to a dispute; and the resolution of such legal questions by the

351. The power of judicial review is discussed in Section VI below.

Court may be an important, and sometimes decisive, factor in promoting the peaceful settlement of the dispute.[352]

210. In the same case, having considered whether the fact that a Special Commission appointed by the Secretary-General was engaged in attempting to resolve the dispute could be seen as a bar to its jurisdiction, the Court decided[353] that the work of the Special Commission, being an "instrument for mediation, conciliation or negotiation to provide a means of easing the situation of crisis", could not be considered in itself as in any way incompatible with the continuance of parallel proceedings before it. The terms of the judgement seem to imply, however, that if the dispute had already been referred to a tribunal empowered to decide matters of fact or law in dispute between the parties, the Court might have taken a different view while those proceedings were pending.

211. It has been urged[354] that although the UN is equipped with a range of organs capable of dealing with the political, legal and enforcement aspects of international disputes, the tendency for those organs to function independently of one another may have had negative consequences. Accordingly, its effectiveness in this field could be enhanced if linkage were to be established between the responsibilities exercised by these organs so as to cover various phases of a dispute. This is intended to result in an automatic reaction to a particular crisis by each organ. Thus, if in practice, efforts undertaken under Chapter VI in order to prevent a conflict should fail, there would be an automatic transition to some form of collective action under Chapter VII. Such linkage could enhance the effectiveness of the various settlement methods employed in early phases, since the

352. *United States Diplomatic and Consular Staff in Tehran,* ICJ Reports 1980 p. 3, at p. 40. The Court reaffirms this opinion in subsequent cases: *Military and Paramilitary Activities in and against Nicaragua,* ICJ Reports 1986, p. 14; *Questions of Interpretation and Application of the 1971 Montreal Convention arising from the Aerial Incident at Lockerbie,* ICJ Reports 1992, p. 114, and in (1998) ibid.

353. Ibid., para. 42.

354. Orrego Vicuña, loc. cit. note 298, p. 41, developing an idea of Sir Brian Urquhart in *The United Nations: from Peace-Keeping to a Collective System?* (1991).

parties would be on notice that, if those methods were to fail, sanctions or the use of force by the United Nations could follow. It would also strengthen the role of the Security Council, since its decisions would gain in cogency from awareness that they were taken following exhaustive efforts at settlement, and on the basis of experience derived from them.

212. These arrangements for sequential action would need to be supplemented by increased interaction between the Secretary-General acting pursuant to Article 99 of the Charter, and the Security Council; substantially augmented facilities for information and intelligence gathering; better machinery for contingency planning, and the availability of standing forces and logistical facilities. The possibility discussed in Section IV that the Secretary-General might himself, within the scope of his functions, be authorized to request advisory opinions of the ICJ, would become a part of this new interlinkage between the main organs of the United Nations.[355]

## VI. New specialized courts and tribunals: some influences on the outlook for the ICJ

213. At the beginning of the 20th century, when efforts to institutionalize the judicial settlement of international disputes began in earnest, statesmen tended to adapt the models of their respective domestic judiciaries to the needs of a then relatively circumscribed collectivity of States. Since the establishment of the Permanent Court of International Justice in 1920 a range of international tribunals of varying scope and duration have been established. The Court of Justice of the European Union, a permanent institution given comprehensive jurisdiction under the Treaties of Rome, surely is institutionally the most advanced of these. Other ones like the Tribunals for the prosecution of war crimes in the former Yugoslavia and in Rwanda, have just begun the discharge of their important but highly

355. Orrego Vicuña, ibid., at p. 44-45.

specialized mandates. A new specialized tribunal, the International Tribunal for the Law of the Sea, dealt with its first case at the end of 1997. A number of so-called Mixed Arbitral Tribunals established in the main to decide claims against governments by foreign private parties, have completed their mandates and been wound up. Another one, the Iran-United States Claims Tribunal, is now in its 18th year. Two intergovernmental institutions, the PCA and ICSID, and an international institution of a private character, the International Chamber of Commerce, maintain arbitration facilities for governments and private commercial enterprises on a permanent basis. Other permanent institutions, like the ILO Administrative Tribunal and the Administrative Tribunals of the UN and the World Bank, are maintained to decide disputes between intergovernmental organizations and their employees. The main features of some of these tribunals have been outlined in Sections II and III above.

214. Examination of the experience of major international courts and tribunals provides an interesting outlook for their own role in the future development of international dispute settlement and inevitably suggests a number of areas in which the function of the ICJ itself might be enhanced. Ideas for enhancement of its role have been compiled before, and it is unlikely that any new compilation would be very different from that based upon the responses to the Secretary-General's questionnaire addressed to Governments,[356] and discussed by the Sixth Committee between 1971-1974, or proposed from time to time in symposia such as those edited by Leo GROSS (1976)[357] or Lori DAMROSCH (1987)[358] and in individual essays.[359] However, the

356. Responses were compiled in a Report of the Secretary-General presented to the GA at its 26th Session, UN Doc. A/8382. For a summary and comment, see L. Gross: "Review of the Role of the International Court of Justice", 66 AJIL (1972) pp. 479-490.

357. L. Gross (ed.): *The Future of the International Court of Justice* (1976).

358. L. Damrosch (ed.): *The International Court of Justice at the Crossroads* (1987).

359. E.g.: S. Rosenne: "The changing role of the International Court", 20 *Israel Law Review* (1985) p. 182-205; Weeramantry, op. cit. note 337, pp. 309-346; L. B. Sohn: "Important improvements in the functioning of the Principal Organs of the United

(continued...)

emergence of other courts and tribunals with responsibilities in areas into which the Court has not yet entered, invites the question whether renewed consideration should not be given to recognizing in or conferring upon it a wider range of competences more consistent with that implied by acceptance of it by virtually all States as their "principal judicial organ". Observations in that direction, at first inspired by analogies with the powers of domestic courts, may today be related directly to the structure and functions of contemporary international tribunals. Three categories of such observations will be considered briefly here: (1) concerning the scope of its jurisdiction in respect of the power of judicial review; (2) concerning its composition, and (3) concerning the facilities and services available to it. Questions concerning broader access to its jurisdiction and advisory functions, and referrals to it by other national or international tribunals have already been discussed in Section IV above.

## VI.1 The Court's power of judicial review

215. Few issues touching the Court have attracted such scholarly attention recently[360] as has the question of its power to review the legality of acts of UN organs.[361] Should the existence of such a power

359. (...continued)
Nations that can be made without Charter Revision", 91 AJIL (1997) pp. 658-661.

360. Professor Caflisch, noting that in the past, judicial review of decisions within international organizations had not been the subject of detailed consideration, mentions two important exceptions: W. Wengler: "Recours judiciaire à instituer contre les décisions d'organes internationaux", 44 (I) *Annuaire* (1952) pp. 224-292 (including a draft resolution); and J. Rideau: *Juridictions internationales et contrôle du respect des traités constitutifs des organisations internationales* (1969). See also 47 (II) *Annuaire* (1957) p. 275.

361. Recent studies of the question include: J. E. Alvarez: "Judging the Security Council", 90 AJIL (1996) p. 1; M. Bedjaoui: *The New World Order and the Security Council: Testing the Legality of its Acts* (19940 p p. 77-91; id.: "Du contrôle de la légalité des actes du Conseil de sécurité", in *Recueil d'études en l'honneur du professeur François Rigaux* (1993) pp. 69-110; D. Bowett: "The impact of Security Council decisions on dispute settlement procedures", 89 *European Journal of International Law* (1994) p. 5; I. Brownlie: "The decisions of political organs of the United
(continued...)

be recognized? Could the Court exercise such a power when it is not expressly conferred by its Statute? Should the power be conferred by amendment of the Statute, and what chance would such a proposal have of successfully traversing the steps prescribed by Article 108 of the Charter? Would the effects of the Court's review be effective *inter partes* only? *Erga omnes*? Prospective? Retroactive? What should be the consequences of the Court's determination of illegality? Would the action determined to be illegal be void, or voidable? Would damages be payable by the organ concerned? Could the Court prescribe other remedial measures? By what means would such measures be enforced? All such issues have of course a significant influence on the functioning of the United Nations as a dispute-settlement system.

216. At least one international court, the Court of Justice of the European Union, actually has both the power and the duty of judicial review of the legality of acts and failures to act of Union institutions (Articles 173 and 175 of the EEC Treaty). If the action instituting review is well founded, the Court is empowered to declare the illegal act void (Article 174). In addition, the Court may require the institution whose act has been declared void or whose failure to act has been declared contrary to the Treaty "to take the necessary measures to comply" with its judgement (Article 176), and in certain circumstances call upon the institution concerned, or its employees, to make good any damage caused in the performance of their duties (Article 215). Specific provision is made for enforcement of the Court's judgements (Articles 187, 192).

217. The Sea-bed Disputes Chamber of the International Tribunal for the Law of the Sea is expressly precluded from exercising jurisdiction

361. (...continued)
Nations and the Rule of Law", in R. St. J. Macdonald (ed.): *Essays in Honour of Wang Tieya* (1994) p. 91; L. Caflisch: "Is the International Court entitled to review Security Council resolutions adopted under Chapter VII of the United Nations Charter?", in N. Al-Nauimi and R. Meese (eds.): *International Legal Issues arising under the United Nations Decade of International Law* (1995) p. 633; D. Akande: "The International Court of Justice and the Security Council: Is there room for Judicial Control of Decisions of the Political Organs of the United Nations?", 46 ICLQ (1997), pp. 309-343.

"with regard to the exercise by the [International Sea-Bed] Authority of its discretionary powers", from substituting its discretion for that of the Authority, and from annulling rules, regulations and procedures of the Authority on the grounds that they are not in conformity with the parent Convention (UNCLOS). However, the same provision empowers the Chamber to decide claims "concerning excess of jurisdiction or misuse of power", as well as for damages for, *inter alia*, failure of a party to comply with its obligations under the Convention (UNCLOS, Article 189).

218. European States with close cultural affinities with one another, relatively affluent and politically stable, have moved in more or less deliberate steps from co-operation in specific areas of economic activity, through the stage of considering themselves an economic community, up to the point where the goal of complete union seems within their grasp. In the process they have established basic political institutions - an Assembly, a Council, a Commission and a Court of Justice - which share legislative, executive and judicial powers regulating to some extent a broad range of economic and social activity within their borders. While not yet completely "united" in the sense a federal State might be, the common avowed objective of these States is "ever closer union", or integration. In the hands of their political institutions including, and perhaps especially, the Court of Justice, are the powers necessary to achieve that result. The European Court is a court with compulsory, and for some cases exclusive, jurisdiction (Article 170 of the EEC Treaty). Express provision for judicial review by such a court, functioning as it does in the midst of democratic communities with a common policy directed toward "ever closer union" would seem both natural and logical. The implications of the Sea-Bed Disputes Chamber's power to decide claims "concerning excess of jurisdiction or misuse of power" in an action, say, against the International Sea-Bed Authority, have yet to be determined, but in

any event relate to a highly specialized and technically circumscribed context.[362]

219. The ICJ operates in a much broader and much less clearly delineated context than do either the European Court or the Sea-bed Disputes Chamber. In the first place, the almost 190 parties to its Statute vary widely in matters of political and social organization and outlook. They do not constitute a "community", although the term is sometimes loosely applied in referring to all of them. Secondly, although anti-majoritarian in concept, the origins and nurturing context of the power of judicial review are essentially democratic,[363] and the collectivity of States is not yet a democracy. Third, the UN Charter lacks the comprehensive, definitive and peremptory nature of a State constitution, or for that matter, of the "foundation" and supplemental treaties of the European Union. It would seem to provide a less-than-adequate regulatory and administrative infrastructure to sustain a power of judicial review as in a domestic context. Fourth, the General Assembly is not a legislative body, nor the Security Council an "executive" to which the Court could be opposed as a "judiciary" in the domestic sense, lacking as it does a comprehensive legal code, compulsory jurisdiction, and enforcement powers. For, after all, the "power of judicial review" is power in any sense only when it is recognized, accepted and obeyed. Fifth, each UN organ is allotted its own field of competence, none subordinate to the other, and often poorly delineated, making its limits more than usually difficult to determine.

220. The modern power of judicial review, originating in the fertile democratic traditions of the United States, and given form in Chief Justice MARSHALL's path-breaking judgement in *Marbury* v.

362. See L. B. Sohn: "Special Limitations on the Review of the Decisions of the International Sea-Bed Authority by the Sea-Bed Disputes Chamber of the International Tribunal for the Law of the Sea", in *Liber Amicorum for Günther Jaenicke* (1999).

363. E. Rostow: "The democratic character of judicial review", 66 *Harvard Law Review* (1952) p. 193 et. seq.

*Madison*[364] spread rapidly within Europe, and thence to colonial territories overseas. Since the end of the Second World War and the return to independence of former European colonies, the mechanism may now be found in one form or another in domestic jurisdictions across all continents.[365] Given a transnational dimension by incorporation into the treaties of the European Union, one may even speculate as to whether the power has gained enough support as to emerge as a general principle of law, ripe for adaptation in the wider international context.

221. Issues concerning the capacity of the Court to examine and determine the legality of action taken by other UN organs, touched upon in scholarly discourse in relation to some of its more recent pronouncements, have been brought into sharper focus by judgements and opinions in the *Lockerbie* and *Bosnia v. Serbia/Montenegro*[366] cases. Such issues have arisen in particular with regard to the actions of one UN organ, the Security Council which, in connection with its "primary responsibility for the maintenance of international peace and security", is authorized under Article 25 of the Charter to take decisions which all UN Members are obligated to carry out, making it the prime (if not the only) UN organ to wield substantial power. Yet, the power is a delegated one (Article 24, paragraph 1), and as noted above is to be exercised "in accordance with the Purposes and Principles of the United Nations" (Article 24, paragraph 2). The issues reflect concerns that are related not so much to the limited composition of the Council (it is, after all, in the main, a "democratically" constituted body), but to the fact that its power is essentially a power belonging to a very few States, and is exercised or mitigated by interaction among five of them.

364. 5 U.S. (1 Cranch), p. 137 (1803).

365. For a description of this development see M. Cappelletti: "The expanding role of judicial review in modern societies", in S. Shetreet (ed.): *The Role of Courts in Society* (1988) pp. 79-96.

366. ICJ Reports 1993, p. 325.

222. A mechanism that may well be used for the formal but non-binding determination of the legality of acts of UN organs already exists in the procedure for requesting advisory opinions of the ICJ (Charter, Article 96, paragraph 1; Statute, Article 65, paragraph 1). But the authority to make such requests is strictly circumscribed: besides the Assembly and the Council, authorized by the Charter to request advisory opinions "on any legal question", only other organs of the UN and those specialized agencies authorized by the Assembly may do so, and then only "on legal questions *arising within the scope of their activities*". This would seem to indicate that an opinion may be sought by "other organs" only in relation to their respective activities. It would, of course, be open to the Security Council to request an opinion concerning a "legal question" of relevance to one of its own decisions, but it may well be that time constraints and other circumstances, and its own informed judgement as to urgency might preclude this, in which case no other organ would have the authority to do so.[367] No other provisions of the Charter or the Court's Statute seem to offer a basis for judicial review. The suggestion, discussed in Section IV, of an amendment to the advisory opinion procedure permitting its use by the Secretary-General (subject to the safeguards explained), by a substantial minority of the members of an organ and by Member States in some cases, and the expanded use of these procedures, could offer a viable route enabling the ICJ to determine the legality of Security Council action. Occasions for review might continue to arise in concrete cases, as it happened in the past, and it would be for the Court to decide each time whether the circumstances warrant judicial action of that kind. It might even be open to the parties to a contentious case so to frame the issues as to move the Court to declare the legality or illegality of some action by the Council.

223. Not all would agree that in the absence of specific textual authorization in the Charter, the ICJ may make a determination of the legality of Security Council actions. In that connection it is often recalled that the Belgian proposal at the San Francisco Peace Con-

367. Possibly the General Assembly?

ference to accord the ICJ a general power to resolve disputes concerning interpretation of the Charter was not adopted.[368] One authority, having concluded from a survey of several jurisdictions that domestic courts may not undertake a review of legislative or executive acts if not expressly empowered to do so by the constitution, suggests in this respect that "... if the existence of a channel of *ex post* judicial review cannot be presumed on the domestic level, this must be even more true in the context of international organizations ...".[369]

224. On the other hand it might be suggested that the ICJ has already exercised a power of review, as evidenced by its pronouncements not unsupportive of Council action in the *Lockerbie* and *Bosnia* cases, which must have been rendered after the usual careful consideration of the issues involved. The Court's action in deliberating upon some act of the Council and concluding formally that the Council had acted in accordance with the Charter, appears to be no less "judicial review" than if such deliberation had resulted in the conclusion that the Council's action was inconsistent with the Charter and thus invalid.

225. The Appeals Chamber of ICTY rejected dicta of the Trial Chamber in the *Tadic* case that (a) the Tribunal lacked authority to review its establishment by the Security Council (citing the dictum of the ICJ in the *Namibia* case[370]) and (b) in any event, the question whether the Council in establishing the Tribunal had complied with the Charter raised "political" questions that were "non-justiciable". It held, in contrast, that the Tribunal's "jurisdiction to determine its own jurisdiction" was among residual powers which "derive from the requirements of the 'judicial function' itself", and that limitation of such powers "cannot be inferred without an express provision allowing the

368. See generally Bedjaoui, loc. cit. note 361, pp. 9-10, and documents reproduced at p. 149 et seq.

369. Caflisch, loc. cit. note 361, atp. 637.

370. ICJ Reports 1971, para. 89.

waiver or shrinking of such a well-entrenched principle of general international law".[371]

226. Citing dicta of the ICJ in the *Namibia* and *Effects of Awards of the United Nations Administrative Tribunal* cases, the Appeals Chamber concluded that ICTY did have jurisdiction to examine the plea against its jurisdiction based on the invalidity of its establishment by the Security Council, a case of what it termed "incidental" jurisdiction in order to distinguish it from "exercising judicial review as a matter of 'primary' jurisdiction", as to which it expressed no opinion. Having discussed in detail the "constitutionality" of the establishment of ICTY as a measure under Chapter VII of the Charter, the Chamber concluded that it had, in fact, been established *inter alia* "in accordance with the appropriate procedures under the United Nations Charter ..."; and "lawfully established as a measure under Chapter VII of the Charter".[372]

227. Does this "judicial review" by a judicial organ of the UN, in spite of its "incidental" character, provide precedential support for the view that the "principal judicial organ" is similarly empowered? It would seem so, although it could be argued that this was rather a case of "self-monitoring" known in some domestic jurisdictions,[373] carried out by the Security Council through an organ that it has itself established, and thus not necessarily of precedential weight.

228. As suggested in Section IV above, in spite of the potential conflict of jurisdiction that may arise between the main organs of the UN, every effort to ensure an harmonious relationship should be

371. The Prosecutor v. Dusko Tadic (Case No. IT-94-1-AR72). Decision on the defence motion for interlocutory appeal on jurisdiction, para. 19.

372. Ibid., paras. 21 and 40.

373. Swiss practice, as referred to in Caflisch, op. cit. note 361, at p. 637: "... the Parliament acts as its own watchdog".

undertaken,[374] and some specific mechanisms for resolving contradictions have been considered in respect of the decisions of the Security Council and the International Criminal Court.

## VI.2 Composition of the ICJ

229. The essential elements of the composition of the ICJ have remained unchanged from its inception nearly 75 years ago. It appears difficult to maintain that a membership of 15 judges, thought to be adequately "representative" of the "main forms" of civilization and "principal" legal systems in 1921 when the League's membership was less than 30,[375] should still be considered adequately representative of a UN membership of nearly double that number in 1946, and of nearly four times the latter number today. Moreover, if on the ILC a membership of no less than 34 is currently considered necessary for representation of "civilizations" and "legal systems", it is difficult to see how a membership of 15 could be adequate for the same purpose on the ICJ.

230. Under existing practice, geographical distribution rather than representation of civilizations and legal systems seems to be the guiding factor.[376] Although no formal agreement governs the allocation of

374. Comments by the Government of China on the Preliminary Report, at p. 5.

375. It should be noted that even the Advisory Committee of Jurists charged by the League of Nations in 1920 with making recommendations concerning the structure and functions of the Permanent Court of International Justice, when proposing a bench of 11 judges and 4 "deputy judges", would have provided for expansion of the bench to 15 judges and 6 "deputy judges". See Art. 9 of the text adopted by the Committee, *Proces-verbal of the Proceedings of the Committee*, June 16-July 24, 1920, at pp. 709-711.

376. Some regions feel particularly uneasy about the fact that these arrangements do not ensure adequate representation for the various legal traditions of those regions; see, e.g., Inter-American Juridical Committee of the OAS, Report cit. note 104, p.7.

seats on the Court[377] to geographical regions recognized by the General Assembly, there are now three seats for Asia, three for Africa and two for Latin America, whereas four seats are held by Members from West Europe, two by the Members of East Europe and one by the United States. Although the five Permanent Members of the Security Council are not guaranteed seats on the Court, they are, as a matter of practice, invariably elected to it, each usually receiving a very high plurality of votes both in the General Assembly and in the Security Council. The membership of the organization as a whole is thus sensitive to the need for the presence of judges from the Five, not merely because of their intrinsic political influence, but also because of the important relationship between the Court and the Security Council established *inter alia* by Article 36, paragraph 3, and Article 94, paragraph 2, of the Charter, as well as by Article 41, paragraph 2, of the Statute of the Court. However, the *de facto* reservation of seats for Permanent Members of the Security Council does take away five of the possible seats that might be available to qualified candidates from other countries, and the number so lost may be increased with the admission of more Permanent Members to the Security Council.

231. In contrast to the Court's membership of 15, every Member State of the European Union may nominate a judge on the Court of Justice of the Union, and every Member State of the Council of Europe may nominate a judge on the European Court of Human Rights; testimony, it seems, to the value of a broad range of national participation in the judicial process even where substantial cultural affinity subsists. Another recent international judicial body, the International Tribunal for the Law of the Sea, consists of 21 judges, provision being made for the election of at least three from each geographical region recognized by the General Assembly. In the first election the seats

377. By contrast, in the case of the ILC, the geographical distribution of members (34) is governed by GA Res. 36/39 of 1981 which calls for the election of 8 members from Africa, 7 from Asia, 3 from East Europe, 6 from Latin America and the Caribbean, and 8 from West Europe and Other States, 1 from Asia/Latin-Caribbean and 1 from Africa/East Europe in rotation. Similarly, the geographical distribution of seats on the Security Council is provided for in GA Res. 1991A (XVIII), 17 December 1963.

were allocated as follows: 5 seats to Asia, 5 to Africa, 4 to Latin America, 4 to West Europe and 3 to East Europe.[378]

232. These developments suggest that consideration might be given to the desirability of an increase in the number of Judges of the ICJ, and perhaps some modification of current election practices, in order to make it more "representative" of a UN membership now vastly expanded, but likely to grow more slowly in future. Thus, the number of judges might be increased to, say, 23, taking into account *inter alia* that the prospective increase in the number of Permanent Members of the Security Council will probably mean a corresponding increase in the number of informally "reserved" seats on the Court, reducing still further the number of places to which the generality of States could be elected. In addition, a new "gentlemen's agreement" should seek to promote opportunities for all States to have their qualified candidates elected to the Court, abandoning practices that restricted those opportunities in the past. Thus, States could agree to show restraint in the matter of successive candidacies of sitting judges, or of candidacies of their other nationals to succeed them; and a State could agree not to "claim" for one of its nationals the remainder of a term of a judge of its nationality who had died in office (a practice that seems inconsistent with the letter and spirit of the Statute), if one of its nationals had in the past completed a full nine-year term. Just as expansion and variability of the membership of the Security Council is declared by many States to be conducive to the maintenance of confidence in the Council's actions, expansion and variability of the membership of the Court could enhance confidence in, and support for, the Court in the discharge of its important responsibilities. An understanding about restricting reelection of judges to just one occasion and to require that regional groups or permanent members of the Security Council nominate more candidates that the allocated vacancies so as to allow a real

378. See *Report of the Preparatory Commission for the International Sea-bed Authority and ITLOS* (LOS/PCN/152), Vol. I, Doc. LOS/PCN/SNC.4/WP.16/Add.10, p. 223; see also the *Interim Report prepared by the Tribunal*, Doc. SPLOS/21, 9 May 1997, p. 3.

choice has also been proposed.[379] In any event, full professional dedication, independence and accountability of judges are also important elements to enhance confidence in the Court.

233. An increase in the number of judges would, of course, require an amendment of the Statute, and that could not be achieved without *inter alia* the agreement of the Permanent Members of the Security Council, as prescribed by Article 108 of the Charter. While such an increase would seem to find an independent basis in the need for broader "representation", it would already be welcome just to *maintain* operational efficiency if the Court's jurisdiction would in fact be expanded to permit access by qualified international organizations and other entities. The system of creating chambers to hear cases instituted by individuals or corporate parties, followed by the Court of Justice of the European Union might then be a model worthy of study.[380] In view of the likely increase in the number of disputes submitted to the ICJ, the organization of its work in chambers of a binding nature discussed above might find justification irrespectively of the additional access by new actors of the international system.

234. The enhanced functions of the ICJ that can be expected in the future pose two further sets of issues in respect of its structure. First, if States are no longer the sole actors of international society but share this task with international organizations of various kinds and eventually with other entities for some purposes, there no longer appears

379. Rosenne, Comments cit. note 226, pp. 16-17.

380. In this connection it may be noted that the Single European Act of 1986 amended the EEC Treaty so as to authorize the Council, acting unanimously, at the request of the Court and after consultation with the Commission and the European Parliament, to "attach to the Court of Justice a court with jurisdiction to hear and determine at first instance, subject to a right of appeal to the Court of Justice on points of law only ..., certain classes of action or proceeding brought by natural or legal persons"; Art. 11 of the Act, adding Art. 168 A to the EEC Treaty and making an addition to Art. 188. The new court is not to have competence with respect to actions brought by Member States or by Union institutions or questions referred for preliminary rulings. Since the commencement of its operation in 1990 and until the end of 1994, the CFI had dealt with over 800 cases. See L.N. Brown and T. Kennedy: *The Court of Justice of the European Communities*, 1994-1995, 1995 Up-date, at p. 12.

to be a good reason for having only State-sponsored and -elected judges. Other entities might be similarly entitled to make nominations by means of some arrangement. In this respect the intention of the original drafters to have independent nominations, that ended up badly distorted, could find a genuine meaning in this new context if the system of nominations is made broader so as to include international organizations, learned institutions and so on. This step in itself would result in a much broader representation on the Court and in facilitating the performance of its tasks.

235. Second, if the ICJ is no longer exclusively a UN organ but makes its services available to the international community as a whole, particularly in terms of the constitutional function discussed above, there would appear to be no good reason for having only the Security Council and the General Assembly intervening in the electoral process. This has been a useful procedure in the past but has ended up heavily politicized, lending a political character to the appointment of judges and to some extent to the Court itself, thus reinforcing the reluctance of States to submit a number of disputes to it. Perhaps other entities should be entitled to elect judges as well. A multi-tiered Court might better respond to the needs of the growing number of institutions likely to request its services under a new role. As with some domestic judicial systems, it is suggested in addition that the Court itself should be able to nominate or appoint a limited number of judges to the bench. Whatever the details of these new arrangements might be, the 21st century is likely to see important developments in this respect.

236. The enlargement of the number of seats on the Court has so far proven a controversial issue. There is a body of opinion that finds ample reason to support this enlargement,[381] but the justification of such an initiative has also been questioned on the ground that it would be extremely difficult to organize deliberations of 23 judges if it is

381. See, e.g., Inter-American Juridical Committee, Report cit. note 104, at p. 7.

difficult enough to do so with the present number.[382] In another view, the ILC has suffered from the enlargement of its membership,[383] and the fact that other judicial bodies work in chambers responds rather to their different nature, nor has it helped to the uniformity of their thinking; in the case of the Court it is thought that working in chambers would not muster support if their composition is not known in advance to the parties. A number of these practical or technical difficulties, however, can be solved by means of specific mechanisms or arrangements. More importantly, these practical questions do not seem to alter the fact that there is a need to ensure a better representation of an expanding international community if the Court is to remain an effective body for the judicial settlement at a global level.

## VI.3 Facilities and services available to the ICJ

237. A third and last category of observations prompted by an examination of the Court in relation to other international tribunals concerns the facilities and services made available for the performance of the Court's important mission. Though at first sight perhaps not likely to evoke substantial interest at the conceptual level, the subject is of fundamental importance because of its intimate connection with that unfailing and relentless indicator of governmental policy priorities, money. While the Court must surely be the envy of other tribunals for its access to both its own library and that of the Peace Palace, together one of the most extensive collections of works on international law anywhere in the world, it seems comparatively less well served as regards availability of legal research staff. According to a recent

382. Guillaume, Comments cit. note 226, pp. 3-4. See also C. G. Weeramantry: "Some Practical Problems of International Adjudication", 17 *Australian Year Book of International Law 1966* (1997) p. 1; and S. M. Schwebel: "Fifty Years of the World Court: A Critical Appraisal", *ASIL Proceedings 1996* (1997) p. 339.

383. Guillaume, loc. cit. note 382, p. 4; see also S. M. Schwebel: "The influence of the International Court of Justice on the work of the International Law Commission and the influence of the Commission on the work of the Court", Keynote speech, UN: *Making better International Law, The International Law Commission at 50*, Proceedings of the UN Colloquium on Progressive Development and Codification of International Law, 1998, p. 161, at p. 164.

*Yearbook* of the Court, besides the Registrar and Deputy Registrar who have a wide range of responsibilities, its legal staff comprised one Principal Legal Secretary, two First Secretaries, two Secretaries and one Legal Officer, none of them assigned to assist a particular judge on a regular basis.

238. By contrast each of the 15 judges of the Court of Justice of the European Union has three legal secretaries permanently assigned to him. In addition, the judges for each case are furnished with a thoroughly researched opinion by the Advocate-General assigned to the case. Each of the nine Advocates-General is himself assisted by three legal secretaries. Each judge of the International Criminal Tribunal for the former Yugoslavia is assigned one legal assistant. The judges of the Iran-United States Claims Tribunal each had two legal assistants and the President three, during much of the Tribunal's existence. The purpose of providing legal assistance to judges is, of course, to enable them to devote as much of their time and resources as possible to the task which they alone may perform, viz. the delicate task of judging, of deliberating and reaching conclusions on the often complex issues before them, leaving research and other preparatory work to be done by others.

239. It would seem only fitting for the judges of the "principal judicial organ" of the United Nations to have access to legal assistance on an appropriate scale. It should also be possible to consider the possibility of creating one or more posts of Advocate-General, an institution that has done much for the development of the law in several domestic jurisdictions, and of European law. But expansion of staff at these levels would require a substantially augmented budget and corresponding increases in contributions by Member States - now anathema to the handful of Members that are the main contributors to the UN regular budget. A similar attitude of those States during preparatory work for the newly constituted International Tribunal for the Law of the Sea has resulted in its 21 judges being granted the assistance of but two legal secretaries. How then might the judges of the ICJ be provided with appropriate legal research assistance? Negative responses may be expected from most governments, influenced

mainly by perceptions of the functions of the domestic judiciary. It may thus be necessary to provide such assistance without seeking an increase in its budget. Should the practice of seconding government officials to the staffs of international tribunals to assist judges of their nationalities (which apparently has been found to be consistent with Article 100 of the Charter) be permitted for the Court as well? Such officials could be compensated directly by their government (or through some regional organization) on mutually agreed terms, and would not be an item on its budget. While there is always some risk of the political independence of the research or the work being compromised by national viewpoints, this can be minimized by ensuring that no such assistant is entrusted with the consideration of matters related to that interest, a process that in any event would be controlled by the Registrar of the Court.

## VII. Continuity and Change in Dispute Settlement: Prospects for the 21st Century

240. At the dawn of the 21st century, the dispute-settlement system of the international community incorporates almost all the elements required for the adequate performance of its traditional functions and the incorporation of new functions in response to emerging needs. This has been the result of a long and continuing evolution since the 1899 Peace Conference, a process that has provided the present system with the solid foundations of both tradition and experience. A number of these elements, however, are still largely unorganized or based on rather isolated arrangements. One important task lying ahead is therefore the development of an adequately interrelated dispute settlement system providing the necessary integration of all these aspects in a broad framework of world justice.

241. At present it is possible to find a traditional system of dispute settlement for questions of international law generally, a more recent and specialized system of dispute settlement for trade and investment,

regional systems, and emerging systems in respect of criminal justice and the settlement of disputes in environmental and other matters. However, these systems have tended to develop in isolation from one another. Their interrelation, while maintaining the freedom of choice that States and parties will wish to safeguard, would provide for appropriate integration of the law and its interpretation. The constitutional function discussed above should at its time become available to all such mechanisms.

## VII.1 A dispute-settlement system in harmony with the new structure of international law

242. As international society and international law reach new stages of integration and decentralization, so the administration of international justice and dispute settlement generally will need to follow a path in full harmony with the nature of the law governing international society. This means, first, that functions of a constitutional nature will be required for the identification, interpretation and application of the governing principles of international law, a task which as suggested above can provide new opportunities for the role of the ICJ. It also means that a decentralized system of dispute settlement will always need to be available. It is only through the combination of both systems that the demands for dispute settlement will be adequately attended to, and this combination is precisely the kind of interrelations that to a large extent is still missing.

243. Two additional developments certainly ought to be encouraged in this context. The first, already well under way, is the organization of dispute settlement arrangements in specialized areas. The cases discussed above in respect of trade, investment, international organizations and other will spread over a number of other activities. The second development is the need for regional courts that might provide for the administration of justice in respect of the main regions of the world. Except for the case of Western Europe where regional courts have attained an important function, even though still largely attached to given areas of co-operation such as economic integration and

human rights, the experience in other regions has been very limited, in most cases of sectoral nature, and in not a few occasions unsuccessful.

244. Both regional courts and specialized dispute settlement arrangements could be interrelated with the ICJ for the purpose of the governing principles of international law discussed above, while keeping with their decentralized nature. The possibility of requesting advisory opinions from the Court is one integrative mechanism that might perform this task. All such arrangements in turn should be supplemented by the ADR global system that has been suggested. A fully integrated and decentralized system of international dispute settlement would thus become available to the international community.

## VII 2 Change and innovation in response to new needs

245. Besides the organizational aspects of dispute settlement, elements of change and innovation are also to be expected in response to the new needs and realities of the international community. An important new element, still based on few precedents, is the need to ensure appropriate access to international dispute settlement for other actors of the international system, in particular international organizations. The case of individuals, corporations and other non-State entities might have to be considered in due course as they become duly recognized and established actors of such a system. This will probably be the most salient feature of the system as the 21st century unfolds.

246. A second change of significance is that because the line separating international from domestic law is also fading away, international mechanisms will increasingly apply and review national legislation, as in the NAFTA Chapter 19 arrangement, just like domestic courts will also increasingly apply and rely on international law for their decisions.

247. As demands for international dispute settlement increase, other considerations will acquire importance. Expeditious procedures and prompt decisions are relevant considerations, particularly when the nature of the matter does not allow for much time, as in the case of exports, investments or other business. The cost of international justice is another important consideration. Above all, there is the question of ensuring transparency and professionalism so that trust and fairness will guide the system and it is perceived to be so guided, a goal that has on occasion proven elusive in the past.

## VII 3 Establishing a special committee of independent legal experts

248. While arrangements to perfect the system of international dispute settlement are carried out, a process that necessarily will require time and effort, some proposals might be implemented from the outset. A first such proposal concerns the establishment of the Special Committee of Independent Legal Experts discussed in Section IV above, attached to but independent from the ICJ or the UN Organization as a whole. The tasks of the Committee, as outlined above, would facilitate the performance of expanded functions by the Court, the UN Legal Counsel and other bodies, and would help to organize some aspects of a broader policy of access to the Court. Linkages with the alternative dispute resolution procedures discussed could also be facilitated by such a body.

249. Another proposal, dealing specifically with conciliation arrangements, is discussed below.

## VII.4 Ensuring the availability of options

250. The experience gathered in a century of efforts to perfect dispute settlement arrangements shows that conflicts and disputes arise between States because their governments pursue interests that are inconsistent with, or opposed to, one another. As rightly noted by one

author, "the fact of the matter is that states are often less interested in settling a dispute than in having their view prevail."[384] As governments act out of a sense of mission, often related to a *raison d'état*, and supported by public opinion, most international disputes are likely to be political, even if they are presented in terms of legal "rights" and "responsibilities". While the situation may be different in respect of disputes involving non-State entities, an attempt to deny or ignore an inter-State dispute's political character, or to "depoliticize" it by forcing it into a legal straitjacket might oversimplify the issues involved, and may not help to resolve the dispute, let alone serve the ends of justice. Thus, while the Charter correctly reminds States that "legal disputes should as a general rule be referred to the ICJ", it preserves the disputants' traditional choices as to the means by which disputes should be settled.

251. Whether or not a State will engage in a particular method of dispute settlement is a matter for decision by the government of the day, and the central motivating factor behind that decision is likely to be the government's need or desire to be shown to be *in the right*. Any decision by a third party that a government's position is untenable may be seen as unwarranted criticism of the quality of its governance and not be welcome. A government's initial reaction upon dealing with a dispute could thus be to remain secure in its sovereignty and belief in the correctness of its view of the matter, and not to contemplate *any* method of settlement. However, if the cost of a continuing dispute were to outweigh the risk of the government's being shown to be wrong, the next option is to choose a method of settlement that explores possibilities for adjustment of the situation without reaching conclusions as to the rights involved, thus leaving the disputant's freedom of action intact. A government may thus choose among negotiation, good offices, and mediation. Inquiry and conciliation, as methods which usually conclude with reports and recommendations as to terms of settlement, i.e. the opinions of neutral third parties on how the dispute might be resolved, represent a step nearer the risk of restriction on freedom of action. However, since such

384. Merrills, p. 57.

reports and recommendations will not, in the absence of agreement to the contrary, be treated as binding on the disputants, a government could still retain its freedom of action, including, most importantly, the freedom to declare itself to be in the right, regardless of any conclusion reached, and to act accordingly.

## VII.5 Reducing uncertainty and risk

252. Submission of a dispute to arbitration or judicial settlement, the outcome of which is an award or judgment binding upon the disputants, deprives them of the right to act in a manner inconsistent with the award or judgement, whether or not it accords with their own views of their respective rights and interests. This is a course which many States consider fraught with uncertainties that generate an unacceptable level of risk, a situation that helps to explain why the prospects for compulsory arbitration or judicial settlement are rather limited. In the first place, the court or tribunal will decide the issues "in accordance with international law" (a court) or "on the basis of respect for law" (an arbitral tribunal), and many rules of international law are open to broad spectra of interpretation, besides being not yet adequately informed by generally accepted convictions as to what constitutes the "general good" that they are intended to protect. Moreover, what one might conceive as the "angle" of the judicial "lens" used to observe the dispute, would be a narrow one, allowing into view all that was legally relevant according to norms which might themselves be open to question, and excluding political factors not clearly within that category, unless the parties agreed to a decision *ex aequo et bono*.

253. A second element of uncertainty contributing to the perception of risk may be the existence of a substantial difference between the legal cultures of the disputants, e.g. civil law/common law, inquisitorial/ adversarial procedures. A third element that may be thought of as increasing uncertainty (and risk) to an unacceptable level, is disparities of *power* or wide differences between the capacities of the disputants to project themselves beyond their borders and to ensure

that the conduct of others will accord with, or serve its interests. The fear is then that justice will be to the strong.

254. Moreover, in this last situation the tendency is likely to be for the powerful State to favour settlement mechanisms that may be expected to apply rules of international law created under the guidance of powerful States and which it recognizes as valid, and to produce binding decisions that are readily, if not automatically, enforceable. In such cases, the weak "losing" party must comply or risk becoming the object of sanctions enacted by the powerful winner. On the other hand, should the powerful State "lose", it still has the option to refuse to comply with the settlement order, convinced that the decision against it was incorrect, if not biased. It may do this with impunity because it need not fear significant or prolonged retaliation from the weak "winner". It may be anticipated that the latter may eventually welcome settlement through negotiation, in which event the superior bargaining capacity of the powerful State will inevitably prevail.

255. Uncertainty as to outcome, compounded when disparities of power are present, leads the great majority of States, each of which needs to retain its freedom of action including, in particular, the freedom to re-affirm its "rightness" notwithstanding a third party's determination to the contrary, to lean away from arbitration and judicial settlement when there is a likelihood of a narrow angle of vision, and to favour methods with a broader angle of vision resulting in merely recommendatory outcomes, which could be the foundation of a negotiated settlement.

## VII.6 Exploring the prospects for conciliation

256. Taking into account the record to date of the numerous instances in which States have been prepared to accept some form of third-party-directed settlement, it appears that conciliation could be the favoured method of choice for most States in the foreseeable future. It has also been successfully applied in international disputes involving individuals, corporations and other non-State entities.

Questions of administration and cost are minimized when resorting to the services of institutionalized procedures offered by intergovernmental organizations, such as the PCA and the UN, or by well-established private institutions. While the ICJ would remain pre-eminent in its field, and arbitration or other means of judicial settlement could always be agreed upon, to give the PCA or the UN a pro-active role in conciliation might be a modest but useful step towards a more ordered world.

257. While the UN, as the organization with the broadest membership, may be the most appropriate to provide such an initiative with the institutional support it requires, it is clear that the purposes set forth in the Charter confer on that Organization, its Secretary-General and Staff, an almost infinite variety of functions and responsibilities. On the other hand, the International Bureau of the PCA is a specialized organ able to direct its full attention to dealing with the delicate issues involved in dispute prevention and resolution. The location of the latter at The Hague, away from the arena of international political controversy and the glare of publicity which attends initiatives undertaken by the UN, could be an advantage. To combine the capabilities of these two organizations could produce useful results.

258. In such an arrangement, it might be proposed that if disputants fail to consider or agree upon a method of settlement, or an agreed method has not been implemented or has remained without success for a specific period, the dispute is referred to a *Permanent Conciliation Committee* to be established by Resolution as a subsidiary organ of the General Assembly.[385] This referral might be made at the request of any UN Member or the Secretary-General, accompanied by the pertinent background note and statement of facts. Such a body could be composed of a limited number of States with equal geographical distribution, say, 20 States, with five each representing Africa, Asia,

385. While conciliation is generally favoured, doubts have been expressed about the convenience of establishing a new permanent organ that could restrict the freedom of choice inherent in this method, Comments by the Government of China on the Preliminary Report, pp. 5-6.

Europe and the Americas; designations would follow a strict order of rotation on the basis of the alphabetical list of the UN Members, and service would be limited to a number of months, for example six months. A proposed alternative to avoid the problems of excessive rotation is to use for this purpose the members of the Bureau of the General Assembly, which are available for a whole year.[386] The Chairman would also be elected on a rotational, monthly basis. The Committee could meet in private each month to review situations occurring worldwide on the basis of information supplied by any Member State or the Secretary-General.

259. Upon receipt of the request for conciliation, the Chairman would designate a Conciliation Team of a limited number of members, i.e. two members from the region of the dispute, three from outside, and the Chairman. This Team could be organized and assisted by the International Bureau of the PCA as the "executing agency",[387] provided with the necessary specialized staff by the UN Secretary-General acting in consultation with his colleague of the PCA, and have all expenses met from the regular budget of the United Nations. The Team could travel to the region of the dispute and to the countries concerned, and prepare within a strict time limit a report to the Permanent Conciliation Committee, setting out the facts as well as making recommendations for settling the dispute. The Committee would decide, again within strict time limits, whether or not to adopt the report, if necessary to require further evidence, and submit the adopted report to the disputants. These procedures could be combined with a request for an Advisory Opinion of the ICJ on any relevant legal question arising in connection with the implementation of the Report. If either party does not accept the recommendations, the failure of the conciliation would be reported to the Security Council.

386. L. B. Sohn: "Broadening the Role of the United Nations in Preventing, Mitigating or Ending International or Internal Conflicts that Threaten International Peace and Security", *International Rule of Law Center Occasional Papers*, Second series, No. 1, 1997, at 35-37.

387. The International Bureau of the PCA has expressed its willingness to performs these functions; see the Initial Comments on the Preliminary Report, June 1998, pp. 2-3.

If recommendations are accepted they could eventually be recorded in a formal agreement between the parties, the implementation of which might be assisted by the UN if required. The procedures in the Committee would be kept strictly confidential until the recommendations are eventually accepted by the disputants.

260. The proposed Permanent Conciliation Committee would seem to meet a number of aspects which have been favoured by States in past and recent experiences, particularly in terms of conciliation giving due weight to legal principles while also taking into account a range of political considerations and equities, and minimizing the impact of power.[388] The objective of conciliation in bringing the disputants together and recommending a course of action likely to restore amicable relations is also fully ensured by means of a process of "quiet diplomacy" conducted with utmost discretion and confidence. No party would be seen as being "at fault" and neither the sovereignty nor even the sensitivities of a State would be affected by the efforts of the Committee. The pro-active role performed by such a body would permit the undertaking of early initiatives on the basis of institutionalized vigilance.

261. The location of this Committee within an existing intergovernmental organization would greatly facilitate its establishment, since this could be done by Resolution of the UN General Assembly under Articles 10-12, 14, 22, 34 and 35 of the Charter, and by action of the Permanent Administrative Council under Articles 47-49 of the 1907 Hague Convention for the Pacific Settlement of International Disputes. The generality of States would be offered opportunities for participation in the work of the Committee. Delays would be minimized in the context of strict time-bound operations and costs would be held to a minimum. Institutionalized "peer pressure" might be legitimately exercised in the procedure for the adoption of reports and

388. For comments about the influence of this proposal on the objective of reducing tensions and bringing the disputants together with a view to the conclusion of an agreement, see generally Consortium on International Dispute Resolution, Consultation on the Peaceful Resolution of Major International Disputes, Report on the Preparatory Meeting, 27-28 March 1998.

assistance might be provided in the implementation of the agreement reached between disputants. The eventual association of the ICJ in terms of advisory opinions is an added institutional safeguard.

262. As discussed in Section III above, conciliation and other options also appear prominently in the ambit of Alternative Dispute Resolution, applicable to both inter-State disputes and disputes involving other public and private entities. All such developments would significantly contribute to a more ordered management of international disputes resolution.

## VIII. Summary of Proposals

263. In the course of this Report, the authors have put forward a number of proposals and suggestions. By way of conclusion these are now summed up, with reference between brackets to the paragraphs where they occur.

1. *Objective.* To develop dispute settlement mechanisms responsive to the needs of an evolving international society and international law (12), while ensuring a broad availability of methods and freedom of choice (13).

2. *Prevention.* Emphasize the prevention of international disputes (97), making available appropriate preventive methods (84), with particular reference to international peace and security (201) and peace-making (84). Increased interaction between the Security Council and the Secretary-General is suggested here with regard to information gathering and contingency planning (212).
The model of dispute prevention in environmental regimes (92) is also recommended in view of its reliance on the intention and capability to perform and on co-operation to this end (93).

3. *Institutionalization and privatization.* Provide for the institutionalization of dispute-settlement methods (99), bearing in mind the new requirements of market economies in terms of ensuring individual rights and private property (100). Develop the supplementary role of a privatized system of international justice (101). Consider the principle of subsidiarity so as to establish a kind of priority in recourse to settlement methods (108).

4. *Negotiations and consultations.* Encourage the settlement of disputes by means of negotiations and other non-adversarial methods (84). Strengthen consultations (102) by means of requirements of notification and the association of relevant interests (103), as well as by appropriate monitoring (104).

5. *Conciliation.* Establish a Permanent Conciliation Committee (258) with the participation of the PCA and the United Nations (257, 259). Establish a roster of conciliators and enlarge the appointing authority to this end (107). Develop simultaneously the role of good offices (108) and the link between these methods and arbitration (108). Develop institutionalized forms of inquiry and fact-finding (106).
Consider the new kinds of disputes arising from internal conflict with international implications (84) and provide for a broader approach in the handling of these disputes (97). Consider in particular the eventual establishment of Truth and Reconciliation Commissions with international participation (110).

6. *Mediation and the role of technical bodies.* Encourage flexible forms of mediation (111) and consider making available the role of an intermediary between disputants (112). Develop the procedures for referring disputes to technical bodies where appropriate (115). Consider the updating of treaties as to these and other methods for dispute settlement (114).

7. *Specialized methods and procedures.* Consider GATT/WTO type procedures for dispute settlement in areas involving special interests, including the variety of choices (124) and the inverted

consensus rule for the adoption of panel reports (125). In particular consider the opening of GATT/WTO procedures to individuals and corporations under a system of optional rules (126). Also consider the international control of domestic legislation available under NAFTA and other arrangements (127), with particular reference to its availability to private parties (128).
Encourage the access by affected private entities to international dispute settlement arrangements of a specialized nature, as available under ICSID (130), the UNCC (131), the World Bank Inspection Panel (132) and the International Administrative Tribunals (133).

8. *A Global ADR system.* Develop an integrated international ADR system supplementary to the public court system (139), under the guidance of the ICJ and other tribunals (136).

9. *Arbitration.* Strengthen international arbitration by means of a greater institutionalization (117), including an International Court of Appeals or an International Court of Arbitral Awards (44). Consider the submission of issues of arbitrability to an independent body, with particular reference to the President of the ICJ (118). Provide for the enforcement of arbitral awards following the relevant precedent of ICSID (119). Consider the development of compulsory arbitration in specialized matters (117) or in respect of lists of agreed subjects (117).

10. *Developing the role of the PCA.* Strengthen the development of a wider scope of PCA involvement in arbitration (52), particularly in order to handle the tidal wave of submissions in general matters of international law that can be expected in the future (120). Enlarge the choice of arbitrators (121). Encourage the ratification of the 1907 Convention (155). Establish a mechanism for the request of advisory opinions from the PCA (160).
Further revise some of the rules of the PCA with participation of experts from the World Bank and other relevant institutions so as to increase the application of such rules (120). Facilitate services of the PCA to other arbitral systems lacking adequate institutional support

(121). Provide for the participation of the PCA in the Permanent Conciliation Committee discussed above (257).

11. *A Constitutional Court.* Consider in due course the establishment of a Constitutional Court for the world community (140) so as to identify and develop the basic principles of international law governing international society (148, 150). Consider the possible role of the ICJ in this respect in addition to its normal dispute settlement functions (141), so as to establish it as the central judicial body of the international community (146).

12. *Consensual and compulsory jurisdiction of the ICJ.* Keep the system of present consensual jurisdiction as a general rule, while considering the alternative of compulsory jurisdiction in respect of a list of agreed subjects (152) and special agreements or specialized arrangements (155) and perfecting the mechanism of reservations to the optional clause (155). Consider withdrawing reservations to major multilateral treaties and include appropriate dispute settlement clauses in new treaties (155). Consider the type of jurisdiction appropriate for the exercise of a constitutional role (157).

13. *Advisory functions.* Expand the advisory functions of the ICJ (158), enabling the UN Secretary General to request advisory opinions within agreed limits (159), as well as selected UN organs and other international organizations (160). Provide a similar authorization to qualified regional organizations (160) and, in the future, to non-governmental organizations and individuals to the extent that they become recognized subjects of international law (161). Consider the request of advisory opinions by States in the context of dispute settlement arrangements (162), by individuals in institutionalized procedures such as those that were available under the UN Administrative Tribunal (163), and by some organs of international organizations in respect of the conformity of given proposals with their constitutive instruments (164). Also consider the role of advisory opinions in the context of the Permanent Conciliation Committee (261).

14. *The ICJ in institutionalized dispute settlement.* Encourage the referral of disputes to the ICJ by the Security Council (168) in institutionalized dispute settlement under the UN (167). Encourage political and judicial organs to work together with a view to effective dispute settlement and the resolution of differences by means of advisory opinions (169). Consider making available a kind of *actio popularis* in respect of fundamental interests, with appropriate safeguards (171).

15. *Access to the ICJ.* Broaden access to the ICJ: for international organizations (173), as well as through a broader interpretation of statehood (175). Consider mechanisms for the appropriate appearance or participation by individuals in State-sponsored proceedings (175), without prejudice to a broader role of individuals in the future (176). Encourage the use of chambers and consider the establishment of binding chambers (175), including one for the eventual access of individuals and corporate parties (233).
Broaden the role of the Trust Fund established under the UN and under the PCA for attending the costs of proceedings, and establish similar funds for other international tribunals such as the International Tribunal for the Law of the Sea (61).

16. *Referrals to the ICJ.* Establish a mechanism for referrals of international law issues to the ICJ by other international tribunals (178) and by national courts (179). Consider the appointment of judges *ad hoc* to this end (180).

17. *Enlargement of the ICJ.* Increase the number of judges in the ICJ and promote opportunities for all States to have their qualified nationals elected (232). Require that permanent members of the Security Council and regional groups nominate more than one candidate to allow for an election (232). Provide for a mechanism of nomination by international organizations and key learned institutions (234). Consider the possibility for other entities to elect judges and for the Court to itself make some appointments to the bench (235).

18. *Advocate General.* Consider the appointment of an Advocate General to work with the ICJ (172).

19. *Independent Committee of Jurists.* Establish an independent Committee of Jurists to facilitate the role of the ICJ and the UN in dispute settlement functions (165). Provide for independent advice on the appropriateness of requests for advisory opinions (165), particularly in respect of requests by the UN Secretary General and other entities (166). Require from the Committee a report on legal issues involved in such requests, the preparation of *amicus curiae* briefs and its views on the legal opinions of the UN Legal Counsel (166). Provide for the Committee to advise on issues raised under referrals to the ICJ (180), to advise on Court-directed ADR procedures (137) and to support the role of an eventual Advocate General (172).

20. *Budget and services of the ICJ.* Increase the budget of the ICJ (239), particularly with a view to providing greater facilities and services (237). Increase the number of legal research staff (237), if necessary and appropriate, through secondment of legal experts from governments or international organizations (239).

21. *Judicial review.* Discuss the power of judicial review (215, 223) in a diverse international society (219). Consider the role of the Security Council, the Secretary-General, minority members of an organ or States as to the eventual request of an advisory opinion in this respect (222), as well as the relevant decisions of international tribunals (224).

22. *International Peace and Security.* Enhance the role of the Security Council in the maintenance of international peace and security in the context of the UN dispute-settlement functions, particularly by developing fact-finding and other activities (202). Develop the role of the UN Secretary-General in reducing tensions and dispute prevention (206). Link up Chapters VI and VII of the Charter so as to ensure an automatic or expedient transition from one to the other (211).

23. *Regional organizations.* Enable regional organizations to request advisory opinions from the ICJ (83). Consider the establishment of an Inter-American Court of Justice (83) and similar suggestions in

respect of the Afro-Asian region (84) and the League of Arab States. Consider an Inter-American understanding to refer some types of disputes to the ICJ, the revision of the Pact of Bogotá and the strengthening of fact-finding in the region (83).

24. *Research needs*. Consider the establishment of an international law research centre under the ILC in respect of multilateral treaties and their effectiveness (187, 188, 189).

25. *Code of International Law*. Develop a Code of International Law using the facilities of the internet (194).

26. *A World School of International Law*. Establish a World School of International Law at The Hague for the advanced teaching and research at the frontiers of international law (190).

# THE HAGUE AGENDA FOR PEACE AND JUSTICE FOR THE 21ST CENTURY

Conference Edition
UN Document A/54/98/Annex

This Hague Agenda for Peace and Justice for the 21st Century has emerged from an intensive process of consultation among the seventy-two members of the Hague Appeal for Peace Organizing and Co-ordinating Committees, and the hundreds of organizations and individuals that have actively participated in the Hague Appeal for Peace process. The Agenda represents what these civil society organizations and citizens consider to be some of the most important challenges facing humankind as it prepares to embark upon a new millennium.

The Agenda reflects the four major strands of the Hague Appeal:

1 Root Causes of War / Culture of Peace
2. International Humanitarian and Human Rights Law and Institutions
3. Prevention, Resolution and Transformation of Violent Conflict and
4. Disarmament and Human Security.

## PREAMBLE

The world is emerging from the bloodiest, most war-ridden century in history. On the eve of the new century, it is time to create the conditions in which the primary aim of the United Nations, "to save succeeding generations from the scourge of war", can be realized. This is the goal of The Hague Appeal for Peace.



*F. Kalshoven (ed.),*
*The Centennial of the First International Peace Conference,* 419–454.

Skeptics will say that it cannot be done. The Hague Appeal challenges this assumption. This century has seen unimagined changes. Society now has the means to cure disease and eliminate poverty and starvation. The twentieth century has also seen the creation of a set of universal norms which, if implemented, would go a long way toward making war unnecessary and impossible. We have witnessed inspiring and successful experiments with active non-violence in struggles for independence and civil rights by unarmed peoples' movements. And this century has seen the replacement of authoritarian forms of government by democratic governance and the increasing role of civil society in the affairs of humanity.

Recent years have seen outbreaks of genocide in Cambodia, Bosnia, Rwanda and Kosovo, brutal attacks against civilians and the spread of horrendous weapons of mass destruction capable of ending life on much or all of the planet. Indigenous populations continue to be denied their rights to self determination. In a great many cases, the world's governments have manifestly failed to fulfill their responsibility to prevent conflict, protect civilians, end war, eradicate colonialism, guarantee human rights and create the conditions of permanent peace.

Therefore, this historic mission and responsibility cannot be entrusted solely to governments. The Hague Appeal proposes a citizens' *Agenda for Peace and Justice for the 21st Century*. This will entail a fundamentally new approach, building on the recent model of New Diplomacy in which citizen advocates, progressive governments and international organizations have worked together for common goals. We will embrace the moral imagination and courage necessary to create a 21st century culture of peace and to develop national and supranational institutions which ultimately must be the guarantors of peace and justice in this world.

There is already much to choose from. Civil society has flourished since the end of the Cold War and launched campaigns aimed at eradicating landmines, reducing the traffic in small arms, alleviating third world debt, ending violence against women, abolishing nuclear weapons, protecting the rights of children, stopping the use of child soldiers and building an independent International Criminal Court. These grassroots efforts are having a major impact. They are succeeding because they mobilize ordinary people, because they integrate different sectors (human rights, the environment, humanitarian assistance, disarmament, sustainable development, etc.) and because they invite the full participation of women, youth, indigenous peoples, minorities, the disabled and other affected groups.

These campaigns have generated unity and cohesion and demonstrate what can be done when people are listened to instead of talked at. The Hague Appeal for Peace intends to listen, learn and then to build. Out of this process will emerge a new citizens' Agenda for Peace and Justice for the 21st Century. It is a vital and realisable goal.

## THEMES

Components of the Hague Appeal, from the conference program to the campaigns, are motivated by the following main themes.

### Traditional Failure

Traditional approaches to preventing war and building peace have by and large failed disastrously. This is evidenced by the growing brutality of warfare, and the callous disregard for civilian life in such conflicts as the Congo, Sierra Leone and Kosovo. Impunity for ethnic cleansing and for crimes against humanity is not compatible with international law. Big-power bullying tactics are not diplomacy. Sanctions that starve the poor are not solidarity. Fire brigade peacekeeping efforts are no substitute for sophisticated early warning and conflict prevention systems.

## Human Security

It is time to redefine security in terms of human and ecological needs instead of national sovereignty and national borders. Redirecting funding from armaments to human security and sustainable development will establish new priorities leading to the construction of a new social order which ensures the equal participation of marginalized groups, including women and indigenous people, restricts use of military force, and moves toward collective global security.

## Soft Power

We are profoundly encouraged that civil society and progressive governments are choosing 'soft power' paths, utilising negotiation, coalition building and new diplomacy methods of settling disputes, while rejecting the 'hard power' dictates of major powers, militaries and economic conglomerates.

## All Human Rights for All

The violation of human rights is one of the root causes of war. These violations include the denial of economic, social and cultural rights, as well as political and civil rights. The artificial distinction between these two sets of rights can no longer be tolerated. We affirm the universality and indivisibility of human rights and call for stronger mechanisms to implement and enforce human rights treaties and to afford redress to victims for the violation of their rights.

## Replacing the Law of Force with the Force of Law

The rule of law has been contemptuously ignored in contemporary conflicts. The Hague Appeal seeks to develop and promote universal adherence to and implementation of international law. It also seeks to invigorate existing institutions of international law like the International Court of Justice and to create new institutions like the International Criminal Court. Knowledge of and recourse to international law must also be made more accessible to individuals.

## Taking the Initiative in Peace-Making

It is time for people to assert their commitment to peace and - if necessary - to wrest peace-making away from the exclusive control of politicians and military establishments. Too often, peace initiatives are proposed as a last resort, with negotiations restricted to the warmongers, and imposed on those most affected, particularly women and children. Those who have suffered the most must have a place at the table when peace agreements are drawn up, with equal representation for women. If necessary, civil society should also convene peace initiatives before crises get out of control and lives are lost. This can help to turn early warning from a slogan into a reality.

## Bottom-Up Globalization

The alarming concentration of economic power and the irresponsible imposition of neo-liberal, macro-economic policies are destroying the environment, generating poverty and desperation, widening divisions and fomenting war. The Hague Appeal encourages efforts to challenge this destructive model of globalization through community-based coalitions such as the Jubilee 2000 call for debt forgiveness and through campaigns to eradicate poverty and to economically empower women.

## Democratic International Decision-Making

The United Nations system and other multilateral institutions have the capacity to be a unique and universal force for peace. Too often, however, they have been treated with cynicism, politicized and underfunded. The international system must be revived, democratized and provided with resources if it is to realise its potential in peacebuilding. In particular, we call for a Security Council that can serve human security rather than Great Power interests, and for a radical reorientation of international financial institutions to make them more transparent and accountable and to serve human rather than corporate needs.

## Humanitarian Intervention

The Hague Appeal demands the speedy and effective intervention of humanitarian forces, subject to the prescriptions of the United Nations Charter, when civilians are threatened by genocide, war crimes, crimes against humanity and extreme national disasters. It is extraordinary that so little attention has been paid to the idea of establishing a standing intervention force. Civil society should consider new forms of civilian intervention as a matter of urgency.

## Finding the Money for Peace and Starving the Funds for War

The allocation of resources is seriously distorted. Many of today's conflicts are fueled by economic greed and the grab for raw materials, while billions are spent on the arms trade and other forms of militarization. At the same time, many worthwhile peace initiatives and programs for human security suffer from a lack of funds even though governments have adopted an extraordinary series of global action plans at the historic world conferences convened during the last ten years. These priorities must be reversed. In addition to eliminating weapons of mass destruction and drastically curbing the arms trade, military budgets must be progressively reduced.

# MAIN ACTIONS - Implementing the Hague Agenda

The Hague Appeal for Peace will serve as a launch pad for several major initiatives and campaigns. Following are some of the key actions that will be highlighted at the Hague. They represent initiatives by civil society and coalitions who are looking for new partners to join their global networks. Many other actions will emerge from the conference itself.

## International Action Network on Small Arms (IANSA)

The International Action Network on Small Arms (IANSA) is a global network of NGOs dedicated to preventing the proliferation and unlawful use of small arms by pushing forward the boundaries for international action. The IANSA launch at the Hague Appeal for Peace will look at the devastating impact of the spread and misuse of small arms, outline the need for a global campaign and encourage civil society organizations to join together to tackle one of the greatest humanitarian challenges of our times.

## Global Campaign for Peace Education

A culture of peace will be achieved when citizens of the world understand global problems, have the skills to resolve conflicts and struggle for justice non-violently, live by international standards of human rights and equity, appreciate cultural diversity, and respect the Earth and each other. Such learning can only be achieved with systematic education for peace.

The Hague Appeal for Peace conference will launch a call and a campaign to support the United Nations Decade for a Culture of Peace and Non-violence for the Children of the World and to introduce peace and human rights education into all educational institutions, including medical and law schools. The campaign will be conducted through a global network of education associations and regional, national and local task forces of citizens and educators.

## Global Ratification Campaign for the International Criminal Court

At the Hague Appeal for Peace, The NGO Coalition for an International Criminal Court (CICC) will launch its global campaign for the ratification of the Rome Statute of the International Criminal Court. The ICC will be a permanent court for bringing to justice individuals accused of genocide, war crimes and crimes against humanity. To reach the target of 60 ratifications the campaign will concentrate on raising awareness and understanding of the ICC among the general public, all sectors of civil society, the news media and decision makers around the world.

## International Campaign to Ban Landmines

The International Campaign to Ban Landmines (ICBL) will unveil its first report on implementation of the Ottawa mine ban treaty and renew the call for its universal ratification. The next steps in the ICBL include universalization, ratification and implementation of this treaty which bans the use, production, stockpiling and transfer of anti-personnel mines. The ICBL also seeks to hold States Parties to the treaty to their commitment to increase mine clearance and victim assistance efforts around the world.

## Abolition of Nuclear Weapons

In June, 1998, the New Agenda Coalition (NAC) which includes seven courageous governments - Brazil, Egypt, Ireland, Mexico, New Zealand, South Africa and Sweden - challenged the Nuclear Weapons States to implement several immediate practical steps, including de-alerting all nuclear forces. They presented their agenda in a UN resolution, which was adopted in December 1998 by 114 votes to 18.

Building on this momentum, a campaign to get nuclear and non-nuclear weapon states to commence negotiations toward the rapid conclusion of a convention to abolish nuclear weapons, as mandated by Article VI of the Non-Proliferation Treaty and by the International Court of Justice, will be launched at the Hague Appeal for Peace by IALANA, INESAP, IPB, IPPNW, Abolition 2000 and Middle Powers Initiative.

## Global Action to Prevent War

At the Hague Appeal, the Institute for Defense and Disarmament Studies, Union of Concerned Scientists and World Order Models Project will launch a Global Action Plan to Prevent War. This is a comprehensive, multi-stage program for moving toward a world in which armed conflict is rare.

Global Action urges a mix of enhanced conflict prevention, peace-keeping, disarmament, and measures promoting human rights, non-violent solutions, and the rule of law. Global Action seeks to contribute to the formation of a coalition, including those concerned with non-violent means of conflict resolution and peace education, with tackling root causes of war arising from social and economic injustice, with humanitarian aid, economic development, conflict prevention, peacekeeping, and disarmament, both "conventional" and nuclear.

## Stop the Use of Child Soldiers

The Coalition to Stop the Use of Child Soldiers was formed in May 1998 by leading international Non-Governmental Organizations seeking an end to the military recruitment and use as soldiers of all children under 18 years of age, whether by governmental armed forces or armed opposition groups. At the Hague Appeal for Peace conference, the international Coalition, in cooperation with UNICEF and the Dutch Coalition to Stop the Use of Child Soldiers, will renew its call for an end to the use of children as soldiers around the world and to promote increased action by government and civil society, particularly in countries where child recruitment and participation in armed conflict continues.

## Introduction to Strand Agenda Points for *The Hague Agenda for Peace and Justice*

The agenda items for the four strands of the Hague Appeal - Root Causes of War/Culture of Peace, International Humanitarian and Human Rights Law and Institutions, Prevention, Resolution and Transformation of Violent Conflict, and Disarmament and Human Security - attempt to represent, as accurately as possible, the issues, initiatives and principles enunciated by the participating organizations. In several instances the specific language or style used for a given agenda item has been proposed by a coalition of organizations or has been reached after lengthy discussions with groups involved. In order to achieve maximum responsiveness to the many contributions received, we have neither attempted uniformity of style among the four strand sections nor eliminated a certain amount of duplication.

# ROOT CAUSES OF WAR / CULTURE OF PEACE

## 1. Educate for Peace, Human Rights and Democracy

In order to combat the culture of violence that pervades our society, the coming generation deserves a radically different education - one that does not glorify war but educates for peace and nonviolence and international cooperation. The Hague Appeal for Peace seeks to launch a world-wide campaign to empower people at all levels with the peacemaking skills of mediation, conflict transformation, consensus-building and non-violent social change. This campaign will:

- Insist that peace education be made compulsory at all levels of the education system.
- Demand that education ministries systematically implement peace education initiatives at a local and national level.
- Call on development assistance agencies to promote peace education as a component of their teacher training and materials production.

## 2. Counter the Adverse Effects of Globalization

Economic globalization has marginalized broad sections of the world's population, further widening the gap between rich and poor. The Hague Appeal for Peace supports the creation of a just global economy with special emphasis on:

- An international campaign among local, national, international and intergovernmental organizations promoting respect for labour rights.
- Democratic reform of the World Bank, the International Monetary Fund, the World Trade Organization and other international financial institutions.
- Regulation of the international financial system.

- Accountability of multinational corporations, including proposals for the granting of international charters and their revocation in cases of gross abuse and for abiding by international marketing codes and standards.
- Financing economic development from new sources, such as modest levies on international transfers of arms or funds (the Tobin tax).
- Expanding the G8 to G16 or creating an economic or environmental security council to include countries from the developing world.
- Cancellation of the crushing debts of the world's poorest countries and the odious debts inherited by democratic governments from the previous corrupt, undemocratic governments they have replaced.
- Recognition and implementation of economic, social and cultural rights, including the right to development, child rights and women's rights.

## 3. Advance the Sustainable and Equitable Use of Environmental Resources

As stated in the 1998 United Nations Development Program Human Development Report, "The world's dominant consumers are overwhelmingly concentrated among the well-off - but the environmental damage from the world's consumption falls most severely on the poor." The Hague Appeal for Peace supports initiatives to:

- Strengthen international environmental law and its implementation by, i.a., promoting the concept of a basic right to a clean and healthy environment.
- Address the problems of overconsumption and misallocation of environmental resources.
- Consider the increasingly serious problem of the inequitable allocation of water.
- Support the campaigns to save the world's forests and species (including the human kind) from environmental degradation.

- End the military destruction of the environment and in particular, the militarisation of indigenous lands.
- Identify alternative approaches to sustainable development.

## 4. Eradicate Colonialism and Neocolonialism

Indigenous and unrepresented peoples are suffering from the suppression of their right to self-determination, ethnic and cultural genocide, the violation of their cultural, language and religious freedoms, and the militarisation and nuclearisation of their lives, lands and waters. The Hague Appeal for Peace endorses:

- The efforts of colonised peoples towards the exercise of their right to self-determination.
- The eradication of colonisation, as stated under numerous international agreements including the "Declaration on the Granting of Independence to Colonial Countries and Peoples" and the "Declaration on the Rights of Indigenous Peoples".
- The maintenance of the UN Decolonisation Committee, until all non-self governing territories have implemented their right to self-determination and independence.
- The establishment of a permanent forum for indigenous peoples within the United Nations.
- An end to the dumping of the industrialized countries' toxic materials in developing countries.
- Closing down foreign military bases.

## 5. Eliminate Racial, Ethnic, Religious and Gender Intolerance

Ethnic, religious and racial intolerance and nationalism are among the principal sources of modern armed conflict. The Hague Appeal for Peace supports:

- Efforts to eliminate the political manipulation of racial, ethnic, religious and gender differences for political and economic purposes.
- The implementation of the Convention on the Elimination of All Forms of Racial Discrimination.
- Preparations for the United Nations World Conference on Racism and Racial Discrimination, Xenophobia and Related Intolerance (2001).
- The inclusion of hate crimes in the world's judicial systems.
- Education and legislation designed to overcome homophobia.
- The promotion of affirmative action until the consequences of past discrimination have been redressed.

## 6. Promote Gender Justice

The costs of the machismo that still pervades most societies are high for men whose choices are limited by this standard, and for women who experience continual violence both in war and in peace. The Hague Appeal for Peace supports:

- The active participation of women in significant numbers in all decision and policy-making forums.
- Efforts to recognise and engage the capacities of women as peace-makers.
- The implementation of the Convention on the Elimination of All Forms of Discrimination Against Women.
- The redefinition of distorted gender roles that perpetuate violence.

## 7. Protect and Respect Children and Youth

Children and youth continue to be exploited and victimized, particularly in violent conflict situations where harming children has become not only a consequence, but frequently a strategy of war. The Hague Appeal for Peace supports initiatives to:

- Ensure the universal adoption and implementation of the Convention on the Rights of the Child including the elimination of child labour and the use of child soldiers.
- Ensure humanitarian assistance and protection to children in situations of armed conflict.
- Rehabilitate and reintegrate children who have been exposed and traumatized by violent conflict.
- Recognize the role of children and youth as peacemakers by including young people in peace-building.

## 8. Promote International Democracy and Just Global Governance

The promotion of democracy at all levels of society is a prerequisite for replacing the rule of force with the rule of law. Establishing more representative and democratic decision-making processes, is a prerequisite to achieving limited, accountable regional and global governance with binding, enforceable, and equitable legislative mechanisms. The Hague Appeal for Peace endorses:

- The reform and democratization of the United Nations, including democratic strengthening of the General Assembly and extending consultative rights to civil society representatives, non-governmental organizations and parliamentarians at all levels of the UN.
- The promotion of regional institutions to advance peace through adherence to international law.
- The modification of the weighted voting formulas utilised by the International Financial Institutions (IFIs) to protect the interests of small nations.
- The recommendations of the Commission on Global Governance, including the participation of civil society in global governance.
- The reform of the United Nations Security Council to make its composition more representative and its decision-making process more transparent.

## 9. Proclaim Active Non-Violence

It is commonly assumed but has never been proved that violence and warfare are inherent in human nature. In fact, many traditions and examples show that active non-violence is an effective way to achieve social change. The Hague Appeal for Peace supports:

- Replacing the glorification of militarism with models of active non-violence.
- A campaign to eliminate, or at least reduce, violence in the media and in everyday language.
- Activities surrounding the United Nations Year for the Culture of Peace (2000) and Decade for a Culture of Peace and Non-Violence for the Children of the World (2001-2010).

## 10. Eliminate Communal Violence at the Local Level

Violence in local communities paves the way for conflicts at national and international levels. The Hague Appeal for Peace supports initiatives to:

- Reintegrate into society the young people and some of their elders who have been marginalized, often as a result of limited economic opportunities, and whose marginalization has led them into violent behaviour.
- Promote local peace initiatives, including gun exchanges, peace camps and conflict resolution training.

## 11. Enlist World Religions in Transforming the Culture of Violence into a Culture of Peace and Justice

Religions have been a cause of war but also have the potential to enable the development of a culture of peace. They must be engaged to implement paths of peace. The Hague Appeal for Peace supports:

- Interfaith, inter-religious cooperation in disarmament and global peace work.
- The promotion of religious co-existence and reconciliation.

# INTERNATIONAL HUMANITARIAN AND HUMAN RIGHTS LAW AND INSTITUTIONS

## 12. Advance the Global Campaign for the Establishment of the International Criminal Court

The Hague Appeal for Peace will support the work of the NGO Coalition for an International Criminal Court (CICC) in expanding upon its global efforts to establish the permanent International Criminal Court, through an intensive education and ratification campaign, and through active participation in the sessions of the United Nations Preparatory Commission for the International Criminal Court. The CICC will be seeking new NGO partners at the Hague Appeal and building upon valuable advocacy and networking lessons from other international treaty campaigns, such as the International Campaign to Ban Landmines.

## 13. Encourage Close Cooperation Between the Converging Fields of International Humanitarian and Human Rights Law

The Hague Appeal for Peace recognizes the increasing convergence between the fields of international humanitarian and human rights law, a development critical to the effective protection of victims of both human rights and humanitarian law violations. The Hague Appeal will advocate changes in the development and implementation of laws in both of these fields, in order to close critical gaps in protection and to harmonize these vital areas of international law.

## 14. Reinforce Support for the International Criminal Tribunals

The international criminal tribunals for the former Yugoslavia and Rwanda represent the first steps which the international community has taken since the end of World War II towards holding individuals criminally accountable for violations of international humanitarian and human rights law. The Hague Appeal will call for the indictment and arrest of alleged war criminals who remain at large. The Hague Appeal will also focus on the practices and working methods of the tribunals and the need to address accusations that they are partisan and to support a mutually constructive working relationship between the tribunals and civil society, regional and international organizations. The Hague Appeal supports the efforts of the United Nations to establish an international criminal tribunal to investigate and prosecute genocide and crimes against humanity in Cambodia.

## 15. Enforce Universal Jurisdiction for Universal Crimes: Building Upon the Pinochet Precedent

It is now generally recognized that war crimes, crimes against the peace and violations of universally recognized human rights principles are matters of global rather than merely national concern. Not every person committing a universal crime can or should be tried by the International Criminal Court once it is established, or by an ad hoc tribunal such as those for Rwanda and the former Yugoslavia. Civil society and domestic courts must do their part, as those of Spain are endeavouring to do in the case of Pinochet. The Hague Appeal will call upon national legislative and judicial systems worldwide to incorporate the principle of universal jurisdiction for such crimes as well as torts into their laws in order to ensure that serious violations of human rights, especially against children, are not treated with impunity.

## 16. Reform and Expand the Role of the International Court of Justice in the Context of a More Comprehensive System of Global Justice

The International Court of Justice must serve as the locus of a more effective, integrated system of international justice. The Hague Appeal will advance proposals for strengthening interrelationships between national, regional and international legal institutions, with the aim of fostering a more comprehensive global system of justice. Initiatives which further this aim include expanding the advisory opinion and conflict resolution functions of the court to provide access for civil society, regional and international organizations; instituting compulsory jurisdiction for states; and encouraging co-operation among international legal institutions and alternate fora for dispute resolution.

## 17. Strengthen Protection of and Provide Reparation for the Victims of Armed Conflict

Since World War Two, the focus of conflict has dramatically shifted, with the result that civilians are frequently targeted and the number of civilians wounded and killed in conflict now vastly outnumbers that of combatants. The Hague Appeal for Peace will advocate greater protection for the most vulnerable and frequent victims of conventional arms proliferation and armed conflict, including internally displaced persons, refugees, women and children. The Hague Appeal will also seek more consistent adherence to the standards of international humanitarian and human rights law by non-State combatants and quasi-state paramilitary forces and will examine the role of the United Nations in situations of armed conflict. Finally, the Hague Appeal will demand that victims of armed conflict and human rights violations be made whole through the establishment of national, regional and international victim compensation funds and other reparation measures, which address the needs of victims in a timely way.

## 18. End Violence Against Women in Times of Armed Conflict

Today, war, armed conflict and the presence of military bases impact women, adolescents and children as never before in history. Women and their families are increasingly targets of violence and war crimes including rape, sexual assault, enforced prostitution and sexual slavery. They also confront a host of problems as victims and survivors who are internally displaced, made refugees or pressured by their governments to refrain from pursuing their rights against violations committed by foreign military personnel. The Hague Appeal endorses the integration of basic protections for women into the statute of the International Criminal Court and will advocate additional changes in the development and implementation of international law, in order to secure the rights and dignity of women in armed conflict.

## 19. Stop the Use of Child Soldiers

More than 300,000 children under 18 years of age are believed to be currently participating in armed conflicts around the world. Hundreds of thousands more are members of armed forces or groups and could be sent into combat at almost any moment. The Coalition to Stop the Use of Child Soldiers, UNICEF and the ICRC are actively campaigning to increase the age of recruitment to 18. They are also appealing to governments and all armed groups to prevent the recruitment of children under the age of 18, to immediately demobilise child soldiers, and to incorporate their needs into peacekeeping, peace agreements and demobilization programs, and for the end of this unconscionable practice and for the rehabilitation and social reintegration of former child soldiers. The Hague Appeal will provide other non-governmental organizations the opportunity to contribute to these campaigns and to explore other methods by which children's rights may be protected.

## 20. Help Victims to Hold Abusers Accountable Under International Humanitarian and Human Rights Law

Recent trends in national and regional litigation and prosecution make it possible for victims of gross human rights and humanitarian law violations to hold abusers accountable. This right exists in some domestic courts and regional tribunals, including the European and Inter-American Courts of Human Rights, and has led to litigation against members of the private sector, such as mercenaries and arms manufacturing and other corporations. The Hague Appeal for Peace will advocate for the extension of this right throughout the international legal order.

## 21. Protect Human Rights Defenders, Humanitarian Workers and Whistleblowers

The year 1998 saw more civilian representatives of the United Nations killed in action than military peacekeepers. In addition, countless human rights defenders and humanitarian workers from national, regional and international organizations have been injured or killed in the course of their work. The Hague Appeal will propose and demand improvements in protection for human rights defenders and humanitarian workers in the field and mechanisms by which violations of these individuals' rights may be monitored and lessened. The Hague Appeal will also call for strengthened protection for whistleblowers; individuals who expose international law violations or other illegal actions of governments, corporations and other institutions at the risk of their careers, and sometimes their lives.

## 22. Train Grassroots Organizations to Use National, Regional and International Mechanisms in the Enforcement of International Law

There are increasing opportunities for grassroots organizations to seek remedies for violations of humanitarian and human rights laws at the local or national level through regional and international mechanisms. The Hague Appeal will provide training and awareness programs, which will heighten understanding of these remedies and how grass-roots organizations may work together or singly to ensure that access to these mechanisms is unrestrained and utilised. The Hague Appeal will also provide an opportunity for activists to learn how they may be involved in identifying violators in their communities and bringing them to account for their actions.

## 23. Promote Increased Public Knowledge, Teaching and Understanding of International Humanitarian and Human Rights Law

The increasing likelihood of international involvement in armed conflicts underscores the need for effective human rights and humani-tarian training for peacekeepers, in parallel with similar training for national military institutions, in order to promote awareness of and adherence to the requirements of international law. There is also a need for greater awareness of international humanitarian and human rights law among national lawmakers and law enforcers. The Hague Appeal for Peace will call for mandatory training in international humanitarian and human rights law for lawyers, legislators, judges and politicians.

## 24. Integrate Human Rights Protections into Conflict Prevention, Resolution and Post-Conflict Reconstruction

International and regional interventions in conflicts is a growing phenomenon in the world of conflict resolution and post-conflict reconstruction. Increasingly, the international community has taken on responsibility for political, legal, social and economic institution-building in post-conflict societies. The Hague Appeal will advocate for measures to ensure that long-term, systematic protection of human rights is central to these processes.

## 25. Build Upon the Successes and Failures of Truth Commissions and Political Amnesties

The field of post-conflict reconstruction has seen remarkable new developments over the last few decades, in particular the use of truth commissions and political amnesties as in South Africa as tools for mending societies torn apart by war, armed conflicts and apartheid. The Hague Appeal will examine the failures and successes of past truth commissions and political amnesties, as well as proposals for new truth commissions in Bosnia, East Timor and elsewhere.

## 26. Establish a Universal and Effective System of Habeas Corpus

The thousands of individuals arrested each year on political, ethnic and other illegal grounds need an effective system by which they or their representation can call attention to their plight before they are killed, tortured or disappeared. Article 9 of the International Covenant on Civil and Political Rights must be given teeth by providing for a rapid and effective system of habeas corpus, with the right of appeal to regional or supra-regional human rights commissions or courts.

## 27. Subject War-making to Democratic Controls

Nothing is more subversive of democracy than allowing the power to take a country to war to reside exclusively in the hands of the executive or military branches of government. The Hague Appeal for Peace will call on all countries and international organizations to take constitutional or legislative action requiring parliamentary approval to initiate armed conflict, except in extreme cases requiring immediate action for self-defence.

# PREVENTION, RESOLUTION AND TRANS-FORMATION OF VIOLENT CONFLICT

## 28. Strengthen Local Capacities

Too often, violent conflict is "resolved" by external actors with little or no reference to the wishes of those who must live with the solution. As a result, the solution reached is often short-lived. If efforts to prevent, resolve and transform violent conflict are to be effective in the long-term, they must be based on the strong participation of local civil society groups committed to building peace.

Strengthening such "local capacities" is vital to the maintenance of peace and may take many forms from education and training and nurturing the volunteer spirit in society, to increased funding of local peace-building initiatives and highlighting the work of local peace-makers in the media.

## 29. Strengthen the United Nations' Capacity to Maintain Peace

The United Nations still constitutes the best hope for achieving world peace through multilateral cooperation. Now more than ever, strong civil society support of the aims and purposes of the United Nations is vital to achieving its full potential as the guardian of international peace and security. In particular, this support should be directed towards the reform of the UN, leading to its greater democratisation, and towards the strengthening of the UN's capacity to prevent violent conflict, mass violations of human rights and genocide, for example, through the creation of standing UN peace forces for use in humanitarian interventions, and through the identification of alternative sources of finance for UN peace operations.

## 30. Prioritise Early Warning and Early Response

The resources expended by governments and intergovernmental bodies in efforts to prevent violent conflict are insufficient, especially when compared with the resources expended on activities that become necessary once violent conflict breaks out; humanitarian intervention, emergency relief, peace enforcement operations, and the general rebuilding of war-torn societies. Civil society must take a lead role in demonstrating that conflict prevention is possible and that it is preferable; in terms of human lives and suffering, as well as cost; to reacting to violent conflict. In particular, priority should be given to: (1) dedicating more resources to conflict prevention, (2) creating and further developing conflict early-warning networks, and
(3) generating the political will necessary to responding quickly to warnings received.

## 31. Promote the Training of Civilian Peace Professionals

The demand for civilian peace-builders, be they election monitors, human rights workers or general observers, is growing fast; the pool from which such specially trained civilians can be drawn is not. There is a strong need to further promote the specialized training of civilian women and men in the techniques of conflict resolution, mediation, negotiation, etc., and to promote their deployment in conflict areas in order to order to carry out peace-building tasks. The long-term aim should be the development of an international body of specially trained "civilian peace professionals" that can be called upon to intervene in conflict areas at short notice.

## 32. Refine the Use of Sanctions

The imposition of economic sanctions is one of the bluntest tools of international diplomacy. Sanctions have the capacity to destroy the fabric of the society against which they are aimed, as well as to inflict terrible hardship on the innocent members of that society. UN Secretary-General, Kofi ANNAN, has demanded that economic sanctions become "more effective and less injurious". To meet this demand, we must develop ways of better targeting economic sanctions so that their effect cannot be transferred from the leaders whose behaviour they are intended to change, on the one hand, to innocent civilians, on the other. In the interest of children, sanctions should not be imposed without obligatory, immediate and enforceable humanitarian exemptions, along with mechanisms for monitoring the impact on children and other vulnerable groups.

## 33. Strengthen Mechanisms for Humanitarian Intervention

In order to help avoid future acts of genocide and gross violations of human rights, it is necessary to develop mechanisms that will allow for humanitarian intervention to protect the lives of people in danger.

## 34. Engender Peace Building

Conflict and war are gendered events. After reproduction, war is perhaps the arena where the division of labour along gender lines is most obvious. Therefore, women and men experience conflict and war differently and have different access to power and decision-making. There is a need for (1) specific initiatives aimed at understanding the interrelationships between gender equality and peace building, (2) strengthening women's capacity to participate in peace building initiatives and (3) equal participation of women in conflict resolution at decision-making levels. To meet these needs, governments must commit to including women representatives of civil society in all peace negotiations; peace and security institutions must incorporate gender-sensitive perspectives into their activities and methods; and civil society must build and strengthen women's peace networks across borders.

## 35. Empower Young People

Wars are initiated by irresponsible leaders, but it is young people who are their most vulnerable victims, both as civilians and as conscripts. Their experience, fresh perspectives and new ideas must be heard, integrated and acted upon at all levels of society. There is ample evidence that young people in conflict situations can find ways to overcome traditional prejudices, to creatively resolve conflicts and to engage in meaningful reconciliation and peace-building processes. The opportunity for youth to participate in peace building is essential for breaking the cycle of violence, for reducing and avoiding conflict. Let us all share our vision, open-mindedness, solidarity and willingness to learn in a truly inter-generational exchange based on mutual respect, trust and responsibility.

## 36. Support Unrepresented Peoples' Right to Self-Determination

Many of today's violent and persistent conflicts are between states and unrepresented peoples and are characterized by an extreme power imbalance. As a result, unrepresented peoples, by themselves, often are unable to engage states in negotiations for peaceful conflict resolution. Consequently, these conflicts tend to continue for decades and result in grave suffering and cultural annihilation. To counteract the power imbalance which drives these conflicts, it is necessary for the international governmental and non-governmental community to actively support peoples' right to self-determination, to prioritise these conflicts and to promote their non-violent resolution.

The denial of the right to self-determination has led to numerous long-term conflicts, most of which remain unresolved. It is important to recognize that it is not the right to self-determination which leads to conflict, but rather the denial of this right. It is therefore imperative that the internationally recognized right to self-determination be actively promoted as a tool of conflict prevention and conflict resolution.

## 37. Strengthen Coalition-Building Between Civil Society Organizations

The diversity of civil-society activity in the area of conflict prevention, resolution and transformation is one of its main strengths. However, the effectiveness of civil society activity is often hampered by a lack of coordination between groups operating in similar fields.

The result is often that scarce resources are wasted through the duplication of tasks and the failure to achieve synergy. To increase effectiveness in this area, it is vital to create networks that promote coalition- and constituency-building between Civil Society Organizations.

## 38. Strengthen Regional and Sub-Regional Capacities for Peace

Strengthening regional capacities for peace, for example, in the form of the Organization for Security and Cooperation in Europe (OSCE), the Organization for African Unity (OAU), the Association of South East Asian Nations (ASEAN), the Organization of American States (OAS), etc., would help to ensure that largely ignored conflicts receive the attention, and efforts at resolution, that they deserve.

## 39. Mainstream Multi-Track Diplomacy

In the next century, we must aim to make "multi-track diplomacy" the standard approach to preventing, resolving and transforming violent conflict. Multi-Track Diplomacy involves the cooperation of numerous sectors of society, governments, non-governmental organizations, religious groups, the media, business, private citizens, etc., in preventing conflict and building peace. It is a multi-disciplinary view of peace-building that assumes that individuals and organizations are more effective working together than separately and that conflict situations involve a large and intricate web of parties and factors that requires a systems approach. Each "track" in the system brings with it its own perspective, approach and resources; all of which must be called upon in the peace-building process.

## 40. Utilise the Media as a Pro-active Tool for Peace-building

The media play a vital, and controversial, role in situations of violent conflict. They have the capacity to exacerbate or to calm tensions and, therefore, to play an essential role in preventing and resolving violent conflict and in promoting reconciliation. Apart from their traditional role in reporting on conflict, the media may also be used to build peace in a wide variety of alternative ways. Special attention needs to be directed towards (1) promoting objective, non-inflammatory reporting of conflict situations so that the media serves the cause of peace rather than war and (2) to further explore the use of the media in creative new ways to build peace and promote reconciliation.

## 41. Promote the Conflict Impact Assessment of Policies

Civil society must encourage national, bilateral and international agencies and international financial institutions to infuse their policy formulation and implementation with conflict prevention dimensions that include (1) conflict impact assessment of proposed economic policies and development projects and (2) the introduction of institution-building and human resources-strengthening elements into various forms of dispute resolution and peace-building, i.e., mediation centres, training in negotiation skills, conflict resolution education, tolerance-building and the promotion of coexistence.

# DISARMAMENT AND HUMAN SECURITY AGENDA

## 42. Implement a Global Action Plan to Prevent War

The Hague Appeal for Peace supports the "Global Action Plan to Prevent War" that will complement measures to protect human rights and strengthen nonviolent conflict resolution with the following major steps: (1) strengthening global and regional security institutions; (2) replacing unilateral military intervention with multilateral defence against aggression and genocide; and (3) negotiating deep, phased reductions in military Forces, weapons, and budgets, aiming for a global defensive security system.

## 43. Demilitarize the Global Economy by Reducing Military Budgets and Shifting Resources Toward Human Security Programs

Peace in the 21st century demands a shift from this century's expenditures on the military to civilian programs that safeguard human security. Disarmament will entail making drastic cuts in weapons, forces and military budgets. Demilitarization will require transforming the military economy to a peace economy by allocating resources for programs that ensure the well being of the world's citizens - that provide for the basic human rights of food, shelter, education, work, health, security and peace. It will require global adherence to United Nations Charter and to the development of non-military security structures and peacemaking institutions.

As a first step toward disarmament and demilitarization, the Hague Appeal for Peace endorses the Women's Peace Petition, which calls for a 5 % reduction a year for 5 years in military spending and the re-allocation of these substantial resources toward human security programs and peace education.

## 44. Negotiate and Ratify an International Treaty to Eliminate Nuclear Weapons

The continued existence of nuclear weapons and their threat or use by accident, miscalculation or design threaten the survival of all humanity and life on earth.
In order to comply with their legal obligations under Article VI of the Non-Proliferation Treaty and the mandate of the International Court of Justice, all states should negotiate and conclude within five years a Nuclear Weapons Convention, which would prohibit the production, use and threat of use of nuclear weapons and would provide for verification and enforcement of their destruction.

The New Agenda Coalition's resolution, adopted by the 53rd General Assembly of the United Nations, calls on the nuclear weapons states to take immediate practical steps to reduce the danger of nuclear war and commence negotiations toward total nuclear disarmament.

Transitional steps toward nuclear disarmament include: ratification of the Comprehensive Test Ban Treaty; adherence to the Anti-Ballistic Missile Treaty; de-alerting; no-first use; de-nuclearization of regional security arrangements; extension of nuclear free zones; transparency of nuclear arsenals and facilities; and a ban on fissile materials and subcritical tests.

## 45. Prevent Proliferation and Use of Conventional Weapons, Including Light Weapons, Small Arms and Guns and Safeguard Personal Security

Small arms, light weapons and landmines pose a big threat to human security; their use results in the majority of civilian deaths and has made it easier to exploit young children as soldiers. Full fledged demobilization programs must reclaim and destroy weaponry and also provide former soldiers with other material benefits and vocational alternatives. The Hague Appeal for Peace endorses the campaign of the International Action Network on Small Arms and calls on all states to negotiate and implement a comprehensive global code of conduct for exports of all types of conventional weapons, including light weapons, small arms and guns.

Steps toward stopping the flow of weapons include: controlling legal transfers between states; monitoring the use and storage of small arms within states; preventing illicit transfers, including transfers to human rights violators; collecting, removing and destroying surplus weapons from regions of conflict; increasing transparency and accountability; reducing demand by reversing cultures of violence; reforming public security institutions; creating norms of non-possession; promoting more effective and sustainable demobilization and reintegration of former combatants.

## 46. Ratify and Implement the Landmine Ban Treaty

All states should sign, ratify and adhere to the 1997 Land Mine Ban Treaty, which opened for signature in December 1997 and entered into force on 1 March 1999.

In addition to the vital and urgent task of de-mining, the International Campaign to Ban Landmines puts a high priority on governments destroying their stockpiles of mines as a form of "preventive mine action." It also puts pressure on all States to develop de-mining activities. Transparency on stockpiles and other mine-related matters is essential. Increased funding should be made available for victim assistance, de-mining, mine-awareness education and rehabilitation for children and their communities.

## 47. Prevent the Development and Use of New Weapons and New Military Technologies, Including a Ban on Depleted Uranium and the Deployment of Weapons in Space

The Hague Appeal for Peace calls for mechanisms to assess the impact of new weapons (e.g. depleted uranium) and technologies and to determine if new weapons violate international law. Depleted uranium weaponry has been listed among weapons of "mass destruction or with indiscriminate effect" by the United Nations Human Rights subcommittee on the prevention of discrimination and protection of minorities. The Hague Appeal calls upon the international community to address the issue of banning the production, transfer and use of such weapons.

The Outer Space Treaty (1967) bans deployment of weapons of mass destruction in space by any nation. The treaty, ratified by 91 countries, states that nations should avoid activities that could produce harmful contamination of space as well as adverse changes in the environment of earth. This treaty requires universal adherence to prevent the deployment of weapons in space.

## 48. Encourage Universal Adherence To and Implementation Of the Biological Weapons Convention and the Chemical Weapons Convention

All States should ratify the Biological Weapons Convention (BWC) and the Chemical Weapons Convention (CWC) as part of a global effort to abolish all weapons of mass destruction. All countries should adopt strong national legislation implementing these treaties without qualifications and should participate in current efforts to enhance compliance with them. No state should take executive or legislative action that dilutes implementation of these treaties.

All state parties that are in compliance with the BWC and CWC should receive equal treatment with respect to trade in dual-purpose agents and equipment covered by these treaties. To insure international accountability, export controls should be managed by organizations established within the framework of the two conventions.

Parties to the BWC should strengthen article X, encouraging the exchange of bacteriological information and materials for peaceful purposes. Research organizations, professional societies, and individual scientists should pledge not to engage knowingly in research or teaching that furthers the development and use of chemical and biological warfare agents. The development of novel biological and chemical agents that to not have unambiguously peaceful purposes should be prohibited, even if these activities are promoted for defensive purposes.

## 49. Hold States and Corporations Accountable for the Impact of Military Production, Testing and Use on the Environment and Health

The nuclear weapons states, in particular, must acknowledge their responsibility for the health and environmental impacts of nuclear testing, production and use. The Hague Appeal calls for greater transparency and accountability of all military activities and their impact on the environment and on health. Governments must introduce or extend programs for monitoring, cleanup and rehabilitation of former military test sites and for compensation to former test site workers and civilian and military personnel at the sites and in neighbouring local communities.

The decommissioning of nuclear and chemical weapons in industrialized countries should not lead to the export of toxic chemical and nuclear wastes to developing countries. States and corporations must make information on the impact of all military production, testing and use at military bases and other sites available to ensure transparency and to facilitate restoration.

## 50. Build a Civil Society Movement for the Abolition of War

Abolishing war will require building the institutions and the capacity to safeguard and fully implement the profound achievements of the past (such as the treaties banning chemical and biological weapons, landmines and nuclear testing) as well as to bring about the difficult negotiations to eliminate all nuclear weapons and to stop the flow of small arms and light weapons. The Hague Appeal envisions a world without violence through a new code of international conduct, which restricts military power and embraces non-violence and adherence to international law.

Civil society has a central role to play in democratizing international relations and strengthening international peacemaking mechanisms. Civil society organizations and citizens have brought the demands of people directly to the international level and have created a "new diplomacy". The Hague Appeal for Peace affirms the necessary role of civil society in the 21st century in international and transnational disarmament and security negotiations.

# OUTCOME OF THE CELEBRATIONS OF THE CENTENNIAL OF THE FIRST INTERNATIONAL PEACE CONFERENCE

## REPORT ON THE CONCLUSIONS

UN Document A/54/381 and Corr.1

Report presented by the Governments of the Kingdom of the Netherlands and the Russian Federation on the conclusions of the expert discussions on the three "Centennial themes"; Peace Palace, The Hague, 18-19 May 1999, and Smolny Palace, St. Petersburg, 22-25 June 1999

## I. GENERAL OBSERVATIONS

### I.1 Introduction

1. Pursuant to United Nations General Assembly Resolutions 51/157, 52/154 and 53/99,[1] regarding the Action dedicated to the 1999 Centennial of the First International Peace Conference of 1899 and to the closing of the United Nations Decade of International Law, the Governments of the Kingdom of the Netherlands and the Russian Federation called meetings of experts for consideration of the reports and comments pertaining to the themes of the 1899 First International Peace Conference and its 1999 Centennial celebrations: disarmament questions, humanitarian law and laws of war, and peaceful settlement

1. A/RES/53/99
1. *Welcomes* the programme of action dedicated to the centennial of the first International Peace Conference, presented by the Governments of the Netherlands and the Russian Federation, which aims at contribution to the further development of the themes of the first and the second International Peace Conference and could be regarded as a third international peace conference;



*F. Kalshoven (ed.),*
*The Centennial of the First International Peace Conference*, 457–501.

of disputes. These activities were undertaken within the framework of the United Nations Decade of International Law, with a view to serving as a useful basis for carrying the results of the Decade of International Law into the next millennium.

2. The present report has been drawn up under the authority of the chairmen of the meetings at The Hague, the Netherlands, (18-19 May 1999) and St. Petersburg, Russian Federation, (22-25 June 1999) and, in Part II, reflect the outcome of the discussions on the three Centennial themes.[2] The conclusions of the expert discussions do not purport to formulate any particular formal position taken on the matter under discussion, nor are they meant to commit any delegation to a particular point of view. The report is presented by the Governments of the co-hosts "as-is", without prejudice to the position of any delegation.[3]

## I.2 Discussions on the Centennial Themes

3. On 18 and 19 May 1999 delegates, legal advisers[4] of United Nations Member States, observer States and of relevant international organizations, assembled at the Peace Palace, The Hague, to consider the legislative and normative aspects of the Centennial themes, contained in the reports conceived and revised[5] by the rapporteurs: Francisco ORREGO VICUÑA and Christopher PINTO on peaceful settle-

2. The thematic conclusions were drawn up with the help of the chairmen of the expert discussions.

3. A/RES/53/99

4. *Requests* the Governments of the Netherlands and the Russian Federation to prepare reports on the outcome of the centennial celebrations at The Hague and St. Petersburg for submission to the General Assembly at its fifty-fourth session, with a view to their consideration at the closing of the United Nations Decade of International Law.

4. Several States were represented by their Ambassador to the Kingdom of the Netherlands.

5. Based on comments posted on www.minbuza.nl/english/conferences/peace_1.html.

ment of disputes, Christopher GREENWOOD on humanitarian law and laws of war, and Hans BLIX on disarmament questions. The Centennial meeting at the Peace Palace was chaired by Hans VAN MIERLO.[6] The opening session was attended by Her Majesty Queen BEATRIX of the Netherlands, patron of the Centennial celebrations at the Peace Palace, Her Royal Highness Princess MARGRIET, chairman of the Standing Commission of the Red Cross and Red Crescent Movement, the Prime Minister, Wim KOK, and the Mayor of the city of The Hague, Wim DEETMAN.

4. Her Majesty Queen BEATRIX marked the long standing commitment of the Dutch Royal Family to the 1899 Peace Conference, which was hosted by her grand-mother, Queen WILHELMINA, and to the 1999 celebration of its Centennial with her presence at the opening session and with a reception at Noordeinde Palace for participants to the expert discussions. In her capacity as Chairman of the Standing Commission, preparing for the 27$^{th}$ International Red Cross and Red Crescent Conference, Her Royal Highness Princess MARGRIET also attended the opening session. This royal presence testifies to the commitment of the Dutch Royal Family and of Dutch society as a whole to the concepts of the international Rule of Law set by the First International Peace Conference, as well as to the position of the city of The Hague as judicial capital of the world, dating back to the days of Queen WILHELMINA. That position was also underlined at the Mayor's reception at the close of the celebrations at The Hague.

5. At the opening session delegates heard speeches[7] by the Secretary-General of the United Nations, Kofi ANNAN; the Minister for Foreign Affairs of the Kingdom of the Netherlands, Jozias VAN AARTSEN; the

6. Former Vice-Prime-Minister and Minister for Foreign Affairs of the Kingdom of the Netherlands, presently Minister of State of the Kingdom of the Netherlands, and Chairman of the Netherlands National Organizing Committee for the Centennial of the First International Peace Conference.

7. Speeches have been forwarded to member/observer States through diplomatic channels and published at the Centennial internet web-site of the Ministry of Foreign Affairs of the Kingdom of the Netherlands: www.minbuza.nl/english/conferences/peace_1.html.

former Minister for Foreign Affairs of the Kingdom of the Netherlands, chairman of the Organizing Committee, Hans VAN MIERLO; the President of the International Committee of the Red Cross (ICRC), Cornelio SOMMARUGA; the Director-General of the Organization for the Prohibition of Chemical Weapons (OPCW), José BUSTANI; the Under Secretary-General for Legal Affairs and Legal Counsel of the United Nations, Hans CORELL; the President of the International Federation of Red Cross and Red Crescent Societies (IFRC), Astrid HEIBERG; the Secretary-General of the Permanent Court of Arbitration (PCA), Hans JONKMAN; and the Peace Palace historian, Arthur EYFFINGER.[8] A message from the Vatican was also read.

6. These interventions pointed to the continued need for an international order based on the Rule of Law, and the continued duty of the international community to build peace and to prevent and suppress violations of international rules, which aim at safeguarding peace and human rights, with all appropriate means.

7. The Ambassador of the Russian Federation to The Hague, Alexander G. KHODAKOV, spoke about the Russian initiatives of 1899 and 1999, with regard to the calling of the First International Peace Conference, and to the celebration of the Centennial of that Conference.

8. Sir Ninian STEPHEN and William PACE presented the conclusions of the commemorative session of the Members of the Permanent Court of Arbitration (Peace Palace, 17 May 1999) and of the HAGUE APPEAL FOR PEACE civil society campaign (The Hague, 11-15 May 1999), respectively.

9. On the eve of its one hundredth anniversary the Permanent Court of Arbitration held a commemorative session of its members on 17 May

8. At the Peace Palace meeting, a third book by his hand was introduced, especially focussed on the 1899 Peace Conference: Arthur EYFFINGER *The 1899 Hague Peace Conference: The Parliament of Man, the Federation of the World*, published by Kluwer International.

1999, at which a resolution was adopted. The following operative paragraphs were included in that resolution:

> 1. Invites Governments of States not Parties to accede to the 1907 Hague Convention for the Peaceful Settlement of International Disputes;
> 2. Acknowledges the important role of the Government of The Netherlands, as depositary of the Conventions;
> 3. Invites Governments and International Organizations to include in treaties, agreements and commercial contracts, where appropriate, clauses referring disputes for resolution through fact-finding, mediation, conciliation or arbitration under the auspices of the Permanent Court of Arbitration;
> 4. Invites Governments, as well as intergovernmental organizations, non-governmental organizations, foundations and others who share a commitment to the peaceful solution of international disputes, to contribute to the Financial Assistance Fund, and to render to the [Permanent] Court [of Arbitration] such financial and other assistance as may be necessary to enable it effectively to maintain and enhance its capacity to administer, promote and assist in the resolution of international disputes, to act as repository of information concerning alternative methods of dispute resolution and, through seminars, conferences, studies and publications, disseminate information relating thereto.

The Chairman of this commemorative session was given the opportunity to present the conclusions of this session at the opening session of the expert meeting. Members of the PCA were encouraged to share their expertise and participate at the expert discussions on 18 and 19 May 1999.

10. On 17 May 1999 the signing ceremony took place of the Additional Protocol to the 1954 Convention on the protection of cultural goods in times of armed conflict[9] in the presence of Colin POWER, Assistant Director-General for Education of UNESCO, Adriaan BOS, Chairman of the Diplomatic Conference, and Lyndel PROTT, Chief of

9. 26 States signed the Protocol at the Peace Palace, The Hague, on 17 May 1999: Albania, Austria, Belgium, Cambodia, Côte d'Ivoire, Croatia, Estonia, Finland, Germany, Ghana, Greece, the Holy See, Hungary, Indonesia, Italy, Luxembourg, Madagascar, the Kingdom of the Netherlands, Nigeria, Pakistan, Qatar, Spain (*ad referendum*), Sweden, Switzerland, Syria, Yemen.

the International Standards Section of the Division of Cultural Heritage of UNESCO. The representatives of States assembled at the signing ceremony heard speeches of Colin POWER and Adriaan BOS, explaining the results of the Diplomatic Conference and the importance of the adoption of this Additional Protocol for the protection of cultural property in times of armed conflict.

11. With a view to the co-ordination of the expert discussions, on 17 May 1999 a meeting was called of the "Friends of 1999" together with the officials of the expert meeting of 18 and 19 May. This meeting was hosted by the Ambassador of the Russian Federation to the Kingdom of the Netherlands.

12. The thematic expert discussions on 18 and 19 May 1999 were chaired by: Dr. Keith HIGHET (peaceful settlement of disputes), Dr. P.S. RAO (disarmament questions), and professor Tim MCCORMACK (humanitarian law and laws of war).

13. The organisation of the Centennial events in the Netherlands benefited greatly from the fact that the Peace Palace, seat of the Permanent Court of Arbitration and the International Court of Justice, was available as venue for expert discussions on the legislative and normative aspects of the Centennial of the First International Peace Conference. A debt of gratitude is due to the Carnegie Foundation and its General Director, Willem HAMEL.

14. From 22 to 25 June 1999 delegates, legal advisers[10] of United Nations Member States, observer States and relevant international organizations assembled at the Smolny Palace in St. Petersburg, Russia, to continue expert discussions and consider the implementation aspects of the Centennial themes, contained in the reports conceived and revised by the rapporteurs: Hans BLIX on disarmament questions, Christopher GREENWOOD on humanitarian law and laws of war, and Francisco ORREGO VICUÑA and Christopher PINTO on

10. Several States were represented by their Ambassadors to the Russian Federation.

peaceful settlement of disputes. The Centennial meeting at Smolny was chaired by Anatoly L. KOLODKIN.[11]

15 The president of the Russian Federation, Boris N. YELTSIN sent participants a massage of greetings in which he stressed that, on the eve of the XXI$^{st}$ century, the main task is to ensure strict compliance with international law and, in particular, with the Charter of the United Nations. This message testifies to the firm commitment of the Russian Federation to the rule of law in international relations.

16. At the opening session participants heard speeches of the Secretary-General of the United Nations, Kofi ANNAN; the Governor of St. Petersburg, Vladimir A. YAKOVLEV; the Deputy Minister of Foreign Affairs of the Russian Federation, Serguey A. ORDZHONI-KIDZE; the Chairman of the Organizing Committee of the Centennial Meeting in The Hague, Hans VAN MIERLO; the Vice-President of the International Committee of the Red Cross, Pierre KELLER; the Deputy Secretary-General of the Permanent Court of Arbitration, Phyllis HAMILTON; the Vice-President of the International Federation of Red Cross and Red Crescent Societies, Luidmila G. POTRAVNOVA; and the President of the HAGUE APPEAL FOR PEACE, Cora WEISS.

17. These interventions stressed the need for strengthening the role of international law. They pointed out the continued duty of each state or group of states to strictly comply with the rules of international law, since it was a *conditio sine qua non* for maintaining peace and security, preventing and suppressing violations of norms of international law and safeguarding human rights.

18. The thematic expert discussions were held from 22 to 25 June 1999 and were chaired by: Jaap RAMAKER (disarmament questions), Hans-Wilhelm LONGVA (international humanitarian law and laws of war) and P. S. RAO (peaceful settlement of disputes).

11. President of the Russian Association of International Law and Association of Maritime Law, Chairman of the National Committee of the Russian Federation on the UN Decade of International Law, Judge at the UN International Tribunal for the Law of the Sea.

19. The organization of the Centennial events in Russia benefited greatly from the fact that Smolny, seat of the St. Petersburg's Administration, was available as venue for the expert discussions on the implementation aspects of the themes of the Centennial of the First International Peace Conference. A debt of gratitude is due to the administration of St. Petersburg and to the Governor of St. Petersburg, Vladimir A. YAKOVLEV.

20. The revised reports discussed at these meetings, the conclusions of the discussions pertaining to each of those reports and the follow-up given to those conclusions will be published by Professor Frits KALSHOVEN, editor in chief of THE CENTENNIAL OF THE FIRST INTERNATIONAL PEACE CONFERENCE: REPORTS AND CONCLUSIONS.[12]

## I.3 Non-Governmental Participation

21. Close co-ordination was called for between the organisers of the governmental expert meetings at the Peace Palace (18-19 May 1999) and the non-governmental HAGUE APPEAL FOR PEACE citizens' conference a week earlier (11-15 May 1999).[13] As representative of the host country, the Minister for Foreign Affairs of the Kingdom of the Netherlands was present at the opening and closing sessions of the HAP and delivered one of the key note speeches. Representatives of the HAP were invited to present the conclusions of the NGO campaign at the opening session of the governmental meetings and to take part in the expert discussions.[14] At the HAP citizens' conference the "Hague Agenda for Peace and Justice for the 21st Century" was adopted,[15] which includes the following campaigns:
- to abolish nuclear weapons;
- global action plan for the abolition of war;

12. To be published by Kluwer Law International in co-operation with UNITAR.

13. See the Hague Appeal for Peace internet web-site: www.haguepeace.org.

14. Due to Peace Palace seating restrictions five NGO experts were invited to the discussions on each of the "Hague themes".

15. A/54/98.

- international action network on small arms;
- implementation of the landmine treaty;
- ratification of the ICC statute;
- to stop child soldiers;
- for peace education at all levels; and
- against poverty.

22. The early ratification and entry into force of the Rome Statute of the International Criminal Court; opened for signature at Rome on 17 June 1998[16] was also referred to frequently during the governmental expert discussions. References to small arms and landmines were frequently made, whereas nuclear disarmament also figured prominently in the governmental expert discussions in The Hague and St. Petersburg. The dialogue between governmental and non-governmental experts was open and constructive, both thematically and organizationally.

## I.4 General organizational matters

23. As endorsed by consecutive resolutions of the General Assembly,[17] the co-hosts of the centennial celebrations, the Kingdom of the Netherlands and the Russian Federation, had, in the earliest stages of their preparations,[18] agreed that these celebrations should, on the one hand, not interfere with the mandates and efforts of contemporary international fora which might be considered heirs to the 1899 Peace Conference, while, on the other hand, the centennial debates on the Centennial themes should be meaningful and comprehensive, as well as universally carried.

16. A/CONF.183/9.

17. Referred to at the top of this document, para. 1.

18. From those earliest stages the factual organization of the Centennial of the First International Peace Conference was in the hands of Thijs BÜCHLI of the Ministry of Foreign Affairs of the Kingdom of the Netherlands and Serguey V. CHATOUNOVSKY DE BYRNOUGH of the Ministry of Foreign Affairs of the Russian Federation.

24. Consequently, a four phased format was chosen, starting with expert reports on each of the Centennial themes,[19] followed by expert discussions on those reports at relevant global,[20] regional,[21] national[22] and even individual levels. In order to facilitate these exchanges and discussions, an Internet web-site[23] was created, enabling arguments to be exchanged freely without the need for extensive mailing or labourious co-ordination.

25. In the third phase, experts met in The Hague, the Netherlands, and in St. Petersburg, Russia, for consideration of the reports on the Centennial themes, as revised taking into account the outcome of the various discussions as reflected at the internet web-site. These expert meetings refrained from taking political decisions, allowing for frank, open and in-depth discussions of the topics at hand. The conclusions of the expert meetings were faithfully recorded by experts from the co-hosts,[24] and are reproduced in Part II, below.

26. The fourth phase called for the conclusions of these expert meeting to be forwarded to the relevant international fora for consideration in

19. Originally, two rapporteurs were invited for each of the Centennial themes. Two rapporteurs decided to issue a joint report, whereas two other rapporteurs were not in a position to finalize their reports.

20. *e.g.* seminar on dispute resolution, London.

21. *inter alia*: Inter-American Juridical Commission, Rio de Janeiro; Asian-African Legal Consultative Committee, New Delhi; Asia-Pacific Region Centennial Conference, University of Melbourne; for a complete list of Centennial related activities, see A/C.6/53/11.

22. *e.g.* by the Netherlands Advisory Board on International Legal Affairs, by the Foreign and Commonwealth Office, United Kingdom, and by the Treaties Bureau of the Ministry of Foreign Affairs of the Republic of Korea.

23. www.minbuza.nl/english/conferences/peace_1.html, click on "downloaded".

24. As verified by the chairmen at the thematic discussions and presented by the national chairmen at the concluding plenary sessions.

accordance with their respective mandates.[25] The present document serves that purpose.

27. As emblem of the Centennial of the First International Peace Conference the ancient Egyptian hieroglyph of *ma-at* was chosen to underline the long lasting heritage of the 1899 Peace Conference. Symbolized in the oldest written language, *ma-at* represented the divine majesty of the rule of law and cosmic harmony, and was heralded as foundation of the earliest civilization known to man.

28. In the implementation of this innovative decentralized conferencing format ("roaming conference") certain aspects had to be taken into account.

29. Due to the innovative character of the conferencing model, the various expert conferences had to be made aware of their special role in the chain of Centennial activities. Moreover, it was felt that regional comments deserved to be collected by the co-hosts, rather than to be delivered to the Executive Secretariats. To these ends the rapporteurs and representatives of the co-hosts attended (or were represented at) those conferences as observers. This approach has yielded very positive results.[26] These visits had implications for the respective agenda's and travel budgets.

30. Certain expert conferences had some difficulties in including consideration of the reports on the Centennial themes in their current schedule of meetings. Since most of these schedules operate on an annual basis, the reports and the invitation for their consideration might have been issued a year earlier. This would have allowed preparatory expert conferences and seminars to include such considerations in their regular schedule more easily. On the other hand,

25. As for the United Nations: cf. Article 13 of the Charter:
13 (1) The Géneral Assembly shall initiate studies and make recommendations for the purpose of:
a. [...] encouraging the progressive development of international law and its codification; [...].

26. Annex lists all documents distributed on the Internet Centennial web-site.

such long period of discussions might have lead to the loss of political momentum. The co-hosts of the Centennial celebrations are grateful to officials of and participants to these expert conferences for their flexibility in this respect.

31. As a consequence of tights scheduling of regional expert conferences, only very little time was left for the rapporteurs to revise their initial reports in the light of the comments made in respect of these reports. Only by their strenuous efforts and dedication have they been able to finalize the revision of their reports in time. The co-hosts cannot but express their profoundest gratitude to the rapporteurs for all their efforts.

32. The establishment of the "Friends of 1999"[27] platform allowed the co-hosts to verify their ideas as to the organisation and coordination of the Centennial events with interested delegations and relevant international organisations, both governmental and non-governmental, thus ensuring broad support both at United Nations level, at the regional levels, as well as among civil society. Co-ordination meetings were called during General Assembly sessions and inter-sessionally.

33. With regard to possible future use of this decentralized conferencing format, the co-hosts of the 1999 centennial celebrations would like to draw attention to the following specific aspects and caveats.

1. Careful consideration as to which topic(s) might be suitable for decentralized preparatory consideration;

27. Australia, Austria, Brazil, Chile, Cyprus, Denmark, Egypt, France, Ghana, India, Indonesia, Malaysia, Mexico, Kingdom of the Netherlands, Nicaragua, Poland, Republic of Korea, Russian Federation, Senegal, South Africa, Sri Lanka, Switzerland, Thailand, Trinidad and Tobago, Ukraine, United Kingdom of Great Britain and Northern Ireland, Permanent Court of Arbitration, International Court of Justice, International Committee of the Red Cross, Carnegie Foundation, Hague Appeal for Peace.

2. Clear coordination with and separation of mandates in relation to the international institution(s) bearing primary responsibility for the subject-matter at hand;
3. Visible advantage of broadening participation of discussions;
4. Definite and long term commitment of the hosting government(s) and/or institution(s) to the organizing of such events, both in terms of maintaining the political momentum, and of the availability of money and personnel.[28]

# II. CONCLUSIONS ON THE CENTENNIAL THEMES

34. The conclusions of the discussions on the Centennial themes refer to the revised report, and are, consequently, best read in conjunction with these reports. Since discussions were held under time constraints, not all points raised by the introductory speakers were actually discussed; whereas certain participants did not have the opportunity to express themselves on the points they would have liked to bring up.

## II.1 Disarmament questions

35. The expert discussions on the legislative and normative aspects of disarmament questions had under consideration the revised report by Dr. Hans BLIX.[29] The discussions in The Hague were chaired by Dr. P. S. RAO,[30], those in St. Petersburg by Jaap RAMAKER,[31]who, each, also introduced the conclusions at the final plenary sessions. The discussions were opened with the introduction of the revised

28. *e.g.* national celebrations of a major event with international dimensions.

29. Director-General Emeritus of the IAEA.

30. of India, chairman of the AALCC-meeting; New Delhi, February 1999.

31. Ambassador of the Kingdom of the Netherlands.

report[32] and, in The Hague, with comments by Dr. Julie DAHLITZ[33]; in St. Petersburg by B. R. TUZMUKHAMEDOV .[34] Delegates identified the following elements and drew the following conclusions as to this Centennial theme.[35]

*International context*

36. The view was expressed that, although since the end of the Cold War new opportunities in the field of disarmament and arms control had led to significant results and substantial reductions in over-all military budgets, the euphoria, that seemed to exist in the early 1990's and which was reflected in the report, had swiftly evaporated and that, at present, the disarmament process seemed to slow down, the level of armament still causing unacceptable financial burdens on society.

*International law / United Nations*

37. Views were expressed that disarmament and arms control efforts were conducted in a fragmentary way and that the universal application of international law in disarmament matters did not play the role it perhaps should. More over-all direction and co-ordination would seem warranted in this respect. In this regard, discussions on the international legal aspects of disarmament and security matters within the Sixth Committee of the United Nations General Assembly were also suggested.

38. A number of participants expressed the view that both legitimacy and success of international actions require that such action be decided upon or authorized by the United Nations. At the same time, the view was expressed that discussions are needed within the United

32. Due to circumstances which prevented Director-General Emeritus BLIX from attending the Peace Palace meeting,, Ambassador Jaap RAMAKERof the Kingdom of the Netherlands took his place in the discussions.

33. Co-ordinator of CIDIR, organizer of the London seminar, December 1998.

34. Constitutional Court of the Russian Federation.

35. The chairman of the discussions on disarmament questions drew the attention of experts to the specific views expressed at regional conferences, notably the AALCC-meeting in New Delhi of February 1999.

Nations as to which reforms could strengthen the United Nations' capacity to cope, on behalf of the international community, with possible violations of agreements on disarmament and arms control, e.g. by enhancing the Security Council's effectiveness by making it more representative while reducing the use of veto, by giving a greater role to regional organizations, and/or by establishing military rapid deployment forces of the United Nations.[36]

*Regional Security Organizations*

39. The view was expressed that greater emphasis should be placed on the role of regional arrangements and agencies,[37] as envisaged under Chapter VIII of the UN Charter using political rather that military tools for conflict resolution.

*Nuclear disarmament/non-proliferation*

40. The need for further progress in nuclear disarmament and in particular in implementation of Article VI of the Nuclear Non-Proliferation Treaty (NPT) was stressed.

41. Some expressed the opinion that the Conference on Disarmament should start work within a special subcommittee, aimed at nuclear disarmament. Nuclear disarmament, according to some, should take place within a time-bound framework, while others expressed the view that nuclear disarmament did not lend itself to be confined within such a time-bound framework. The latter view held that a step by step approach to nuclear disarmament was the only realistic and viable approach.

42. The importance was stressed of early ratification and entry into force of START 2 Agreement and early start of negotiations on START 3 to further reduce the nuclear arsenals of the United States and the Russian Federation, while some others stressed that the pro-

36. See also speeches delivered at the ceremonial opening of the Peace Palace meeting.

37. Such as OSCE.

gress in bilateral negotiations should not be stopped by blockage in one area.

43. Some believed that the progress in nuclear disarmament will require rejection of the nuclear deterrence principle.

44. The need for the early entry into force of the Comprehensive Test Ban Treaty (CTBT) as an important step towards nuclear non-proliferation and disarmament was generally felt.

45. Some suggested that nuclear weapons should be taken off alert status and be withdrawn to the territories of the nuclear states to which they belong.

46. The need for an urgent start of substantive negotiations within the Conference on Disarmament on a Fissile Material Cut-off Treaty (FMCT) was widely supported.

47. A view was expressed that the closure and monitoring of the nuclear weapons infrastructure should begin at the earliest possible time in the process of nuclear disarmament.

48. The need for an effective mechanism to monitor the irreversibility of the process of nuclear disarmament was underlined.[38]

49. In connection with obligations under the NPT a number of participants pointed out the need for unhampered transfer of technology and funds for peaceful uses of nuclear energy to developing countries.

50. A suggestion was raised for a study on nuclear weapon free zones or zones free of weapons of mass destruction in areas of special tension, like the Middle East and South Asia. A call was made for nuclear weapon states giving suitable support to such zones.

38. "Trilateral initiative": the ongoing IAEA-Russia-US efforts to put nuclear weapons material withdrawn from nuclear weapons under IAEA verification could constitute a good example of such mechanism.

*Anti-ballistic missiles*

51. The need to control and regulate development and proliferation of missile technology was indicated.

52. A number of participants emphasized the key role of the Anti-Ballistic Missiles (ABM) Treaty of 1972 as a corner stone of strategic stability in the world, and a pre-requisite for further nuclear weapons reduction. Some expressed the opinion that the Theatre Missile Defence project could seriously jeopardize the viability of the ABM Treaty.

*Non-Proliferation of missiles and missile technology*

53. The proposal was made that negotiations should be undertaken within the Conference on Disarmament on a multilateral convention on the non-proliferation of missiles and missile technology.

*Biological and Chemical weapons*

54. Various participants emphasized the importance of early completion of an effective Protocol regarding verification of the Biological and Toxin Weapons Convention (BTWC) as well as of effective implementation of the verification measures under the Chemical Weapons Convention (CWC).

55. A view was expressed that both the BTWC and the CWC should reflect a true balance between gains and sacrifices, in particular for developing countries. It was also mentioned that the influence of stakeholders (like biotechnical industry) in negotiations should not lead to a weakening of verification regimes.

*Anti-personnel landmines*

56. A number of participants stressed that ratification of the Ottawa Convention on Anti-Personnel Landmines should be accelerated. Attention was also paid to the importance of Protocol II to the Conventional Weapons Convention of 1980.

*Conventional arms / small arms*

57. Particular attention was paid to small arms, as this category of weapons had been responsible for most casualties in recent conflicts. It was recognized that there was no one simple solution to this problem; although various recommendations were made:

1. the scope of the UN weapons register might be extended to include small arms;
2. more attention should be paid to the illicit trafficking of weapons and the arsenals of small arms; links with international humanitarian law and human rights law were warranted in this respect;
3. an international code of conduct might be developed, including, *inter alia*, criteria for export of small arms, in addition to existing regional arrangements;

58. With regard to conventional weapons in general, it was noted that:

1. development of new weapons should be in conformity with international humanitarian law;[39]
2. States were invited to give consideration to the criteria developed by the ICRC in its SIrUS project;[40]
3. the importance was stressed of ratification of Protocol IV[41] to the Conventional Weapons Convention.

59. Some participants felt that there is a need to extend and strengthen the UN Arms Register to cover small arms.

60. Some emphasized the need for the early conclusion of an agreement to adapt the Treaty on Conventional Armed Forces in Europe.

39. In this respect it was questioned in general whether humane use of modern weapons was possible at all.

40. Helping to assess which weapons by their design cause superfluous injury or unnecessary suffering.

41. On blinding laser weapons.

*Conference on Disarmament*

61. A well-functioning Conference on Disarmament (CD) was considered of great importance for the future of multilateral arms control and disarmament. Important results had been achieved by the CD in recent years with the conclusion of the Chemical Weapons Convention and the Comprehensive Test Ban Treaty. However, views were expressed that, in order to secure the CD's position as an important forum for multilateral arms control and disarmament, its working procedures need to be revised:

1. the consensus rule on procedural matters should be modified;
2. the practice of yearly renewal of mandates of existing ad-hoc committees should be abandoned; and
3. the possibility should be created to establish preliminary committees to discuss possible mandates for future negotiations.

*Control / Verification Mechanisms*

62. Views were expressed that there is a need for exchange of experience between various control mechanisms of the existing and future multilateral legal instruments in the field of non-proliferation and disarmament, *inter alia* NPT, CTBT, CWC, BTWC. One should also bear in mind the aspect of cost effectiveness and control techniques.

63. Verification and compliance are essential to the further progress in disarmament. Verification is not an aim in itself, but without adequate verification, progress in disarmament is not very likely.

*Civil Society*

64. The view was expressed that civil society could play a greater role in, what was called, "societal verification" of nuclear weapons free regimes ("whistleblowing") and in disarmament negotiations.

65. The view was also expressed that the international community should pay more attention to the protection of peace activists.

66. Some recommended that civil society should be allowed access to various forums, negotiating nuclear and other disarmament and arms control treaties.

*General remarks*

67. A plea was made for a war-free future, and a transformation of the culture of war into a culture of peace and consultation. In this regard, special attention was called to the recognition of the role of civil society. The view was also expressed that attention be given to ways and methods to diminish the wishes of states to possess and acquire weapons.

## II.2 Humanitarian law and laws of war

68. The expert discussions on humanitarian law and laws of war had under consideration the revised report by professor Christopher GREENWOOD.[42] The discussions at The Hague were chaired by professor Tim MCCORMACK,[43] those at St. Petersburg by Hans-Wilhelm LONGVA,[44] who, each, also introduced the conclusions at the final plenary session. The discussions were opened with the introduction of the revised report and with comments by professor Georges ABI-SAAB[45] at The Hague and Y. M. KOLOSOV[46] at St. Petersburg.

69. The sessions noted with approval the recent adoption of a new Protocol to the 1954 Hague Convention on Cultural Property, the Ottawa Landmines Convention and the Rome Statute of the International Criminal Court. In the light of these developments, there was

42. of the United Kingdom, London School of Economics.

43. of Australia, organizer of the Asia-Pacific Centennial conference, Melbourne, February 1999.

44. Legal Adviser of Norway.

45. of Egypt, former Centennial rapporteur.

46. Moscow State Institute of International Relations of the Ministry of Foreign Affairs of the Russian Federation

agreement with the Rapporteur's general proposition that the urgent need was for measures to promote compliance with existing law rather than for new laws, although some development of existing law remained desirable.

70. Delegates identified the following elements and drew the following conclusions.

*Ius in bello, ius ad bellum*
71. Acts of warfare must not only to be in conformity with relevant rules of the laws applicable in armed conflict; they must also be necessary for and proportionate to the achievement of objectives permitted under international law. There was a difference of opinion regarding the circumstances under which the use of force might be permitted, in the context of which repeated reference was made, *inter alia*, to the UN Charter as sole basis for the use of force. These was, however, agreement that the use of force in all circumstances must meet these requirements of necessity and proportionality. The implications of this principle on features such as the duration and geographical delimitation of hostilities and the choice of targets and means and methods of warfare, including their long-term effects, must have the close attention of political and military decision makers.

*Neutrality*
72. In particular, the impact of armed conflict on relations between parties to the conflict and neutral parties should be made the object of further study as a matter of priority.

*Naval Warfare*
73. The law of naval warfare as stated in the Conventions of 1907 being largely outdated, a full-scale revision of this body of law may be called for. The 1995 *San Remo Manual on International Law Applicable to Armed Conflicts at Sea* provides a starting point for such revision. A diplomatic conference on the subject should, however, only be convened after further thorough preparation and with the active support of major naval powers.

*Belligerent Occupation*

74. While in general the law of belligerent occupation, as elaborated in the 1899 (1907) Hague Regulation on Land Warfare, the 4th Geneva Convention of 1949 and Additional Protocol I of 1977, may be regarded as sufficiently elastic to allow for a degree of adaptation to changing circumstances in society, any such adaptation must respect the core principle that, even in the event of a prolonged occupation, the occupying power may not exploit the occupied territories for the benefit of its own population. By contrast, the provisions of the Hague Regulations on the taking of property in occupied territories are deemed so archaic as to warrant an enquiry into the possibility of modernization of those rules.

*United Nations Military Operations*

75. There was an extensive discussion of the law applicable to UN military operations and responsibility for acts of UN forces.[47] To achieve the highest possible level of conformity of United Nations military operations with applicable principles and rules of international humanitarian law, the legal instruments applicable to such operations need to be reconsidered. In particular, priority should be given to:

1. clarification of the circumstances in which a United Nations force is to be regarded as a party to an armed conflict and reconfirmation that such United Nations force, under such circumstances, is subject to the whole of international humanitarian law; and, as a minimum,
2. extending the greatest possible content to the obligation to observe the principles and spirit of humanitarian law in cases in which a United Nations force is not a party to an armed conflict, but nevertheless engaged in hostilities.

47. Note by the co-hosts: cf. Secretary-General's Bulletin: Observance by United Nations forces of international humanitarian law, ST/SGB/1999/13, of 6 August 1999.

*Internal Armed Conflicts: scope*

76. International humanitarian law applicable in internal armed conflicts binds both the government and other parties to such conflicts. While Additional Protocol II of 1977 has been given a higher threshold of application as compared to Article 3 common to the Geneva Conventions of 1949, this higher threshold does not really appear warranted. Accordingly, to enhance the protection afforded to those not taking part in hostilities in a situation of an internal armed conflict, the international community should undertake steps:

1. to set the threshold for the application of Protocol II at the same level as presently applied under the terms of common Article 3;
2. to ensure that the resulting lower threshold is faithfully applied in all cases (notwithstanding reluctance of governments in recognizing the existence of a situation of internal armed conflict);
3. to recognize the relationship between the law of internal armed conflict and the law of human rights, for example by identifying applicable common standards.

*Internal Armed Conflicts: substantive law*

77. Many principles applicable in international armed conflicts - on the protection of the wounded and sick, the protection of the civilian population from the effects of hostilities and the law of weaponry - should be applicable in internal armed conflicts. One way to achieve this, is through the development of customary law. The enquiry, undertaken by the International Committee of the Red Cross, into the content of customary international humanitarian law especially as applicable in internal armed conflicts, may be expected to clarify the state of affairs in this regard. It may also provide the basis for efforts towards a more systematic revision of the law.

*Compliance*

78. The record of compliance with the law of armed conflict urgently needs to be improved. This would require:

1. measures to be taken in time of peace;
2. preventive measures to be taken in armed conflict;
3. measures at national and international level to repress violations of international humanitarian law.

79. Important practical steps which would contribute to enhancing compliance with international humanitarian law and which all states and other relevant entities should be encouraged to take included the following:

1. Measures of education and training designed to ensure that the principles of international humanitarian law are widely understood and to create a "culture of compliance" with international humanitarian law;
2. Practical preparation for armed conflict, such as the establishment of mechanisms for handling Prisoners of War and civilian detainees; and in time of armed conflict, constant awareness of the need to apply the rules of international humanitarian law to concrete cases;
3. The adoption of the legislative and administrative mechanisms necessary to enable states to comply with their obligations to prosecute and punish grave breaches of the Geneva Conventions and Protocols;
4. Enhancing the role of external monitoring during armed conflict, in particular:
    a. encouraging all states involved in armed conflict to nominate, and to accept the nomination of, protecting powers;[48]
    b. reaffirming and strengthening the right of initiative of the ICRC;
    c. encouraging all states to accept the competence of the International Fact-Finding Commission[49] and all parties to armed conflicts to make use of the Commission. The competence of the Commission to perform its functions in internal armed conflicts should formally be recognized;
    d. having recourse to the monitoring mechanisms of human rights conventions.
5. Considering the possibility of establishing, in regions of conflict, areas for the protection of civilians and other qualified persons ("protected areas"), either as "humanitarian zones" in accordance

48. cf. Article 8 of the Geneva Conventions I, II and III, Article 9 of Geneva Convention IV, Article 5 of Additional Protocol I.

49. established pursuant to Article 90 of Additional Protocol I.

with the relevant provisions of the 1949 Geneva Conventions and Additional Protocol I of 1977, or as militarily enforced "security zones"; in the latter case, on the basis of a clear understanding regarding (I) the demilitarization of such areas and (II) the level of protection to be accorded to them.
6. Encouraging all states to honour their obligations to prosecute and punish violations of international humanitarian law wherever and whomsoever they are committed.
7. Encouraging all states to ratify the Statute of the International Criminal Court and to participate fully in its work.

80. It was noted that the Rome Statute of the International Criminal Court also applies to crimes within the jurisdiction of the Court when committed in the context of an internal armed conflict.

81. In addition, those participating in the discussions considered that thought should be given to developing:
1. a system of reporting in which states give notice of the steps taken in peacetime to comply with their obligations under international humanitarian law;
2. an individual complaints mechanism.

## II.3 Peaceful settlement of disputes

82. The expert discussions on peaceful settlement of disputes had under consideration the revised report by professor Francisco ORREGO VICUÑA[50] and Dr. Christopher PINTO.[51] The discussions in The Hague were chaired by Dr. Keith HIGHET,[52] those in St. Petersburg by Dr. P. S. RAO, who, each, also introduced the conclusions at the final plenary session. The discussions in The Hague were opened with the introduction of the revised report and, in The Hague, with

50. University of Santiago de Chile.

51. Secretary-General of the US-Iran Claims Tribunal.

52. of the USA, chairman of the IAJC expert conference, Rio de Janeiro, August 1998.

comments by Judge Gilbert GUILLAUME[53]; in St. Petersburg by K. G. GUEVORGUIAN.[54] Delegates identified the following elements and drew the following conclusions as to those elements.

*Prevention and resolution*

83. Attention should be given to continuing to develop appropriate methods of resolving international disputes. To the greatest extent possible, disputes should be prevented from occurring or continuing, and to this end the institutionalization of new techniques of assisting this process would be useful. On the other hand, the flexibility of ad hoc solutions should not be lost in the process of too much institutionalization of mechanisms for the peaceful settlement of disputes.

84. Care must be taken to develop existing institutions and not to create new institutions for their own sake. A balance should be struck between the optimal use of existing mechanisms and considering the establishment of new machinery. The fact that available mechanisms do not function properly might be caused by the lack of political will, rather than by inherent deficiencies of such mechanisms.

85. Peace and security are not necessarily achieved by techniques of "dispute resolution" as such. The role of the judiciary, after all, is limited to deciding on particular cases, rather than developing law or institutions.[55] On the other hand, the view was expressed that the role of the International Court of Justice was becoming increasingly normative.

86. The peaceful solution of disputes depended in final analysis on the strict compliance with the principles of non-use of force and sovereign equality of states.

87. It was emphasized that the proliferation of actors on the international scene should not detract from the primary function of inter-

53. Judge at the International Court of Justice.

54. Deputy Legal Adviser at the Russian Ministry of Foreign Affairs.

55. See also below: Codification of international law.

national law, which is, and should remain, the regulation of inter-state relations.

*Negotiations and consultations*

88. Negotiation and consultation are considered to be, still, the most fruitful methods of dispute resolution. It must be remembered that specific legal and political methods of dispute resolution are both part of a larger picture.

89. The obligation to continue to seek peaceful solution to disputes remains, even after negotiations break down.

90. Third party intervention does not prevent negotiations continuing simultaneously.

*Permanent Court of Arbitration*

91. The Permanent Court of Arbitration's services for dispute resolution are available both under the traditional terms of the 1899 and 1907 Hague Conventions for the Pacific Settlement of International Disputes, and as part of a global "alternative dispute resolution" system.[56] Its new Rules[57] give the Court broad competence.[58]

92. The Security Council should also consider referral to the Permanent Court of Arbitration, when making recommendations under Article 36, para. 1, of the Charter, given the Court's broad competence.

56. "Alternative dispute resolution" is proposed by the rapporteurs as supplementary to the public court system for the administration of international justice.

57. Available at www.law.cornell.edu/icj/pca/eng/home.html; see also operational para. 4 of A/RES/53/100.

58. Already, the Permanent Court of Arbitration acts to "rescue" stalled alternative dispute resolution under the UNCITRAL Rules.

*International Court of Justice*

93. Universal acceptance of the compulsory jurisdiction of the International Court of Justice[59] was perceived as a long term goal. For this to be achieved:

1. existing problems of requesting interim measures of protection should be solved;
2. due regard should be had to potential abuse of the system;
3. solutions should be found for the high costs of, and length of time involved with litigation.

94. Caution was expressed with regard to possible unexpected results from the formation of Chambers,[60] for example the possible imbalance in the assignment of judges.

95. Diverse and strongly felt views were expressed with regard to possible enlargement of the bench of the Court.

96. The Court's Trust Fund deserves further support.

97. Broad support was expressed for increasing the resources of the Court,[61] for example by providing well-trained professional assistance to the International Court of Justice, although care should be taken in the selection process of such personnel.

98. With regard to the suggested broader access to the Court, it was pointed out that there is precedent for Non-Independent States as parties to the Statute.

99. An emerging trend was recognized for accepting the need for international organizations to have access to the Court.

59. cf. Article 36, 2 of the ICJ Statute.

60. Allowing for a greater work load of the Court.

61. Note by the co-hosts: see in this respect: Annexes to "Report of the International Court of Justice: 1 August 1997 - 31 July 1998" (A/53/4).

100. The need was felt for careful consideration of various aspects of the expansion of the advisory function of the Court and its complex consequences, e.g.:

1. channel for a possible *actio popularis*;[62]
2. possible introduction of an "Advocate-General" at the Court, especially in connection with a possible *actio popularis*;
3. possible filtering of requests for advisory opinion, e.g. by an "Independent Committee of Jurists";
4. referrals to the Court by other tribunals or by regional organizations.[63]

101. Attention should be given to the issues arising from the bilateral nature of litigation in cases involving *erga omnes* obligations.[64]

102. The possibility of division of cases into small and large, or important and less important matters, drew spirited debate.

*Role of Security Council and Secretary-General*

103. The role of the Security Council and/or the Secretary-General[65] in reducing tension and dispute prevention should be further developed.

104. The role of the Security Council in the maintenance of international peace and security in the context of the United Nations dispute settlement function should be enhanced, particularly by developing fact-finding and other activities.

105. Members of the Security Council should discharge their responsibilities for the Council's primary responsibility for international peace and security by seeking agreement and taking the appropriate decisions within the Council. Some referred, in this connection, to the Council's practice in the early 90's.

62. Caution was expressed about possible politicization.

63. As suggested by the rapporteurs; not specifically discussed.

64. cf. *Barcelona Traction, Light and Power Company, Ltd* case, ICJ Reports 1970, p. 3: para's 33 and 34.

65. See also below, Permanent Conciliation Committee.

106. For the Security Council to be able credibly to perform such functions as representative of the international community, enlargement of the membership of the Council was advocated by some.

107. The effectiveness of the various settlement methods employed in early phases of a dispute might be enhanced by ensuring an automatic or expedient transition from Chapter VI to Chapter VII of the Charter. Activities under these Chapters should be better correlated with UN bodies focussing on the prevention of disputes.

108. In this connection attention was drawn to the sometimes disastrous effects of economic sanctions on the civilian population. Others advocated entrusting peace keeping solely to United Nations contingents, to be put at the Organization's disposal in advance.

109. On the other hand, the opinion was also voiced that compliance might best be induced by also including incentives, notably at the economic level.

*Regional courts*

110. More frequent recourse to regional courts would facilitate the coherence and uniformity of regional community law, which often shows a greater measure of compliance than general dispute settlement systems.

111. As to suggestions for regional courts to apply general international law, regional instruments, such as the Pact of Bogotá and the Latin American Collective Security Arrangements, should be carefully regarded. In this respect the idea was advanced, that regional courts should be somewhat specialized in their activities, so as not to compete with the International Court of Justice in the application of general international law.[66]

66. See above: International Court of Justice's advisory functions; and below: International Court of Appeals.

*International Court of Appeals*

112. There was little support for the suggestion in the report that the International Court of Justice could also act as an International Court of Appeals. As for arbitral awards, it was felt that these benefited from finality.[67] Moreover, an appeals system could not be imposed from the outside, since it is for the parties to the dispute to accept or not an appeal in such a case.[68]

*International Constitutional Court*

113. The report requests the interesting possibility of an international constitutional court to be studied. Partly, the International Court of Justice is already fulfilling a constitutional role within the UN-system,[69] protecting that system from disintegration. In many domestic legal systems a Constitutional Court as well as a Supreme Court exist side by side.[70] The view was expressed, however, that in order to have a Constitutional Court, a Constitution would be a pre-requisite.

*Specialized methods and procedures*

114. A multiple combination of political and legal methods might be made available to settle disputes in areas involving special interests. As to the legal methods a variety of choices might be included and the introduction of the "inverted consensus" rule for the adoption of panel reports might be considered.

115. A system of optional rules might be developed to open GATT/ WTO procedures to individuals and corporations.

116. The availability to private parties of mechanisms for international control of domestic legislation, such as are currently in place under NAFTA and other arrangements, might be considered for wider use.

67. See also above: Regional Courts.

68. e.g. in private commercial arbitration.

69. e.g. by allowing UN organs and specialized agencies to ask advisory opinions on legal questions, cf. Article 65 ff of the ICJ Statute.

70. See above: International Court of Appeals.

117. Access by affected interested private entities to international dispute settlement arrangements of a specialized nature[71] might be encouraged and might be followed in other types of arrangements involving individual rights and interests.

*Permanent Conciliation Committee*

118. Questions were raised about the need for or the advisability of a Permanent Conciliation Committee, as well as regarding:

1. the function and role of mediation/conciliation;
2. whether a Permanent Conciliation Committee would enjoy the confidence of parties, essential to the conciliation process and
3. whether such functions might be better co-ordinated with the Permanent Court of Arbitration[72] or entrusted to the Secretary-General of the United Nations; and
4. the appointment and rotation of the members of such Committee.

*Codification of international law*

119. The development in publication by the UN of authoritative volumes and compendia on the law, e.g. regarding human rights, disarmament, etc.,[73] was noted with satisfaction. The same was true for studies on the work of the International Law Commission.

120. It was felt that codification alone is not enough; law creation is also needed.

71. Such as ICSID, the UNCC, the World Bank Inspection Panel and the International Administrative Tribunals.

72. See above, Prevention and Resolution, on institutionalization, and Permanent Court of Arbitration, on the Court's broad competence under its Rules.
Note by the co-hosts: see also the coordinating role of the UN Legal Counsel in the "Lockerbie-affair": cf. letter dated 5 April 1999 from the Secretary-General addressed to the President of the Security Council (S/1999/378).

73. Note by the co-hosts: see also the new electronic database for the United Nations Treaty Collection, access to information concerning United Nations activities in the field of international law, and the Internet access to the United Nations Treaty Series and the Multilateral Treaties Deposited with the Secretary-General, all referred to in A/RES/54/100.

*World school of international law*
121. As to the proposal, expressed in the report, for the creation of a "world school of international law" it was suggested to study such proposals in conjunction with the Hague Academy of International Law.

122. The following points of the report, although tabled, were not specifically discussed during the expert meetings.

*Mediation and the role of technical bodies*
123. Mediation might be used with great flexibility, while a special role of a mediator might be considered in particular sensitive disputes.

124. In the context of specialized areas of cooperation, procedures might be developed for referring such disputes to technical bodies where appropriate.

125. Treaties as to these and other methods for dispute settlement that have fallen into disuse might be updated.

# Annex
## Reports, comments and speeches

The following reports and comments have been contributed[74] to the Centennial discussions by experts and posted on the internet by the Executive Secretariat.[75]

74. In the Peace Palace languages: English or French.

75. www.minbuza.nl/english/conferences/c_peace_docs.html
All documents were posted as Adobe® Acrobat® files (✶.pdf) in order to allow cross-platform accessibility and guarantee integrity of the documents. For reading and printing Acrobat® Reader® software was offered as free download.

| *document title* | *file name* |
|---|---|
| PRELIMINARY REPORT<br>The Peaceful Settlement of Disputes: Prospects for the Twenty-first Century<br>by: Francisco ORREGO VICUÑA and Christopher PINTO | settle1.pdf |
| PRELIMINARY REPORT<br>Development of International Law Relating to Disarmament and Arms Control since the First Hague Peace Conference in 1899<br>by: Hans BLIX | arms1.pdf |
| PRELIMINARY REPORT<br>International Humanitarian Law and the Laws of War<br>by: Christopher GREENWOOD | human1.pdf |
| Commentaires sur le rapport préliminaire de MM. F. Orrego Vicuña et C. Pinto<br>by: Gilbert GUILLAUME | guilaum.pdf |
| Initial comments of the International Bureau of the Permanent Court of Arbitration on the report by F. Orrego Vicuña and C. Pinto<br>by: the International Bureau | PCAcom.pdf |
| Observations on the document by F. Orrego Vicuña and C. Pinto<br>by: Dr. Eduardo VÍO GROSSI | IAJCSetl.pdf |
| Comments on the preliminary report by F. Orrego Vicuña and C. Pinto<br>by: Dr. Keith HIGHET | IAJCHigh.pdf |
| The Fridtjof Nansen Memorial Lecture<br>by: Knut VOLLEBÆK | small1.pdf |
| Peaceful Settlement of Disputes - an Overview<br>by: Dr. Galo LEOROF. | SetAJC.pdf |
| Comments on sections III + V of the preliminary report by F. Orrego Vicuña and C. Pinto<br>by: Prof. Barbara KWIATKOWSKA | Kwiatkow.pdf |
| Two Other Ideas<br>by: Roy S. LEE | Lee.pdf |

| *document title* | *file name* |
|---|---|
| General Comments on "Peaceful Settlement of Disputes" by: Shabati ROSENNE | Rosenne1.pdf |
| Comments on the International Court of Justice by: Shabati ROSENNE | Rosenne2.pdf |
| Comments on the preliminary report by F. Orrego Vicuña and C. Pinto by: the Netherlands Advisory Committee on International Issues | cavveng1.pdf |
| Comments on "International Humanitarian Law and the Laws of War" by Christopher Greenwood by: the Netherlands Advisory Committee on International Issues | cavveng2.pdf |
| Comments on "Development of International Law Relating to Disarmament and Arms Control since the First Hague Peace Conference in 1899" by Hans Blix by: the Netherlands Advisory Committee on International Issues | cavveng3.pdf |
| Informal Comments on the draft report by Hans Blix by: ICRC | ICRCarms.pdf |
| "The Feasibility of Implementing The Hague/St. Petersburg Centennial Recommendations under the UN System" by: Hans CORELL, as distributed in New Delhi, 11-12 February 1999 | Corell.pdf |
| Statement by the President of the 37th Session of the Asian-African Legal Consultative Committee by: P. S. RAO | Rao.pdf |
| Report by the Rapporteur of the Second Session on "International Humanitarian Law and the Laws of War", New Delhi, 11 February 1999 | delhihum.pdf |
| Draft Report of the Rapporteur of the First Session on "Peaceful Settlement of Disputes", New Delhi, 11 February 1999 by: S. M. CONFIADO | delhistl.pdf |

| *document title* | *file name* |
|---|---|
| Speech by the Chinese Representative at the Expert Meeting of AALCC on the Preliminary Reports on the Commemoration of the Centennial of the 1st Hague Peace Conference | delhichn.pdf |
| International Law and the Clarification of the Right of Self Defence<br>by: Zahra NOPARAST | delhiirn.pdf |
| The International Law of Disarmament: a Centennial Overview<br>by: V. S. MANI | delhmani.pdf |
| Comments on the Preliminary Reports of Special Rapporteur Prof. Christopher Greenwood on International Humanitarian Law and the Laws of War<br>by: B. S. CHIMNI | delhchim.pdf |
| Point of Correction to the report by Hans Blix<br>by: G. BOZKURT | Ottoman.pdf |
| Arms control and disarmament: One of the main themes of the Hague Peace Conference of 1899<br>by: Hans BLIX | melbbli.pdf |
| Prospects for Nuclear disarmament: Sir Kenneth Bailey Memorial Lecture<br>by Jayantha DHANAPALA | melbdha.pdf |
| Asia-Pacific Approaches to Disarmament, The Peaceful Settlement of Disputes and International Humanitarian Law<br>by: The Hon. Alexander DOWNERMP, Minister for Foreign Affairs of Australia | melbdow.pdf |
| Achieving peace in Cambodia<br>by The Hon. Gareth EVANSMP | melbeva.pdf |
| Session on Cambodia<br>by: Tony KEVIN | melbkev.pdf |
| Speech at the Commemoration of the Centenary of the 1899 Hague Peace Conference<br>by: Rashit L. KHAMIDULIN | melbkha.pdf |

| *document title* | *file name* |
|---|---|
| The 1899 Hague Peace Conference and the Development of the Laws of War: Asia's Contribution to the Quest for Humanitarianism<br>by: Vitit MUNTARBHORN | melbmun.pdf |
| Arms Control and Disarmament: The Development in the Asia-Pacific Region<br>by: Nugroho WISNUMURTI | melbwis.pdf |
| China and Peaceful Settlement of Disputes<br>by: Kening ZHANG | melbzha.pdf |
| Statement on the legacy of the 1899 Peace Conference<br>by; Hans VANMIERLO | melbmlo.pdf |
| Excerpts from "Peaceful Resolution of Major International Disputes", Summaries and Recommendations<br>edited by: Julie DAHLITZ | London.pdf |
| Improving the System of Settlement of Disputes<br>by: Roy S. LEE | Roy.pdf |
| Report on the Asia-Pacific Conference to Commemorate the Centenary of the First Hague International Peace Conference of 1899<br>by: Tim MCCORMACK | melb.pdf |
| UK Government Comments on the Preliminary Report by Mr. Hans Blix concerning Disarmament and Arms Control<br>by: The Foreign and Commonwealth Office | FCOarms.pdf |
| UK Government Comments on the Preliminary Report by Professor Christopher Greenwood for The Hague Centennial Commemoration<br>by: The Foreign and Commonwealth Office | FCOhum.pdf |
| UK Government Comments on the Preliminary Report by Professor Orrego Vivuña and Mr. Pinto on "The Peaceful Settlement of Disputes: Prospects for the Twenty-First Century"<br>by: The Foreign and Commonwealth Office | FCOsettl.pdf |

| *document title* | *file name* |
|---|---|
| Seminar Commemorating the First International Peace Conference of 1899<br>by: The South African Department of Foreign Affairs | SADC.pdf |
| Comments regarding the preliminary report by Hans Blix, "Development of International Law Relating to Disarmament and Arms Control since the First Hague Peace Conference in 1899"<br>by: CHOI Seung-hoh, Director-General of the Treaties Bureau, Republic of Korea | ROKBlix.pdf |
| Comments regarding the preliminary report by Christopher Greenwood, "International Humanitarian Law and the Laws of War"<br>by: CHOI Seung-hoh, Director-General of the Treaties Bureau, Republic of Korea | ROKGreen.pdf |
| The Peaceful Settlement of Disputes: the Role of International Law and tha International Court of Justice<br>by: Cheryl A. THOMPSON-BARROW | jamaica.pdf |
| REVISED REPORT<br>The Peaceful Settlement of Disputes: Prospects for the Twenty-first Century<br>by: Francisco ORREGO VICUÑA and Christopher PINTO | settle3.pdf |
| REVISED REPORT<br>International Humanitarian Law and the Laws of War<br>by: Christopher GREENWOOD | human3.pdf |
| REVISED REPORT<br>Development of International Law Relating to Disarmament and Arms Control since the First Hague Peace Conference in 1899, especially the rules and practices regarding verification and compliance<br>by: Hans BLIX | arms3.pdf |
| Draft conclusions of the Centennial discussions at the Peace Palace, The Hague, 18-19 May, 1999 | 99concl3.pdf |
| Some Observations on the Revised Blix Reoprt on Disarmament<br>by: John BURROUGHS Lawyers' Committee on Nuclear Policy | lcnp.pdf |

| *document title* | *file name* |
|---|---|
| CONCLUSIONS<br>Outcome of the celebrations of the Centennial of the First International Peace Conference<br>Report submitted to the 54th United Nations General Assembly by the Governments of the Kingdom of the Netherlands and the Russian Federation | 1999ccl8.pdf<br>A/54/381 |

The following (key-note) speeches were delivered[76] at the Peace Palace sessions of the celebration of the Centennial of the First International Peace Conference (18 and 19 May 1999) and posted on the internet by the Executive Secretariat.[77]

| *document title* | *file name* |
|---|---|
| On the Cutting Edge<br>by: Jozias VAN AARTSEN, Minister for Foreign Affairs of the Kingdom of the Netherlands | speech1.pdf |
| The International Rule of Law Established at the 1899 Peace Conference<br>by: Hans VAN MIERLO, Chairman of the Centennial celebrations at the Peace Palace | speech2.pdf |
| The Effectiveness of the International Rule of Law in Maintaining International Peace and Security<br>by: Kofi ANNAN, Secretary-General of the United Nations | speech3.pdf<br>UN Press Release<br>SG/SM/6997 |
| International Humanitarian Law: from the Hopes of 1899 to the Challenges of 1999<br>by: Cornelio SOMMARUGA, President of the International Committee of the Red Cross | speech4.pdf |

76. In the Peace Palace languages: English or French.

77. www.minbuza.nl/english/conferences/peacespeeches/c-speeches.html
All documents were posted as Adobe® Acrobat® files (*.pdf) in order to allow cross-platform accessibility and guarantee integrity of the documents. For reading and printing Acrobat® Reader® software was offered as free download.

| *document title* | *file name* |
|---|---|
| The Disarmament Legacy of the First International Peace Conference<br>by: José BUSTANI, Director-General of the Organization for the Prohibition of Chemical Weapons | speech6.pdf<br>www.opcw.org/dg-hap.htm |
| The United Nations as Successor to the International Rule of Law Established at the 1899 First International Peace Conference<br>by: Hans CORELL, Under Secretary-General and Legal Counsel of the United Nations | speech5.pdf |
| The Humanitarian Legacy of the First International Peace Conference<br>by: Astrid HEIBERG, President of the International Federation of Red Cross and Red Crescent Societies | speech11.pdf |
| Possible Ways Ahead with regards to Peaceful Settlement of Disputes<br>by: Hans JONKMAN, Secretary-General of the Permanent Court of Arbitration | speech12.pdf |
| Report of the Commemorative Conference of the Members of the Permanent Court of Arbitration<br>by: Sir Ninian STEPHEN, Chairman of the Commemorative Session | speech9.pdf |
| Report on the Conclusions of the Hague Appeal for Peace citizens' conference<br>by: Bill PACE, Secretary-General of the Hague Appeal for Peace | speech10.pdf |
| The Beginning, Not the End: an Appraisal of the 1899 Hague Peace Conference<br>by: Arthur EYFFINGER, Peace Palace Historian | speech13.pdf |
| The Hague Peace Conference of 1899: an Historical Introduction<br>by: Robin SHARWOOD, University of Melbourne | speech8.pdf |
| Le Règlement pacifique des différends: perspectives pour le 21e siècle<br>by: Gilbert GUILLAUME, introductory speaker | guilopp.pdf |

| *document title* | *file name* |
|---|---|
| Comments on the Report by Hans Blix entitled "Development of International Law Relating to Disarmament and Arms Control"<br>by: Julie DAHLITZ, introductory speaker | dltzopp.pdf |
| Closing Remarks of the Discussions on the Legislative and Normative Aspects of the Themes of the First International Peace Conference<br>by: Hans VAN MIERLO, Chairman of the Centennial celebrations at the Peace Palace | speech7.pdf |

The following (key-note) speeches were delivered[78] at the Smolny Palace sessions of the celebration of the Centennial of the First International Peace Conference (22-25 June 1999) and posted on the internet by the Executive Secretariat.

| *document title* | *file name* |
|---|---|
| Opening speech<br>by: Anatoly L. KOLODKIN | SPkolop.pdf |
| To the International conference "100th anniversary of the Russian initiative: from the First Peace Conference of 1899 to the third of 1999", welcome address by: Boris YELTZYN, President of the Russian Federation | SPyeltzyn.pdf |
| Speech by Deputy Minister for Foreign Affairs of the Russian Federation, Mr. S.A. ORDZHONIKIDZE | SPordzh.pdf |
| Speech by the Secretary-General of the United Nations, Kofi A. ANNAN | Spsgun.pdf |
| Speech by the Governor of St. Petersburg, Mr. V.A. YAKOVLEV | Spyakov.pdf |
| Speech by the Deputy Secretary-General of the Permanent Court of Arbitration, Mrs. Phyllis HAMILTON | Sphamil.pdf |

78. In: English, French or Russian.

| *document title* | *file name* |
|---|---|
| "La mise en oeuvre du droit international humanitaire: le grand défi", par: M. Pierre KELLER, Vice-Président du Comité international de la Croix-Rouge | Spicrc.pdf |
| Speech by the President of the Russian Organization of the Red Cross and Vice-president of the International Federation of Red Cross and Red Crescent Societies, Mrs. L.G. POTRAVNOVA | SPpotra.pdf |
| Speech by the President of the Hague Appeal for Peace, Mrs. Cora WEISS | SPweiss.pdf |
| "One Aspect of Implementation: Small Arms Control", speech by Minister of State and Chairman of the National Centennial Organizing Committee of the Kingdom of the Netherlands, Hans VANMIERLO | SPhafmo.pdf |
| "Disarmament questions", introduction by Hans BLIX | Spblix.pdf |
| "Disarmament questions", by Mr. TUZMUKHAMEDOV Constitutional Court of the Russian Federation | Sptouz.pdf |
| "International Humanitarian Law: Urgent Need for Preventing Vionaltions" by Professor Yury KOLOSOV | SPkolos.pdf |
| "Non-judicial methods of settling disputes: Some thoughts on implementation", introduction by Christopher PINTO | SPpinto.pdf |
| "Peaceful settlement of conflicts: Forecast for XXIst Century - Implementation aspects", by Kiril GUEVORGUIAN Deputy Director of the Legal Department of the Ministry of Foreign Affairs of the Russian Federation | SPguev.pdf |
| "Comments Regarding the Revised Report ... The Peaceful Settlement of Disputes: Prospects for the twenty-first Century ...", by CHO Jung-won, Director of the Treaties Division II, Ministry of Foreign Affairs and Trade, Republic of Korea | Spkorea.pdf |
| Address by Mr. Viraphand VACHARATHIT Deputy Director General, Department of Treaties and Legal Affairs of Thailand | Spthail.pdf |
| "Conclusions on the Peaceful Settlement of Disputes", remarks by Dr. P.S. RAO | Sprao.pdf |

| *document title* | *file name* |
| --- | --- |
| Closing speech by Mr. A.L. KOLODKIN | Spkolcl.pdf |

The following historical contributions relating to the 1899 Peace Conference have also been placed on the internet by the Executive Secretariat.

| *document title* | *file name* |
| --- | --- |
| Austria<br>Austria-Hungary and the First Hague Peace Conference, 1899<br>by: Claudia HAM | 1899a.pdf |
| Belgium<br>La Belgique et la Première Conférence de la Paix de La Haye (1899)<br>by: Rik COOLSAET | 1899b.pdf |
| Bulgaria<br>La Première Conférence de la Paix à La Haye et la Participation de la Bulgarie à la Conférence<br>by: Katia TODOROVA | 1899bul.pdf |
| China<br>China and the First Hague Peace Conference<br>by: LI Yongsheng | 1899chin.pdf |
| Denmark<br>Denmark and the Hague Peace Conference of 1899<br>by: Frede P. JENSEN | 1899dk.pdf |
| Germany<br>The German Reich at the Hague Peace Conference of 1899<br>by: Christophe EICK | 1899d.pdf |
| Greece<br>Greece's part at the First International Peace Conference of 1899<br>by: Photini CONSTANTOPOULOU | 1899hel.pdf |

| *document title* | *file name* |
| --- | --- |
| Italy<br>Participation de l'Italie à la Première Conférence pour la Paix de La Haye de 1899<br>by: Umberto LEANZA | 1899it.pdf |
| Japan<br>The encounter of Japan with International Law and International Adjudication<br>by: Hisashi OWADA | 1899jap.pdf |
| Mexico<br>Mexico and the First Hague Peace Conference<br>by: Miguel Angel GONZÁLEZ FÉLIX | 1899mex.pdf |
| The Netherlands<br>In the Midst of the Throng and Crush - The Dutch Policy at the First Hague Peace Conference<br>by: Arthur EYFFINGER | 1899nl.pdf |
| Norway<br>"... was Norway mentioned specifically?" Norway and the Hague Peace Conference of 1899<br>by: Nils Ivar AGOY | 1899nor.pdf |
| Russian Federation<br>Russia in the 1899 and 1907 Hague Peace Conferences<br>by: Anatoly L. KOLODKIN and Serguey V. CHATOUNOVSKY DE BYRNOUGH | 1899rus.pdf |
| Spain<br>The Role of Spain in the Hague Peace Conference of 1899<br>Carlos GIMENEZ PIERNAS | 1899esp.pdf |
| Sweden<br>The 1899 Peace Conference in The Hague - The Swedish view<br>by: Love KELLBERG | 1899sw.pdf |
| Thailand<br>Siam and the First Hague Peace Conference of 1899 : A Preliminary Note<br>by: Chalong SOONTRAVANICH | 1899thai.pdf |

# OUTCOME OF THE ACTION DEDICATED TO THE 1999 CENTENNIAL OF THE FIRST INTERNATIONAL PEACE CONFERENCE

United Nations General Assembly Resolution 54/27
of 17 November 1999

*The General Assembly,*

*Reaffirming* the commitment of the United Nations and its Member States to the adherence to and the development of international law as a basis for conducting international relations,

*Recognizing* the historical importance of the 1899 first International Peace Conference for the rule of international law, the peaceful settlement of disputes, the development and codification of international law and the practice of multilateral diplomacy,

*Recalling* that, in accordance with its previous resolutions,[1] the centennial of the first International Peace Conference coincides with the closing of the United Nations Decade of International Law and could be considered as a third international peace conference,

*Recalling also* that the United Nations Decade of International Law will be closed at a plenary meeting of the General Assembly on 17 November 1999,

*Recalling with gratitude* the initiatives[2] for the celebration of the centennial of the first International Peace Conference by the Governments of the Russian Federation and the Kingdom of the Netherlands with regard to the themes of the Conference: development of international

1. Resolutions 44/23, 51/157, 52/153 and 53/100.
2. Resolutions 51/159, 52/154 and 53/99; A/C.6/52/3, A/C.6/53/10, A/C.6/53/11.



*F. Kalshoven (ed.),*
*The Centennial of the First International Peace Conference*, 503–506.

law relating to disarmament and arms control, humanitarian law and laws of war, and peaceful settlement of disputes,

*Recalling further* that these initiatives called for, *inter alia*, discussions on these themes on the basis of in-depth reports at the global, regional and national levels by intergovernmental, governmental, diplomatic, academic, and civil society[3] experts at conferences, seminars and other meetings as well as through the Internet, to be reported on to the General Assembly for consideration at its fifty-fourth session,

*Noting* that the general outcome of these discussions was that, while progressive development and codification of international law remains important, the furtherance of the rule of international law would best be served by the faithful compliance of States with existing international obligations, focusing more on the timely implementation of these obligations,

*Noting also* that the year 1999 marks the fiftieth anniversary of the adoption of the four Geneva Conventions of 12 August 1949,

*Noting further* that the Permanent Court of Arbitration was established as a result of the first International Peace Conference in 1899,

*Convinced* that the legacies of the first International Peace Conference have been enhanced by the centennial initiatives and by the plenary meeting of the General Assembly at the closing of the United Nations Decade of International Law,

3. cf. The Hague Agenda for Peace and Justice in the Twenty-first Century (A/54/98, Annex).

1. *Takes note with interest* of the outcome of the centennial of the first International Peace Conference, reported by the co-hosts, the Governments of the Kingdom of the Netherlands and the Russian Federation;[4]

2. *Commends* all who, through their efforts, wisdom and expertise, contributed to the success of the celebration of the centennial of the first International Peace Conference;

3. *Commends* the International Committee of the Red Cross for its work in promoting adherence to and compliance with the four Geneva Conventions of 12 August 1949 and other instruments of international humanitarian law;

4. *Congratulates* the Permanent Court of Arbitration on its one hundredth anniversary;

5. *Expresses its appreciation* to the Secretary-General for bringing the outcome of the centennial of the first International Peace Conference to the attention of the relevant international forums;

6. *Invites* States, organs of the United Nations, international organizations and other relevant international forums to take note of the outcome of the centennial of the first International Peace Conference and to consider, where appropriate:
(a) Giving attention to the outcome of the thematic discussions within the sphere of their respective competences and mandates;
(b) Making use in the future of the format of discussions of the centennial of the first International Peace Conference in accordance with any relevant rules and procedures;

4. A/54/381, annex.

7. *Invites*:
(a) The Governments of the Russian Federation and the Kingdom of the Netherlands to file the records of the centennial of the first International Peace Conference in their archives and to provide access to these records to interested parties;
(b) All who contributed to the centennial of the first International Peace Conference to file their records in this respect with either of these Governments.

# UNITED NATIONS DECADE OF INTERNATIONAL LAW

United Nations General Assembly Resolution 54/28
of 17 November1999

*The General Assembly,*

*Recalling* its resolution 44/23 of 17 November 1989, by which it declared the period 1990-1999 the United Nations Decade of International Law,

*Recalling also* that the main purposes of the Decade, according to its resolution 44/23, should be, *inter alia*:
(a) To promote acceptance and respect for the principles of international law,
(b) To promote means and methods for peaceful settlement of disputes between States, including resort to and full respect for the International Court of Justice,
(c) To encourage the progressive development of international law and its codification,
(d) To encourage the teaching, study, dissemination and wider application of international law,

*Noting* the conclusion of the United Nations Decade of International Law,

*Reaffirming* its resolution 53/101 of 8 December 1998, entitled "Principles and guidelines for international negotiations, adopted within the framework of the Decade,



*F. Kalshoven (ed.),*
*The Centennial of the First International Peace Conference,* 509–515.

*Greatly encouraged* by the significant achievements in the development and promotion of international law which occurred during the Decade, which has contributed to the strengthening of the rule of international law,

*Recognizing* that, *inter alia*, the establishment of the International Tribunal for the Former Yugoslavia in 1993, the International Tribunal for Rwanda in 1994 and the International Tribunal for the Law of the Sea in 1996 and the adoption of the Rome Statute of the International Criminal Court in 1998 constitute significant events within the Decade,

*Recognizing also* efforts made during the Decade by Legal Advisers of the Ministries of Foreign Affairs worldwide to create a common understanding of their role through annual informal consultations at the Headquarters of the United Nations,

*Convinced* that the end of the Decade affords the international community an opportunity to reflect on those achievements and that States, international organizations and educational organizations should continue to encourage and promote activities in the legal field aimed at contributing to its main purposes,

*Convinced also* of the need to continua aiming towards the implementation of the main purposes of the Decade,

*Welcoming* the significant increase in the recourse to the International Court of Justice by States for the settlement of disputes,

*Noting* that international humanitarian law has been an important topic during the United Nations Decade of International Law, and mindful of the contributions made in this field by the International Committee of the Red Cross and the International Red Cross and Red Crescent Conferences,

*Noting also* that the year 1999 marks the fiftieth anniversary of the adoption of the four Geneva Conventions of 12 August 1999,

*Expressing its appreciation* to the Governments of the Russian Federation and the Kingdom of the Netherlands for their efforts in realization of the programme of action dedicated to the first International Peace Conference which could be regarded as a significant contribution to the United Nations Decade of International Law,

*Taking note with interest* of the consideration of the outcome of the actions dedicated to the 1999 centennial of the first International Peace Conference in the General Assembly during its fifty-fourth regular session,

*Expressing its gratitude* to the rapporteurs and all organizations, groups and individuals who contributed to the discussion of the centennial themes,

*Having considered* the report by the Secretary-General,[1] and expressing its appreciation therefor,

*Noting* the deposit by the Secretary-General, on 21 December 1998, of an act of formal confirmation, on behalf of the United Nations, of the Vienna Convention on the Law of Treaties between States and International Organizations or between International organizations of 21 March 1986,

*Welcoming* the progress that has been made towards eliminating the backlog in the publication of the United Nations *Treaty Series* by the implementation of a plan to be completed in 2001, and stressing the need for the elimination of such backlog, as well as for comprehensive electronification of the work of the Treaty Section of the Office of Legal Affairs of the Secretariat,

*Recalling* that, at the forty-fifth session of the General Assembly, the Sixth Committee established the Working Group on the United Nations Decade of International Law,

1. A/54/362 and Add.1.

*Noting* that the Working Group continued its work during the fifty-fourth session in accordance with resolution 53/100,

*Having considered* the oral report of the Chairperson of the Working Group to the Sixth Committee,

1. *Expresses its appreciation* for the work done by the Working Group on the United Nations Decade of International Law;

2. *Acknowledges* that the Decade has contributed significantly to the strengthening of the rule of international law;

3. *Reaffirms* the continued validity of the main objectives of the Decade, the fulfilment of which is essential to achieve the purposes of the United Nations;

4. *Expresses its appreciation* to States and international organizations and institutions that have undertaken activities in the implementation of the programme for the activities for the final term (1997-1999) of the Decade;

5. *Requests* the Secretary-General to continue developing the Treaty Section electronic database, with a view to providing Member States expeditiously with a wider range of easily accessible treaty-related information on the electronic medium, and to keep the list, now established on the Internet, of the titles of the multilateral treaties deposited with him updated in all official languages of the Organization;

6. *Urges* States and international organizations, in particular depositaries, to continue assisting the Secretariat of the United Nations in its efforts to expedite the registration of treaties and their publication by providing it with paper copies of treaties, or electronic copies, including maps, for registration and, wherever possible, translations of treaties in English or French;

7. *Requests* the Secretary-General to implement vigorously the plan to eliminate the backlog in the publication of the United Nations *Treaty Series*, and highlights, in this context, the relevance of timely translation;

8. *Expresses its appreciation* to the Office of Legal Affairs of the Secretariat for the establishment during the Decade of various Internet Web sites and the United Nations Audiovisual Library in International Law, and takes note of its efforts to maintain those sites and the Library;

9. *Notes* the publication by the Office of Legal Affairs of the Secretariat of the *Collection of Essays by Legal Advisers of States, Legal Advisers of International Organizations and Practitioners in the Field of International Law* and its intention to issue in 2000 two publications entitled *International Instruments related to the Prevention and Suppression of International Terrorism* and *The United Nations and the Development of International Law during the 1999s* to highlight the work accomplished in this area during the Decade;

10. *Invites* States, organs of the United Nations, international organizations and other relevant international forums to continue to give attention to the themes and outcome of the centennial of the first International Peace Conference;

11. Congratulates the Permanent Court of Arbitration on its one hundredth anniversary, commends that organization for its role in the international system of peaceful dispute resolution, and invites States to consider making full use of the facilities of the Court and to support its work;[2]

12. *Expresses its appreciation* to the International Committee of the Red Cross for the activities undertaken in the field of international humanitarian law, including with regard to the protection of the environment in times of armed conflict;

2. A/54/381, annex, para.9.

13. *Invites* States and international organizations to continue promoting the acceptance of and respect for the rules and principles of international law;

14. *Welcomes* the achievements during the Decade in the codification and progressive development of international law, and calls upon States, in order to contribute further to the rule of international law, to consider, if they have not yet done so, becoming parties to the multilateral treaties adopted during the Decade, including those listed in the annex to the report of the Secretary-General;[3]

15. Invites States and international organizations to continue promoting the strengthening of the use of means and methods of peaceful settlement of disputes;

16. *Recalls* that States have the obligation to solve their disputes by peaceful means, including resort to the International Court of Justice, and that one of the main purposes of the Decade is to promote the full respect for the Court in accordance with the relevant provisions of the Charter;

17. *Invites* States to continue to pay attention to the identification of areas of international law that might be ripe for progressive development or codification, and to promote discussion thereon in the competent forums;

18. *Invites* States and international organizations to continue encouraging the publication of books or other materials on subjects of international law and the holding of symposia, conferences, seminars or other meetings aimed at promoting a wider appreciation of international law;

19. *Invites* States to continue encouraging educational institutions to introduce or increase the number of courses of international law;

3. A/54/362 and Add.1.

20. *Requests* the Secretary-General to bring the present resolution to the attention of States, international organizations and institutions working in the field of international law;

21. *Decides* to continue considering developments in the progress made in the implementation of the purposes of the Decade beyond its conclusion, in the framework of the agenda item entitled "United Nations Programme of Assistance in the Teaching, Study, Dissemination and Wider Appreciation of International Law".